Handbook of
Prescriptive Treatments for Adults

Handbook of
Prescriptive
Treatments for
Adults

Edited by
Michel Hersen
Nova Southeastern University
Fort Lauderdale, Florida

and
Robert T. Ammerman
Western Pennsylvania School for Blind Children
Pittsburgh, Pennsylvania

Plenum Press • New York and London

Library of Congress Cataloging-in-Publication Data

Handbook of prescriptive treatments for adults / edited by Michel
  Hersen and Robert T. Ammerman.
        p.   cm.
    Includes bibliographical references and index.
    ISBN 0-306-44682-0
    1. Mental illness--Treatment--Handbooks, manuals, etc.
  I. Hersen, Michel. II. Ammerman, Robert T.
    [DNLM: 1. Mental Disorders--therapy. 2. Drug Therapy.
  3. Behavior Therapy.   WM 400 H2356 1994]
  RC480.H2856 1994
  616.89'1--dc20
  DNLM/DLC
  for Library of Congress   94-15528
                                                          CIP

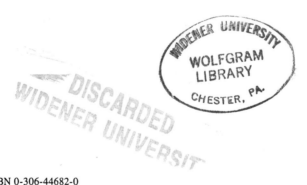

ISBN 0-306-44682-0

©1994 Plenum Press, New York
A Division of Plenum Publishing Corporation
233 Spring Street, New York, N.Y. 10013

Printed in the United States of America

To

VICKI, JONATHAN, AND NATHANIEL

—MH

and to

JOANNE JOHNSTON AND CHARLES BENNETT

—RTA

Contributors

Ron Acierno • Center for Psychological Studies, Nova Southeastern University, Fort Lauderdale, Florida 33314.

Robert T. Ammerman • Western Pennsylvania School for Blind Children, Pittsburgh, Pennsylvania 15213-1499.

Stewart A. Anderson • Department of Psychiatry, Western Psychiatric Institute and Clinic, Pittsburgh, Pennsylvania 15213.

Gavin Andrews • Clinical Research Unit for Anxiety Disorders, University of New South Wales, Sydney 2010 Australia.

Susanne Bailey • Department of Psychology, University of Houston, Houston, Texas 77204-5341.

T. D. Borkovec • Department of Psychology, The Pennylvania State University, University Park, Pennsylvania 16802.

Heather Breiter • Department of Psychology, University of South Carolina, Columbia, South Carolina 29208.

Michael P. Carey • Department of Psychology, and Center for Health and Behavior, Syracuse University, Syracuse, New York 13244-2340.

Gary Alan-Hue Christenson • Department of Psychiatry, University of Minnesota, Minneapolis, Minnesota 55455.

Gerard J. Connors • Research Institute on Addictions, Buffalo, New York 14203.

Philip M. Coons • Larue D. Carter Memorial Hospital, Indiana University, Indianapolis, Indiana 46202.

Michelle G. Craske • Department of Psychology, University of California, Los Angeles, Los Angeles, California 90024-1563.

Conor Duggan • Department of Psychiatry, The University of Nottingham, Nottingham NG3 6AA England.

Lisa M. Fisher • National Center for PTSD—Behavioral Science Division, VA Medical Center, and Tufts University School of Medicine, Boston, Massachusetts 02130.

Diane R. Follingstad • Department of Psychology, University of South Carolina, Columbia, South Carolina 29208.

Charles V. Ford • Department of Psychiatry and Behavioral Neurobiology, School of Medicine, University of Alabama at Birmingham, Birmingham, Alabama 35294-0018.

Grant T. Harris • Mental Health Centre, Penetanguishene, Ontario L0K 1P0 Canada.

Michel Hersen • Center for Psychological Studies, Nova Southeastern University, Fort Lauderdale, Florida 33314.

Terence M. Keane • National Center for PTSD—Behavioral Science Division, VA Medical Center, and Tufts University School of Medicine, Boston, Massachusetts 02130.

Robert D. Kerns • Psychology Service, West Haven VA Medical Center, West Haven, Connecticut 06516, and Department of Psychiatry, Neurology, and Psychology, Yale University, New Haven Connecticut 06520.

Matcheri S. Keshavan • Department of Psychiatry, Western Psychiatric Institute and Clinic, Pittsburgh, Pennsylvania 15213.

Dennis J. Krauss • Urology Section, Surgical Service, Syracuse Department of Veterans Affairs Medical Center, and Department of Urology, SUNY Health Science Center at Syracuse, Syracuse, New York 13210.

Karen E. Krinsley • National Center for PTSD—Behavioral Science Division, VA Medical Center, and Tufts University School of Medicine, Boston, Massachusetts 02130.

Larry J. Lantinga • Psychology Service, Syracuse Department of Veterans Affairs Medical Center, and Department of Psychiatry, SUNY Health Science Center at Syracuse, Syracuse, New York 13210.

James P. LePage • Department of Psychology, University of Houston, Houston, Texas 77204-5341.

Kenneth L. Lichstein • Department of Psychology, Memphis State University, Memphis, Tennessee 38152.

Thomas Brooke Mackenzie • Department of Psychiatry, University of Minnesota, Minneapolis, Minnesota 55455.

Richard P. Mattick • National Drug and Alcohol Research Centre and Clinical Research Unit for Anxiety Disorders, University of New South Wales, Sydney 2033 Australia.

Nathaniel McConaghy • Psychiatric Unit, Prince of Wales Hospital, Randwick, New South Wales 2031 Australia.

F. Dudley McGlynn • Department of Psychology, Auburn University, Auburn, Alabama 36849-5214.

Benoit H. Mulsant • Western Psychiatric Institute and Clinic, and Department of Psychiatry, University of Pittsburgh School of Medicine, Pittsburgh, Pennsylvania 15213.

Barbara L. Niles • National Center for PTSD—Behavioral Science Division, VA Medical Center, and Tufts University School of Medicine, Boston, Massachusetts 02130.

Pamela E. Parker • Department of Psychiatry, College of Community Health Sciences, University of Alabama, Tuscaloosa, Alabama 35487-0326.

Robert A. Philibert • Department of Psychiatry, University of Iowa College of Medicine, Iowa City, Iowa 52242-1057.

Lynn P. Rehm • Department of Psychology, University of Houston, Houston, Texas 77204-5341.

Marnie E. Rice • Mental Health Centre, Penetanguishene, Ontario L0K 1P0 Canada.

Brant W. Riedel • Department of Psychology, Memphis State University, Memphis, Tennessee 38152.

Lizabeth Roemer • Department of Psychology, The Pennsylvania State University, University Park, Pennsylvania 16802.

Jules Rosen • Western Psychiatric Institute and Clinic, and Department of Psychiatry, University of Pittsburgh School of Medicine, Pittsburgh, Pennsylvania 15213.

Shannon B. Sebastian • Department of Psychology, Louisiana State University, Baton Rouge, Louisiana 70803.

Ralph M. Turner • Department of Psychiatry, Temple University School of Medicine, Philadelphia, Pennsylvania 19140.

Petronilla Vaulx-Smith • Department of Psychiatry, Western Psychiatric Institute and Clinic, and Department of Psychiatry, University of Pittsburgh School of Medicine, Pittsburgh, Pennsylvania 15213.

Sachin V. Waikar • Department of Psychology, University of California, Los Angeles, Los Angeles, California 90024-1563.

Kimberly S. Walitzer • Research Institute on Addictions, Buffalo, New York 14203.

Donald A. Williamson • Department of Psychology, Louisiana State University, Baton Rouge, Louisiana 70803.

George Winokur • Department of Psychiatry, University of Iowa College of Medicine, Iowa City, Iowa 52242.

Preface

This book could not have been conceptualized or published 20 years ago. Indeed, it is doubtful that we could have organized the material for this handbook 10 years ago. Over the last 20 years, however, the painstaking efforts of many clinical researchers working with a variety of resistive psychopathologies have resulted in specific psychotherapies and pharmacotherapies that are effective with a significant proportion of patients, at least for some of the disorders. Much clinical research remains to be carried out in the forthcoming decades. But now that we are nearing the 21st century, at least some statement about efficacy can be made.

In 1967, Gordon Paul succinctly stated that the ultimate goal of treatment outcome research is to determine "*What* treatment, by *whom*, is most effective for *this* individual with *that* specific problem, and under *which* set of circumstances" (p. 111). At that time, empirical evaluations of psychosocial and pharmacologic treatments were few and far between. Methodological strategies for determining treatment effectiveness were also in the formative stage, as exemplified by introduction of control groups that received inactive interventions (i.e., placebo) and the relatively recent practice of comparing two or more treatments in addition to placebo. In the almost three decades since Paul's oft-quoted dictum, both the quantity and the quality of treatment outcome research with adults have increased dramatically. Improved selection criteria, more valid assessment approaches, and more clearly delineated intervention techniques have all contributed to a greater understanding of which treatments are most effective for a given disorder.

As our research sophistication has increased, however, it has also become evident that there are a variety of impediments to a successful therapeutic outcome. For example, many patients present with comorbid psychiatric conditions. For these individuals multiple interventions may be required, and the prognosis for a full recovery may be diminished. Other types of patients exhibit chronic disorders (e.g., schizophrenia, personality disorders) and often require frequent clinical contact to maintain stable functioning. Furthermore, in some cases the "treatment of choice" will be ineffective, necessitating use of second- and third-order interventions.

The *Handbook of Prescriptive Treatments for Adults* is based on the premise that although there are ample data documenting the efficacy of behavior therapy, pharmacotherapy, and alternative therapies for disorders in adults, nowhere is it documented for all the disorders discussed herein how one decides which treatment strategy (or strategies) to choose first and what one does when the first-line option does not work out. This book, then, has marked implications for the therapist (psychologist, psychiatrist, social worker, nurse practitioner) who is intent on making treatment decisions given what documentation is now available in the empirical literature. We have structured the chapters with considerable care to elicit from the respective experts the problem areas that are likely to be encountered. Thus, in addition to documenting the status of the empirical literature for that adult disorder, each chapter presents a comprehensive clinical case that takes the reader into a real or hypothetical clinical situation that highlights differential diagnosis and assessment, treatment selection, treatment course, outcome and termination, and follow-up and maintenance.

The chapters in this book examine, by disorder, the most effective treatments for adults that have emerged from the empirical literature. Chapters in Part II and Part III use a highly structured format to enhance readability and maximize usefulness of the material for the empirically minded clinician. The authors have particularly focused on behavior therapy and pharmacotherapy, given the proportionally greater research attention directed toward these interventions, although alternative treatments are also reviewed. The authors have also addressed obstacles to treatment (e.g., poor response, nonadherence to treatment), and they have provided guidelines for clinician response to such challenges. In addition, they offer recommendations for how to proceed if the optimal treatment choice is unsuccessful or impractical to implement.

We will now briefly summarize each chapter, highlighting new developments in the field and important considerations for clinicians.

The book begins with an overview of prescriptive approaches to assessment and treatment (Chapter 1) by Acierno, Hersen, and Ammerman. The authors review the relatively recent transition from use of theoretically derived treatments implemented indiscriminately across disorders, to empirically based interventions differentially applied to a given disorder. They point out that a prescriptive approach requires flexibility in treatment, whereby periodic assessments are conducted to monitor progress and determine whether changes in strategy are required. The authors suggest that continued research will further refine our abilities to match specific treatments with specific disorders (and their subtypes).

Alzheimer's disease is examined by Mulsant and Rosen in Chapter 2. Dementia affects between 5 and 15% of individuals over the age of 65 years. Alzheimer's disease, the most common form of dementia, is a pervasively disabling and degenerative condition resulting in cognitive deficits, mood and personality disturbances, neurologic impairments, and behavioral problems. The etiology is unknown, although the most promising avenue of research supports a genetic basis for the disorder. Unfortunately, treatment options are limited and primarily consist of management of specific symptoms with pharmacologic agents. The cholinesterase inhibitor tacrine, for example, appears to be helpful in the improvement of cognitive and memory deficits. Likewise, antidepressants and neuroleptics may be helpful for depression and psychosis, respectively. Environmental manipulations and structured behavioral programming are often beneficial for the patient who is agitated, confused, or aggressive. The authors note that the fluctuating status of Alzheimer's disease necessitates treatment that is individually tailored to the unique needs and clinical presentation of the patient. Moreover, the database in this area is insufficient to provide universal guidelines for treatment.

In Chapter 3, Walitzer and Connors consider the prescriptive treatment of psychoactive substance use disorders. These disorders have attracted considerable attention because of their deleterious impact on the patient, his or her family, and the community. Despite prominence of psychoactive substance use disorders in the clinical setting, identification of consistently efficacious treatments has been elusive. This is, in large part, because of the heterogeneity of such disorders in terms of severity, duration and type of symptoms, etiology, and comorbidity. Treatment must be comprehensive, flexible, and ongoing. Frequent assessment is recommended to guide shifts in treatment strategy as the clinical picture changes. Moreover, ancillary social and vocational services are required to maximize the likelihood of recovery and maintenance of gains.

In Chapter 4, Anderson, Vaulx-Smith, and Keshavan discuss the prescriptive treatment of schizophrenia. This condition is characterized by a chronic and often highly debilitating course, affecting cognitive, affective, and social functioning. Although the etiology of schizophrenia is not fully understood, research has implicated disturbances in several neurophysiologic and neuroanatomic systems as the source of the disorder. Pharmacotherapy is the mainstay of treatment for schizophrenia. Neuroleptics are typically the first treatment of choice, although potential short- and long-term side effects necessitate careful monitoring and may prompt changes in dosage or type of medication. Recent evidence also supports use of other agents, in particular clozapine, for patients who do not respond to neuroleptics. Combined social skills training and family therapy have been found to be important adjuncts to pharmacotherapy, resulting in lower relapse rates. For the majority of schizophrenics, however, the unstable course of the disorder will require frequent contact with clinicians, often involving intermittent hospitalizations.

In adult psychopathology, few disorders have received as much empirical attention as major depression. Rehm, LePage, and Bailey review this sizable literature in Chapter 5. The assessment of depression is highly developed, and a variety of self-report, interview, and clinician-report assessment approaches are available to assist in making the diagnosis and measuring symptomatology. The literature points toward the interaction of biological and environmental factors in the emergence of the disorder. Accordingly, several types of medications (particularly those affecting the norepinephrine and serotonin neurotransmitter systems) and psychosocial interventions (particularly cognitive therapy, self-management therapy, and interpersonal skills training) have been shown to be efficacious. For severe depression, medication appears to be the treatment of choice. Likewise, psychosocial interventions are useful in preventing relapse. There is some evidence supporting the combined use of pharmacologic and psychosocial interventions over either form of treatment alone.

The prescriptive approach as applied to bipolar disorder is outlined in Chapter 6 (Philibert and Winokur). This disorder, consisting of alternating episodes of mania and depression interspersed with asymptomatic intervals, has a lifetime prevalence of approximately 0.5 to 1%. Twin adoption studies have strongly implicated a genetic etiology in bipolar disorder. Lithium is the first-order treatment for acute mania and the sine qua non of prophylaxis between episodes. For patients who do not respond to lithium, a second line of intervention consists of the anticonvulsants (particularly carbamazepine) or the neuroleptics. The authors note that psychosocial interventions show promise in reducing morbidity and increasing medication compliance if implemented between episodes, although this area awaits further empirical attention.

Considerable advances have been made in the past decade in the treatment of panic disorder, and these are reviewed by Craske and Waikar in Chapter 7. Although agoraphobia (the fear of open spaces) was once viewed as the hallmark of this condition, it is now recognized that panic attacks constitute the primary feature of panic disorder. The prescriptive treatment of panic disorder involves concurrent attention directed toward the panic attacks and the pervasive avoidance that typically accompanies them. The cognitive-behavioral approach to panic disorder incorporates cognitive restructuring to address irrational fears and beliefs about anxiety and panic, in vivo exposure to agoraphobic situations, and exposure to bodily sensations that may trigger a panic response (i.e., interoceptive exposure). Well-controlled outcome research has shown that from 70 to 90% of patients who undergo cognitive-behavioral therapy are panic free after treatment; an additional 70 to 80% show significant reductions in agoraphobia. Moreover, treatment gains have been shown to be maintained at up to 4 years posttreatment. Pharmacotherapy, too, is an effective intervention for panic disorder. Alprazolam is useful for the acute treatment of panic, although relapse rates are high, and the potential for addiction precludes the use of this agent on a long-term basis. The antidepressants, in particular imipramine, are more suitable for long-term treatment. Preliminary evidence supports use of anti-depressants and cognitive-behavioral therapy in combination, although the authors caution that pharmacotherapy may interfere with the learning processes thought to be essential for exposure-based behavioral interventions.

Social phobia, reviewed by Mattick and Andrews in Chapter 8, is a recently recognized anxiety disorder affecting between 1 and 2% of the population. This condition, which can be quite disabling and chronic, is characterized by a fear of public scrutiny and humiliation. The authors point out that there continue to be disputes about appropriate diagnostic criteria, reflecting the early stage of our understanding of the disorder, which is underscored by the paucity of assessment instruments available that specifically measure features of social phobia. Empirical evaluations of treatment have been conducted only in the past decade. Research supports the effectiveness of in vivo exposure to feared situations, although evidence has emerged in favor of cognitive therapy in combination with exposure to achieve maximum benefits. Pharmacotherapy has emphasized the monoamine oxidase inhibi-tor phenelzine, particularly in the treatment of more pervasive and severe social phobia. As with the other anxiety disorders, relapse is common following discontinua-tion of medication. The authors recommend that further research address: (a) the effects of combined behavior therapy and pharmacotherapy, (b) the long-term effects of treatment, and (c) the differential impacts of treatment given the high rate of morbidity and complicating features (e.g., substance abuse) in social phobia.

In contract to most of the other anxiety disorders, simple phobia (reviewed by McGlynn, Chapter 9) has generated a sizable and rich empirical treatment literature. Etiological formulations underscore the role of classical conditioning and modeling in the development of the disorder. It has also been suggested that certain individuals exhibit biological vulnerabilities that make them more susceptible to phobia-inducing situations. Prescriptive assessment strategies comprise both self-report of fear and behavioral approach to feared stimuli. Exposure, desensitization, and modeling have all demonstrated efficacy when subjected to empirical evaluation. Pharmacotherapy, however, appears to play a minor role in the treatment of simple phobia. Given the proven success of behavioral interventions, and the possible interference of benzo-diazepines in the extinction process, medications should be reserved for especially severe and resistant cases.

In Chapter 10, Duggan reviews exciting new developments in the assessment and treatment of obsessive-compulsive disorder (OCD). This condition, once thought to be highly resistant to treatment, is responsive to behavior therapy (incorporating exposure as the primary intervention) in up to 70% of cases. In addition, specific serotonergic reuptake inhibitors, especially clomipramine, have been empirically demonstrated to be highly effective in the remediation of OCD symptoms. Despite these promising treatments, for many patients OCD is a chronic condition in which the chances of eventual relapse are high. Long-term contact and periodic booster sessions are often needed to maintain treatment gains.

In Chapter 11, Christenson and Mackenzie look at trichotillomania, once viewed as an extremely rare disorder but now thought to occur in up to 0.6% of the population. Research on trichotillomania is in its earliest stages, but a surprising amount of information has been gathered in the past decade. The etiology of trichotillomania is not well understood, although several authors have proposed a link between the condition and obsessive-compulsive disorder. Christenson and Mackenzie, however, caution against the premature acceptance of this association, given the differences between trichotillomania and obsessive-compulsive disorder on several important clinical features. Currently, the prescriptive treatments for trichotillomania involve habit reversal (a behavioral intervention using competing responses to hair pulling) and clomipramine. Unfortunately, habit reversal requires a high degree of patient motivation and self-monitoring and is difficult to carry out with patients who are easily frustrated or reluctant to participate actively in treatment. With clomipramine use, uncomfortable side effects may result in premature termination of a medication trial. Moreover, relapse has been reported to be common following discontinuation of the drug. Clearly, assessment and treatment of trichotillomania is an area with several promising interventions that await further empirical examination.

Advances in the assessment and treatment of posttraumatic stress disorder (PTSD) are documented by Keane, Fisher, Krinsley, and Niles in Chapter 12. This disorder develops in response to a severe stressor, leading to heightened physiologic arousal, reexperiencing of the traumatic event, and emotional numbing and avoidance. In its most severe form, PTSD can be chronic and significantly disabling. Comorbidity (e.g., substance abuse) is relatively common. The authors agree that individuals with preexisting psychopathology or a biological vulnerability are at particular risk for developing PTSD in response to a high-magnitude stressor. Assessment has become considerably more sophisticated in recent years and is composed of clinician interviews, psychologic testing, and physiologic measurements. The optimal treatment approach incorporates multiple components, including emotional and behavioral stabilization, education, stress management, and exposure. Empirical research supports this treatment model, although the relative efficacy of specific components remains to be examined. The newly developed intervention, eye movement desensitization, appears to be effective, but it awaits controlled outcome research. Pharmacotherapy, consisting primarily of antidepressant and anxiolytic administration, is widely used despite the paucity of empirical studies on its effectiveness. Treatment of PTSD is often long term, requiring continued follow-up to prevent relapse.

Borkovec and Roemer, in Chapter 13, discuss generalized anxiety disorder (GAD). Diagnostic criteria for GAD have been in a state of flux over the years, and, in all likelihood, additional changes have been made in DSM-IV. Essentially, GAD consists of chronic and persistent worry and anxiety that is not triggered by easily identifiable stimuli and does not involve panic attacks. The research literature on GAD is small but of high quality and level of sophistication. Cognitive-behavioral therapy, comprising self-monitoring, applied relaxation, self-centered desensitization, and cognitive restructuring, is the treatment of choice for GAD. Almost 60% of patients receiving this integrated package report significant improvement at one year post-treatment. The authors suggest that individuals currently experiencing a significant stressor, or those with characterologic features of anger and entitlement, respond poorly to this form of treatment. Benzodiazepines have been used to treat GAD, although the high relapse rate and potential for addiction make these medications a poor choice for the long term. Buspirone and the antidepressants have also been used, with apparent success. The empirical literature on pharmacotherapy for GAD is sparse, however, thereby precluding the recommendation of any particular medicine at this point.

In Chapter 14, Parker and Ford discuss difficulties inherent in diagnosing and treating somatization disorder. Patients with somatization disorder present with multiple physical symptoms that cannot be explained physiologically. They often go from physician to physician, seeking new diagnostic tests and medical procedures. Polysubstance use is common, often involving addictive medications. Once identified, these patients are challenging to treat. Comorbidity is often evident, and the authors recommend addressing such concurrent conditions (most often including anxiety, depression, and substance abuse). Research in this area is sparse, although several researchers recommend behavioral interventions to reduce the secondary gain associated with the family's responses to the patient's symptom complaints, and to teach patients more effective communication skills. Somatization disorder requires long-term treatment, and there is always a risk that the patient will terminate prematurely and seek alternative medical interventions.

Coons covers the growing literature on multiple personality disorder (MPD) in Chapter 15. It is only recently that MPD has become widely accepted as a distinct diagnostic entity. It is characterized by a dissociative state in which there are two or more personalities that alternately take control of the patient's behavior. Often, "amnesia" is a core feature of the disorder, whereby different personalities are unaware of each other or of experiences had during times when alternate personalities are dominant. The majority of patients with MPD are women, and they typically report traumatic abuse in childhood. Several assessment measures (e.g., Dissociative Experience Scale) and interviews (e.g., Structured Interview for Dissociative Disorders) have been developed for MPD and other dissociative disorders. There are a number of case reports on the treatment of MPD, although controlled outcome research is lacking in this area. Behavior therapy is, for the most part, unexplored. Pharmacotherapy may be useful in addressing concurrent disorders or symptom status (e.g., depression). The author indicates that long-term psychodynamic therapy is currently the treatment of choice, in which the ultimate goal is to integrate the personalities. Firm recommendations about the selection of optimal treatments awaits empirical evaluation of the long-term impacts of various treatment modalities.

The paraphilias include several different sexual deviations and that on gender identity disorders, including exhibitionism, voyeurism, and pedophilia. McConaghy reviews this literature in Chapter 16. Etiological formulations have emphasized stimulus control models in which deviant stimuli are associated with sexual arousal. The author, in turn, expands upon this model to account for the frequently compulsive nature of most paraphilias. The assessment of paraphilias is controversial. Much of the research in this area has used physiologic measures of penile responses to sexual stimuli, although serious reservations have been voiced about the validity of these procedures. Despite this shortcoming, the prescriptive treatment of sexual deviations primarily consists of the behavioral interventions of covert sensitization, imaginal desensitization, and satiation therapy. Medroxyprogesterone acetate (MPA), which lowers levels of testosterone, has also been successfully used to diminish sexual urges and decrease deviant sexual behavior. The author calls for more controlled research in this area, particularly examining the long-term effects of various treatments.

Carey, Lantinga, and Krauss evaluate male erectile disorder in Chapter 17. Although solid empirical data on the epidemiology of this condition are unavailable, it is generally accepted that male erectile disorders are common and account for a large number of physician visits. The authors reject the simplistic notion that such problems are usually either psychologically or organically based in favor of a more complex biopsychosocial model, in which emotional, social, and physical factors interact synergistically to bring about erectile dysfunction. Accordingly, they recommend a comprehensive assessment approach that includes a physical examination, clinical interview (with particular attention focused on interpersonal relationships), and psychophysiologic measurement. Preliminary research supports use of cognitive-behavioral interventions incorporating sensate focus exercises, education, stimulus control procedures, relationship enhancement techniques, cognitive restructuring, and health promotion. Comorbidity, substance use, rigid beliefs about masculinity, and poor relationship quality are associated with poorer treatment responses. Somatic therapies are widely employed, and a limited research base supports use of such interventions as self-injected papaverine and phentolamine, and external suction/constriction devices and penile prostheses. The authors recommend that psychosocial interventions be carried out concurrently if somatic treatments are used.

With between 10 and 20% of adults reporting severe and chronic insomnia, this sleep disorder must be viewed as a significant and prevalent health concern. Riedel and Lichstein cover this topic extensively in Chapter 18. Insomnia is a heterogeneous disorder that relies heavily on the patient's subjective reports of sleep quality. Numerous factors can interfere with sleep, including poor sleep hygiene, psychopathology, environmental stressors, maladaptive sleep habits, and medications. Accordingly, the authors recommend a careful and comprehensive clinical interview to identify the parameters of and potential contributors to insomnia. Additional assessment strategies include self-monitoring, physiologic monitoring of sleep at home, and the more involved monitoring of sleep in the laboratory. Research has established efficacy of several interventions, including relaxation training, stimulus control therapy, sleep restriction therapy, and improvement of sleep hygiene. Benzodiazepines are the most frequently prescribed medications for insomnia. They are best utilized for the short term, however, given the risk of tolerance, addiction, and rebound insomnia following discontinuation of the medication.

In Chapter 19, Turner discusses the prescriptive approach to the treatment of three of the dramatic-impulsive personality disorders: borderline, narcissistic, and histrionic. Much of the chapter focuses on borderline personality disorder (BPD), given the comparatively more extensive research literature available for this diagnosis. Borderline personality disorder is characterized by chronic patterns of impulsivity, emotional lability, and interpersonal problems. Depression and anxiety are common complaints of patients with BPD. Additionally, brief psychotic episodes, self-mutilation, and suicide attempts are common. Because the core features of BPD include emotional disturbances, treatment has (until recently) consisted almost exclusively of psychodynamic therapy, which, in turn, has rarely been subjected to empirical evaluation. Newly developed interventions, however, such as Linehan's dialectical behavior therapy, Turner's dynamic cognitive behavior therapy, and Beck's cognitive therapy, show considerable promise in the treatment of this challenging disorder. Their interventions draw upon traditional tenets of behavioral and cognitive therapy but also incorporate insights derived from developmental theory. Preliminary research using methodologically rigorous experimental designs supports the use of cognitive-behavioral interventions in reducing BPD symptoms. In addition, dialectical behavioral therapy stands out in reducing the rate of premature termination, which is so often a problem with this population. Pharmacotherapy is often employed, although identifying optimal medications can be an arduous process for the psychiatrist. Patient compliance may be poor, and the frequent risk of suicide poses limitations on what drugs can be used. Borderline personality disorder is chronic, and intermittent contact with clinicians is often required for at least several years posttreatment.

Under the rubric of special issues in Part III Williamson and Sebastian (Chapter 20) examine treatment of three psychophysiologic disorders: headaches, irritable bowel syndrome, and cardiovascular disease. In the case of migraine and tension headaches, relaxation training and biofeedback are effective in reducing headache frequency and severity of pain. Similarly, propranolol and amitriptyline were successful in 40 to 60% of cases for migraine and tension headaches, respectively. In irritable bowel syndrome, relaxation training, stress management training, and cognitive-behavioral therapy have been shown to reduce the gastrointestinal symptoms associated with this condition. Biofeedback, on the other hand, appears to be of limited utility. Changes in diet and use of anxiolytics are potentially useful adjuncts to psychosocial treatment for this condition. Cardiovascular disease often develops as a function of several health risks, such as obesity and cigarette smoking. Modest gains in reducing hypertension have been found with biofeedback and relaxation training, and the authors advocate use of these interventions in conjunction with medication. Behavioral interventions targeting weight loss and smoking cessation show encouraging short-term success, although relapse rates are quite high. In all likelihood, most psychophysiologic disorders will have a chronic course in which effective management rather than cure is the ultimate goal.

In Chapter 21, Kerns reviews new developments in pain management. It is readily acknowledged that pain is a complex phenomenon, involving neurophysiologic, psychosocial, and environmental components. Therefore, assessment is comprehensive, targeting both physical and psychological domains. Kerns argues that the primary purpose of assessment is to generate hypotheses about factors that cause and maintain pain. These, in turn, can be used to formulate a treatment plan. In general, research supports a multidisciplinary approach to pain treatment, in which psychosocial interventions and pharmacotherapy are implemented concurrently. Research studies in this area, however, exhibit several shortcomings in design, thereby providing little guidance to the clinician in selecting optimal treatments for specific types of pain. Kerns points out that a significant impediment to treatment is the reluctance of patients to accept a biobehavioral model of pain, resulting in lowered levels of motivation and participation in psychosocial interventions.

Harris and Rice (Chapter 22) cover prescriptive approaches to managing the violent patient. Such patients are particularly challenging for the clinician, in terms of both inpatient management and outpatient treatment. In their own research, the authors employ an actuarial approach to predicting violence in psychiatric patients. Employing 12 variables, of which a measure of psychopathy was the most influential, they developed an actuarial table for predicting risk of future violence. Furthermore, Harris and Rice advocate use of such a system in identifying individuals who are appropriate for treatment or, for chronically violent patients, incarceration. Treatment must take into account factors that may contribute to the emergence of violence, such as substance abuse, antisocial personality, and deviant sexual activities. In general, treatment should be intensive, target needs that directly contribute to the expression of violence, and incorporate cognitive-behavioral approaches. Unfortunately, long-term outcome studies of the treatment and prevention of violence are lacking. Until further investigations are conducted, clinicians must make do with broad approaches to treatment in lieu of specific, optimal interventions.

The treatment of men who batter their partners is reviewed in Chapter 23 by Follingstad and Breiter. Now recognized as a major public health problem, battering in couples has attracted considerable attention in the past decade. Initially, services focused almost exclusively on the female victim of battering. More recently, however, interventions for male perpetrators have emerged. The predominant mode of treatment is cognitive-behavioral therapy with groups of batterers. Typically, a variety of topics is addressed, including anger control, attitudes and beliefs about male and female roles, and self-esteem. Several other types of programs are also used, reflecting insight-oriented theoretical viewpoints and the feminist model. Unfortunately, research in this area is in its infancy, and controlled outcome studies are scarce. Several studies suggest that relapse rates are high, particularly for men who are also substance abusers.

When taken together, the chapters in this volume document the considerable progress that has been made in developing optimal interventions for a variety of adult disorders. The authors have shared their collective expertise to provide clear guidelines for assessment and treatment. Working from the existing empirical literature, they have recommended procedures to be followed in the clinical setting. Moreover, they have directly addressed the problems and impediments to treatment that are so often encountered by clinicians. As the quality of research on treatment efficacy improves, further refinements in prescriptive approaches to assessment and treatment can be anticipated.

Many individuals have contributed to the fruition of this project, and we would like to acknowledge their respective efforts. First, we thank our friend and editor at Plenum Press, Eliot Werner, who once again has been forward-looking in this editorial decision. Second, we thank our eminent contributors for their willingness to share with us particular conceptualizations of their segments of the field. Finally, we thank Burt G. Bolton, Ann Huber, Angela Dodson, Christine Ryan, and Nancy Simpson for their gracious technical assistance.

MICHEL HERSEN

ROBERT T. AMMERMAN

Fort Lauderdale, Florida

Pittsburgh, Pennsylvania

Reference

Paul, G. H. (1967). Strategy of outcome research in psychotherapy. *Journal of Consulting Psychology, 31,* 109–118.

Contents

I

INTRODUCTION

1

Overview of the Issues in Prescriptive Treatments

Ron Acierno, Michel Hersen, and Robert T. Ammerman

Introduction: Historical Perspectives

Four decades of increased empiricism in the field of clinical psychology have served to yield several confident responses to Paul's "ultimate" question: "What treatment, by whom, is most effective for this individual with that specific problem under which set of circumstances?" (1967, p. 111). Paul's call for specification of the conditions under which an intervention will be effective is consistent with the notion ·of a "prescriptive" approach to the treatment of psychopathology (i.e., the prescription of a highly specified, thoroughly evaluated treatment regimen in order to ameliorate a highly specified, thoroughly assessed complaint). Application of prescriptive interventions to psychological problems is not entirely novel. Indeed, this has been the approach followed by the psychopharmacological field for some time (albeit with somewhat limited success, the causes of which will be discussed below). Reasons for psychologists' delay in deriving and applying prescriptive psychological treatments to psychopathology become apparent through examination of early 20th century trends in theory and conceptualization.

Initial developments in clinical psychology were largely the result of deduction and "experimentation" in the form of descriptive case studies (e.g., Freud's Anna O.). Precedence for employing this form of reasoning in the derivation of psychological interventions is easily traced to Hippocrates, who hypothesized that psychopathology was grounded in a somatic substrate: namely, an imbalance among an individual's four

Ron Acierno and **Michel Hersen** • Center for Psychological Studies, Nova Southeastern University, Fort Lauderdale, Florida 33314.   **Robert T. Ammerman** • Western Pennsylvania School for Blind Children, Pittsburgh, Pennsylvania 15213-1499.

Handbook of Prescriptive Treatments for Adults, edited by Michel Hersen and Robert T. Ammerman. Plenum Press, New York, 1994.

bodily humours. Treatment, therefore, called for purging of those humours found to be in excess. Along similar lines, and somewhat more relevant to contemporary psychology, Freud ingeniously deduced the existence of a system of intrapsychic constructs (also ultimately based in the somatic substrate) to account for mental illness. By combining a priori psychological dispositions with environmental events, Freud arrived at a seemingly integrated theory with specific treatment correlates. Consistent with the mode of its genesis, evaluation of this theory in the clinical realm proceeded according to the rules of deductive logic. Unfortunately, the validity of these evaluations was suspect (Eysenck, 1952), because the act of supporting a construct (or intervention) developed through deductive reasoning with further deduction is tautological. One is led, for example, to the statement: A patient is cured once his oedipal conflict is resolved; if a patient still evidences pathology, then his oedipal conflict must not yet be resolved. Because treatments were deduced on the basis of rational (rather than empirical) examination of information upon which a particular theoretical framework had been superimposed, interventions were rather unidimensional (nonprescriptive)—that is, treatments were theory consistent rather than problem specific.

Although "deductive research" dominated the clinical field in the early 20th century, empiricists were not wholly absent. "Bottom-up research" with animals and nonclinical populations proceeded in the laboratories of Watson, Thorndike, Pavlov, and Skinner. Work of these experimenters followed the tenets of inductive reasoning, in that all possible assumptions were evaluated via the scientific method prior to their incorporation into theory. Operant and associative laws of learning were discerned, rather than deduced, and the importance placed upon empirical objectivism resulted in the conceptual approach to psychology known as behaviorism. Conclusions were now to be based on data rather than on beliefs or inferences (Bellack & Hersen, 1985). As a result of the nature of the inductive approach, however, application of empirical constructs to clinical psychology was necessarily delayed. In 1958, however, Joseph Wolpe bridged the gap between experimental and clinical realms with his landmark work, *Psychotherapy by Reciprocal Inhibition*. Here for the first time was an experimentally constructed and verifiable intervention, the origins of which were precisely traced to empirically revealed laws of learning. Indeed, Wolpe's technique of reciprocal inhibition represented the first prescriptive treatment in the field of clinical psychology in that its intended application was by no means universal but, rather, required precise and thorough assessment and verification of the existence of a learned, maladaptive neurotic habit for which relearning could occur.

The demonstrated success of experimentally based interventions, combined with increased disillusionment (e.g., Eysenck, 1960) with deductively based treatments (e.g., psychoanalysis), provided the impetus for researchers and clinicians to adopt an attitude of increased empiricism. Indeed, psychology's acceptance of the inductive approach is evident in an informal survey the first author conducted of the content of the 1953, 1963, 1973, 1983, and 1992 volumes of the *Journal of Consulting and Clinical Psychology*. In 1953, 3% of this publication's treatment-related articles achieved some level of experimental control. An additional 5% of the papers were related to treatment in some manner but were uncontrolled. Fully 92% of the articles were concerned with nontreatment topics (e.g., personality assessment via the Rorschach Ink Blot test). In 1963 (following publication of Wolpe's *Psychotherapy by Reciprocal Inhibition*), interest in the clinical realm had grown: 11% of the articles were treatment related; only 1%, however, were experimental in nature. By 1973, empiricism, too, was on the rise: 7% of the articles were experimental evaluations of psychological interventions, and an additional 19% were treatment related in some way. Still, 73% of the articles in this issue were not related to treatment. Increased empiricism was readily evident in the 1983 volume, within which 15% of the articles were controlled treatment evaluations. Articles related to uncontrolled treatment composed 17% of this volume, and papers not directly related to treatment (largely intelligence and neuropsychological assessment topics) accounted for 68% of the contents. The trend toward increased clinical empiricism continues today: 19% of the articles published in the 1992 volume of the *JCCP* were controlled, treatment-related studies, 39% were related to treatment in some manner, and 43% covered nontreatment topics.

Clearly, interest in psychological interventions has grown remarkably in the last 50 years, with a concomitant growth in the number of empirical evaluations of these interventions. The result (and intent) of these empirical endeavors has been to predict and specify which treatment, given by whom, will be most effective for which individual, with which problem, under what circumstances. Furthermore, Omer and Dar (1992) note that, within the context of clinical research, the focus upon pragmatism (over blind empiricism) has intensified. The emphasis on clinical utility over empirical theorizing is evident in the increased employment of clinical, rather than college student subject populations; a reduction in analog research; increased attention to the enduring nature of therapeutic effects; and a relatively greater interest in clinical than in statistical significance. It is from this context that prescriptive treatments are specified, implemented, and evaluated.

Prescriptive Assessment

Successful implementation of focused prescriptive treatments requires multi-faceted, focused assessment of (a) symptom presentation, (b) maintaining factors, (c) etiological factors, and (d) subject characteristics and history. Thorough assessment across each area permits the informed selection of those treatments found to be most effective in ameliorating well-defined problems. Exclusive assessment along only one parameter (e.g., symptoms) ignores the existence of diagnostic subtypes and increases the likelihood that an inappropriate or ineffective treatment will be applied to an individual's pathology. Psychopharmacologists have been most guilty of inadequate, unidimensional assessment prior to treatment selection, but they are by no means alone in their errant ways. Behaviorists, likely in response to an inherited predisposition to flee unsubstantiated etiological theorizing, also often fall short of performing encompassing assessments.

Most disturbing is the assumption by clinical researchers of homogeneity across individuals sharing the same symptom presentation (see Beutler, 1979; Hersen, 1981). Wolpe (1977) has referred to this practice as "the Achilles heel of outcome research in behavior therapy." Assumptions of homogeneity are problematic in that conclusions reached regarding the efficacy of a particular treatment are meaningless when one is not fully aware of the nature of the disorder (or disorders) treated. (This criticism is particularly relevant to meta-analytic endeavors, in which the blurring effects of multiple inappropriate assumptions of homogeneity are compounded.)

The weakness of unidimensional assessment is illustrated by a case of cocaine-induced psychosis. The symptomatic presentation of this condition (severe agitation, hallucinations, and bizarre thinking) is identical to that of paranoid schizophrenia. Applying the appropriate prescriptive treatment for paranoid schizophrenia to this case, however, would be ineffective and potentially dangerous. Rather, additional assessment of etiology and maintaining variables provides the clinician with sufficient information to implement the appropriate intervention.

The diagnosis of major depression in the *Diagnostic and Statistical Manual of Mental Disorders*, Third Edition, Revised (DSM-III-R) serves as another informative example. As a result of its flight from etiological controversy, the DSM-III-R now separates depression into only two symptom-defined categories: major depressive disorder and bipolar disorder. (Although the DSM-IV will likely increase the number of categories to three, each category will be solely symptom defined [Barlow, 1993].) It is unlikely, however, that the category of major depression is homogeneous, as the DSM implies. Indeed, both symptomatic and etiological subtypes have been shown to exist (Wolpe, 1977, 1986). Unfortunately, empirical evaluations of treatments for depression rarely recognize probable heterogeneity among subjects. As a result, conclusions based upon these studies are "rendered nugatory by the imprecision of the data" (Wolpe, 1977). In the prescriptive diagnosis of depression, however,

> the label, depression, would serve to cue the therapist as to which factors [in each of the four areas mentioned] need to be included in the assessment. Treatment would then be designed to match the problem area(s). If the problem is a lack of social skills, then the client should receive social skills training; if the problem is a distortion of environmental feedback, then cognitive therapy for the particular problem should be undertaken; if the problem is excessive standard setting, then more realistic standard setting should be taught . . . and so on (Craighead, 1980, p. 126).

Clearly, inadequate assessment or assumptions of homogeneity result in the non-prescriptive assignment of treatment to poorly defined disorders (Burke & Silverman, 1987).

Symptoms

Assessment of symptom presentation precedes assessment in other areas, includes measurement of cognition, motoric behavior, and physiology, and is most often accomplished through subject self-report, behavioral observation, and physiological monitoring. Comprehensive assessment at the symptom level will address each of the response channels proposed by Lang (1968). Thorough assessment of symptoms across each response channel enhances the degree to which prescriptive treatments can be "fine-tuned." To demonstrate this point, Ost, Johansson, and Jerremalm (1982) divided 34 claustrophobic subjects into groups of "physiological" or "behavioral" responders on the basis of a tripartite assessment battery. Half of each group received a behavior-based intervention, while the other half received a treatment which was largely physiological. Results indicated that physiological responders who received a physiologically based treatment benefitted to a relatively greater extent than did physiological responders who received a behavior-based treatment. Analogously, behavioral responders who received a behavior-based treatment showed more improvement than did behavioral responders who received a physiologically based treatment. Ost, Jerremalm, and Johansson (1981) found that a similar pattern existed in social phobics, indicating that for these disorders, symptom-specific subtypes are present and respond differentially to treatment.

Ley (1992) reported that comparable symptom subtypes of panic exist. Through tripartite symptom assessment, Ley demonstrated that, in some panic disordered individuals, attacks are characterized by large increases in heart rate accompanied by sharp decreases in end-tidal CO_2 pressure. In others, heart rate increases and end-tidal CO_2 decreases are absent, but apprehensive anxiety and catastrophic cognitions are found to precede panic. The former attacks are characterized by hyperventilation, while the latter are characterized by exceptionally frightening thoughts. Therefore, the prescriptive treatment of the former (panic characterized by hyperventilatory symptoms) will emphasize the relative importance of breathing retraining, whereas the latter ("cognitive" panics) will require a prescriptive treatment that features decatastrophizing (Ley, in press) (a third subtype of "conditioned" panic will be addressed in the etiological assessment section below).

Analogous findings are evident in the depression literature. Symptom subtypes of depression correspond to etiological subtypes and have been shown to respond differentially to treatment (e.g., lithium carbonate for bipolar disorder). Furthermore, the importance of tripartite assessment of anxiety symptoms in individuals suffering from depression has been illustrated repeatedly by Wolpe (1977, 1979, 1986) and is reflected in the likely "readmittance" in DSM-IV of the anxious-depression subtype. Indeed, in addition to subjective reports of anxiety, anxious depression can be physiologically differentiated from nonanxious depression on the basis of sedation thresholds or the amount of sodium amobarbital required to produce certain EEG and behavioral nonresponding effects (Wolpe, 1986). Individuals suffering from anxious depression evince higher sedation thresholds than is the norm (as do individuals suffering from anxiety disorders), whereas nonanxious depressed individuals show *lower*-than-average sedation thresholds. These depressive subtypes, therefore, are qualitatively, rather than simply quantitatively, different and as such require markedly different prescriptive treatments. Indeed, Conti, Placidi, Dell'Osso, Lenzi, and Cassano (1987) found that nonanxious depressives responded well to antidepressant medication, whereas anxious depressives responded no better to antidepressants than to placebo. The prescriptive treatment for anxious depression, therefore, will include procedures that foster anxiety reduction (Hersen, 1981; Wolpe, 1986) as well as techniques that reduce depressive affect.

In addition to the process of intracategorical differential diagnosis discussed thus far, thorough tripartite symptom assessment also facilitates intercategorical differential diagnosis (Hersen, 1973). In other words, precise symptomatic evaluation contributes to the clinician's ability to distinguish (and thereby prescriptively treat) dementia from depression, social from simple phobia, and posttraumatic stress disorder from generalized anxiety disorder. As mentioned, however, prescriptive assessment must not end at the symptom level. Rather, the context within which symptoms present (i.e., the variables which serve to maintain the symptoms) must also be precisely measured.

Maintaining Variables

Functional analysis entails identification of contingencies and/or discriminative stimuli found in a patient's natural environment that serve to perpetuate or elicit the target pathological behavior. Whereas delineation of the actual target behavior is accomplished through symptom assessment, functional assessment often reveals the purpose a particular set of symptoms serve, or reasons for their perpetuation. With this knowledge, prescriptive treatments can be chosen that address symptomatic variables as well as provide more appropriate means by which to achieve a given purpose.

The process by which a functional analysis, or assessment of maintaining variables, is carried out is determined, to a large extent, by the symptomatic presentation of the client. However, every assessment should include (a) delineation of the antecedents and consequences of the target behavior; (b) specification of the effects the target behavior has upon the patient's significant others, and their responses to these effects; and (c) determination of the environmental stimuli that vary as a function of the target behavior. The difficulty in performing a functional assessment depends largely upon the type of presenting disorder (e.g., functional assessment of school refusal in a child will likely entail less effort than functional assessment of major depression in a married adult). Data garnered in each case will be integral to selecting an appropriate prescriptive treatment, however.

In their treatment of hysterical paralysis in a 42-year-old man, Kallman, Hersen, and O'Toole (1975) illustrate the necessity of complementing symptom assessment with a functional analysis of maintaining variables. In the 5 years prior to his presentation for treatment, the patient had experienced several 1- to 2-week periods during which he was unable to walk or even move his legs. Assessment revealed that onset of these symptoms occurred soon after the subject's early retirement and assumption of what were formerly his wife's household duties. Furthermore, the investigators determined that episodes of past paralysis coincided with exacerbations of familial discord. In addition, it was evident that during periods of paralysis, the patient received a considerable amount of social reinforcement from family members (e.g., breakfast in bed) as well as relief from household duties. The patient was hospitalized and a focused prescriptive treatment was derived in which standing and walking behaviors were differentially reinforced through social praise provided by attractive research assistants. As predicted, standing and walking abilities returned quickly. The authors noted that, with few exceptions, both frequency and duration of standing and walking behaviors were directly related to the amount of reinforcement the assistants provided. The patient was discharged; gains were maintained for only 4 weeks, whereupon he was readmitted to the hospital, again unable to walk. Since previous functional assessment revealed antecedents or discriminative stimuli that served to trigger hysterical paralysis (familial stress), as well as consequences that served to maintain and increase the likelihood of future hysterical paralytic events (social reinforcement and relief from household duties), comprehensive prescriptive treatment was implemented in which family members were trained to differentially reinforce standing and walking behaviors and ignore (extinguish) hysterical paralysis behavior. Appropriate social reinforcement from the family (rather than from only the nurses) resulted in lasting therapeutic gains. Clearly, comprehensive prescriptive treatment demands an assessment beyond the symptomatic level in order to achieve enduring effects.

Often, the operants and resulting consequences that serve to maintain a pathological behavior are significantly less obvious than those in the preceding illustration. Barlow (1993) reported a case of recurring panic disorder for which symptomatic and functional assessment served to yield a treatment with effects limited to about 12 months. In his initial functional analysis, Barlow noted that the client's panics were triggered by interoceptive cues, such as rapid heart rate and upset stomach. Furthermore, it was apparent that this subject was negatively reinforced for avoidance of these interoceptive cues in much the same way that phobics are negatively reinforced for avoiding their feared object (Mowrer, 1947). As a result of continued avoidance, no learning (extinction) occurred, and the interoceptive stimuli retained their anxiety-eliciting power. Barlow's prescriptive treatment, therefore, involved exposure to, rather than avoidance of, subtle interoceptive cues through such physically exerting activities as planned exercise. As mentioned, panic attacks were successfully eliminated through this procedure for a short time but eventually returned in full force. A thorough assessment of maintaining variables was again performed, and it was discovered that, in addition to triggering panic, interoceptive stimuli were also discriminitive cues for some particularly frightening cognitions. Specifically, each time the client perceived his heart to be beating rapidly, he experienced the belief that he might be going insane and would be institutionalized, as his brother had been. This cognition, which had not been directly addressed in the previous intervention, eventually became sufficiently anxiety-producing to elicit a panic attack. Therefore, a comprehensive prescriptive treatment was implemented (resulting in lasting therapeutic gains) that combined (a) procedures specifically designed to desensitize the client to the subjective fear produced by thoughts of impending insanity with (b) interoceptive exposure techniques designed to eliminate the autonomically generated panic response.

This example supports the position that to comprehensively assess the variables that maintain a pathology, one should address both the contingencies that sustain an operant, as well as subtle (second-order) discriminative stimuli that repeatedly elicit the behavior. In other words, knowledge of both instrumental and associative properties of the environment facilitates the application of encompassing, multidimensional prescriptive treatments. Yet the assessment must not end here, for, as Wolpe (1986) notes, "The most effective treatments of diseases are usually based on knowledge of their etiology" (p. 499).

Etiological Factors

The highly focused nature of prescriptive treatment demands the added therapeutic precision that etiological assessment provides. Indeed,

> on an a priori basis, it would seem that in cases where faulty habits have been conditioned, a therapeutic strategy directed toward their deconditioning would be most appropriate. On the other hand, where cognitive misperceptions predominate, a therapeutic strategy directed toward correcting such misperceptions would seem warranted (Hersen, 1981, p. 21).

In contrast to many clinical endeavors, etiological assessment is rarely employed to guarantee subject homogeneity in empirical evaluations of psychological interventions (Hersen, 1981; Wolpe, 1977, 1979). As a result, treatment conditions are composed of heterogeneous individuals, and noted effects (or the lack thereof) are potentially attributable to the intervention, to etiological differences among subjects, or to some interaction of the two. Neglect of etiological assessment in research is traced, in large part, to the DSM's rejection of etiological specification in diagnostic classification as a means to avoid theoretical baggage. However, the baby thereby has been thrown out with the bathwater; in any prescriptive treatment, etiological assessment is essential in that it directs the clinician to those aspects of an intervention most relevant to a particular client's presenting problem.

The treatment literature on depression clearly illustrates the relevance of etiological assessment to prescriptive interventions. In a recent meta-analysis of treatment outcome studies evaluating the relative effectiveness of newer antidepressants, standard antidepressants, and placebo, Greenberg, Bornstein, Greenberg, and Fisher (1992) found that medication was not significantly more effective than placebo in the treatment of depression. These results are potentially misleading, however, because subjects in the studies were not consistently differentiated on the basis of etiology. (Of the studies, 59% did not attempt etiological differentiation; the remainder of the studies employed varying criteria for differentiation.) As a result, treatment effects were potentially confounded by etiological differences across conditions. Similarly, Taylor and McLean (1993) found that specific treatment "outcome profiles" (i.e., proportions of patients displaying recovery, recovery followed by remission, and no recovery) produced by behavior therapy, amitriptyline, psychodynamic therapy, and relaxation training did not differ at 3 months posttest. Although behavior therapy resulted in the largest overall mean improvement, each condition had relatively equal proportions of treatment responders, nonresponders, and responders who experienced relapse. Again, however, subjects were not differentiated on the basis of etiology, and reported results were confounded by a possible interaction between etiological subtype and treatment condition. Evidence for the validity of this concern is provided by a number of studies that demonstrate (a) etiological subtypes of depression do, in fact, exist; and (b) these subtypes respond differentially to treatment.

Several investigators have reported data that support the existence of a biologically based, "endogenous" depressive syndrome differentiated from nonendogenous depression on the basis of several reliable indices (Conti, Placidi, Dell'Osso, Lenzi, & Cassano, 1987; Feinberg, 1992; Kupfer & Thase, 1983; Thase, Hersen, Bellack, Himmelhoch, & Kupfer, 1983; Wolpe, 1986). As mentioned, endogenous depressives evince below-average sedation thresholds, as well as abnormal EEG, REM latency, and REM density patterns during sleep (Feinberg, 1992; Jones, Kelwala, Bell, & Dube, 1985; Kupfer & Thase, 1983). In addition, nonsuppressors on the dexamethasone suppression test are almost exclusively endogenous depressives. Furthermore, endogenous depressives are more likely than are nonendogenous depressives to present with early morning awakening, motor retardation, reduced coordination, ideas of guilt or self-reference, and little or no anxiety (Gunther, Gunther, Streck, & Ronig, 1988; Wolpe, 1979).

Whereas the origin of endogenous depression is, by definition, biological, Wolpe (1986) identifies four etiological subtypes of nonendogenous (he prefers the term *neurotic*) depression: depression (a) as a consequence of severe conditioned anxiety, (b) as a consequence of devaluative cognitions, (c) as a consequence of interpersonal inadequacy or social skills deficits, and (d) as a consequence of severe bereavement. As is the case with endogenous depression, reliable differentiation among these four subtypes is achieved through a comprehensive behavioral analysis (see Wolpe, 1986).

Several authors have provided support for the contention that subtypes of depression, particularly endogenous and nonendogenous subtypes, respond differentially to treatment. Raskin and Crook (1976) found that endogenous depressives responded well to antidepressant medication but poorly to placebo, whereas nonendogenous depressives responded depressives responded well to both treatments. In a follow-up to a separate study, Kiloh, Ball, and Garside (1977) found that endogenous depressives treated with antidepressants maintained gains to a significantly greater extent than did nonendogenous depressives undergoing identical treatment. In contrast, Rush (1983) found that none of the subjects in his study diagnosed with endogenous depression responded to cognitive therapy. In a second, related experiment, however, eight of nine nonendogenous depressives responded well to the identical cognitive intervention. Demonstrating the differential effectiveness of treatments on the subtypes of nonendogenous depression, McKnight, Nelson, Hayes, and Jarrett (1992) found that depressed subjects who evinced social skills deficits but not depressogenic cognitions improved to a relatively greater extent on measures of both depression and social skills following skills training than did similarly classified subjects receiving cognitive therapy. In contrast, depressed subjects who displayed depressogenic cognitions but not social skills deficits improved to a relatively greater extent on measures of both depression and irrational cognitions following cognitive therapy than did similar subjects who received social skills training. Clearly, assessment of etiological factors in depression potentiates increasingly effective application of prescriptive interventions. Furthermore, empirical evaluations of the efficacy of both psychological and pharmacological treatments designed to eliminate depression must assure subject homogeneity in order to achieve meaningful results.

Analogous findings exist in the phobia literature, in that origins of circumscribed fears with identical symptom presentations are not necessarily homogeneous across subjects (Ost, 1991). Indeed, Wolpe (1981) and Rachman (1977) have proposed that, whereas some phobias are acquired through conditioning experiences, others may result from misinformation or faulty logic—or, in the case of social phobias, skills deficits. Wolpe, Lande, McNally, and Schotte (1985) and Ost and Hugdahl (1983) have demonstrated reliable methods to determine phobic etiologies. Wolpe et al. (1985) classify phobias as having a cognitive or misinformational origin "when a patient's beliefs lead him to conclude that the feared situation presents or predicts real and present danger in the sense that it is likely to produce damage to his physical or mental well being" (p. 289). In contrast, the fear is classified as having a conditioned basis if the subject reports feeling "as if" he or she will be danger but does not actually *believe* the stimulus will be harmful, or reports fearing the panic associated with the phobic object rather than the object itself (McNally & Steketee, 1985; Wolpe et al., 1985). Similarly, Ost and Hugdahl (1983) employ a Phobic Origins Questionnaire to differentiate conditioned from cognitive fear etiologies on the basis of subject self-report of either traumatic conditioning experiences or negative information and instruction. Reliability of etiological classification with respect to phobias is further enhanced by combining the two assessment strategies.

Ost (1985) has demonstrated an interaction between mode of phobia acquisition and method of treatment employed. In his study, subjects with conditioned fears who received treatments aimed at counterconditioning or extinguishing anxiety responded positively to a greater extent than did subjects with conditioned fears who received cognitive restructuring. Along similar lines, Trower, Yardley, Bryant, and Shaw (1978) found that socially phobic subjects who evinced social skills deficits improved significantly more after receiving social skills training than did comparable subjects receiving systematic desensitization. However, socially anxious subjects who did not manifest skills deficits responded equally well to both treatments. Consistent with findings in the depression literature, it appears that thorough etiological assessment of phobic subjects, particularly those with identical symptomology, facilitates prescription of an effective intervention.

Further research will likely yield similar findings with panic disorder. Indeed, Ley (1992) has outlined three etiological subtypes of panic and notes that responses to treatment among the subtypes are not consistent. In "Type I," or hyperventilatory, panics, hyperventilation plays a causal role *each* time a panic attack is experienced. In "Type II," or conditioned, panics, hyperventilation or some other discrete event causes an initial panic but contiguous interoceptive stimuli become higher-order conditioned elicitors of future panics. In "Type III," or cognitive, panics, unfamiliar or unexpected interoceptive stimuli are erroneously interpreted as evidence of imminent physical and mental breakdown. This misinformed conclusion results in additional anxiety, which further exacerbates somatic cues, thereby reaffirming the disastrous nature of the initial missattribution, and so on until the vicious cycle results in a panic attack. Clearly, the prescriptive treatment for Type I panics will necessarily include breathing retraining procedures so that incidence of hyperventilation in the patient is reduced (e.g., Ley, 1993). Prescriptive interventions for Type II panics must entail interoceptive exposure so that learned anxiety responses can be extinguished or counterconditioned (e.g., Griez & van den Hout, 1986). Finally, prescriptive treatments for Type III panics demand cognitive restructuring techniques so that somatic symptoms are no longer catastrophically missattributed (e.g., Beck, Sokal, Clark, Berchick, & Wright, 1992). Again, it is evident that thorough etiological assessment contributes significantly to effective prescription of psychological interventions for specific problems.

Subject Characteristics and History

The implicit relevance of subject characteristics and history to effective prescriptive interventions is evident from the methods section of every treatment outcome study. Indeed, the *Journal of Consulting and Clinical Psychology* (*51*[6]) devoted a multipage editorial to delineating several subject characteristics that must be assessed and reported in any papers accepted for publication on the topic of depression. Assessment of age, gender, socioeconomic status, level of social support, and ethnicity provides essential diagnostic information that is often highly relevant to treatment selection and outcome. For example, initial presence of actively psychotic symptoms in an 18-year-old man is highly indicative of schizophrenia. Identical symptoms appearing for the first time in a 60-year-old man, however, probably implicate an organic disorder, such as delirium, rather than schizophrenia.

Clinician's employing prescriptive treatments must also be aware that prevalence of many disorders varies as a function of a patient's sociocultural characteristics. Indeed, posttraumatic stress disorder (PTSD) is relatively more prevalent in African Americans and Hispanics than in European Americans (Lonigan, Shannon, Finch, & Daugherty, 1991). Alcoholism is relatively less common in Italians and Jews than in the Irish, Russian, or French (Swinson & Eaves, 1978). Patients from lower socioeconomic levels are at a greater risk for almost any psychological disorder than are individuals from middle and upper socioeconomic ranges (Dohrenwend & Dohrenwend, 1974). Young Native Americans are at a significantly greater risk for suicide than are those of any other ethnic group (May, 1987). Organic disorders are significantly more likely to occur in older (than younger) adults. And anorexia and simple phobias, but not obesity and social phobia, are significantly more prevalent in females than in males.

In addition to providing some direction to the process of diagnosis, varying subject characteristics are associated with differential treatment responses and requirements. For example, Bupp and Preskorn (1991) found that older adults maintained on set levels of nortriptyline had higher steady-state blood plasma levels than did younger adults receiving the same dosage. Older adults, therefore, require relatively less of the medication to achieve the same potency. Failure to reduce dosage accordingly subjects the patient to unwarranted side effects from the drug. In a second example, George, Blazer, Hughes, and Fowler (1989) reported that depressed elderly subjects (particularly males) with poor social networks were significantly more likely to reexperience depression at 6 to 32 months posttreatment than were similarly treated depressed elderly subjects with more intact social supports. Therefore, successful and enduring prescriptive treatments for elderly depressed men will necessarily include components that function to increase the quality and extent of their social networks as well as techniques to reduce depressive affect.

In addition to predicting diagnostic categories or response to treatment, subject characteristics and history often speak to the appropriateness of a particular therapy for a given individual. For example, systematic desensitization may not be entirely suitable for very young children who have not attained the level of cognitive development required to generate affective imagery. Furthermore, flooding might be contraindicated with frail or elderly patients suffering from anxiety disorders. Treatments that have proven to be ineffective for a particular individual in the past should be discarded in favor of interventions which have produced positive results.

It is evident from the above review that the highly focused nature of prescriptive treatment requires thorough, multidimensional assessment. In contrast to general "psychotherapy" (e.g., psychoanalysis or supportive counseling), which is applied to a vast number of problems, prescriptive treatments entail specified procedures that change according to the disorder and client. Indeed, prescriptive treatments vary as a function of symptoms, maintaining factors, etiology, and subject characteristics. Note, however, that the effects of prescriptive treatments are intentionally circumscribed. While exceptionally potent, the therapeutic results of these techniques are limited to targeted problems. Rarely, however, do patients present with only a single, well-defined complaint. Rather, their problems are complex and, as such, require complex solutions (Hersen, 1981). Often, therefore, prescription of multiple treatments will be appropriate and necessary to eliminate suffering in an individual. The scope of an intervention package employed with a given client is determined by repeated evaluation of the variables specified above. At no time during the clinician's involvement with the patient is the assessment completed. In contrast, measurement is continuous and dynamic, yielding prescriptive treatments that are refined and changed according to the needs of the client.

Effectiveness of Prescriptive Treatments

Pharmacological Interventions

Application of prescriptive treatments to psychopathology presupposes experimental demonstration that such interventions are effective. In contrast to the state of affairs at the time of Eysenck's review (1952), several such demonstrations have now been conducted, largely through the efforts of behavioral and psychopharmacological investigators. The following is a partial review of the "what works" prescriptive treatment literature—first that describing pharmacological interventions, and then that concerning psychological treatments.

Pharmacological approaches have been shown to successfully ameliorate distressing symptoms of major depression (particularly the endogenous subtype), bipolar disorder, several anxiety disorders, bulimia, insomnia, the positive signs of schizophrenia, and seizure disorders. In a review of 30 controlled trials of imipramine versus placebo, Rogers and Clay (1975) found that "the benefit of the drug in patients with endogenous depression . . . is indisputable" (p. 599). However, it is evident from the meta-analysis performed by Greenberg et al. (1992) that indiscriminate inclusion of subjects with nonendogenous depression in blind placebo trials mitigates this effect. While clearly effective in the treatment of endogenous depression, antidepressant medications may be no more effective than placebo in the treatment of non-endogenous depression.

In contrast to mixed results regarding the effectiveness of antidepressants with unipolar mood disorders, "there is excellent evidence that lithium carbonate is more effective than placebo in preventing the recurrence of affective episodes, either manic or depressive, in bipolar patients" (Schatzberg & Cole, 1991, p. 155). Furthermore, the temporary addition of neuroleptics to a regimen of lithium has been found to be effective in treating severe manic presentations (Goodwin & Zis, 1979). Electroconvulsive therapy has proven very effective in countering psychotic and melancholic symptoms, as well as suicidal obsessions found in severely depressed individuals.

Several recent reviews of the controlled treatment literature (Insel & Zohar, 1987; Marks, 1987; Perse, 1988) and a meta-analysis (Christensen, Hadzi-Pavlovic, Andrews, & Mattick, 1987) indicate that clomipramine, a potent serotonin reuptake inhibitor, is moderately effective in the treatment of obsessive-compulsive disorder (OCD). Specifically, subjects in studies by Insel et al. (1983) and Thoren, Asberg, Cronholm, Jornestedt, and Traskiman (1980) who received clomipramine reported a 34% and 42% mean improvement on ratings of obsessions, respectively, in comparison to a mere 7% improvement in subjects receiving a placebo. Furthermore, Gitlin (1990) noted that, although not completely improved, 60 to 70% of OCD subjects receiving clomipramine respond positively to some degree (compared to the same percentages of subjects reporting nearly complete improvement in response to exposure/response prevention behavior therapy) (Foa et al., 1983). Of note, Marks (1987) reported that presence of depression in individuals with OCD predicts an increased antiobsessional response to clomipramine. Similarly acting drugs, such as fluoxetine, also show promise in the treatment of OCD.

Individuals suffering from panic disorder with agoraphobia respond to imipramine, particularly when the drug is accompanied by programmed, in vivo exposure (note that both biological and learning etiologies are addressed in this intervention) (Mavissakalian, Michelson, & Dealy, 1983; Zitrin, Klein, & Woerner, 1980). Failure to incorporate adjunctive exposure into pharmacological treatment of panic disorder with agoraphobia severely compromises potential gains. Indeed, Telch, Agras, Taylor, Roth, and Gallen (1985) found that imipramine without exposure, while improving client's mood, had no effect on panic or phobic avoidance. Along similar lines, alprazolam has recently proven effective in reducing panic in roughly 50% of individuals suffering from panic disorder without agoraphobia (Klosko, Barlow, Tassinari, & Cerny, 1990). Although alprazolam is beneficial for its immediate calming effects, tolerance and dependence in response to its continued use are major concerns. These findings are particularly relevant when one considers that positive effects of the drug typically disappear when its use is discontinued (Fyer et al., 1987). Therefore, prescriptive use of alprazolam should be limited to short-term reduction of acute panic exacerbations.

The results of a large-scale NIMH collaborative study indicate that imipramine is often effective in the treatment of generalized anxiety disorder (GAD) (Kahn et al., 1986). Indeed, this study found imipramine to be more effective in reducing self-ratings of anxiety and interpersonal sensitivity than the more commonly prescribed benzodiazepine chlordiazepoxide, thus indirectly supporting the validity of DSM-IV's "new" diagnosis of anxious depression. Poor reliability associated with the diagnosis of GAD has impeded treatment-outcome research of greater depth.

With schizophrenics, neuroleptics have been evaluated to the extent that "the drug placebo difference . . . is so clear and well established that it would be unethical to conduct further experiments with any of the standard anti-psychotics" (Gitlin, 1990, p. 131). Although the efficacy of the major tranquilizers in reducing actively psychotic or "positive" schizophrenic signs (e.g., hallucinations) is clear, it is, however, apparent that negative schizophrenic signs (e.g., flat affect, social withdrawal) respond to medication to a much lesser extent (Lydiard & Laird, 1988). Furthermore, Kane and Lieberman (1987) note that 33% of schizophrenics maintained on a regimen of antipsychotics will experience a relapse after 1 year, and Cheung (1981) reports that 66% of medicated patients who do not relapse for 3 to 5 years will do so within 18 months after medication is withdrawn, indicating that positive effects are contingent upon continued use.

Several short-term outcome studies support the efficacy of antidepressants in the treatment of bulimia, particularly when depression is a comorbid diagnosis. In these evaluations, bulimics maintained on antidepressants evinced an average decrease in binge frequency of 75% relative to subjects receiving a placebo (Walsh, 1987). Pharmacological treatment of bulimia in isolation, however, is not recommended.

Finally, benzodiazepines, particularly triazolam and temazepam, have been shown to effectively alleviate symptoms of transient insomnia. However, the indicated use of benzodiazepines for sleep onset problems is limited to three weeks' duration (Schatzberg & Cole, 1991), after which time nonpharmacological approaches are more appropriate.

Psychological Interventions

In addition to the aforementioned pharmacological interventions, there exist several psychological approaches with demonstrated efficacy in ameliorating the symptoms of anxiety, depression, insomnia, sexual dysfunction, substance use disorders, pain, and schizophrenia. Prior to reviewing these prescriptive treatments, however, a brief discussion of relevant meta-analytic conclusions is warranted. In essence, several meta-analyses have failed to support the contention that a particular type of intervention is *considerably* more efficacious in treating psychopathology than any other (with the exception of a statistical, though not clinical, advantage for "cognitive-behavior therapy") (Shapiro & Shapiro, 1982). Meta-analyses yielding such conclusions employ grossly defined dependent and independent variables (e.g., "presence of psychopathology" and "theoretical treatment orientation"). As such, the methods used in these studies are antithetical to prescriptive approaches to assessment and treatment described thus far: objective averaging of "effect sizes" produced by multiple studies that routinely fail to examine the interactions among highly specified forms of treatment, well-defined psychological complaints, and subject characteristics and history serve to obliterate precisely those effects that are of interest to prescriptive therapists (Beutler, 1991; Stiles, Shapiro, & Elliott, 1986). Indeed, lack of a clear advantage for any vaguely defined intervention across vaguely defined disorders is exactly what is predicted by the prescriptive approach. In effect, because each treatment is applied to all disorders, large benefits produced by appropriately "matched" interventions and pathologies are inevitably offset by small or negative effects produced by interventions that are not "matched" to pathologies. Beutler (1991) and Shadish and Sweeney (1991) offer suggestions to increase the relevance and validity of meta-analytic evaluations to prescriptive treatments. These include careful and continuous assessment of both subject and pathology characteristics (treatment mediators), as well as evaluation of specific patterns of treatment effects (treatment moderators). Until these factors are considered, controlled group and single-case research will provide the most appropriate evaluations of prescriptive interventions. To date, the majority of this research has been performed by behaviorally oriented investigators.

Behavior therapy's first and firmest foothold in the arena of prescriptive interventions involved treatment of phobic disorders, in which exposure (both in vivo and in vitro) played a central role (Barlow, 1988). Systematic desensitization (Wolpe, 1990) is exceptionally effective with phobic individuals who have attained the requisite cognitive development, do not wish to endure intense anxiety, and/or fear conditioned circumscribed stimuli that are not easily presented in vivo. In contrast, flooding (Marks, 1975) has been found to be an effective intervention for phobics who are highly motivated, desire rapid improvement, and are willing to endure heightened levels of anxiety. Additionally, participant modeling (Bandura, Jeffery, & Gajdos, 1975), or graded exposure, falls somewhere between flooding and systematic desensitization in terms of rapidity of effect and level of experienced fear and is the appropriate prescriptive treatment for individuals who evince deficits in self-efficacy or mastery and avoid easily reproducible, circumscribed stimuli. Social skills training is an effective prescriptive treatment for social phobia when phobia anxiety is the result of performance failures stemming from skills deficits (Curran, 1977). In contrast, impressive reductions in social anxiety in the absence of skills deficits have been shown to result from graduated exposure complemented with anxiety management training (Butler, Cullington, Munby, Arnies, & Gelder, 1984). Along similar lines, exposure-based interventions have been shown to effectively ameliorate agoraphobic symptoms in 60 to 70% of treated subjects (Jansson & Ost, 1982). Again, parameters of exposure trials vary with the mode of prescriptive treatment chosen. Highly motivated individuals desiring relatively rapid improvement require massed and intensive, rather than spaced and graduated, exposure episodes (Feigenbaum, 1988; Marshall, 1985). Finally, the addition of coping strategies to exposure is justified with agoraphobic individuals who would otherwise be unable to endure prolonged intense anxiety.

Effectiveness of psychological interventions with anxiety disorders other than phobias has also been established. Barlow, Craske, Cerny, and Klosko (1989) have devised a componential prescriptive treatment for panic, panic control training (PCT), which includes interoceptive exposure, breathing retraining, muscle relaxation, and cognitive restructuring. In a long-term study of PCT's effectiveness, Craske, Bran, and Barlow (1991) found that 80% of subjects evinced significant improvement at both 12-week posttest and 2-year follow-up. Beck et al. (1992) have devised and evaluated focused cognitive therapy (FCT) for individuals with panic resulting from catastrophic missattributions. Fully 85% of the subjects in this study who received FCT remained panic free at the 1-year point (note that this intervention contains exposure components similar to that of Barlow et al., 1989). Additionally, Ost (1988) found progressive muscle relaxation effective in eliminating panic when specifically applied to interoceptive stimuli that trigger attacks; failure to apply relaxation to interoceptive cues severely mitigates this effect. Along similar lines, Borkovec and Mathews (1988) have found therapist-guided, comprehensive relaxation training to be effective in reducing the symptoms of GAD. Furthermore, Barlow (1993) indicates that individuals with GAD characterized by obsessive worry respond well to treatments involving exposure to anxiety-eliciting stimuli (content of worry) combined with prevention of escape responses normally employed to alleviate worry. Exposure plus response prevention has also been shown to be the treatment of choice for OCD (Foa et al., 1983). Indeed, 80-90% of OCD subjects undergoing exposure plus response prevention evince improvement, with 77% maintaining gains at 3-year follow-up. Prolonged, anxiety-eliciting exposure (albeit imaginal) is also the primary component of Keane et al.'s (1989) demonstratedly effective intervention for PTSD. However, Foa, Rothbaum, Riggs, and Murdock (1991) reported that a nonaversive package that combines exposure with anxiety management techniques was as effective as flooding in removing the symptoms of PTSD. Indeed, this intervention is considerably more appropriate than flooding when treating individuals for whom intense or prolonged anxiety is contraindicated (e.g., children).

As mentioned, empirically evaluated psychological interventions for nonendogenous depression exist and include activity scheduling, social skills training, cognitive restructuring, and interpersonal psychotherapy. Lewinsohn, Sullivan, and Grosscup (1982) provided evidence that increasing the frequency of positively reinforcing experiences and concomitantly decreasing aversive experiences through positive activity scheduling reduces depression. Additionally, Hersen, Bellack, Himmelhoch, and Thase (1984) reported that providing depressed subjects with the social skills necessary to elicit positive reinforcement, while reducing punishment from others, is effective in eliminating depression in individuals who lack such skills. Furthermore, several studies support the efficacy of Beck's cognitive therapy in the treatment of depression (Beck, Hollon, Young, Bedrosian, & Budenz, 1985; Rush, Beck, Kovacs, & Hollon, 1977). Indeed, short-term therapeutic effects of cognitive restructuring equal, and long-term effects exceed, gains noted in response to antidepressant medications, in that significantly fewer relapses are noted following cognitive therapy (Blackburn, Eunson, & Bishop, 1986; Simons, Murphy, Levine, & Wetzel, 1986). Along slightly different lines, several investigators (Elkin et al., 1989; Frank et al., 1990; Weissman et al., 1979), including those involved in the major 1989 NIMH collaborative study, have demonstrated that interpersonal therapy is highly effective in reducing depression. Furthermore, subjects receiving interpersonal therapy are at a decreased risk for future depressive episodes when monthly "booster" sessions are provided following formal treatment (Frank et al., 1990). Finally, and in contrast to earlier concerns, Rounsaville, Klerman, and Weissman (1981) and Weissman et al. (1979) report that addition of antidepressant medication to psychotherapy does not diminish the effectiveness of the latter; rather, the combination is potentially more effective than either treatment in isolation.

Psychological treatments for insomnia include progressive muscle relaxation (PMR), lifestyle management, and stimulus control procedures. Borkovec (1982) noted that in controlled trials PMR consistently reduced latency of sleep by an average of 45%. Stimulus control procedures aimed at reestablishing bed and bedroom as discriminitive stimuli for sleep are relatively more effective than relaxation, averaging a 50% reduction in latency of sleep onset (Bootzin, 1973).

Several empirically validated, prescriptive psychological treatments for sexual dysfunctions exist and include general anxiety reduction techniques as well as specific performance enhancement strategies. Obler (1973) has demonstrated the efficacy of systematic desensitization in alleviating performance-inhibiting anxiety related to sexual interactions. In contrast to imaginal exposure, graded in vivo trials and reinforced practice have been found to reduce erectile problems in men (Everaerd, 1977) and secondary orgasmic dysfunction in women (Everaerd & Dekker, 1982). In addition, Riley and Riley (1978) found that 90% of their previously inorgasmic subjects achieved orgasm following training in directed masturbation, compared to the 47% success rate resulting from sensate focus exercises. Finally, 95% of men suffering from premature ejaculation have been successfully treated with "stop-and-go" or "squeeze" techniques (Seamens, 1956).

Prescriptive interventions for paraphilias include aversion techniques designed to reduce inappropriate arousal patterns, and conditioning procedures designed to increase appropriate arousal behaviors. Covert sensitization has been successfully employed by Brownell, Hayes, and Barlow (1977) to reduce urges of exhibitionism, sadism, pedophilia, and transvestitism, and by Harbert, Barlow, Hersen, and Austin (1974) in the treatment of incestuous pedophilia. Appropriate redirection of sexual arousal in paraphiliacs has been achieved through orgasmic reconditioning by Van Deventer and Laws (1978). Controlled outcome studies in this area are few, and as a result additional prescriptive interventions have not yet been validated.

Empirically evaluated interventions for substance use disorders include techniques to control urges and improve interpersonal skills, as well as strategies to reduce marital distress and increase employment opportunities (Hersen, 1981). Azrin's (1976) community reinforcement program combines a disulfiram assurance procedure with behavioral marital therapy and vocational training in an effective comprehensive prescriptive treatment for married alcoholics. Behavioral self-control training, emphasizing stimulus control and self-reinforcement to reduce urges, has demonstrated long-term effectiveness in reducing alcohol abuse (Hester & Miller, 1989). Individuals who abuse alcohol in response to interpersonal stress or unassertiveness evince improvement following social skills training (Chaney, O'Leary, & Marlatt, 1978; Van Hasselt, Hersen, & Milliones, 1978). Specific conditioning procedures employed to reduce urges to use alcohol include taste aversion therapy (Cannon & Baker, 1981) and covert sensitization (Olson, Ganley, Devine, & Dorsey, 1981). Azrin, McMahon, Lapinsky, Besalel, and Donohue (1991) reported preliminary success in reducing cocaine and marijuana use in substance abusers through a componential treatment that includes behavioral marital therapy, stimulus control, covert sensitization, and vocational ("Job-Club") procedures.

Effective psychological treatments for pain include relaxation techniques, operant procedures, and cognitive restructuring strategies. As is the case with panic disorder, *applied* muscle relaxation (as opposed to the simple training in PMR) has been found effective in controlling pain exacerbations (Linton, 1982). In operant procedures (e.g., Fordyce, 1976), ingestion of pain medication is not contingent on the presence of discomfort (i.e., PRN) but instead follows a predetermined hourly schedule, thereby removing negative reinforcement acquired through "pain behaviors." Alternately, "non-pain behaviors," such as exercise or social interactions, are differentially reinforced so that physical health is improved while "sick" behavior is minimized. Finally, cognitive procedures, such as stress inoculation training (Meichenbaum & Turk, 1976), serve to "close the pain gate" by engaging patients in mental activities incompatible with the perception of pain (e.g., positive imagery).

In the treatment of schizophrenia, efficacy of behavioral family therapy and social skills training has been supported by controlled and replicated research. Falloon, McHill, Boyd, and Pedersen (1987) found that only 17% of schizophrenic patients maintained on a regimen of antipsychotics and treated with behavioral family therapy relapsed within 2 years, compared to an 83% rate of relapse in patients who received antipsychotic medication alone. Bellack, Turner, Hersen, and Luber (1984) have demonstrated the efficacy of social skills training in the short-term alleviation of schizophrenic symptoms, while Liberman, Mueser, and Wallace (1986) reported that intensive skills training (12 hours per week) resulted in better functioning and fewer hospitalizations and relapses in patients 2 years after treatment than found in a comparable group receiving a "holistic health" intervention. Furthermore, Hogarty et al. (1986) found that a combination of somatic maintenance therapy, behavioral family therapy, and skills training prevented relapse in 100% of treated schizophrenic patients at the 1-year point. Prescriptive psychological interventions with demonstrated effectiveness also exist for trichotillomania (Azrin & Peterson, 1987), bulimia (Wilson, Rossiter, Kleifield, & Lindholm, 1986), anorexia (Agras, Barlow, Chapin, Abel, & Leitenberg, 1974), obesity (Craighead, Stunkard, & O'Brien, 1981), and marital discord (Hahlweg & Markman, 1988). (See Table 1.1 for a summary of both validated and possible prescriptive treatments for a number of disorders.)

Relevance of Single-Subject Research to Prescriptive Interventions

Clearly, the effectiveness of prescriptive psychotherapy and pharmacotherapy has been established with the majority of psychopathologies to the extent that continued use of nonprescriptive approaches (e.g., psychoanalysis) for specific problems is hardly justified. As mentioned, however, the clinician employing prescriptive treatments must be aware of the intentionally circumscribed nature of their effects, particularly when considering the fact that most individuals do not present with only one simple or circumscribed complaint. Unfortunately, this fact is often overlooked in group studies cited in support of the efficacy of an intervention, because within-subject variability is assigned minimal importance relative to overall group scores on the dependent variable. Indeed, random assignment of subjects to treatment conditions enables conclusions to be drawn concerning an intervention *despite* subject differences on variables deemed irrelevant to the topic at hand; these differences are averaged out, and "findings are not readily translatable or generalizable to the practicing clinician since . . . the clinician cannot determine which particular patient characteristics are correlated with improvement [in response to which treatment]" (Barlow & Hersen, 1984, p. 16).

Therefore, results of controlled group studies serve to suggest general directions for prescriptive interventions. Subsequent refinement of prescriptive treatments will occur through methods of empirical evaluation that purposefully highlight through specification, rather than nullify through randomization, subject differences. Replicated single case experimental designs (e.g., withdrawal, multiple baselines), which regularly provide detailed elaboration of both subject and pathology characteristics, are extremely useful in delineating precise parameters within which prescriptive interventions will be effective (Persons, 1991). Reciprocally, the highly structured nature of prescriptive treatments makes them particularly suited for evaluation through single case experimental methods.

Babbitt and Parrish's (1991) study using multiple baselines across settings

TABLE 1.1. **Disorders and Prescriptive Treatments**

Disorder class	Disorder subtype	Indicated treatment	Possible treatment
Bipolar disorder		Lithium carbonate	
Major depression	Endogenous/melancholic	Antidepressants/electro-convulsive therapy	
Major depression	Anxious		Desensitization
Major depression	Cognitive	Cognitive restructuring	
Major depression	Skills deficit	Social skills training	
Major depression	Reduced reinforcement	Reinforcement planning	
Major depression	Interpersonal relations	Interpersonal therapy	
Panic disorder	Hyperventilatory		Breathing retraining
Panic disorder	Conditioned	Interoceptive exposure	
Panic disorder	Cognitive	Focused cognitive therapy	
Panic disorder	Mixed	Panic control training	Alprazolam (acute tx)
Panic disorder w/agoraphobia		Panic control training + graded exposure	Imipramine
Obsessive-compulsive disorder		Exposure + response prevention	Clomipramine
Obsessive-compulsive disorder	Primarily obsessions		Thought stopping
Simple phobia	Conditioned	Desensitization	
Simple phobia	Cognitive	Self-efficacy training	
Social phobia	Skills deficit	Social skills training	
Social phobia	Anxious	In vivo desensitization	
Sexual dysfunction	Premature ejaculation	Stop-go/squeeze method	Desensitization
Sexual dysfunction	Anxious/aversion	Desensitization	
Sexual dysfunction	Primary inorgasmia	Directed masturbation	
Sexual dysfunction	Vaginismus	Applied relaxation/dilators	
Sexual dysfunction	Inhibited desire	Behavioral marital therapy	
Sexual dysfuntion	Psychogenic erectile	Graduated exposure	
Sexual dysfunction	Organic erectile	Penile implant	
Paraphilias	Inappropriate arousal	Covert sensitization	
Paraphilias	Low appropriate arousal	Orgasmic reconditioning	
Substance abuse		Community reinforcement	Disulfiram/social skills training
Pain	General/reinforced	Contingency restructuring	
Pain	Anxious	Applied relaxation	
Schizophrenia	Positive signs	Antipsychotics	
Schizophrenia	Negative signs	Social skills training	
Insomnia	Sleep onset	Stimulus control	Progressive muscle relaxation
Bulimia		Exposure + response prevention	Antidepressants
Anorexia	Very low body weight	Contingency restructuring	
Generalized anxiety disorder		Applied relaxation	Imipramine
Posttraumatic stress disorder		Anxiety management training	Flooding

illustrates this point nicely. The subject was a mildly retarded, 6-year-old girl with spastic diplegia cerebral palsy who was referred for treatment of a "phone phobia." She was very verbal, attentive to adults, and sociable. Her parents reported that the "phobia" had begun 1 year earlier and typically involved the client's ceasing all activity, gasping, crying, and finally screaming in response to a ringing phone or adults making phone calls. This behavior continued until the call was terminated. She showed no such fear when playing with her own toy phone. Her parents had altered their behavior to minimize phone use during her waking hours. The authors established that parental use of the phone interrupted the ongoing reinforcement they had been providing to the child. In response, the child had a tantrum until phone was terminated and reinforcement density was again increased.

Note that the authors addressed and reported each level of assessment required of prescriptive interventions: Symptoms were observed and defined (e.g., screaming); variables that maintained and elicited the behavior were elucidated (e.g., parental attention); etiology, while not explicitly verified, was hypothesized and supported (e.g., operant conditioning); and subject characteristics were noted and specified (e.g, mentally retarded, female child). Treatment was initially limited to the clinic and involved exposure to planned adult phone calls with systematic implementation of time-out periods contingent on crying or similar behavior. The frequency of target behaviors displayed at the clinic was reduced by 80%, in contrast to a 0% reduction noted at home. Implementation of similar contingencies in the home resulted in a 90% reduction of displayed target behaviors, providing strong support for the conclusion that "phone-phobic" behavior was determined by existing reinforcement contingencies.

Although repeated replication of any experiment (particularly single case designs) is necessary to firmly demonstrate the efficacy of an intervention, suggestions for therapists confronted with a mildly retarded, highly social, and attentive 6-year-old girl who evinces tantrum-like behavior upon removal of attention are clear: contingency restructuring, rather than play therapy, is demanded. Controlled group studies suggest general treatment directions, but many controlled single case experiments involving a wide variety of pathologies have been conducted and are potentially useful in further directing and refining prescriptive interventions. Indeed, information garnered from both modes of research provides answers to Paul's (1967) ultimate inquiry and tells us definitively what treatment, by whom, is most effective for this individual with that specific problem under which set of circumstances.

Summary

Initial endeavors in clinical psychology were largely the result of deductive reasoning. Consequently, evaluation of early treatments took the form of uncontrolled clinical case studies. Unfortunately, the act of supporting a rationally derived construct with further deduction is tautological and provides little direction to clinicians interested in refining or improving a given technique. Instead, "general" interventions result and are applied indiscriminately to a number of pathologies. In effect, deductively derived treatments are theory consistent rather than problem specific. As such, their effectiveness is limited.

In response to disillusionment with deductive approaches, such as psychoanalysis, clinicians have turned increasingly to inductively derived, cognitive-behavioral and pharmacological interventions. As a result of this increased empiricism, several prescriptive treatments currently exist for well-defined, specific problems (see, e.g., American Psychiatric Association, 1993). While exceedingly potent, however, prescriptive interventions are intentionally circumscribed. Therefore, highly focused and ongoing assessment of presenting pathologies is necessary. Specifically, prescriptive treatments require thorough assessment of (1) symptoms, (2) maintaining factors, (3) etiological factors, and (4) subject characteristics and history.

Measurement across each variable facilitates the informed selection of those treatments found to be most effective in ameliorating well-defined problems. Assessment along only one parameter, to the exclusion of others, disregards the possible existence of diagnostic subtypes and thereby increases the possibility that an inappropriate or ineffective treatment will be applied to an individual's pathology. Indeed, several investigators have reported that patients who manifest similar symptoms often differ in etiology or maintaining factors—and will respond differentially to treatment.

There exist experimentally validated interventions, both pharmacological and psychological, with demonstrated effectiveness across several areas of psychopathology. Pharmacological approaches have been shown to alleviate the distressing aspects of endogenous major depression, bipolar disorder, several anxiety disorders, bulimia, insomnia, and the positive signs of schizophrenia. Additionally, successful prescriptive psychological interventions exist for almost every anxiety disorder, nonendogenous depression, insomnia, sexual dysfunction, substance use disorders, pain, and the skills deficits often found in schizophrenics.

Whereas group outcome studies suggest general directions for therapy, the detailed nature of controlled single case research enables clinicians to further refine and focus prescriptive treatments. Additionally, prescriptive interventions are well suited to evaluation through single case methodology. Future directions include further delineation of the parameters (e.g., symptoms, etiology) within which particular prescriptive treatments are effective with particular disorders.

References

Agras, W. S., Barlow, D. H., Chapin, H. N., Abel, G. G., & Leitenberg, H. (1974). Behavior modification of anorexia nervosa. *Archives of General Psychiatry*, *30*, 279–286.

American Psychiatric Association (1993). Practice guideline for major depressive disorder in adults. *American Journal of Psychiatry*, *150*(Suppl.), 1–26.

Azrin, N. H. (1976). Improvements in the community-reinforcement approach to alcoholism. *Behaviour Research and Therapy*, *14*, 339–348.

Azrin, N. H., McMahon, P., Lapinsky, K., Besalel, V., & Donohue, B. (1991). *Behavior therapy for drug abuse*. Paper presented at the meeting of the Association for the Advancement of Behavior Therapy, New York.

Azrin, N. H., & Peterson, A. L. (1987). Habit reversal for the treatment of Tourette syndrome. *Behaviour Research and Therapy*, *26*, 347–351.

Babbitt, R. L. & Parrish, J. M. (1991). Phone phobia, phact or phantasy? An operant approach to a child's disruptive behavior induced by telephone usage. *Journal of Behavior Therapy and Experimental Psychiatry*, *22*, 123–129.

Bandura, A., Jeffery, R. W., & Gajdos, E. (1975). Generalizing change through participant modeling with self-directed mastery. *Behaviour Research and Therapy*, *13*, 141–152.

Barlow, D. H. (1988). *Anxiety and its disorders: The nature and treatment of anxiety and panic*. New York: Guilford.

Barlow, D. H. (1993, February). *The diagnosis and treatment of anxiety and panic disorders: New developments*. Workshop presented at Nova University, Fort Lauderdale, Florida.

Barlow, D. H., Craske, M. G., Cerny, J. A., & Klosko, J. S. (1989). Behavioral treatment of panic disorder. *Behavior Therapy*, *20*, 261–282.

Barlow, D. H., & Hersen, M. (1984). *Single case experimental designs: Strategies for studying behavior change* (2nd ed.). New York: Pergamon.

Beck, A. T., Hollon, S. D., Young, J. E., Bedrosian, R. C., & Budenz, D. (1985). Treatment of depression with cognitive therapy and amitriptyline. *Archives of General Psychiatry*, *42*, 142–158.

Beck, A. T., Sokal, L., Clark, D., Berchick, R., & Wright, F. (1992). A crossover study of focused cognitive therapy for panic disorder. *American Journal of Psychiatry*, *149*, 778–783.

Bellack, A. S., & Hersen, M. (1985). General considerations. In M. Hersen and A. S. Bellack (Eds.), *Handbook of clinical behavior therapy with adults* (pp. 3–19). New York: Plenum.

Bellack, A. S., Turner, S. M., Hersen, M., & Luber, R. F. (1984). An examination of the efficacy of social skills training for chronic schizophrenic patients. *Hospital and Community Psychiatry, 35,* 1023–1028.

Beutler, L. E. (1979). Toward specific psychological therapies for specific conditions. *Journal of Consulting and Clinical Psychology, 47,* 882–897.

Beutler, L. E. (1991). Have all won and must all have prizes? Revisiting Luborsky et al.'s verdict. *Journal of Consulting and Clinical Psychology, 59,* 226–232.

Blackburn, I. M., Eunson, K. M., & Bishop, S. (1986) A two-year naturalistic follow-up of depressed patients treated with cognitive therapy, pharmacotherapy and a combination of both. *Journal of Affective Disorders, 10,* 67–75.

Bootzin, R. R. (1973). *Stimulus control of insomnia.* Paper presented at the meeting of the American Psychological Association, Montreal, Quebec, Canada.

Borkovec, T. D. (1982). Insomnia. *Journal of Consulting and Clinical Psychology, 50,* 880–895.

Borkovec, T. D., & Mathews, A. M. (1988). Treatment of nonphobic anxiety disorders: A comparison of nondirective, cognitive, and coping desensitization therapy. *Journal of Consulting and Clinical Psychology, 56,* 877–884.

Brownell, K. D., Hayes, S. C., & Barlow, D. H. (1977). Patterns of appropriate and deviant sexual arousal: The behavioral treatment of multiple sexual deviations *Journal of Consulting and Clinical Psychology, 45,* 1144–1155.

Bupp, S. J., & Preskorn, S. H. (1991). The effect of age on plasma levels of nortriptyline. *Annals of Clinical Psychiatry, 3,* 61–65.

Burke, A. E., & Silverman, W. K. (1987). The prescriptive treatment of school refusal. *Clinical Psychology Review, 7,* 353–362.

Butler, G., Cullington, A., Munby, M., Amies, P., & Gelder, M. (1984). Exposure and anxiety management in the treatment of social phobia. *Journal of Consulting and Clinical Psychology, 52,* 642–650.

Cannon, D. S., & Baker, T. B. (1981). Emetic and electric shock alcohol aversion therapy: Assessment of conditioning. *Journal of Consulting and Clinical Psychology, 49,* 360–368.

Chaney, E. F., O'Leary, M. R., & Marlatt, G. A. (1978). Skill training with alcoholics. *Journal of Consulting and Clinical Psychology, 46,* 1092–1104.

Cheung, H. K. (1981). Schizophrenics fully remitted on neuroleptics for 3–5 years: To stop or continue drugs. *British Journal of Psychiatry, 139,* 490–494.

Christensen, H., Hadzi-Pavlovic, D., Andrews, G., & Mattick, R. (1987). Behavior therapy and tricyclic medication in the treatment of obsessive-compulsive disorder: A quantitative review. *Journal of Consulting and Clinical Psychology, 55,* 701–711.

Conti, L., Placidi, G. R., Dell'Osso, L., Lenzi, A., & Cassano, G. B. (1987). Therapeutic response in subtypes of major depression. *New Trends in Experimental and Clinical Psychiatry, 3,* 101–107.

Craighead, L. W., Stunkard, A. J., & O'Brien, R. (1981). Behavior therapy and pharmacotherapy of obesity. *Archives of General Psychiatry, 38,* 763–768.

Craighead, W. E. (1980). Away from a unitary model of depression. *Behavior Therapy, 11,* 122–128.

Craske, M. G., Bran, T. A., & Barlow, D. H. (1991). Behavioral treatment of panic disorder: A two-year follow-up. *Behavior Therapy, 22,* 289–304.

Curran, J. P. (1977). Social skill training as an approach to the treatment of heterosexual social anxiety. *Psychological Bulletin, 84,* 140–157.

Dohrenwend, B. P., & Dohrenwend, B. S. (1974). Social and cultural influences upon psychopathology. *Annual Review of Psychology, 25,* 417–452.

Elin, I., Shea, M. T., Watkins, J. T., Imber, S. D., Sotsky, S. M., Collins, J. F., Glass, D. R., Pilkonis, P. A., Leber, W. R., Docherty, J. P., Fiester, S. J., & Parloff, M. B. (1989). National Institute of Mental Health treatment of depression collaborative research program: General effectiveness of treatments. *Archives of General Psychiatry, 46,* 971–982.

Everaerd. W. (1977). Comparative studies of short-term treatment methods for sexual inadequacies. In R. Gemme & C. C. Wheeler (Eds.), *Progress in sexology.* New York: Plenum.

Everaerd, W., & Dekker, J. (1982). Treatment of secondary orgasmic dysfunction: A comparison of systematic desensitization and sex therapy. *Behaviour Research and Therapy, 2,* 269–274.

Eysenck, H. J. (1952). The effects of psychotherapy: An evaluation. *Journal of Consulting Psychology, 16,* 319–324.

Eysenck, H. J. (1960). The effects of psychotherapy. In H. J. Eysenck (Ed.), *Handbook of abnormal psychology: An experimental approach.* London: Pittman.

Falloon, I. R., McHill, C. W., Boyd, J., & Pedersen, J. (1987). Family management in the prevention of morbidity of schizophrenia: Social outcome of a two-year longitudinal study. *Psychological Medicine*, *17*, 59–66.

Feigenbaum, W. (1988). Long-term efficacy of ungraded versus graded massed exposure in agoraphobics. In I. Hand & H. Whittchen (Eds.), *Panic and phobia: Treatments and variables affecting course and outcome*. Berlin: Springer-Verlag.

Feinberg, M. (1992). Comment: Subtypes of depression and response to treatment. *Journal of Consulting and Clinical Psychology*, *60*, 670–674.

Foa, E. B., Grayson, J. B., Steketee, G. S., Doppelt, H. G., Turner, R. M., & Latimer, P. R.(1983). Success and failure in the behavioral treatment of obsessive-compulsives. *Journal of Consulting and Clinical Psychology*, *51*, 287–297.

Foa, E. B., Rothbaum, R., Riggs, D., & Murdock, T. (1991). Treatment of PTSD in rape victims: A comparison between cognitive behavioral procedures and counseling. *Journal of Consulting and Clinical Psychology*, *59*, 715–723.

Fordyce, W. E. (1976). *Behavioral methods for chronic pain and illness*. St. Louis: Mosby.

Frank, E., Kupfer, D. J., Perel, J. M., Cornes, C., Jarrett, D. B., Mallinger, A. G., Thase, M. E., McEachran, A. B., & Grochocinski, V. J. (1990). Three-year outcomes for maintenance therapies in recurrent depression. *Archives of General Psychiatry*, *47*, 1093–1099.

Fyer, A., Liebowitz, M., Gorman, J., Campeas, R., Leven, A., Davies, S. O., Goetz, D., & Klein, D. F. (1987). Discontinuation of alprazolam treatment in panic patients. *American Journal of Psychiatry*, *144*, 303–308.

George, L. K., Blazer, D. G., Hughes, D. C., & Fowler, N. (1989). Social support and the outcome of major depression. *British Journal of Psychiatry*, *154*, 478–485.

Gitlin, M. J. (1990). *The psychotherapist's guide to psychopharmacology*. New York: Free Press.

Goodwin, F. K., & Zis, A. P. (1979). Lithium in the treatment of mania: Comparison with neuroleptics. *Archives of General Psychiatry*, *36*, 840–844.

Greenberg, R. P., Bornstein, R. F., Greenberg, M. D., & Fisher, S. (1992). A meta-analysis of antidepressant outcome under "blinder" conditions. *Journal of Consulting and Clinical Psychology*, *60*, 664–669.

Griez, E., & van den Hout, M. (1986). CO_2 inhalation in the treatment of panic attacks. *Behaviour Research and Therapy*, *24*, 145–150.

Gunther, W., Gunther, Streck, P., & Ronig, H. (1988). Psychomotor disturbances in psychiatric patients as a possible basis for new attempts at differential diagnosis and therapy: III. Cross validation study on depressed patients: The psychotic motor syndrome as a possible state marker for endogenous depression. *European Archives of Psychiatry and Neurological Sciences*, *237*, 65–73.

Hahlweg, K., & Markman, H. J. (1988). Effectiveness of behavioral marital therapy: Empirical status of behavioral techniques in preventing and alleviating marital distress. *Journal of Consulting and Clinical Psychology*, *56*, 440–447.

Harbert, T. L., Barlow, D. H., Hersen, M., & Austin, J. B. (1974). Measurement and modification of incestous behavior: A case study. *Psychological Reports*, *34*, 79–86.

Hersen, M. (1973). Developments in behavior modification: An editorial. *Journal of Nervous and Mental Disease*, *156*, 373–376.

Hersen, M. (1981). Complex problems require complex solutions. *Behavior Therapy*, *12*, 15–29.

Hersen, M., Bellack, A. S., Himmelhoch, J. M., & Thase, M. E. (1984). Effects of social skills training, amitriptyline, and psychotherapy in unipolar depressed women. *Behavior Therapy*, *15*, 21–40.

Hester, R. K., & Miller, W. R. (Eds.) (1989). *Handbook of alcoholism treatment approaches: Effective alternatives*. New York: Pergamon.

Hogarty, G. E., Anderson, C. M., Reiss, D. J., Kornblith, S. J., Greenwald, D. P., Javna, C. D., & Madonia, M. J. (1986). Family psycho-education, social skills training and maintenance chemotherapy: I. One year effects of a controlled study on relapse and expressed emotion. *Archives of General Psychiatry*, *45*, 797–805.

Insel, T. R., Murphy, D. L., Cohen, R. M., Alterman, I., Kilts, C., & Linnoila, M. (1983). Obsessive-compulsive disorder: A double-blind trial of clomipramine and clorgyline. *Archives of General Psychiatry*, *40*, 605–612.

Insel, T. R., & Zohar, S. (1987). Psychopharmacologic approaches to obsessive-compulsive disorder. In H. Y. Meltzer (Ed.), *Psychopharmacology: The third generation of progress*. New York: Raven.

Jansson, L., & Ost, L. G. (1982). Behavioral treatments for agoraphobia: An evaluative review. *Clinical Psychology Review*, *2*, 311–336.

Jones, D., Kelwala, S., Bell, J., & Dube, S. (1985). Cholinergic REM sleep induction response correlation with endogenous major depressive subtype. *Psychiatry Research, 14*, 99–110.

Kahn, R. J., McNair, D. M., Lipman, R. S., Covi, L., Rickels, K., Downing, R., Fisher, J., & Frankenthaler, L. M. (1986). Imipramine and chlordiazepoxide in depressive and anxiety disorders: II. Efficacy in anxious outpatients. *Archives of General Psychiatry, 43*, 79–85.

Kallman, W. M., Hersen, M., & O'Toole, D. H. (1975). The use of social reinforcement in a case of conversion reaction. *Behavior Therapy, 6*, 411–413.

Kane, J. M., & Lieberman, J. A. (1987). Maintenance pharmacotherapy in schizophrenia. In H. Y. Meltzer (Ed.), *Psychopharmacology: The third generation of progress*. New York: Raven.

Keane, T. M., Fairbank, J. A., Caddell, J. M., & Zimering, R. T. (1989). Implosive (flooding) therapy reduces symptoms of PTSD in Vietnam veterans. *Behavior Therapy, 20*, 245–260.

Kiloh, L. G., Ball, J. R., & Garside, R. F. (1977). Depression: A multivariate study of Sir Aubrey Lews's data on melancholia. *Australian and New Zealand Journal of Psychiatry, 11*, 149–156.

Klosko, J., Barlow, D. H., Tassinari, R., & Cerny, J. (1990). A comparison of alprazolam and behavior therapy in the treatment of panic disorder. *Journal of Consulting and Clinical Psychology, 58*, 77–84.

Kupfer, D. L., & Thase, M. F. (1983). The use of the sleep laboratory in the diagnosis of affective disorders. *Psychiatric Clinics of North America, 6*, 3–25.

Lang, P. J. (1968). Fear reduction and fear behavior: Problems in treating a construct. In J. M. Shlien (Ed.), *Research in psychotherapy*, (Vol. 3). Washington, DC: American Psychological Association.

Lewinsohn, P. M., Sullivan, J. M., & Grosscup, S. J. (1982). Behavior therapy: Clinical applications. In A. J. Rush (Ed.), *Short-term psychotherapies for depression* (pp 50–87). New York: Guilford.

Ley, R. (1992). The many faces of Pan: Psychological and physiological differences among three types of panic attacks. *Behaviour Research and Therapy, 30*, 347–357.

Ley, R. (1993). Breathing retraining in the treatment of hyperventilatory complaints and panic disorder: A reply to Garssen, De Ruiter, and van Dyck. *Clinical Psychology Review, 13*, 393–408.

Liberman. R. P., Mueser, K. T., & Wallace, C. J. (1986). Social skills training for schizophrenic individuals at risk for relapse. *American Journal of Psychiatry, 143*, 523–526.

Linton, S. J. (1982). A controlled study of the effects of applied relaxation and applied relaxation plus operant procedures in the regulation of chronic pain. *British Journal of Clinical Psychology, 23*, 291–299.

Lonigan, C., Shannon, M., Finch, A., & Daugherty, T. (1991). Children's reactions to a natural disaster: Symptom severity and degree of exposure. *Advances in Behaviour Research and Therapy, 13*, 135–154.

Lydiard, R. B., & Laird, L. K. (1988). Prediction of response to antipsychotics. *Journal of Clinical Psychopharmacology, 8*, 3–13.

Marks, I. M. (1975). Behavioral treatments of phobic and obsessive-compulsive disorders: A critical appraisal. In M. Hersen, R. M. Eisler, & P. M. Miller (Eds.), *Progress in behavior modification* (Vol. 1, pp. 66–158). New York: Academic.

Marks, I. M. (1987). *Fears, phobias, and rituals: Panic, anxiety, and their disorders*. New York: Oxford University Press.

Marshall, W. L. (1985). The effects of variable exposure in flooding therapy. *Behavior Therapy, 16*, 117–135.

Mavissakalian, M., Michelson, L., & Dealy, R. S. (1983). Pharmacological treatment of agoraphobia: Imipramine versus imipramine with programmed practice. *British Journal of Psychiatry, 143*, 348–355.

May, P. (1987). Suicide and self destruction among American Indian youths. *American Indian and Alaska Native Mental Health Research, 1*, 52–69.

McKnight, D., Nelson, R., Hayes, S., & Jarrett, R. (1992). Importance of treating individually assessed response classes of depression. *Behavior Therapy, 15*, 315–335.

McNally, R., & Steketee, G. (1985). The etiology and maintenance of severe animal phobias. *Behaviour Research and Therapy, 23*, 431–435.

Meichenbaum, D., & Turk, D. (1976). The cognitive-behavioral management of anxiety, anger, and pain. In J. Davison (Ed.), *The behavioral management of anxiety, depression and pain*. New York: Brunner/Mazel.

Mowrer, O. H. (1947). On the dual nature of learning—a reinterpretation of "conditioning" and "problem solving." *Harvard Educational Review, 17*, 102–148.

Obler, M. (1973). Systematic desensitization in sexual disorders. *Journal of Behavior Therapy and Experimental Psychiatry, 4*, 93–101.

Olsen, R. P., Ganley, R., Devine, V. T., & Dorsey, G. C. (1981). Long-term effects of behavioral versus insight-oriented therapy with inpatient alcoholics. *Journal of Consulting and Clinical Psychology, 49*, 866–877.

Omer, H., & Dar, R. (1992). Changing trends in three decades of psychotherapy research: the flight from theory into pragmatics. *Journal of Consulting and Clinical Psychology, 60*, 88–93.

Ost, L. G. (1985). Ways of acquiring phobias and outcome of behavioral treatment. *Behaviour Research and Therapy, 23*, 683–689.

Ost, L. G. (1988). Applied relaxation vs. progressive relaxation in the treatment of panic disorder. *Behaviour Research and Therapy, 26*, 13–22.

Ost, L. G. (1991). Acquisition of blood and injection phobia and anxiety response patterns in clinical patients. *Behaviour Research and Therapy, 29*, 323–332.

Ost, L. G., & Hugdahl, K. (1983). Acquisition of agoraphobia, mode of onset and anxiety response patterns. *Behaviour Research and Therapy, 21*, 623–631.

Ost, L. G., Jerremalm, A., & Johansson, J. (1981). Individual response patterns and the effects of different behavioral methods in the treatment of social phobia. *Behaviour Research and Therapy, 19*, 1–16.

Ost. L. G., Johansson, J., & Jerremalm, A. (1982). Individual response patterns and the effects of different behavioral methods in the treatment of claustrophobia. *Behaviour Research and Therapy, 20*, 445–460.

Paul, G. L. (1967). Outcome research in psychotherapy. *Journal of Consulting Psychology, 31*, 109–118.

Perse, T. (1988). Obsessive-compulsive disorder: A treatment review. *Journal of Clinical Psychiatry, 49*, 48–55.

Persons, J. B. (1991). Psychotherapy outcome studies do not accurately represent current models of psychotherapy. *American Psychologist, 46*, 99–106.

Rachman, S. (1977). The conditioning theory of fear-acquisition: A critical examination. *Behaviour Research and Therapy, 15*, 375.

Raskin, A., & Crook, T. H. (1976). The endogenous–neurotic distinction as a predictor of response to antidepressant drugs. *Psychological Medicine, 6*, 59–70.

Riley, A. J., & Riley, E. J. (1978). A controlled study to evaluate directed masturbation in the management of primary orgasmic failure in women. *British Journal of Psychiatry, 133*, 404–409.

Rogers, S. C., & Clay, P. M. (1975). A statistical review of controlled trials of imipramine and placebo in the treatment of depressive illness. *British Journal of Psychiatry, 127*, 599–603.

Rounsaville, B. J., Klerman, G. L., & Weissman, M. M. (1981). Do psychotherapy and pharmacotherapy for depression conflict? Empirical evidence from a clinical trial. *Archives of General Psychiatry, 38*, 24–29.

Rush, A. J. (1983). A phase II study of cognitive therapy in depression. In J. B. Williams & R. L. Spitzer (Eds.), *Psychotherapy research: Where are we and where should we go* (pp. 216–234). New York: Guilford.

Rush, A. J., Beck, A. T., Kovacs, M., & Hollon,S. (1977). Comparative efficacy of cognitive therapy and pharmacotherapy in the treatment of depressed outpatients. *Cognitive Therapy and Research, 1*, 17–37.

Schatzberg, A. F., & Cole, J. O. (1991). *Manual of clinical psychopharmacology*, (2nd ed.). Washington, DC: American Psychiatric Press.

Seamens, J. H. (1956). Premature ejaculation: A new approach. *Southern Medical Journal, 49*, 353–357.

Shadish, W. R., & Sweeney, R. B.(1991). Mediators and moderators in meta-analysis: There's a reason we don't let dodo birds tell us which psychotherapies should have prizes. *Journal of Consulting and Clinical Psychology, 59*, 883–893.

Shapiro, D. A. & Shapiro, D. (1982). Meta-analysis of comparative therapy outcome studies: A replication and refinement. *Psychological Bulletin, 92*, 581–604.

Simons, A. K., Murphy, G. E., Levine, J. L., & Wetzel, R. D. (1986). Cognitive therapy and pharmacotherapy for depression: Sustained improvement over one year. *Archives of General Psychiatry, 43*, 43–48.

Stiles, W. B., Shapiro, D. A., & Elliott, R. (1986). Are all psychotherapies equivalent? *American Psychologist, 41*, 165–180.

Swinson, R. P., & Eaves, D. (1978). *Psychiatric topics for community workers: Alcoholism and addiction*. England: Woburn.

Taylor, S., & McLean P. (1993). Outcome profiles in the treatment of unipolar depression. *Behaviour Research and Therapy, 31*, 325–330.

Telch, M. J., Agras, W. S., Taylor, C. B., Roth, W. T., & Gallen, E. C. (1985). Combined pharmacological and behavioral treatment for agoraphobia. *Behaviour Research and Therapy, 23*, 325–335.

Thase, M. E., Hersen, M., Bellack, A. S., Himmelhoch, J. M., & Kupfer, D. J. (1983). Validation of a Hamilton subscale for endogenomorphic depression. *Journal of Affective Disorders, 5*, 267–278.

Thoren, P., Asberg, M., Cronholm, R., Jornestedt, R. N., & Traskiman, L. (1980). Clomipramine treatment of obsessive-compulsive disorder. *Archives of General Psychiatry, 37*, 1281–1285.

Trower, P., Yardley,K., Bryant, B., & Shaw, P. (1978). The treatment of social failure: A comparison of anxiety reduction and skills acquisition procedures for two social problems. *Behavior Modification, 2,* 41–60.

Van Deventer, A. D., & Laws, D. R. (1978). Orgasmic reconditioning to redirect sexual arousal in pedophiles. *Behavior Therapy, 9,* 748–765.

Van Hasselt, V. B., Hersen, M., & Milliones, J. (1978). Social skills training for alcoholic drug addicts: A review. *Addictive Behaviors, 3,* 221–233.

Walsh, B. T. (1987). Psychopharmacology of bulimia. In H. Y. Meltzer (Ed.), *Psychopharmacology: The third generation of progress.* New York: Raven.

Weissman, M. M., Prusoff, B. A., DiMascio, A., Neu, C., Goklaney, M., & Klerman, G. (1979). The efficacy of drugs and psychotherapy in the treatment of acute depressive episodes. *American Journal of Psychiatry, 136,* 555–558.

Wilson, G. T., Rossiter, E., Kleifield, E. I., & Lindholm, L. (1986). Cognitive-behavioral treatment of bulimia nervosa: A controlled evaluation. *Behaviour Research and Therapy, 24,* 277–288.

Wolpe, J. (1958). *Psychotherapy by reciprocal inhibition.* Stanford, CA: Stanford University Press.

Wolpe, J. (1977). Inadequate behavior analysis: The Achilles heel of outcome research in behavior therapy. *Journal of Behavior Therapy and Experimental Psychiatry, 8,* 1–3.

Wolpe, J. (1979). The experimental model and treatment of neurotic depression. *Behaviour Research and Therapy, 17,* 555–565.

Wolpe, J. (1981). The dichotomy between classically conditioned and cognitively learned anxiety. *Journal of Behavior Therapy and Experimental Psychiatry, 12,* 35–42.

Wolpe, J. (1986). The positive diagnosis of neurotic depression as an etiological category. *Comprehensive Psychiatry, 27,* 449–460.

Wolpe, J. (1990). *The practice of behavior therapy* (4th ed.). New York: Pergamon.

Wolpe, J., Lande, S. D., McNally, R. J., & Schotte, D. (1985). Differentiation between classically conditioned and cognitively based neurotic fears: Two pilot studies. *Journal of Behavior Therapy and Experimental Psychiatry, 16,* 287–293.

Ziltrin, C. M., Klein, D. F., & Woerner, M. G. (1980). Treatment of agoraphobia with group exposure in vivo and imipramine. *Archives of General Psychiatry, 37,* 63–72.

II

SPECIFIC DISORDERS

2

Dementia (Alzheimer's Disease)

Benoit H. Mulsant and Jules Rosen

Description of the Disorder

Clinical Features

"Dementia," derived from the Latin *de* (out of) and *mens* (mind), means literally "out of one's mind." In DSM-III-R (American Psychiatric Association, 1987), this term is restricted to denote only a syndrome characterized by acquired cognitive deterioration involving memory and at least one other higher function, or personality changes with significant impairment of social or occupational functioning. Sjogren, Sjogren, and Lindgren (1952) established the modern concept of Alzheimer's disease (AD), reporting that (a) most cases of AD arise in those in the senile age range, (b) about 10% of patients have a positive family history with an autosomal dominant pattern of transmission, and (c) three stages can be delineated: the confused, demented, and vegetative stages. Sim and Sussman (1962) completed the clinical picture of AD, describing a pattern of amnesia (with, in particular, difficulty in learning new material) preceding aphasia, apraxia, and agnosia—the 4 *A*'s of AD—and confirming the occurrence of neurologic symptoms, particularly in the late stages of the disease. In another landmark study, Blessed, Tomlinson, and Roth (1968) demonstrated that dementia is not part of normal aging but, rather, is usually associated with one of two specific pathologies: either the changes characteristic of AD first described in 1907 by the German neuropathologist Alois Alzheimer or, more rarely, multiple small infarcts.

Benoit H. Mulsant and **Jules Rosen** • Western Psychiatric Institute and Clinic, and Department of Psychiatry, University of Pittsburgh School of Medicine, Pittsburgh, Pennsylvania 15213.

Handbook of Prescriptive Treatments for Adults, edited by Michel Hersen and Robert T. Ammerman. Plenum Press, New York, 1994.

Associated Features

In addition to myoclonic jerks and seizures (Sim & Sussman, 1962), various neurologic findings have been linked to AD: extrapyramidal symptoms (EPS) (Stern, Mayeux, Sano, Hauser, & Bush, 1987), cerebellar signs (Huff et al., 1987), sleep-disordered breathing (Hoch et al., 1989), cardiovascular autonomic instability (Francheschi, Ferini-Strambi, Minicucci, Sferrazza-Papa, & Smirne, 1986; Rezek, 1987; Warner, Peabody, Flattery, & Tinklenberg, 1986), olfactory deficits (Knupfer & Speigel, 1986), visual field deficits (Steffes & Thralow, 1987), and hearing impairment (Grimes, Grady, Foster, Sunderland, & Patronas, 1985).

Of greater clinical significance, AD and other dementias are often associated with major behavioral disturbances. The point prevalence of a major depressive syndrome among patients with AD has been estimated to be as high as 87%, with most estimates approximating 20% (Wragg & Jeste, 1989). Similarly, the point prevalence of psychotic features (delusions or hallucinations) among patients with AD has been estimated to range from 10 to 73%, with most estimates around 30% (Deutsch, Bylsma, Rovner, Steele, & Folstein, 1991; Wragg & Jeste, 1989). Longitudinal studies have reported that, between onset of dementia and death, psychotic symptoms may occur in as many as 50% of patients with AD (Drevets & Rubin, 1989; Rosen & Zubenko, 1991). Behavioral disturbances associated with AD and other dementias exaggerate the functional impairment of patients and increase the burden on their caregivers, and thus they are often a determinant in the institutionalization of demented patients (Morycz, 1985; Mulsant & Thornton, 1990; Steele, Rovner, Chase, & Folstein, 1990; Zubenko, Rosen, Sweet, Mulsant, & Rifai, 1992).

Epidemiology

The demographic characteristics of the American population will make dementia one of the major medical, social, and economic problems of our society during the coming decades. Dementia is a markedly age-dependent condition that affects 5 to 15% of the population over age 65 and has been reported in as many as 50% of those over 85 (Evans et al., 1989), the fastest growing segment of the US population. Epidemiologic studies (e.g., Rocca, Amaducci, & Schoenberg, 1986) have demonstrated that, despite a constant incidence rate, prevalence of AD will continue to increase and more than 8 million people should be affected by the year 2000.

Although families make up the largest group of caregivers, providing 80% of the long-term care received by the extremely impaired elderly (Brody, Johnsen, Fulcomer, & Lang, 1983; Shanas, 1979), dementia is one of the major factors leading to institutionalization (Katzman, 1986). As a result, 40 to 60% of nursing home patients suffer from a dementing disorder—AD in 50 to 80% of cases (Rovner, Kafonek, Filipp, Lucas, & Folstein, 1986; Tariot, Podgorski, Blazina, & Leibovici, 1993).

Etiology

Dementing Disorders. Table 2.1 presents a breakdown of the relative frequencies of the most common dementing disorders. The recognition of these dementing disorders started in 1735, with the attribution of pellagra—characterized by a typical triad of dermatitis, diarrhea, and dementia—to a poor diet, shown two centuries later to result in a deficiency of nicotinic acid (niacin). Since then, causes of

TABLE 2.1. Dementing Disorders and Their Relative Frequencies

Alzheimer's disease	40%
Mixed vascular disorder and Alzheimer's disease	25
Vascular disorder	10
Alcoholism	5
Drug intoxication	3
Intracranial mass	2
Normal-pressure hydrocephalus	2
Huntington's disease	1
Creutzfeldt-Jakob disease	1
Other (include posttraumatic conditions, postsubarachnoid hemorrhage, postencephalitis, neurosyphilis, amyotrophic lateral sclerosis, Parkinson's disease, Pick's disease, thyroidopathy, vitamin B_{12} deficiency, hepatic failure, epilepsy)	8
Uncertain	3

Adapted from Mulsant, B. H., & Thornton, J. E. (1990). Alzheimer disease and other dementias. In M. E. Thase, B. A. Edelstein, & M. Hersen (Eds.). *Handbook of Outpatient Treatment of Adults: Nonpsychotic Mental Disorders* (pp. 353–388). New York: Plenum.

dementia have continued to be regularly identified: Parkinson's disease in 1817; general paresis or dementia paralytica (i.e., chronic syphilitic meningoencephalitis) in 1822; pernicious anemia (due to vitamin B_{12} deficiency) in 1849; Huntington's disease in 1872; myxedema (i.e., hypothyroidism) in 1873; Wernicke-Korsakoff syndrome due to thiamin deficiency associated with chronic alcoholism and malnutrition in 1881–1887; Pick's disease in 1892; Alzheimer's disease in 1907; the autosomal recessive hepatolenticular degeneration described by Wilson in 1911; Creutzfeldt-Jakob disease in 1921; the prototypical subcortical dementia, progressive supranuclear palsy, in 1963; normal-pressure hydrocephalus in 1964; the dementia syndrome of depression (Kay, Roth, & Hopkins, 1955); the various types of vascular dementias (Blessed et al., 1968; Freyhan, Woodford, & Kety, 1951; Hachinski, Lassen, & Marshall, 1974); and, most recently, the dementia associated with infection by the human immunodeficiency virus (HIV) (Navia & Price, 1987; Nielsen, Petito, Urmacher, & Posner, 1984).

Alzheimer's Disease. Over the past 30 years, AD has been demonstrated to be a specific disease distinct from the process of normal aging. Presenile and senile forms of AD have been shown to represent the same entity occurring in different populations, characterized by specific neuropathologic changes (i.e., neurofibrillary tangles and neuritic plaques), occurring in a preferential topographic pattern and associated with a specific biochemical abnormality (i.e., a central cholinergic deficit). This cholinergic deficit has been causally linked to memory impairment, one of AD's clinical hallmarks. Various etiologic hypotheses for the neuropathologic and neurochemical features of AD have been proposed—for example, aluminum intoxication, viral infection, and immune reaction—but none of these hypotheses has been confirmed. The current search for an etiological factor has been focusing on the possible genetic determinants of AD. Epidemiologic studies have suggested that "sporadic" (i.e., nonfamilial) cases of AD may in fact be transmitted in an autosomal dominant fashion (Breitner, 1987). Because it has now been recognized that almost all patients with trisomy 21 (Down syndrome) who survive past age 40 develop AD, recent studies have focused on chromosome 21, but these studies have not yet led to any definite conclusions.

Differential Diagnosis and Assessment

Benoit H. Mulsant
and Jules Rosen

DSM-III-R and DSM-IV Categorization

Dementia. In DSM-III-R, diagnosis of a *dementia syndrome* is "based on clinical factors alone, and carries no connotations concerning prognosis." The diagnostic criteria have three major emphases: (a) there exists an acquired cognitive impairment involving memory and at least one other higher cognitive function (e.g., abstract thinking, judgment, language, constructional abilities) or personality changes; (b) this impairment is not due exclusively to delirium; and (c) it is severe enough to interfere with occupational or social functioning. This last criterion differentiates dementia from the milder cognitive alterations experienced by most elderly individuals, referred to as "benign senescent forgetfulness" in the past and "age-associated memory impairment" more recently.

DSM-III-R grades dementia as mild, moderate, or severe, according to the level of independence the patient can maintain. A mild dementia implies preserved "capacity for independent living"; in a moderate dementia, "independent living is hazardous, and some degree of supervision is necessary"; with severe dementia, "activities of daily living are so impaired that continual supervision is required."

Alzheimer's Disease. According to DSM-III-R, to establish a diagnosis of dementia, a specific causative organic disease must be identified. When no organic disease is identified, if all the nonorganic mental disorders can be ruled out, a clinical diagnosis of "primary degenerative dementia of the Alzheimer type" (PDD-AT) can be made by exclusion. According to the DSM-III-R principle stating that an organic mental disorder preempts diagnosis of another disorder that could produce the same symptoms, patients with behavioral disturbances superimposed on AD should generally be given only a diagnosis of PPD-AT. The associated behavioral disturbance(s) can be indicated by specifying the subtype "with depression," "with delusions," or "with delirium," or by an additional Axis I diagnosis of organic hallucinosis or organic anxiety disorder.

DSM-IV. In DSM-IV the separate definition of the dementia syndrome is eliminated and six types of dementia are considered: dementia of the Alzheimer type (DAT), vascular dementia, dementia due to other nonpsychiatric medical conditions (e.g., dementia due to Parkinson's disease or dementia due to HIV disease), substance-induced persisting dementia, dementia due to multiple etiologies, and dementia due to unknown etiology (American Psychiatric Association, 1991). These six types of dementia share a first diagnostic criterion similar to the definition of the DSM-III-R dementia syndrome (i.e, presence of memory impairment and aphasia, apraxia, agnosia, or disturbance in executive functioning) and a requirement of impairment in social or occupational functioning. Additional criteria specific to each type of dementia define the typical course and how the etiology is to be established (e.g., which disorders must be ruled out to make a diagnosis of DAT). Finally, an expanded subtyping scheme specifies the features associated with DAT: depressed mood, delusions, hallucinations, perceptual disturbance, behavioral disturbance (e.g., violence), communication disturbance, motor skills disturbance, or mixed.

When a patient presents with cognitive decline, the clinician has to engage in a four-step process. First, presence of delirium has to be excluded. Second, presence of a dementia syndrome has to be established and its severity assessed. Third, etiology of the dementia syndrome has to be investigated. Finally, in the presence of AD or another progressive dementing disorder, the clinician must search for associated treatable conditions that could be exacerbating the dementia. Going through these four steps will not only provide data essential to guide selection of an optimal long-term management strategy, but also establish rapport with and a sense of confidence on the part of the patient and his or her family. Later, this relationship will help them accept the working diagnosis, particularly if it carries a grim prognosis. Despite an initial thorough evaluation, etiology of a dementia often remains obscure and only evolution of the patient's condition will reveal his or her dementing disorder. Conversely, the yield of a dementia work-up will be the highest in patients presenting with incipient dementia, since most reversible or arrestable dementing disorders are such only in their early stages (Clarfield, 1988; Meyer, Judd, Tawaklna, Rogers, & Mortel, 1986; Reifler & Larson, 1988).

Ruling Out Delirium. The onset, or an unexpected worsening, of a global cognitive impairment requires that one rule out delirium as a cause. The cardinal features of a syndrome of delirium are fluctuations in level of consciousness, inability to focus and maintain attention, disorganization of thoughts, and rapid onset (over days or weeks). Symptoms commonly associated with delirium are disorientation to time and place (rarely to person), emotional disturbances (frequently marked by inappropriate vocalizations), perceptual disturbances (usually, visual illusions and hallucinations) and abnormal movements (e.g., tremor, asterixis). Symptoms of delirium often worsen at night because of decreased environmental cues. Whereas dementia may be conceptualized as a form of chronic brain failure that can be assessed over a relatively extended period, delirium is equivalent to acute brain failure and warrants immediate evaluation. Unless etiology of delirium is rapidly identified and treated, irreversible damage (i.e., progression to dementia) or death may occur.

Assessing the Dementia Syndrome. The nature and severity of cognitive impairment should be objectively and quantitatively documented. In clinical practice, the Folstein Mini-Mental State Examination (MMSE) (Folstein, Folstein, & McHugh, 1975), an 11-item scale, is widely used. Neuropsychological testing may help document cognitive deterioration in highly educated patients presenting with incipient dementia, or in patients with an uncommon cultural background or with a previously known cognitive impairment (e.g., mental retardation). Repeated testing may be useful in following these patients longitudinally.

Identification of specific clinical patterns of cognitive impairment can also help differentiate various dementing disorders. Cummings and Benson (1992) distinguish three clinical patterns of dementia, named according to the topography of the pathologic process. First, cortical dementias, such as AD and Pick's disease, involve primarily the cerebral cortex; they present with the specific cognitive deficits described earlier (the 4 *A*'s) and almost normal neurologic findings until the late stages. Subcortical dementias include the extrapyramidal disorders (e.g., Parkinson's,

Huntington's, and Wilson's diseases, progressive supranuclear palsy), normal-pressure hydrocephalus, and toxic-metabolic conditions. These subcortical dementias affect the basal ganglia, thalamus, and brainstem and are characterized by a slowing of cognition, forgetfulness, and depression, apathy, or, more rarely, mania. They also are associated with prominent neurologic abnormalities. Finally, global or mixed dementias involve both cortical and subcortical structures and present with both types of features. They include multi-infarct dementia (MID) and various infectious, traumatic, neoplastic, and anoxic dementias. Unfortunately, usefulness of this theoretical conceptualization is limited by the considerable overlap in the clinical presentation of the three types of dementias.

Establishing the Clinical Etiology of Dementia and Identifying Associated Conditions. Whereas AD is considered a diagnosis by exclusion by DSM-III-R, as we have discussed, McKhann et al. (1984) have proposed clinical criteria for a "positive" diagnosis of definite, probable, or possible AD. A definite diagnosis requires a brain biopsy or postmortem examination and is rarely made except in research settings. A probable diagnosis requires presence of a dementia syndrome, with a typical insidious onset after age 40, progressive worsening, and "the absence of systemic disorders or other brain disease that could account for the progressive deficits in memory and cognition." Depression, psychosis, angry or hostile outbursts, incontinence, and weight loss, as well as neurologic abnormalities (including seizures) in the advanced stages, are considered consistent with a probable diagnosis. Conversely, a sudden onset, focal neurologic findings, seizures, and gait disturbance very early in the course of the disease make a diagnosis of probable AD unlikely. A diagnosis of possible AD corresponds to an atypical presentation of progressive dementia when other dementing disorders have been reasonably excluded. Remembering that "atypical presentations of common disorders are more common than classic presentations of rare disorders" (Cutler, 1979), among the more than 60 recognized dementing disorders, the following have to be specifically excluded: mood disorder, Parkinson's disease, MID, drug intoxication, thyroid disease, pernicious anemia, syphilitic meningoencephalitis and other chronic central nervous system infections, normal-pressure hydrocephalus, subdural hematoma, Huntington's disease, Creutzfeldt-Jakob disease, and brain tumors.

In clinical practice, such a differential diagnosis process requires a systematic clinical and laboratory evaluation (Consensus Conference, 1987). Even in the absence of a reversible or arrestable dementing disorder, this "dementia work-up" will often detect a concurrent treatable condition that is exacerbating the dementia (Reifler & Larson, 1988). The clinical history is probably the single most important element in the diagnosis of dementia (Mulsant & Thornton, 1990). It should be obtained both from the patient and from an informant close to the patient. It is essential to characterize the mode of onset and time course of the process, presence of possible precipitants, the patient's psychiatric and medical history, and his or her family history. The physical examination can confirm information obtained during the history taking or, sometimes, reveal additional etiologic clues.

In light of the high social and economic costs involved in the management of a demented patient, the etiologic investigation of dementia usually includes a systematic "battery" of diagnostic tests to exclude as definitely as possible a reversible or arrestable dementing disorder. The following laboratory values are usually obtained: serum electrolyte, glucose, and blood urea nitrogen (BUN)–creatinine levels, liver and metabolic profile findings including calcium level, thyroid function test results including thyroid-stimulating hormone (TSH), vitamin B$_{12}$, and folate levels, and erythrocyte sedimentation rate. Other tests performed include complete blood count, serology for syphilis, urinalysis, chest roentgenogram, electrocardiogram, and central nervous system imaging (either magnetic resonance imaging—MRI—or, when MRI is contraindicated, computed tomography—CT). Other diagnostic tests (e.g., HIV testing, electroencephalogram, lumbar puncture, and radioisotope cisternography) are restricted to specific cases (Mulsant & Thornton, 1990). MR spectroscopy, positron emission tomography, and the study of various peripheral markers are presently limited to research settings.

Treatment

Evidence for Prescriptive Treatments

Cognitive Deficit. Many drugs have been tried to treat or to palliate the cognitive deficit of AD. Some cholinergic enhancers have shown a limited effect in some research studies; these results had been insufficient to justify the clinical use of these drugs until recently. However, since the mid 1980s, several short-term studies have shown that tacrine (tetrahydroaminoacridine), a cholinesterase inhibitor, significantly enhances cognition and functioning in some patients with mild to moderate AD (Small, 1992). Despite absence of long-term studies, the Food and Drug Administration has approved use of tacrine (Cognex). Typically, tacrine dosage is started at 40 mg a day in four divided doses and, if tolerated, is titrated over several weeks up to 160 mg a day. Since 20 to 30% of patients develop reversible elevations of transaminases, liver function tests must be monitored weekly for 4 months and less frequently thereafter. Other adverse effects include nausea, vomiting, diarrhea, and abdominal pain.

Given that the cognitive deficit of most patients with AD will not improve, treatment interventions should focus on reducing the problematic behaviors associated with progression of AD (Eisdorfer et al., 1992). Pharmacologic or behavioral interventions based on a careful assessment may reduce these behaviors and avoid or delay institutionalization (Zubenko et al., 1992).

Agitation and Other Behavioral Problems. We define agitation in demented patients as "vocal or motor behavior that is either disruptive, unsafe, or interferes with delivery of care in a particular environment" (Rosen, Mulsant, & Wright, 1992). This definition is not based on the impact of behavior on others, nor does it require that the observer make assumptions regarding the patient's needs. Rather, this definition relies on observed behaviors that are maladaptive within the patient's setting, since certain behaviors might be considered "agitation" in one environment but not in another. This conceptualization distinguishes "abnormal behaviors" from "agitation." Abnormal behaviors that are not disruptive and do not interfere with the patient's physical health or care need not be the target of pharmacological interventions. However, these "annoying" behaviors may be amenable to behavioral therapy or environmental changes.

Agitation is a nonspecific manifestation of one or more medical or psychiatric processes. When assessing agitation in demented subjects, one should systematically consider six potential etiologic categories: pain/discomfort, delirium, depression, psychosis, anxiety/distress, and caregiver burden (Salzman, 1987a). Since the treatment approach will differ according to etiology, behavioral and pharmacologic interventions will be discussed for each of these specific causes of agitation. Table 2.2 summarizes the clinical features of agitation resulting from these different processes and guidelines for targeted intervention.

Pain/Discomfort. Skin breakdown, urinary tract infection, constipation or fecal impaction, arthritis, compression or long bone fractures, cancers, and angina are common causes of pain and agitation in demented patients. Agitation may be a patient's only way of communicating discomfort. After identification of the etiology of discomfort, judicious use of analgesics may be helpful. Acetaminophen and nonsteroidal anti-inflammatory agents are preferred to narcotics, because the latter often produce delirium and a worsening of agitation. In selected cases, short-term aggressive management with narcotics may be warranted. Behavioral therapy techniques are generally not helpful when agitation is due to pain.

TABLE 2.2. Dementia with Agitation

Etiology	Clinical features	Management guidelines
Pain or discomfort	Associated with urinary retention, constipation or impaction, fractures, cancer, angina, others	Physical examination and medical interventions Judicious use of analgesics (avoid narcotics)
Delirium	Rapid change Fluctuating attention EEG changes Associated with medical changes, pharmacological changes	Medical evaluation Review of medication changes Treatment of underlying problems Behavioral interventions: —frequent reorientation —room with window —physical restraints if needed Avoidance of pharmacological interventions Use of high-potency neuroleptics if necessary
Depression	Sad affect, crying, death wish, food refusal Premorbid or family history of depression	Aggressive antidepressant management: —nortriptyline in therapeutic range —sertraline or paroxetine —consider electroconvulsive therapy
Psychosis	Delusions of simple paranoid nature Visual or auditory hallucinations Usually occurs in later stages	Use of neuroleptics —those of medium potency, such as perphenazine, better tolerated
Anxiety or distress	Repeated requests for help Searching for family members Often relieved by reassurance	Behavioral/milieu interventions Pharmacotherapy: —neuroleptics —benzodiazepines —serotonin reuptake inhibitor, buspirone —other agents
Caregiver burden	Decreased tolerance of an overburdened caregiver	Counseling, support, respite Consider depression in caregiver

Adapted from Rosen, J., Mulsant, B. H., & Wright, B. A. (1992). Agitation in severely demented patients. *Annals of Clinical Psychiatry, 4,* 207–215.

Delirium. Patients with dementia are exceptionally vulnerable to a super-imposed delirium as a result of minor changes in their medical or pharmacologic status (Beresin, 1988; Francis, Martin, & Kapoor, 1990). Delirium in this population often presents as agitation. Appropriate interventions will be dictated by the etiology of the delirium. Until the causes can be corrected, behavior may improve with simple interventions such as the use of one primary nurse, frequent reorientation, the placing of familiar objects in the room, and the removal of extraneous noise or other stimuli. At times, physically restraining a patient is preferable to prescribing sedating medications that may interfere with assessment and impede recovery. A high-potency neuroleptic at a low dosage (e.g., haloperidol 0.5 or 1 mg ever four or six hours) can be used temporarily for safety.

Depression. Depression is usually diagnosed during the early stages of AD, when sad mood and hopelessness are often clearly expressed (Fischer, Simanyi, & Danielczyk, 1990; Mulsant & Zubenko, 1993). It is unclear if as dementia progresses, depression occurs less often or is less frequently recognized (Cohen-Mansfield & Marx, 1988; Emery & Oxman, 1992). Patients with advanced dementia are often not able to provide a verbal description of their mood state, and depression may present as irritability or agitation. In this context, sad affect, crying spells, verbalization of death wish, or food refusal may warrant an antidepressant trial. A history of major depression prior to the onset of dementia, or a family history of mood disorder, increases the probability of response to antidepressant treatment (Pearlson et al., 1990; Rovner, Broadhead, Spencer, Carson, & Folstein, 1989).

Psychotherapeutic and milieu interventions may effectively reduce depressive symptoms in demented patients. Increasing patients' "control" (Rodin & Langer, 1977; Schultz, 1976) improves satisfaction and quality of life in elderly nursing home residents. Adult day care or activity groups may reduce the sense of isolation that demented people feel. Various forms of therapy, such as reminiscence therapy, music and art therapy, and support groups result in improved mood in some demented patients.

Since only a few studies have assessed the efficacy and safety of antidepressant drugs in treating the depressive symptoms of demented patients (Nyth & Gottfries, 1990; Reifler et al., 1989), treatment of a depressive syndrome in the context of dementia should follow the same guidelines as treatment of major depression occurring in late life (Gerson, Plotkin, & Jarvik, 1988; Jenike, 1988). In the absence of contraindications, nortriptyline, because of its efficacy, linear pharmacokinetics, modest anticholinergic effects, limited changes in orthostatic blood pressure, and mild sedative effect, has been considered the antidepressant of choice in late life (Pollock, Perel, & Reynolds, 1990; Roose, Glassman, & Dalack, 1989; Rosen, Sweet, Pollock, & Mulsant, 1993). Plasma levels should be monitored to ensure adequate dosing, and the treatment trial should continue for at least 6 weeks (Preskorn & Fast, 1991). In addition to monitoring of plasma level, regular assessment of side effects (especially increased confusion or lethargy), fall precaution measures, monitoring of orthostatic blood pressure, and serial electrocardiograms should be standard practice in this population.

Although few studies have yet assessed the efficacy of serotonin reuptake inhibitors (SRIs) in the treatment of depression in late life (Cohn et al., 1990; Feighner, Boyer, Meredith, & Hendrickson, 1988; Nyth & Gottfries, 1990), these antidepressants appears promising based on the neuropathologic and neurochemical profile of patients suffering from degenerative dementia with depression (Mulsant & Zubenko, 1993; Zubenko & Moossy, 1988; Zubenko, Moossy, & Kopp, 1990; Zweig et al., 1988). Furthermore, due to their lack of anticholinergic or cardiovascular toxicity and their wide therapeutic index, SRIs are easier to use in older outpatients than are tricyclic antidepressants.

In demented patients with severe depression who fail to respond to an adequate antidepressant trial, electroconvulsive therapy should be considered (Mulsant, Rosen, Thornton, & Zubenko, 1991; Nelson & Rosenberg, 1991)

Psychosis. Delusions or hallucinations occur in about half of patients with AD (Deutsch et al., 1991; Lopez et al., 1991), usually in the middle and late stages of the disease (Drevets & Rubin, 1989; Eisdorfer et al., 1992; Jeste, Wragg, Salmon, Harris, & Thal, 1992; Wragg & Jeste, 1989). Initial interventions should address the environmental and caregiver factors that may contribute to psychosis. A demented patient should be instructed to keep valuables, such as a watch or wallet, in a specific place. This may reduce hiding behaviors that lead to paranoid beliefs when a particular object is misplaced and cannot be found. Caregivers must learn how to respond to the paranoid beliefs. Confrontations or arguments are rarely of benefit. If simple reassurances do not work, tactics of diversion and distraction may be effective in reducing the patient's distress. When delusions or hallucinations result in behaviors that interfere with safety or care, and these nonpharmacological interventions are not effective, medications should be considered.

There is some evidence, albeit inconclusive, that neuroleptics reduce agitation in some demented psychotic patients (Mulsant & Gershon, 1993; Rosen, Bohon, & Gerson, 1990; Salzman, 1987b; Schneider, Pollock, & Lyness, 1990). Haloperidol is being widely used because of its favorable anticholinergic profile. However, neuroleptics of intermediate potency, such as loxapine or perphenazine, also induce relatively low levels of anticholinergic side effects and may be better tolerated than high-potency neuroleptics because they have fewer extrapyramidal side effects at therapeutic dosage (Bolvig-Hansen & Larsen, 1985; Petrie et al., 1982). "As needed" (PRN) dosing obscures the assessment of treatment response by introducing daily variations of drug levels and should be avoided in most cases (Druckenbrod, Rosen, & Cluxton, in press). The clinician should adopt a standardized dosing strategy with repeated assessments of behavior and side effects. Initial neuroleptic dosages should be low (e.g., 4 mg a day of perphenazine), with increases in dosage every 7 to 10 days until the desired therapeutic effect is obtained or side effects emerge. Typically, psychosis in demented patients responds to fairly low dosages (e.g., 4 to 12 mg a day) within a few weeks. However, some demented patients may tolerate and require higher dosages to reduce agitation and paranoia.

Anxiety/Distress. Some demented patients with severe agitation do not fit into any of the above categories. Such patients may present with a sense of distress and bewilderment, attempting to leave in order to "go home" or periodically yelling for help when in no particular distress. Behavioral disturbances occurring during activities, such as toileting or bathing, should be considered in this spectrum (Cohen-Mansfield, Werner, & Marx, 1990). Similarly, disrupted sleep architecture associated with AD (Hoch et al., 1989) may result in poor sleep and nighttime agitation. Such nighttime behaviors that interfere with the caregiver's rest is one of the most frequently cited reason for institutionalization (Pollack & Perlick, 1991).

Environmental manipulations and behavioral techniques may be most helpful in controlling this type of agitation (Fisher & Carstensen, 1990; Mulsant & Thornton, 1990). For instance, a patient who becomes agitated when his wife (whom he no longer recognizes) tries to assist him with toileting may accept assistance from a male. Another patient who becomes hostile when she is given a morning shower may accept a bath in the afternoon. When agitation in the evening is due to tiredness, a structured 1- to 2-hour nap in the afternoon may improve evening behavior. Effectively treating these problems behaviorally requires creative thinking and trial and error.

When behavioral interventions fail, sedating medications such as neuroleptics, trazodone, or benzodiazepines may be tried (Coccaro et al., 1990; Houlihan et al., 1994). Trazodone, 50 to 100 mg at bedtime (less than the dosage required to treat depression), seems to be useful in inducing sleep without residual daytime sedation. However, any sedating medication increases the risk of fall and of hip fracture in elderly patients (Granek et al., 1987; Ray, Griffin, Schaffner, Baugh, & Melton, 1987). Thus dosage of a sedating medication should be low initially and then gradually titrated until the desired effect is obtained or until troublesome side effects occur. Buspirone has a favorable side effect profile but, although its efficacy in treating anxiety in the elderly has been demonstrated (Böhm et al., 1990), its role in treating agitation in demented patients has not yet been established (Herrmann & Eryavec, 1993; Schneider & Sobin, 1991). Similarly, case reports and clinical series have suggested the usefulness of several other agents (e.g., carbamazepine, lithium, propranolol) in reducing nonspecific agitation in some demented patients (Schneider & Sobin, 1991). Controlled studies of these agents in demented patients with agitation are needed before their use can be recommended.

Caregiver Burden. A report of increased agitation in a demented patient may reflect the decreased tolerance of an overburdened, ailing caregiver rather than an acute change in the patient's behavior. More than two-thirds of caregivers report a decline in their physical health due to stress (Snyder & Keefe, 1985), as many may be suffering from major depression (Cohen & Eisdorfer, 1988), and more than one-fifth cite their own ill health as the reason for institutionalization (Chenoweth & Spencer, 1986). When caregiver burden is suspected, the primary intervention to treat "agitation" should target the caregiver rather than the demented patient (Mulsant & Thornton, 1990). Individual and group supportive therapy can improve caregivers' well-being and increase their coping skills. Caregivers can be taught how to reduce the impact of disturbing behavior by becoming aware of the anxiety, frustration, or anger it generates in them. Caregivers can then recognize that they are upset not by the behavior itself but, rather, by how they evaluate it. Perseveration, inoffensive delusions or hallucinations, and failure to perform a simple daily task are examples of symptoms and behaviors that are commonly evaluated as "hostile."

When accumulation of minor stressors rather than one particular problem is the source of a caregiver's frustration, taking time for himself or herself or getting some respite can prevent tensions from building up. In this context, supportive therapy may enable a caregiver to seek more help or to consider institutionalization for a patient whose dementia has progressed beyond the caregiver's ability to continue in that role (Zarit & Zarit, 1982). Finally, interventions aimed at reducing caregiver burden may also involve the demented patient. For instance, adult day care may provide a caregiver with some free time; pharmacologic treatment of a patient's sleep disturbance may enable the caregiver to rest adequately at night.

Selecting Optimal Treatment Strategies

Benoit H. Mulsant
and Jules Rosen

Behavioral disturbances in demented patients present challenging clinical problems. In the absence of definitive empirical data, a thorough assessment of the patient and caregiver will permit rational selection of a behavioral and/or pharmacologic treatment (see Table 2.2). The approach presented in this chapter is based on a careful review of the literature as well as clinical experience. Table 2.3 presents an overview of medications frequently prescribed for demented patients.

Table 2.4 presents common problems occurring at different stages of dementia along with appropriate management techniques for caregivers.

Problems in Carrying Out Interventions

Unsuccessful management of behavioral complications of the dementia patient often results in placement in a more restrictive environment (Zubenko et al., 1992) and financial and emotional burdens on caregivers. Since demented persons tend to respond to and mirror the affective behavior of those around them, caregivers should act as role models by displaying patience, gentleness, and calm (Bartol, 1979). Smiling, touching, or holding hands are often the best ways to soothe the patient. Caregivers should praise desired behaviors, while ignoring undesired behavior when safely

TABLE 2.3. Overview of Medications Prescribed to Demented Patients

Agent	Comments	Dosages
Neuroleptics	Modest benefits supported by literature Elderly vulnerable to extrapyramidal and anticholinergic side effects First choice with delusional patients	Perphenazine: start at 4 mg and titrate up to 24 mg daily as needed and tolerated. Common range: 8–16 mg daily
Benzodiazepines	Avoid drugs with long half-lives that will accumulate Tolerance may develop Very sedating May interfere with memory	Lorazepam: start at 0.25 mg b.i.d. Increase until sedation or confusion emerges. Common range: 0.5–1.5 mg b.i.d.
Tricyclics	Watch for orthostasis, anticholinergic and cardiac side effects May take 4–6 weeks for therapeutic effect	Nortriptyline: Start 25 mg h.s.; titrate to yield plasma level of 80–120 ng/ml Common range: 25–100 mg h.s.
Serotonin reuptake inhibitors	Nausea common during the first few days of therapy May take 4–6 weeks for therapeutic effect	Sertraline: start at 50 mg in A.M and titrate up to 200 mg as needed and tolerated
Trazodone	Very effective to consolidate sleep at low dose Generally well tolerated by elderly Higher doses needed to treat depression are too sedating	Start at 25 mg h.s. and titrate to reach desired effect. Common range to promote sleep: 50–100 mg
Buspirone	Non-benzodiazepine antianxiety agent Requires up to 6 weeks for therapeutic effect	Buspirone: 30–60 mg daily in 2 or 3 divided doses

Adapted from Rosen, J., Mulsant, B. H., & Wright, B. A. (1992). Agitation in severely demented patients. *Annals of Clinical Psychiatry, 4,* 207–215.

TABLE 2.4. Managing Behavior Problems Associated with Dementia: Strategies for Caregivers

Common problems	Recommended management techniques
	I. Early Dementia
Learning and recent memory deficit	Use memory aids and reminders: notes, logs, calendars, clocks.
Losing things	Establish "a place" for things such as keys and wallet.
Communication problems	Use reassurances; speak slowly, distinctly, and softly; avoid open-ended questions; communicate through noverbal cues such as smiling and holding hands.
Attempts to "cover up"	Use respect in response to a person's denial as a coping skill, yet ensure safety.
Depression	Discuss feelings; seek professional help.
Lack of motivation or initiative	Suggest activities or plans.
Fear of losing control	Establish familiar and secure routines; encourage the person to do as much for himself or herself as is safely possible (e.g., prepare simple meals using a microwave); give praise for accomplishments.
Problems in judgment or calculation	Simplify decisions or tasks; help with financial matters; avoid rationalizing or asking, "Why did you do that?"
	II. Moderate Dementia
Confusion and disorientation	Minimize distractions; use repetition.
Safety concerns	Look for safety hazards in and around the home (cooking, bathing, using electrical appliances) and make needed changes; don't hesitate to restrict driving when necessary.
Difficulties with bathing, grooming	Use simple "one-step" directions; employ humor.
Changes in sexual behavior	Initiate intimate and affectionate exchanges; recognize impairments and limitations.
Sleep disturbances	Encourage regular exercise and sleep hygiene (i.e., discourage daytime naps); prevent boredom. Ask physician about medications.
Angry outbursts and agitation	Identify the precipitants and avoid them; respond in a calm, reassuring voice; smile and try touch if this doesn't upset the person further; use distractors; leave the room if necessary. Ask physician about medications.
	III. Severe Dementia
Decreased recognition of family and familiar places	Use links from the past (photo albums, portraits, memories); use reasurance and repetition.
Problems in dressing	First, offer help with choosing clothes, then with actual mechanics of dressing; use "one-step" directions; use special clothing (e.g., shoes with Velcro bands instead of laces).
Eating problems	Do not rush mealtime; serve foods easily broken or eaten with one utensil; use "finger foods"; give one item at a time; instruct when to chew or swallow.
Incontinence	Inform physician; use routine toileting; restrict fluids after evening meal; use special clothing and adult diaper.
Falls	Eliminate throw rugs and other safety hazards; provide adequate lighting (e.g., night lights); provide walker or cane; supervise ambulation; have a plan to pick up fallen person.

Adapted with permission from M. Bozich and S. Housley (1985). Unpublished.

feasible. However, caregivers may be extremely resistant to interventions that require them to change their mode of interacting with the dementing patient. Similarly, caregivers may resist taking time for themselves. Understanding that they are the main resource for their demented dependent and that they must take care of themselves to be able to continue to provide good care may help them to do so without feeling guilty of neglect. As emphasized by Lezak (1978): "This very important issue must be brought up early and often, for the notion of enlightened self-interest runs counter to popular moral equations of self abnegation and duty taught by many religious and social institutions" (p. 595).

As dementia progresses, cognitive impairment may prevent the implementation of behavioral interventions or render previously effective interventions ineffective. The treatment focus may shift to pharmacotherapy. In any medication trial, it is important to adjust dosage slowly. When titration cannot be based on plasma levels, dosage should be increased until either therapeutic effects or adverse effects emerge. A treatment trial should last at least 4 weeks. This will prevent the premature discontinuation of a potentially helpful agent. PRN dispensation of medications and polypharmacy should be avoided in most cases.

Relapse Prevention

Minimal information is available on the course of behavioral disturbances that are associated with dementia. As AD progresses, the degenerative process may exacerbate a previously stabilized problem, thus requiring additional evaluation and treatment. Conversely, some behavioral disturbances may resolve over time, and some medications may no longer be needed.

Case Illustration

Case Description

Mr. M. is a 75-year-old man who presented for outpatient evaluation with his wife. The patient had no complaint, but his wife reported that her husband had become very irritable over the past 6 months. He had been refusing to shower before going to bed, insisting that he had already showered. This had resulted in verbal altercations two or three times per week and, on one occasion 3 weeks prior, he had pushed her into a wall. Since then, Mrs. M had been sleeping in a separate room because of her husband's poor hygiene.

Mrs. M. also reported that over the same period, her husband had lost interest in most activities, including family outings with his grandchildren. He had been sleeping poorly with frequent awakenings and had lost 20 pounds, becoming thin. Mr. M. had been frequently complaining that he "might as well be dead"; however, he has not been expressing suicidal ideation, and there was no history of an attempt.

Upon specific questioning, Mrs. M. reported that her husband had become increasingly forgetful over the past few years. The first definite example of a significant memory problem she could identify had occurred two years earlier, when her husband went to the bank to withdraw money for their vacation, not recalling that he had done so the day before. Since then, his memory had slowly and insidiously continued to deteriorate. Mr. M. had stopped driving 3 months before, when he was stopped by the police for driving the wrong way down a one-way street in his neighborhood.

The patient had no history of psychiatric evaluation or treatment. He had a history of drinking 6 to 8 beers daily for many years but had been abstinent since he retired from working as a salesman, 10 years prior. There had been considerable marital strife over his drinking but no other social or medical sequelae related to excessive alcohol use. There was no history of symptoms of depression, psychosis, or anxiety disorder.

Mr. M. suffered from chronic atrial fibrillation that had been diagnosed 3 years before, when he experienced two episodes of transient ischemic attack (TIA). In addition, he had a history of hypothyroidism that was diagnosed when he retired and he has been treated for hypertension for the past 6 years. There were no other active medical problems. There were no reports of loss of consciousness, TIA, or other neurological events over the past 2 years. There was no history of toxic or industrial exposure. Current medications included digoxin 0.125 mg daily, nifedipine 10 mg t.i.d. levothyroxine (Synthroid) 0.01 mg daily, and one aspirin per day.

Mrs. M. reported that her husband's mother had died in a state hospital at the age of 85 after a 10-year stay due to "senility." His father had been an alcoholic who committed suicide at the age of 68, when he began to "think he had terminal cancer."

On mental status examination Mr. M. appeared mildly apprehensive initially, but was generally congenial and pleasant. He was alert during the course of the evaluation. His speech was clear although somewhat slow and stereotypic. Frequent paraphasic errors were noted. He denied feeling sad or hopeless, and his affect showed a good range. His thoughts were poorly organized with evidence of derailment and perseveration. He had no recollection of fighting with his wife, but complained that she often "nagged" him. He denied delusions or hallucinations; however, his wife reported that on two recent occasions he had thought someone had stolen his wallet. These episodes lasted approximately 30 minutes and resolved when his wallet was found.

On cognitive testing, Mr. M. was able to state his full name but not the date or the day of the week. He was aware that he was in a doctor's office but was unaware of the floor, the address, or the name of the county. He was able to immediately repeat the names of three objects but could not recall any of the three 2 minutes later. He could name a pen and a watch, but not the band, face, or winder of the watch. He could not repeat "No ifs, ands, or buts." He was able to follow a simple three-step command and to write a sentence ("It is a nice day"), but was unable to copy two intersecting figures. He was able to correctly recite the days of the week forward and backward, but was unable to recite the months of the year in reverse order. He could not name the present or previous president of the United States. He did not think there was anything wrong with his memory and attributed his errors to being tired.

Mr. M. was in generally good health. He had an irregular cardiac rhythm with a rate of 82 beats per minute and was asymptomatic, with a 15 mmHg drop in blood pressure upon standing. There were no focal findings on neurologic examination. The rest of his physical exam findings were normal. Laboratory evaluation, including complete blood count, liver and metabolic profile, thyroid function tests and TSH, B_{12}, folate, and electrolyte levels, sedimentation rate, and serological antibody studies were normal. Electroencephalography revealed slowing of alpha rhythm without evidence of focility or seizure activity. Magnetic resonance imaging revealed a small lacunar infarct in the basal ganglia and periventricular white matter lucencies.

Differential Diagnosis and Assessment

Even though Mr. M. presented with symptoms consistent with a major depressive syndrome (irritability, loss of interest, poor sleep, weight loss, and passive death wish), his decrease in functioning and memory problems over the past two years suggest an underlying primary dementia. Based on available information, the primary differential diagnosis consideration consists of an MID versus a primary degenerative dementia of the Alzheimer's type (AD). According to the recently proposed criteria for vascular dementia (Chui et al., 1992), Mr. M. probably does not suffer from this disorder. Although atrial fibrillation is a risk factor for vascular dementia and a lacuna was noted on MRI, the neurologic examination revealed no focal findings. The clinical course was not step-wise, and there was no temporal relationship between a vascular event and cognitive decline. The patient did not have urinary incontinence or gait disturbance. Therefore, although there is definite evidence of cerebrovascular disease, Mr. M.'s dementia is more likely to be caused by a primary degenerative process than by his cerebrovascular illness.

Though alcoholism can result in dementia, abstinent alcoholics who have a progressive dementia are indistinguishable in terms of neuropsychological profile, behavioral symptoms, and outcome from patients with AD (Rosen et al., 1993). Thus, these patients are most likely to suffer from a primary degenerative dementia (AD). Given the normal thyroid function test findings and TSH level, we can assume that the patient's thyroid disease is adequately treated and is not contributing to his dementia or behavioral problems.

Treatment Selection

In this patient with a moderate dementia and a depressive syndrome, the risk/benefit ratio of a tacrine trial was not judged to be favorable, and thus the main goal of treatment was to reduce his behavioral disturbances so that he could be maintained at home. Mrs. M. identified his resistance to showering as the most troublesome problem. Upon learning that Mr. M.'s premorbid habit was to shower in the morning, prior to going to work, we suggested that a schedule restoring the patient's lifelong routine be implemented. We suggested that Mr. M. attend an adult day care program that would give a sense of structure to his day, as well as enable him to participate in activities and socialize. We decided to wait before initiating an antidepressant trial, to see whether his depressive symptoms would resolve with additional environmental stimulation and an increase in socialization. In addition, we provided Mrs. M. with some printed information on AD and we referred her to an on-going psychoeducational group for family caregivers of demented patients.

Treatment Course and Problems in Carrying Out Interventions

Three weeks after initiation of recommended environmental changes, Mrs. M. informed us that her husband's resistance to showering had resolved but that his depressive symptoms were unchanged. In fact, Mr. M. had refused to attend the adult day care during the previous week.

After an electrocardiogram (ECG) was obtained, which confirmed diagnosis of atrial fibrillation, a regimen of nortriptyline 25 mg daily at bedtime was started. After 1 week there were no complaints of side effects, no increase in the orthostatic drop in systolic blood pressure, and a repeat ECG was unchanged. Nortriptyline plasma level was 42 ng/ml. Given the linear level–dose relationship of nortriptyline, its dosage was doubled to 50 mg nightly to increase the plasma level to the middle of the therapeutic range (50 to 150 ng/ml). Two weeks later, Mr. M.'s nortriptyline level was 93 ng/ml. His affect was brighter, and Mrs. M was reporting an improvement in his sleep and increased socialization (he had resumed attendance at adult day care). A repeat ECG showed a new left bundle branch block with a QRS complex of 140 msec. Nortriptyline administration was discontinued. Treatment with sertraline, 50 mg in the morning was initiated. After complaining of mild nausea for 2 days, Mr. M. seemed to tolerate his medication well.

Outcome and Termination

Mr. M. was maintained on a regimen of sertraline for the next 8 months, during which he remained euthymic, without problem with his sleep or appetite. At this point, sertraline administration was discontinued at the patient's wife's request. Over the next 2 years, Mr. M. became increasingly confused, to the point where he became incontinent and needed to be dressed and fed. However, his wife was able to care for him at home, with some assistance from a home-care agency two afternoons a week and from her daughter during weekends. Mr. M. eventually developed pneumonia and died after a short hospitalization.

Summary

Dementia can be caused by a wide variety of neuropathologic processes. Alzheimer's disease is the most common cause of cognitive decline; however, the diagnosis is made primarily by excluding other possible etiologies. Thus, evaluation of dementia includes a thorough psychiatric, neurologic, and medical examination. Laboratory evaluation and brain imaging are also necessary.

At this time there is no broadly effective treatment for the cognitive decline of AD, but associated behavioral problems and psychiatric syndromes can be effectively managed with behavioral and pharmacologic therapies. A thorough characterization of the behavioral presentation is necessary prior to formulating any rational treatment plan. In most cases, if behaviors are not presenting immediate risk to the patient or caregiver, alterations in the environment or in the approach of the caregiver may be sufficient to control aberrant behaviors. When agitation or other behavioral problems persist, pharmacotherapy that is based on the presumed etiology of the behavioral disturbance should be initiated. The treatment should be as specific as possible for a given target symptom or syndrome. Initial low medication dosage should be increased once steady state plasma levels are attained, and dosage titration should continue until a predetermined plasma level is reached, the target symptom resolves, or side effects appear. PRN medications should be avoided.

Each patient must be considered as an individual case study. By working closely with caregivers to effect environmental changes and with the judicious use of medication, the quality of life of many demented patients can be maintained.

Benoit H. Mulsant
and Jules Rosen

References

American Psychiatric Association (1987). *Diagnostic and statistical manual of mental disorders* (3rd ed., rev.). Washington, DC: Author.

American Psychiatric Association (1991). *DSM-IV options book: Work in progress*. Washington, DC: Author.

Bartol, M. A. (1979). Nonverbal communication in patients with Alzheimer's disease. *Journal of Gerontological Nursing, 5*, 21–31.

Beresin, E. V. (1988). Delirium in the elderly. *Journal of Geriatric Psychiatry and Neurology, 1*, 127–143.

Blessed, G., Tomlinson, B. E., & Roth M. (1968). The association between quantitative measures of dementia and of senile changes in the cerebral gray matter of elderly subjects. *British Journal of Psychiatry, 114*, 797–811.

Böhm, C., Robinson, D. S., Gammans, R. E., Shrotriya, R. C., Alms, D. R., Leroy, A., & Placci, M. (1990). Buspirone therapy in anxious elderly patients: A controlled clinical trial. *Journal of Clinical Psychopharmacology, 10*(3), 47S–57S.

Bolvig-Hansen, L., & Larsen, N. (1985). Therapeutic advantages of monitoring plasma concentrations of perphenazine in clinical practice. *Psychopharmacology, 87*, 16–19.

Breitner, C. S. (1987). Genetic factors in the etiology of Alzheimer's disease. In H. Y. Meltzer (Ed.), *Psychopharmacology: The third generation of progress* (pp. 929–938). New York: Raven.

Brody, E. M., Johnsen, P. T., Fulcomer, M. C., & Lang, A. M. (1983). Women's changing roles and help to elderly parents: Attitude of three generations of women. *Journal of Gerontology, 38*, 597–607.

Chenoweth, B., & Spencer, B. (1986). Dementia: The experience of family caregivers. *Gerontologist, 26*, 267–272.

Chui, H. C., Victoroff, J. I., Margolin, D., Jagust, W., Shankle, R., & Katzman, R. (1992). Criteria for the diagnosis of ischemic vascular dementia proposed by the state of California Alzheimer's disease diagnostic and treatment centers. *Neurology, 42*, 473–480.

Clarfield, A. M. (1988). The reversible dementias: Do they reverse? *Annals of Internal Medicine, 109*, 476–486.

Coccaro, E. F., Kramer, E., Zemishlany, Z., Throne, A., Rice, C. M., Giordani, B., Duvvi, K., Patin, B. M., Torres, J., Nora, R., Neufeld, R., Mohs, R. C., & Davis, K. L. (1989). Serotonergic studies in patients with affective and personality disorders. *Archives of General Psychiatry, 46*, 587–599.

Coccaro, E. F., Kramer, E., Zemishlany, Z., Thorne, A., Rice, C. M., Giordani, B., Duvvi, K., Patel, B. M., Torres, J., Nora, R., Neufeld, R., Mohs, R. C., & Davis, K. L. (1990). Pharmacologic treatment of noncognitive behavioral disturbances in elderly demented patients. *American Journal of Psychiatry, 147*(12), 1640–1645.

Cohen, D., & Eisdorfer, C. (1988). Depression in family members caring for relative with Alzheimer's disease. *Journal of the American Geriatrics Society, 36*, 885–889.

Cohen-Mansfield, J., & Marx, M. S. (1988). Relationship between depression and agitation in nursing home residents. *Comprehensive Gerontology Bulletin, 2*, 141–146.

Cohen-Mansfield, J., Werner, P., & Marx, M. S. (1990). Screaming in nursing home residents. *Journal of the American Geriatrics Society, 38*, 785–792.

Cohn, C. K., Shrivastava, R., Mendels, J., Cohn, J. B., Fabre, L. F., Claghorn, J. L., Dessain, E. C., Itil, T. M., & Lautin, A. (1990). Double-blind, multicenter comparison of sertraline and amitriptyline in elderly depressed patients. *Journal of Clinical Psychiatry, 51*, 28–33.

Consensus Conference (1987). Differential diagnosis of dementing diseases. *Journal of the American Medical Association, 258*, 3411–3416.

Cummings, J. L., & Benson, D. F. (1992). *Dementia. A clinical approach*. Boston: Butterworth-Heinemann.

Cutler, P. (1979). *Problem solving in clinical medicine: From data to diagnosis* Baltimore: Williams and Wilkins

Deutsch, L. H., Bylsma, F. W., Rovner, B. W., Steele, C., & Folstein, M. F. (1991). Psychosis and physical aggression in probable Alzheimer's disease. *American Journal of Psychiatry, 148*, 1159–1163.

Drevets, W. C., & Rubin, E. H. (1989). Psychotic symptoms and the longitudinal course of senile dementia of the Alzheimer type. *Biological Psychiatry, 25*, 39–48.

Druckenbrod, R. W., Rosen, J., & Cluxton, R. J. (in press). As needed (PRN) use of antipsychotic drugs: Limitations and guidelines for use. *Annals of Pharmacotherapy*.

Eisdorfer, C., Cohen, D., Paveza, G. J., Ashford, J. W., Luchins, D. J., Gorelick, P. B., Hirschman, R. S., Freels, S. A., Levy, P. S., Semla, T. P., & Shaw, H. A. (1992). An empirical evaluation of the global deterioration scale for staging Alzheimer's disease. *American Journal of Psychiatry, 149*(2), 190–194.

Emery, V. O., & Oxman, T. E. (1992). Update on the dementia spectrum of depression. *American Journal of Psychiatry, 149*(3), 305–317.

Evans, D. A., Funkenstein, H. H., Albert, M. S., Scherr, P. A., Cook, N. R., Chown, M. J., Hebert, L. E., Hennekens, C. H., & Taylor, J. O. (1989). Prevalence of Alzheimer's disease in a community population of older persons. *Journal of the American Medical Association, 262*, 2551–2556.

Feighner, J. P., Boyer, W. F., Meredith, C. H., & Hendrickson, G. (1988). An overview of fluoxetine in geriatric depression. *British Journal of Psychiatry, 153*(3), 105–108.

Fischer, P., Simanyi, M., & Danielczyk, W. (1990).Depression in dementia of the alzheimer type and in multi-infarct dementia. *American Journal of Psychiatry, 147*, 1484–1487.

Fisher, J. E., & Carstensen, L. L. (1990). Behavior management of the dementias. *Clinical Psychology Review, 10*, 611–629.

Folstein, M. F., Folstein, S. E., & McHugh, P. R. (1975). Mini mental state: A practical method for grading the cognitive state of patients for the clinician. *Journal of Psychiatric Research, 12*, 189–198.

Francheschi, M., Ferini-Strambi, L., Minicucci, F., Sferrazza-Papa, A., & Smirne, S. (1986). Signs of cardiac autonomic dysfunction during sleep in patients with Alzheimer's disease. *Gerontology, 32*, 327–334.

Francis, J, Martin, D., & Kapoor, W. N. (1990). A prospective study of delirium in hospitalized elderly. *Journal of the American Medical Association, 263*, 1097–1101.

Freyhan, F. A., Woodford, R. B., & Kety, S. S. (1951). Cerebral blood flow and metabolism in psychosis of senility. *Journal of Nervous and Mental Disease, 113*, 449–456.

Gerson, S. C., Plotkin, D. A., & Jarvik, L. F. (1988). Antidepressant drug studies, 1964 to 1986: Empirical evidence for aging patients. *Journal of Clinical Psychopharmacology, 8*, 311–322.

Granek, E., Baker, S. P., Abbey, H., Robinson, E., Myers, A. H., Samkoff, J. S., & Klein, L. E. (1987). Medications and diagnoses in relation to falls in a long-term care facility. *Journal of the American Geriatrics Society, 35*, 503–511.

Grimes, A. M., Grady, C. L., Foster, N. L., Sunderland, T., & Patronas, N. J. (1985). Central auditory function in Alzheimer's disease. *Neurology, 35*, 352–358.

Hachinski, V. C., Lassen, N. A., & Marshall, J. (1974). Multi-infarct dementia: A cause of mental deterioration in the elderly. *Lancet, 2*, 207–210.

Herrmann, N., & Eryavec, G. (1993). Buspirone in the management of agitation and aggression associated with dementia. *American Journal of Geriatric Psychiatry, 1*, 249–253.

Hoch, C. C., Reynolds, C. F., Nebes, R. D., Kupfer, D. J., Berman, S. R., & Campbell, D. (1989). Clinical significance of sleep-disordered breathing in Alzheimer's disease. *Journal of the American Geriatrics Society, 37*, 138–144.

Houlihan, D. J., Mulsant, B. H., Sweet, R. A., Rifai, A. H., Pasternak, R. E., Rosen, J. & Zubenko, G. S. (1994). A naturalistic study of trazodone in the treatment of demented elderly. *American Journal of Geriatric Psychiatry, 2*, 78–85.

Huff, F. J., Boller, F., Lucchelli, F., Querriera, R., Beyer, J., & Belle, S. (1987). The neurologic examination of inpatients with probable Alzheimer's disease. *Archives of Neurology, 44*, 929–932.

Jenike, M. A. (1988). Assessment and treatment of affective illness in the elderly. *Journal of Geriatric Psychiatry and Neurology, 1* 89–107.

Jeste, D. V., Wragg, R. E., Salmon, D. P., Harris, M. J., & Thal, L. J. (1992). Cognitive deficits of patients with Alzheimer's disease with and without delusions. *American Journal of Psychiatry, 149*, 184–189.

Katzman, R. (1986). Alzheimer disease. *New England Journal of Medicine, 314*, 964–973.

Kay, D. W. K., Roth, M., & Hopkins, B. (1955). Affective disorders arising in the senium: Their association with organic cerebral degeneration. *British Journal of Psychiatry, 101*, 302–316.

Knupfer, L., & Speigel, R. (1986). Differences in olfactory test performance between normal aged, Alzheimer and vascular type dementia individuals. *International Journal of Geriatric Psychiatry, 1*, 3–14.

Lezak, M. (1978). Living with the characterologically altered brain injured patient. *Journal of Clinical Psychology, 39*, 592–598.

Lopez, O. L., Becker, J. T., Brenner, R. P., Rosen, J., Bajulaiye, O. I., & Reynolds, C. F. (1991). Alzheimer's disease with delusions and hallucinations: Neuropsychological and electroencephalographic correlates. *Neurology, 41*, 906–912.

McKhann, G., Drachman,D., Folstein, M., Katzman, R., Price, D., & Stadlan, E. M. (1984). Clinical diagnosis of Alzheimer's disease: Report of the NINCDS-ADRDA work group under the auspices of Department of Health and Human Services task force on Alzheimer's disease. *Neurology, 34*, 939–944.

Meyer, J. S., Judd, B. W., Tawaklna, T., Rogers, R. L., & Mortel, K. F. (1986). Improved cognition after control of risk-factors for multi-infarct dementia. *Journal of the American Medical Association, 256,* 2203–2209.

Morycz, R. C. (1985). Caregiving strain and the desire to institutionalize family members with Alzheimer's disease. *Research on Aging, 7,* 329–361.

Mulsant, B. H., and Gershon, S. (1993). Neuroleptics in the treatment of psychosis in late-life: A rational approach. *International Journal of Geriatric Psychiatry, 8,* 979–992.

Mulsant, B. H., Rosen, J., Thornton, J. E., & Zubenko, G. S. (1991). A prospective naturalistic study of electroconvulsive therapy in late-life depression. *Journal of Geriatric Psychiatry and Neurology, 4,* 3–13.

Mulsant, B. H., & Thornton, J. E. (1990). Alzheimer disease and other dementias. In M. E. Thase, B. A. Edelstein, & M. Hersen (Eds.), *Handbook of outpatient treatment of adults: Nonpsychotic mental disorders* (pp. 353–388). New York: Plenum.

Mulsant, B. H., & Zubenko, G. S. (1993). Clinical, neuropathological, and neurochemical correlates of depression and psychosis in primary dementia. In V. O. B. Emery & T. E. Oxam (Eds.), *The spectrum of dementia* (pp. 336–352). Baltimore: Johns Hopkins University Press.

Navia, B. A., & Price, R. W. (1987). The acquired immunodeficiency syndrome dementia complex as the presenting or sole manifestation of human immunodeficiency virus infection. *Archives of Neurology, 44,* 65–69.

Nelson, J. C., & Rosenberg, D. R. (1991). ECT treatment of demented elderly patients with major depression: A retrospective study of efficacy and safety. *Convulsive Therapy, 7,* 157–165.

Nielsen, S. S., Petito, C. K., Urmacher, C. D., & Posner, J. B. (1984). Subacute encephalitis in acquired immunodeficiency syndrome: A post-mortem study. *American Journal of Clinical Pathology, 82,* 678–682.

Nyth, A. L., & Gottfries, C. G. (1990). The clinical efficacy of citalopram in treatment of emotional disturbances in dementia disorders. *British Journal of Psychiatry, 157,* 894–901.

Pearlson, G. D., Ross, C. A., Lohr, W. D., Rovner, B. W., Chase, G. A., & Folstein, M. F. (1990). Association between family history of affective disorder and the depressive syndrome of Alzheimer's disease. *American Journal of Psychiatry, 147,* 452–456.

Petrie, W. M., Ban, T. A., Berney, S., Fujimori, M., Guy, W., Ragheb, M., Wilson, W. H., & Schaffer, J. D. (1982). Loxapine psychogeriatrics: A placebo- and standard-controlled clinical investigation. *Journal of Clinical Psychopharmacology, 2,* 122–126.

Pollack, C. P., & Perlick, D. (1991). Sleep problems and institutionalization of the elderly. *Neurology, 4,* 201–210.

Pollock, B. G., Perel, J. M., & Reynolds, C. F. (1990). Pharmacodynamic issues relevant to geriatric psychopharmacology. *Journal of Geriatric Psychiatry and Neurology, 3,* 221–228.

Preskorn, S. H., & Fast, G. A. (1991). Therapeutic drug monitoring for antidepressants: efficacy, safety, and cost effectiveness. *Journal of Clinical Psychiatry, 52,* 23–33.

Ray, W. A., Griffin, M. R., Schaffner, W., Baugh, D. K., & Melton, L. J., III (1987). Psychotropic drug use and the risk of hip fracture. *New England Journal of Medicine, 316,* 363–369.

Reifler, B. V., & Larson, E. (1988). Excess disability in demented elderly outpatients: The rule of halves. *Journal of the American Geriatrics Society, 36,* 82–83.

Reifler, B. V., Teri, L., Raskind, M., Veith, R., Barnes, R., White, E., & McLean, P. (1989). Double-blind trial of imipramine in Alzheimer's disease patients with and without depression. *American Journal of Psychiatry, 146,* 45–49.

Rezek, D. L. (1987). Olfactory deficits as a neurologic sign in dementia of Alzheimer type. *Archives of Neurology, 44,* 1030–1032.

Rocca, W. A., Amaducci, L. A., & Schoenberg, B. S. (1986). Epidemiology of clinically diagnosed Alzheimer's disease. *Annals of Neurology, 19,* 415–424.

Rodin, J., & Langer, E. J. (1977). Long-term effects of a control-relevant intervention with the institutionalized age. *Journal of Personality and Social Psychology, 35,* 897–902.

Roose, S. P., Glassman, A. H., & Dalack, G. W. (1989). Depression, heart disease, and tricyclic antidepressants. *Journal of Clinical Psychiatry, 50*(Suppl.), 12–17.

Rosen, J., Bohon, S., & Gerson, S. C. (1990). Antipsychotics in the elderly. *Acta Psychiatrica Scandinavica, 82,* 170–175.

Rosen, J., Colantonio, A., Becker, J. T., Lopez, O. L., DeKosky, S. T., & Moss H. B. (1993). Effects of a history of heavy alcohol consumption on Alzheimer's disease. *British Journal of Psychiatry, 163,* 358–363.

Rosen, J., Mulsant, B. H., & Wright, B. A. (1992). Agitation in severely demented patients. *Annals of Clinical Psychiatry, 4,* 207–215.

Rosen, J., Sweet, R. A., Pollock, B. G., & Mulsant B. H. (1993). Nortriptyline in the hospitalized elderly: Tolerance and side effect reduction. *Psychopharmacology Bulletin, 29*, 327–331.

Rosen, J., & Zubenko, G. S. (1991). Emergence of psychosis and depression in the longitudinal evaluation of Alzheimer's disease. *Biological Psychiatry, 29*, 224–232.

Rovner, B. W., Broadhead, J., Spencer, M., Carson, K., & Folstein, M. F. (1989). Depression and Alzheimer's disease. *American Journal of Psychiatry, 146*, 350–353.

Rovner, B. W., Kafonek, S., Filipp, L., Lucas, M. J., & Folstein, M. F. (1986). Prevalence of mental illness in a community nursing home. *American Journal of Psychiatry, 143*, 1446–1449.

Salzman, C. (1987a). Treatment of agitation in the elderly. In H. Y. Meltzer (Ed.), *Psychopharmacology: The third generation of progress* (pp. 1167–1176). New York: Raven.

Salzman, C. (1987b). Treatment of the elderly agitated patient. *Journal of Clinical Psychiatry, 48*(5), 19–22.

Schneider, L. S., Pollock, V. E., & Lyness, S. A. (1990). A metaanalysis of controlled trials of neuroleptic treatment in dementia. *Journal of the American Geriatrics Society, 38*, 553–563.

Schneider, L. S., & Sobin, P. B. (1991). Non-neuroleptic medications in the management of agitation in Alzheimer's disease and other dementia: A selective review. *International Journal of Geriatric Psychiatry, 6*, 691–708.

Schultz, R. (1976). Effects of control and predictability on the physical and psychological well-being of the institutionalized aged. *Journal of Personality and Social Psychology, 5*, 563–573.

Shanas, E. (1979). Social myth as hypothesis: The case of the family relations of old people. *Geronotologist, 19*, 3–9.

Sim, M., & Sussman, I. (1962). Alzheimer's disease: Its natural history and differential diagnosis. *Journal of Nervous and Mental Disease, 135*, 489–499.

Sjogren, T., Sjogren, H., & Lindgren, G. H. (1952). Morbus Alzheimer and morbus Pick: A genetic, clinical, and pathoanatomical study. *Acta Psychiatrica Scandinavica, 34*(Suppl. 82),

Small, G. W. (1992). Tacrine for treating Alzheimer's disease. *Journal of the American Medical Association, 268*, 2564–2565.

Snyder, B., & Keefe, K. (1985). The unmet needs of family caregivers for frail and disabled adults. *Social Work in Health Care, 10*, 1–14.

Steele, C., Rovner, B. W., Chase, G. A., & Folstein, M. F. (1990). Psychiatric symptoms and nursing home placement of patient with Alzheimer's disease. *American Journal of Psychiatry, 147*, 1049–1051.

Steffes, R., & Thralow, J. (1987). Visual field limitation in the patient with dementia of the Alzheimer's type. *Journal of the American Geriatrics Society, 35*, 198–204.

Stern, Y., Mayeux, R., Sano, M., Hauser, W. A., & Bush, T. (1987). Predictors of disease course in patients with probable Alzheimer's disease. *Neurology, 37*, 1649–1653.

Tariot, P. N., Podgorski, C. A., Blazina, L., & Leibovici, A. (1993). Mental disorders in the nursing home: Another perspective. *American Journal of Psychiatry, 150*, 1063–1069.

Warner, M. D., Peabody, C. A., Flattery, J. J., & Tinklenberg, J. R. (1986). Olfactory deficits and Alzheimer's disease. *Biological Psychiatry, 21*, 116–118.

Wragg, R. E., & Jeste, D. V. (1989). Overview of depression and psychosis in Alzheimer's disease. *American Journal of Psychiatry, 146*, 577–587.

Zarit, S., & Zarit, J. (1982). Families under stress: Interventions for caregivers of senile dementia patients. *Psychotherapy: Theory Research and Practice, 19*, 461–471.

Zubenko, G. S., & Moossy, J. (1988). Major depression in primary dementia: Clinical and neuropathologic correlates. *Archives of Neurology, 45*, 1182–1186.

Zubenko, G. S., Moossy, J., & Kopp, U. (1990). Neurochemical correlates of major depression in primary dementia. *Archives of Neurology, 47*, 209–214.

Zubenko, G. S., Rosen, J., Sweet, R. A., Mulsant, B. H., & Rifai, A. H. (1992). Impact of psychiatric hospitalization on behavioral complications of Alzheimer's disease. *American Journal of Psychiatry, 149*, 1484–1491.

Zweig, R. M., Ross, C. A., Hedreen, J. C., Steele, C., Cardillo, J. E., Whitehouse, P. J., Folstein, M. F., & Price, D. L. (1988). The neuropathology of aminergic nuclei in Alzheimer's disease. *Annals of Neurology, 24*, 233–242.

3

Psychoactive Substance Use Disorders

Kimberly S. Walitzer and Gerard J. Connors

Description of the Disorders

The diagnostic classification of psychoactive substance use disorders in DSM-III-R (American Psychiatric Association, 1987) includes two major categories—substance dependence and substance abuse—for nine classes of drugs (alcohol, amphetamines, cannabis, cocaine, hallucinogens, inhalants, opioids, phencyclidine (PCP), and sedatives).

Clinical Features

The diagnostic definitions of substance abuse and substance dependence have changed as revisions of the DSM have evolved. Generally speaking, substance dependence is characterized by the presence of physical and/or psychological dependence on the substance. The two hallmarks of physical dependence are "marked" tolerance (i.e., increase of *at least 50%* in the amount of substance needed to achieve intoxication or effects) and presence of withdrawal symptoms when substance use is reduced or stopped. The extent of tolerance and symptoms of withdrawal vary as a function of the particular substance. Psychological dependence is characterized by preoccupation in thought and lifestyle with substance use. Substance dependence is usually associated with negative consequences that may include job, family, financial, health, or legal problems. In contrast, substance abuse traditionally has been considered a less severe diagnosis that was used to denote maladaptive or otherwise

Kimberly S. Walitzer and Gerard J. Connors • Research Institute on Addictions, Buffalo, New York 14203.

Handbook of Prescriptive Treatments for Adults, edited by Michel Hersen and Robert T. Ammerman. Plenum Press, New York, 1994.

problematic ingestion of a particular substance that did not meet the criteria for dependence.

Associated Features

Comorbidity. The occurrence of another disorder in conjunction with a substance use disorder has been reported in both community and treatment samples. The results from the Epidemiologic Catchment Area (ECA) survey have described psychiatric comorbidity associated with alcohol and drug problems in the general population. The ECA study entailed over 20,000 interviews with respondents in five major cities and determined the lifetime occurrence of DSM-III (American Psychiatric Association, 1980) diagnoses using the structured Diagnostic Interview Schedule-III (DIS-III). The ECA study found substantial comorbidity with both alcohol and drug disorders as delineated in DSM-III. As reported by Regier et al. (1990), 13.5% of the general population received a lifetime diagnosis of alcohol abuse or dependence; of that subgroup, 36.6% had at least one other DSM-III mental disorder, and 21.5% had another drug abuse or dependence diagnosis. The comorbidity rate for the 6.1% of the population with a lifetime drug abuse or dependence diagnosis was much higher: 53.1% of that subgroup had at least one other DSM-III mental disorder, and 47.3% had an alcohol abuse or dependence disorder (Regier et al., 1990).

Helzer and Pryzbeck (1988) examined mental disorders associated with alcohol disorders based on the ECA data. Individuals with a lifetime alcohol diagnosis were 21 times more likely than those in the general population to meet DSM-III criteria for antisocial personality disorder. Furthermore, they were 7.2 times more likely than the general population to meet criteria for a drug disorder, 6.2 times more likely to meet criteria for mania, and 4 times more likely to meet criteria for schizophrenia (Helzer & Pryzbeck, 1988).

In treatment samples, major depression has been found to co-occur with drug disorders (see Hendriks, Steer, Platt, & Metzgar, 1990) and depression and anxiety disorders have been found to co-occur with alcohol disorders (e.g., Herz, Volicer, D'Angelo, & Gadish, 1990; Hesselbrock, Meyer, & Keener, 1985; Powell, Penick, Othmer, Bingham, & Rice, 1982). The ECA data, however, indicate that anxiety and affective disorders are *not* significantly more prevalent in those with an alcohol disorder than they are in the general population (Helzer & Pryzbeck, 1988). The higher prevalence of psychiatric symptoms with substance use disorders in treatment samples may reflect a tendency for individuals with a comorbid diagnosis to be more likely to seek treatment than individuals with only the alcohol diagnosis (Agosti, Nunes, Stewart, & Quitkin, 1991; Helzer & Pryzbeck, 1988).

Multiple Substance Use. Substance use disorders often co-occur across several drug categories within an individual. The ECA data indicate that an individual with an alcohol disorder diagnosis is 35 times more likely than those in the general population to also have a diagnosis of cocaine abuse or dependence. It is common for patients in substance abuse treatment programs to be using or abusing more than one substance. In one study, Miller, Gold, and Millman (1989) found that 94% of their cocaine-dependent clients also met the criteria for alcohol dependence. Also, multiple abuse often involves drugs with similar actions, such as alcohol, sedatives, and anxiolytics, or cocaine and amphetamines. The DSM indicates that when multiple substances are abused, all diagnoses applicable should be given. This is in contrast to the polysubstance dependence diagnosis, which describes multiple substance use when the use of no single substance meets diagnostic criteria, although criteria are met across substances.

Suicidal Behavior. Suicide is generally considered a risk in affective diagnoses. Suicide attempts and completions are also highly associated with substance use disorders. Sternberg's (1991) review of this literature indicates significantly higher risk of both suicide attempts and suicide completions in individuals with alcohol or drug use disorders than in the general population. Multiple substance use and comorbid psychiatric diagnoses further increase the risk of suicidal behavior.

Physical Complications. A variety of physical complications are associated with chronic alcohol or drug use, or both, several of which are considered in the diagnostic criteria (e.g., tolerance, physical dependence symptoms). Other common physical consequences of chronic use include malnutrition, liver damage, cognitive and memory dysfunction, and organic mental syndrome. Acquired immune deficiency syndrome (AIDS), hepatitis, tetanus, and malaria can be transmitted through intravenous drug use.

Epidemiology

Relative to other DSM disorders, alcohol use disorders and drug use disorders are among the most prevalent (13.5% and 6.1% in the general population, respectively). A 1984 general population survey reported that 76% of men and 64% of women 18 years old and older had consumed alcohol in the previous year (Hilton, 1987). Furthermore, 48% of men and 25% of women were classified as frequent drinkers (i.e., drink at least once per week). Of current drinkers, 14% of men and 6% of women had experienced moderate alcohol problems during the previous year (i.e., at least four tangible consequences from alcohol use).

A survey by the National Institute on Drug Abuse (1988) found that among young adults, 21.9% reported marijuana use, 7.7% cocaine use, and 4% stimulant use during the previous month. The ECA data indicate that marijuana and amphetamines are the most prevalent drugs of abuse (4% and 1.7%, respectively) in the general population (Regier et al., 1990). In sum, whereas clinical substance use problems are prevalent, subclinical problems (i.e., those having occasional negative consequences) affect an even larger percentage of the population.

Etiology

There are many questions and few certainties about the development of alcohol and drug problems. Alcohol problems do tend to recur within families, as has been demonstrated in family, twin, and adoption studies (see Cotton, 1979; Goodwin, 1985). The nature versus nurture argument has been intense in the field of alcoholism, but most experts in the field of addictions view both genetic and environmental factors as potentially crucial etiological variables.

Heritability Theory. The heritability theory is widely held in the alcoholism field. As a result, one interpretation of the prevalence of familial alcohol problems is that alcoholism (i.e., alcohol dependence) is inherited. However, not all offspring of alcoholics develop alcohol problems and individuals without alcoholic relatives can develop such problems. It has been postulated that the heritable component in alcoholism leads to a *predisposition* toward drinking problems. Such predisposition is activated and leads to serious alcohol problems in some individuals and appears to remain dormant in others. Considerable research has been conducted in an attempt to identify the nature of the hypothesized inherited predisposition, including studies of personality, physiologic, neuropsychological, and biochemical traits. Although differences have been documented between individuals "biologically predisposed" to alcoholism (i.e., individuals with biological first-degree alcoholic relatives) and those assumed not to be predisposed (i.e., individuals with no family history of alcohol problems), no simple trait representing the predisposition for alcohol problems has been identified. Thus, although alcohol problems do appear to have some level of genetic loading, it seems unlikely that alcoholism is the simple result of genetics. A similar perspective is evolving in the drug abuse field (Glantz & Pickens, 1992).

Vulnerability Theory. A slightly different perspective on the etiology of addictions is offered by the "vulnerability" theory. In this case, the focus is on identifying characteristics that *increase vulnerability* to addictions, rather than on heritability and genetics. A host of variables has been found to be predictive of alcohol abuse, and these have been combined to construct a complex model of alcoholism, highly heterogeneous as to etiology. Sher (1991), for example, has outlined a comprehensive model of vulnerability that combines family factors, personality, neuropsychological functioning, beliefs about alcohol, academic achievement, and peer influences. Similar models are being developed for drug abuse (see Glantz & Pickens, 1992). Genetic loading may play a role within these factors, but it is theorized that there are multiple pathways to addiction that may and may not include genetic loading.

Differential Diagnosis and Assessment

DSM-III-R and DSM-IV Categorization

The DSM-III-R psychoactive substance dependence diagnosis requires (a) a minimum of three symptoms of a possible nine and (b) the persistence of symptoms for at least 1 month or repeated occurrence of symptoms over time. Generally, a diagnosis of substance dependence indicates impairment in three domains: cognitive (e.g., impaired control over substance), behavioral (e.g., use of substance despite psychosocial consequences), and physiologic (e.g., marked tolerance, withdrawal). A current diagnosis can be described as mild, moderate, or severe, based on the number of symptoms. An inactive diagnosis can be categorized as "in partial remission" when substance use and "some" symptoms have occurred in the previous 6 months, or as "in full remission" when no substance use, or only asymptomatic substance use, has occurred during the previous 6 months. The term "alcoholism" is commonly used to refer to alcohol dependence.

As defined in DSM-III-R, the diagnostic category of psychoactive substance abuse is a residual diagnosis used to document maladaptive use among persons who do not meet (and have never met) the criteria for substance dependence. The substance abuse diagnosis often is applicable to individuals who have recently begun using a substance, and to persons using substances not generally associated with the development of withdrawal.

Nathan (1991) has reported that the DSM-IV Substance Use Disorders Work Group is modifying the criteria for substance abuse and dependence. The proposed substance abuse diagnosis will require the presence of two of eight criteria. Thus, the abuse diagnosis will move from its DSM-III-R residual status to a more meaningful description of harmful or potentially harmful substance use. The proposed DSM-IV substance dependence diagnosis requires the presence of substance abuse *and* either marked tolerance or withdrawal symptoms. According to Nathan's (1991) description of these proposed diagnostic criteria, individuals meeting the DSM-III-R criteria for substance dependence but *not* exhibiting tolerance or withdrawal may well meet DSM-IV criteria for substance abuse as opposed to substance dependence.

Differential Diagnosis

Multiple substance use makes diagnosis more difficult. An assessment that includes an individual's "drug(s) of choice" and chronology of specific drug usage and consequences can aid in diagnosis. According to DSM-III-R, multiple abuse and dependence diagnoses are given when indicated. The polysubstance dependence diagnosis applies only when multiple drugs are used but use of any single drug does not meet criteria for diagnosis.

As discussed earlier, substance use disorders tend to co-occur with other psychiatric disorders, most notably mood and anxiety disorders, schizophrenia, and antisocial personality disorder. When a comorbid diagnosis is present, a helpful differential diagnosis often can be made between a *primary* and a *secondary* substance use disorder. When it can be determined that the substance use disorder existed prior to the comorbid disorder, the substance use disorder is considered primary; when the comorbid disorder was initially present, the substance use disorder is considered secondary. In the latter case, it should be considered that the pathological substance use is potentially a symptom or a consequence of the primary (comorbid) disorder. For example, problematic substance use (e.g., alcohol, sedatives) may result from a primary depression or anxiety disorder when the individual uses the substance to self-medicate. When the substance use disorder is considered secondary, one potential treatment strategy is to focus on alleviating the primary disorder with less immediate attention to the problematic substance use.

In the case of a primary substance use disorder, the reverse situation should be considered. Chronic substance use can produce life stressors and biochemical changes sufficient to contribute significantly to an affective or anxiety disorder. Further, certain substances can produce psychotic symptoms (e.g., amphetamines, hallucinogens). When a primary substance use disorder is thought to be contributing to the secondary, comorbid disorder, it is often effective to treat the substance use disorder first, followed by a reassessment of the secondary disorder. These guidelines, of course, are general, and focusing on the primary problem area does not mean attention should be arbitrarily withheld from the secondary problem. Instead, appropriate and responsive attention to secondary problems is provided as warranted.

Assessment Strategies

Although an assessment for problematic substance use may rely primarily on self-report, a complete assessment will also include collateral reports (those by significant others) and physiological assessment. Although a comprehensive initial assessment is vital to the case formulation and subsequent selection of treatment strategies, ongoing assessment is an important component of the treatment process. Thus, a complete and nonjudgmental survey of factors contributing to the patient's drug use and life consequences resulting from such use should occur prior to and during treatment.

Assessment of Substance Use. An assessment of current substance use should include an identification of the types of substances, the quantity and frequency of use, and information on combined drug intake. Frequency of use is straightforward and usually references the number of times a particular substance is used in a typical day, week, or month. Quantity of use is more complex. With alcohol, care must be taken to account for different "proofs" or ethanol contents of various alcoholic beverages. For example, one "standard drink" is typically defined as 0.5 ounces of ethanol (e.g., 12 ounces of 5% beer, 4 ounces of 12% wine, 1.25 ounces of 80 proof hard liquor). Quantity of other substances is more difficult to assess, as the user is more likely to be unaware of the amount and chemical strength of the drug or drugs being ingested. Urine and blood toxicology procedures that yield quantitative information often are helpful in assessing the type and quantity of substance use.

In addition to amount, the style of substance use is also important to assess. Pathological styles, or methods of ingestion highly associated with abuse, include morning intake, binges, and use to counteract withdrawal symptoms.

Assessment of Negative Consequences. The majority of the DSM-III-R and proposed DSM-IV diagnostic criteria are based on consequences of substance use. Current and lifetime assessment of negative consequences of use should include a variety of areas including social, legal, financial, marital, familial, work, health, and dependence symptoms. Although in practice most of this information can be gathered simply from a patient's spontaneous report, it is worthwhile to inquire into areas not mentioned by the individual.

In addition to current and previous problems, the assessment should include areas where the individual is *at risk* for consequences that have not yet occurred. For instance, although an individual who drinks and drives may not have experienced negative consequences, the risk of physical, legal, and financial consequences is great. An individual may test negative for the presence of HIV, but the possibility that his or her substance use is increasing risk of HIV contact should be explored.

Assessment of Contributing Factors. Various factors that contribute to the development and maintenance of alcohol or drug problems should also be assessed. The individual's family history of alcohol and drug problems is important, both in terms of the possible genetic contribution and as social learning and modeling effects. Beliefs and cognitions regarding drug effects, such as alcohol/drug expectancies, are important in maintaining drug use and in relapse. Assessment of social and lifestyle factors that may encourage or promote alcohol/drug use also is important.

Functional Analysis of Substance Use. A specialized assessment procedure useful in treatment planning is the functional analysis of substance use. This behavioral analysis seeks to identify the way in which substance use "functions" within the patient's life and to identify specific factors that have served to maintain or reinforce substance use. An understanding of how substance use functions in the patient's life will identify areas in which treatment should be focused. Identification of emotions, activities, environments, and people that are strongly associated with substance ingestion will begin to illustrate the manner in which the substance use has functioned. The majority of the functional analysis can be performed during the pretreatment assessment, but it is worthwhile to continue the functional analysis during and after treatment as additional issues become apparent.

Collateral Reports. The assessments described thus far rely solely on self-report. Although research generally has found the self-reports of alcohol and drug users to be reliable and valid (see reviews by Maisto, McKay, & Connors, 1990, and Sobell & Sobell, 1990), valuable insights can be obtained from the perspective of a spouse or significant other of the patient. When collateral contacts are presented as a way of obtaining a different perspective on the patient's functioning—rather than seeking solely to verify the patient's report—most individuals will permit collateral interviews. Important information can be obtained from collaterals concerning home, family, work, and social life as they relate to substance use and factors that maintain or encourage it.

Physiological Assessment. Physiological measurement of drug and alcohol use includes laboratory and biochemical assessments of use, physiological consequences, or both. These measures assess use within a limited time frame and are not necessarily diagnostic, because many test results may be elevated for physiological reasons not associated with alcohol or drug use.

The most common physiological assessment for the presence of alcohol is the breath test. Major factors in the popularity of the breath test are that it is noninvasive, accurate when correctly used, and quick and easy to administer. An advantage of the breath test relative to a urinalysis is the immediacy of results. Urinalysis, however, can also be used to test for the presence of other drugs. Two additional assessments of recent alcohol use, each receiving increasing attention, are the sweat-patch and the "dipstick." The sweat-patch collects perspiration at a steady rate, and the concentration of alcohol in that patch is correlated with the amount of alcohol consumed over the period of time the patch is worn (up to 8 to 10 days). The "dipstick" consists of filter paper that changes color when dipped in blood, urine, or saliva samples that contain alcohol. Although still being refined, each has the potential to be a useful and efficient clinical assessment tool.

Biochemical measures derived from blood samples are another category of physiological assessment. An important feature of these laboratory tests is that they provide an indication of longer-term alcohol use. For example, elevated levels of gamma-glutamyl transferase (GGT) and mean corpuscular volume (MCV) are often associated with recent excessive alcohol consumption. These and other laboratory tests can be especially useful when posttreatment results are compared to pretreatment values, because levels of such variables as GGT and MCV generally return to normal following cessation of heavy drinking.

Treatment

Evidence for Prescriptive Treatments

Empirical outcome studies have examined the efficacy of a variety of treatment strategies for alcohol and drug problems. The present review includes a description of the more frequently used and most promising treatment modalities. Because treatment outcome research is more plentiful for alcohol-abusing populations, the review is weighted in that direction. With only a few exceptions, however, these treatment strategies are equally applicable to drug use disorders.

Behavior Therapy. A number of behavioral strategies to treat alcohol and drug use disorders have been empirically investigated. Four areas of behavioral treatment are reviewed here: social skills training, positive reinforcement, marital therapy, and drinking moderation training.

Social Skills Training. Following a review of alcoholics' social skills, O'Leary, O'Leary, and Donovan (1976) concluded that alcoholics have deficient social skills compared to nonalcoholics and that treatment focusing on increasing their social repertoires would aid in the development and utilization of alternatives to drinking. Thus, social skills training approaches are geared toward teaching individuals to deal more effectively with their environments. Components of skills training include assertion training, communication training, problem solving, and development of drinking/drug use refusal skills.

Numerous controlled treatment outcome studies have examined the efficacy of social skills packages and components, and only a sampling of this research is described here. Oei and Jackson (1980, 1982) noted that inpatient alcoholics reported lower posttreatment alcohol consumption when treatment included social skills training, and that benefits of social skills training may be further enhanced when treatment includes a cognitive restructuring component designed to modify irrational beliefs associated with social skills enhancement. Rohsenow, Monti, Binkoff, Liepman, and Nirenberg (1991) investigated communication skills training (including training in assertiveness, listening skills, enhancing close relationships, and drink refusal) and mood management treatment (coping with negative emotions and desires to drink) and reported that, although mood management training was as effective as the communication skills training for alcoholics with higher education, less anxiety, and less urge to drink, the communication skills training appeared to benefit a broader array of alcoholics.

Positive Reinforcement. Treatment of substance use problems with positive reinforcement relies on principles of operant conditioning. Simply put, the goal of treatment is to alter the consequences of substance use so that abstinence is reinforced and alcohol or drug use is not.

Miller (1975) described a behavioral intervention with chronic alcoholics (i.e., alcoholics with eight or more public drunkenness arrests during the previous year). Subjects were provided with housing, employment, medical care, meals, and so forth, contingent upon their sobriety (assessed by service providers, employers, and random blood alcohol concentration tests). The control group received identical services regardless of their sobriety status. Alcoholics in the behavioral intervention group exhibited more successful 2-month outcome findings than did controls. Despite a small subject size and relatively brief follow-up period, the positive response exhibited in such a chronic population is noteworthy.

Hunt and Azrin (1973) and Azrin (1976) described the development of a community-reinforcement treatment approach. This strategy greatly increases the density of available reinforcers in the sober alcoholic's life (e.g., marital, occupational, and social reinforcers) so that the "time out" and loss of reinforcers that come with alcohol intoxication are more salient and intense. The alcoholics who received the community-reinforcement treatment exhibited significantly improved outcome, enhanced further by the addition of disulfiram therapy.

Similar principles operate in therapeutic communities, an approach used to treat drug problems that includes as a cornerstone a system of clearly specified rewards and punishments for a range of behaviors. Therapeutic communities have been an effective intervention for many drug abusers (Institute of Medicine, 1990).

Marital Therapy. The previous treatment strategies focus solely on the individual with the substance use disorder. The rationale behind marital therapy provides an alternate conceptualization of substance use treatment: both spouses (or partners) in a couple in which one member has an alcohol or drug disorder are involved in the maintenance of the problem behavior. Thus, in order for treatment to be effective, the functioning and interaction of the couple must be examined. Involving the spouse in the treatment process has been found to produce reliably better treatment outcomes for alcohol-dependent individuals than does individual treatment that excludes the spouse (Corder, Corder, & Laidlaw, 1972; McCrady, 1989a).

Behavioral marital therapy (BMT) is a well-researched and effective behavioral technique for alleviating marital distress. Three core components of BMT are increasing marital reinforcement and satisfaction, communication skills, and negotiation skills. The addition of BMT into the treatment of alcohol-dependent patients has been reported to produce better outcomes (McCrady, Stout, Noel, Abrams, & Nelson, 1991; O'Farrell, Cutter, & Floyd, 1985), although a 2-year outcome study suggests that the marital treatment gains may be more stable and lasting than the alcohol treatment gains (O'Farrell, Cutter, Choquette, Floyd, & Bayog, 1992).

Marital therapy has not been extensively studied as a component of treatment for drug abuse. However, the research in the alcohol area indicates that these techniques may be effectively applied to drug problems.

Drinking Moderation Training. The vast majority of treatment approaches for substance use disorders are designed to assist the patient in achieving abstinence. In the last several decades, however, clinical researchers have investigated the efficacy of drinking moderation training with heavy drinkers or problem drinkers not severely dependent on alcohol. Secondary prevention treatment approaches such as these have sought to reduce alcohol consumption and minimize risks associated with drinking among this population of problem drinkers.

A frequently used treatment to moderate drinking is a package of behavioral self-control strategies, including self-monitoring, goal setting, drinking moderation strategies, and functional analysis of drinking (Miller & Munoz, 1982). This package is flexible and can be self-administered or guided by a therapist in individual or group sessions. Treatment outcome research has demonstrated the efficacy of behavioral self-control strategies in the moderation of alcohol consumption in this population (see reviews by Miller & Hester, 1980; Rosenberg, 1993).

Pharmacotherapy. The most common pharmacological treatments are medications to foster abstinence. The best known are disulfiram (Antabuse) in the treatment of alcohol problems and methadone in the treatment of opiate use. When disulfiram is ingested regularly, alcohol consumption leads to a highly discomforting reaction that includes nausea, hypotension, and vasodilation. Fear of this reaction serves to decrease the likelihood of drinking. Disulfiram is probably most effective with persons who fear these consequences and who consistently take the medication. However, compliance can be a problem, and disulfiram's effectiveness is enhanced when administration is fully or partially supervised. Generally, disulfiram is not used as a solitary treatment intervention but, instead, as an adjunct to other treatment approaches.

Methadone is a synthetic opiate used mostly in the treatment of heroin addiction. Administered orally (as opposed to the intravenous route used for heroin), it reduces heroin "craving." Usually administered daily, in decreasing dosages over long periods of time, methadone has been used to treat many heroin addicts. However, methadone itself is addictive, although to a lesser extent than heroin, and has no effect on alcohol and other drugs of abuse. Like disulfiram, methadone is typically used as an adjunctive treatment strategy within a larger treatment plan.

In the case of a comorbid diagnosis, especially a primary comorbid diagnosis (e.g., affective or anxiety diagnosis), a pharmacologic treatment is often used to treat psychiatric symptoms.

Alternative Treatments. Two major alternatives to the just-described treatment strategies for substance use disorders include self-help groups and family therapy.

Self-Help Groups. Alcoholics Anonymous (AA) has been in existence since 1935 and is one of the oldest structured approaches to alcohol problems. The program combines a religious orientation with insight, confrontation, and social support. Members are encouraged to attend meetings daily, work the Twelve Steps of AA, and regularly interact with other members. There has been little research into AA's effectiveness, partially because of its anonymous nature. Studies that have been conducted have yielded the unsurprising but nevertheless important conclusion that AA-oriented programs and groups are generally helpful and effective for individuals who adopt the philosophy and tenets of the organization. The strengths of AA include the social support, structure, and widespread availability of meetings. A potential disadvantage is a rigid adherence to ideology that makes it an unacceptable option for some alcoholics, who disagree with one or more of its tenets.

Other self-help organizations have developed over the years for persons with substance use disorders. These include Secular Organizations for Sobriety (SOS), an organization geared predominantly toward alcohol abusers; Narcotics Anonymous (NA) and Cocaine Anonymous (CA), geared toward drug problems and following tenets similar to those of AA; and Rational Recovery (RR), geared toward abusers of both alcohol and other drugs.

Family Therapy. Family systems theory emphasizes the role of reciprocal determination of behavior among family members and the maintenance of equilibrium in the functional or dysfunctional family. Using this perspective, the behavior of the "identified patient" (i.e., the problem drinker or drug user) is viewed as maintaining the family's interaction style and protecting the family from change. Treatment within this perspective includes the spouse and, often, other important family members in an effort to change the functioning and interactions of the entire family so that the problem behavior is no longer maintained. Unfortunately, there is little controlled research assessing the efficacy of the family systems model (see Collins, 1990; McCrady, 1989b, for reviews).

The development of a substance use disorder treatment package is intimately associated with the assessment process. The characteristics of the individual, the pattern of substance use, and the resources and support available dictate necessary treatment components. The therapist must be prepared to offer a variety of services including education, social work, recreational therapy, vocational counseling, and individual and group psychotherapy.

Type of Substance.   To some extent the selection of a treatment strategy will be influenced by the nature of the substance being abused. Effective treatment for alcohol abuse is not necessarily the same as for heroin abuse, which is not necessarily the same as for marijuana abuse or multiple substance abuse. For example, the severity and intensity of physical and psychological dependence differ across substances, and a goal of moderation is more acceptable in the context of alcohol consumption than it is for illegal substances. Nevertheless, the reality is that there are relatively few specialized treatments for individual substances. Except for several substance-specific pharmacologic treatments, such as disulfiram and methadone, and groups such as AA, NA, and CA, alcohol and drug use disorders are all managed similarly.

Level of Physical Dependence.   Research has found that increasing severity of alcohol physical dependence is predictive of poorer treatment outcome (e.g., Cronkite & Moos, 1978; Miller & Hester, 1980). Thus, the greater the severity of physical dependence, potentially the greater the intensity of treatment and posttreatment aftercare required. For example, high levels of dependence may require the additional therapeutic support available through an inpatient hospitalization program or a longer-term therapeutic community (e.g., halfway house) while the individual learns to function physically and emotionally in a drug-free environment. Outpatient treatment or partial hospitalization (e.g., day hospital) may be more therapeutic for individuals with lower levels of dependence, as these modalities allow individuals to practice skills in their own environment and cope with daily life stressors.

Because alcohol is a legal substance, drinking moderation can in some cases be considered as opposed to the standard goal of abstinence. Individuals low on indices of physical dependence (e.g., "problem drinkers" or "heavy drinkers") have been found to respond more favorably to drinking moderation training than have those with higher levels of physical dependence (Rosenberg, 1993). In fact, research has shown that a moderated-drinking goal is preferred by this group (Sanchez-Craig, Annis, Bornet, & MacDonald, 1984).

Level of Motivation.   Despite the available treatment technology, successful treatment requires the collaboration of the patient. All clinicians in the substance abuse area have had contacts with individuals who appeared to be uninterested in changing their substance use despite the presence of sometimes profound negative consequences. The influence of family members or employers, or other factors, may have lead or coerced the individual to a treatment service, but unwillingness to follow through with treatment (often referred to as "lack of motivation") stymies treatment efforts.

In such cases, the first "treatment strategy" should be to explore, in an accepting and nonjudgmental manner, the reasons behind the unwillingness or hesitancy to enter treatment. Barriers to treatment may exist, such as financial or transportation difficulties, need for child care, and work or other responsibilities. The therapist may be required to reduce the impact of these barriers before the logistics of treatment are viewed as feasible by the individual.

A common issue surrounding motivation is ambivalence regarding substance use versus abstinence. The changing balance between the drug's attractive features and its negative consequences can produce a strong conflict regarding treatment. This phenomenon sometimes has been referred to as denial or resistance and has been interpreted by some as a personal or character flaw. However, this phenomenon might be more therapeutically conceptualized as ambivalence and considered instead as a natural, understandable feature of many patients seeking treatment for a substance use disorder.

Miller and Rollnick (1991) have reviewed this concept in greater detail and have formulated a counseling approach referred to as motivational interviewing. This method acknowledges and normalizes the ambivalence in accepting ways that can cultivate the individual's motivation, or willingness, to change substance use patterns and engage in treatment. This approach has an empathic, nonconfrontational style with a goal of helping the client verbalize and consider the "aversion" side of his or her ambivalence, which is then reflected and reinforced by the therapist. This style is in marked contrast to the "confrontational" approach frequently observed in addiction counseling, in that the therapist using motivational counseling guides the client to describe reasons for change rather than confronting the client with reasons for change.

Other Psychiatric Symptoms.   The presence of other psychiatric symptoms or comorbid psychiatric disorders generally predicts poorer substance abuse treatment outcome (e.g., Ojehagen, Berglund, Appel, Nilsson, & Skjaerris, 1991). Thus, clients presenting with additional psychiatric symptomatology should be considered for supplementary treatment (psychological or pharmacologic) focused on the additional symptoms. With a primary substance use disorder and a secondary psychiatric disorder, a traditional treatment guideline has been to achieve abstinence, because the psychiatric symptoms may remit with abstinence. After an abstinent period, the psychiatric symptoms are reassessed and additional symptom-specific treatment is provided if necessary. In the case of a clearly secondary substance use disorder, treatment guidelines are less clear as to the order in which to address symptoms. However, it is recommended that the drug problem not be ignored while the primary psychiatric disorder is treated. It is important to address the drug use disorder, either prior to or concurrently with treatment of the psychiatric disorder, because the continuing presence of substance use problems may undermine treatment.

Functional Analysis of Substance Use.   The functional analysis of substance use performed during assessment is central to the selection of prescriptive treatment strategies for a given patient. For example, if an individual is using a substance to help cope with feelings of anxiety, depression, or boredom, then strategies to cope with and alleviate these emotions are indicated. An individual who has a social lifestyle involving heavy drinking may require treatment focusing on assertion and communication as well as development of an alternative social network. Vocational counseling, job-finding skills, financial or budgeting counseling, recreational counseling, family therapy, couples counseling, or in-depth psychotherapy on personal issues may be indicated as a result of the functional analysis.

Problems in Carrying Out Interventions

The barriers to successful treatment for substance use disorders can be formidable. As mentioned earlier, the initial phase of treatment may require exploring and addressing the psychological, attitudinal, and logistical barriers to treatment. A variety of problems and issues may need to be addressed during early treatment or even prior to the onset of treatment, such as inability to pay for treatment, lack of transportation to treatment facilities, need for child care, or time away from employment and family responsibilities. Apparent lack of motivation or treatment ambivalence may be addressed via the motivational interviewing described earlier. Attitudes involving stereotypes and concerns about being labeled an "alcoholic" or an "addict" may need to be addressed and overcome prior to an individual's being willing to engage in treatment. Negative experiences with previous treatment (e.g., confrontation) may need to be discussed and explored.

Relapse Prevention

Relapse, or the return to substance use, is the bane of substance use disorders. In their frequently cited review, Hunt, Barnett, and Branch (1971) described 65 to 75% relapse rates (defined as *any use* of the abused substance) in the year following treatment across three substances: heroin, tobacco, and alcohol. Furthermore, two-thirds of all relapses occurred within the first 90 days following treatment. Relapse is so central to substance use disorders that relapse and recovery from relapse have been incorporated in conceptualizations of the disorders, and recovery from substance abuse problems has increasingly been viewed as a cyclical process (e.g., Prochaska, DiClemente, & Norcross, 1992). Thus, prevention and minimization of relapse are crucial components of treatment and posttreatment care.

Relapse prevention in the substance use disorders field has become a comprehensive treatment package in and of itself. Described at length by Marlatt and Gordon (1985), relapse prevention includes cognitive restructuring, skills training, identification of high-risk situations, and problem solving. The goal of relapse prevention training is not only to prevent relapse but, perhaps more important, to cope with a relapse should it occur. Marlatt and Gordon (1985) make a distinction between a "lapse" (or "slip") and a full-blown relapse. Given the prevalence of lapses, or brief returns to substance use, clients are taught cognitive and behavioral strategies to cope successfully with and minimize a lapse so as to avoid a total relapse (a return to pretreatment substance use patterns). There have been relapse prevention programs developed for specific drugs, such as cocaine, as well (Carroll, Rounsaville, & Keller, 1991).

The traditional approach to relapse prevention is lifelong attendance and involvement in self-help groups, such as AA or NA. As discussed earlier, despite the general lack of research on the efficacy of self-help involvement, the availability and natural support of these organizations are such that self-help groups certainly deserve exploration as a component in an individual's relapse prevention package.

Relapse prevention takes on a slightly different meaning in the context of drinking moderation treatments. When the goal is abstinence, relapse is often defined as *any* return to substance use. With a moderated drinking goal, the definition of a relapse becomes more complex. It is important that the individual have clear drinking limits so that the early warning signs of a slip can be detected. Drinking over a client-set limit may define a lapse, and drinking over a higher limit or the occurrence of an alcohol symptom (e.g., hangover, blackout, argument with spouse) may define a relapse.

Case Illustration

N.J. is a 28-year-old, single woman who presented to a psychological clinic with concerns about her drinking. She had been referred by a social services agency for an alcohol abuse assessment. At intake, N.J. stated, "I want to drink less," and, "I don't want to become an alcoholic."

N.J. reported that she was lesbian and living with her partner of several years. She had received a high-school graduate equivalency diploma (school through grade 11) and was currently enrolled in a community college. N.J. was unemployed and had come into contact with social services because of financial difficulties. At intake she appeared slightly nervous, of average intelligence, pleasant, and motivated to change her alcohol use.

Differential Diagnosis and Assessment

Assessment of Substance Use.   N.J. reported consuming alcohol almost daily, typically 3 to 6 12-ounce beers on each drinking day. Approximately 2 days per month, she reported, she drank up to 8 to 10 beers. Her drinking during the prior 6 months had steadily followed this pattern, with two exceptions. The first was 1 month prior to intake, when for 2 weeks she drank daily and more heavily (generally 10 beers per day over an 8- to 10-hour period); she reported being under much pressure during this holiday period. The second atypical period occurred 4 months prior to intake, when she was abstinent for approximately 2 weeks following minor surgery.

N.J. reported a history of marijuana use in her late teens with no evidence of abuse or dependence.

Assessment of Negative Consequences.   N.J. reported that she had been concerned about her drinking during the past 2 years, although she had noted sporadic problems during the prior 5 years. She had experienced mild tolerance and had attempted to reduce her alcohol consumption previously. After drinking, N.J. reported, she was vulnerable to depression, anger, and arguments with her partner. N.J. was at considerable risk because of her alcohol use, especially while driving. She denied previous treatment, alcohol-related arrests, blackouts, morning drinking, binges, withdrawal symptoms, or fits or seizures associated with drinking.

Based on her report of drinking style and consequences, N.J. met three of the nine DSM-III-R criteria for alcohol dependence (substance taken in larger amounts than intended; unsuccessful efforts to cut down; substance use when it was physically hazardous). Thus, she received a diagnosis of alcohol dependence—mild. Note that the "dependence" diagnosis was applicable even in the absence of traditional alcohol dependence symptoms (marked tolerance, withdrawal symptoms). According to the proposed DSM-IV criteria, N.J. would receive the alcohol abuse diagnosis.

Assessment of Contributing Factors. N.J. reported no family history of alcohol, drug, or psychiatric disorders. Her chief expectancy regarding alcohol's effects was that it was calming and relaxing. She believed that alcohol consumption helped her fall asleep as well as calm her when she was angry or anxious. N.J. appeared to hold these expectancies strongly despite the contradictions present in her history (e.g., arguing with her partner after drinking). Her lifestyle appeared generally supportive of treatment. Her partner was encouraging of treatment and was herself a light drinker. In addition to her partner, several close friends were also concerned about her drinking and supportive of treatment.

Functional Analysis of Substance Use. At intake, N.J. reported that alcohol served two main functions in her life: to help her to sleep and to reduce stress. Her typical drinking situations were with acquaintances in a bar in the late afternoon after classes, and at home. During treatment, it became apparent that alcohol consumption also helped her release feelings of frustration with her partner and cope with dissatisfactions with her life (e.g., lack of education, limited occupational opportunities, financial difficulties).

Collateral Report. N.J. willingly provided a release of information, allowing her partner to be interviewed via telephone. During the brief conversation, N.J.'s partner confirmed her drinking pattern and lack of severe alcohol-related consequences; no contradictory information was provided. She expressed concern about the effects of alcohol on N.J.'s mood and her desire for N.J. to stop drinking. She also mentioned the occasions of N.J.'s irritability and anger after drinking and the potential for physical abuse.

Physiological Assessment. Laboratory test findings were within normal limits. A urine drug screen indicated no recent drug use.

Assessment of Psychiatric Comorbidity. The intake assessment included a review of DSM-III-R diagnostic criteria. The interview revealed some indications of occasional panic, but she did not meet diagnostic criteria. "Panicky" feelings occurred during periods of unemployment and inactivity. The interview indicated no history of affective disorder, anxiety disorder, drug disorder, or antisocial personality disorder.

Treatment Selection

The treatment selection process began with a discussion between the therapist and N.J. as to her treatment goals. N.J. strongly wanted to reduce her alcohol consumption but not abstain from alcohol. After assessment and discussion, the therapist and N.J. contracted to work toward drinking reduction rather than abstinence. This decision was based on N.J.'s low level of dependence on alcohol, normal liver function test results and desire to work toward this goal. Included in the treatment contract were 12 weekly 50-minute sessions, occasional conjoint sessions with N.J.'s partner, and a reassessment of goal options (e.g., moderation versus abstinence) in 2 months (or earlier if warranted).

The content of treatment followed the behavioral self-control drinking moderation approach described by Miller and Munoz (1982). This included establishing weekly alcohol consumption goals, daily self-monitoring of alcohol use, and implementation of a variety of drinking reduction strategies. Based on N.J.'s initial functional analysis of drinking, skills training in relaxation techniques and problem solving was provided. Conjoint sessions were included to assess the couple's functioning in relation to alcohol and monitor the level of conflict in the relationship.

Treatment Course and Problems in Carrying Out Interventions

Conjoint Sessions.   N.J. provided a release of information to allow her partner to attend sessions. The first conjoint sessions were scheduled early in treatment in order to discuss N.J.'s treatment plans and goals with her partner. In these sessions her partner voiced considerable concern over N.J.'s goal of moderation as opposed to abstinence. Drinking had become a significant conflict area, and N.J. continued to drink while her partner insisted that N.J. was an alcoholic and must stop drinking. Also, the couple had previously had several major arguments that the partner attributed to N.J.'s drinking. The therapist stated that, while N.J. and her partner disagreed on moderation versus abstinence, the goal they agreed on was to stop the arguments and tension about drinking. The therapist also stated that, while N.J. had characteristics that indicated that drinking moderation might be possible, no one could predict whether she would be successful in cutting down. After discussion, N.J. and her partner made a contract to use the first 2 months of therapy to work toward N.J.'s moderation of alcohol use. Her partner agreed that during these 2 months she would not accuse N.J. of overdrinking and she would attend a conjoint session at least once every 3 weeks to discuss how she felt therapy was progressing. N.J. agreed to attend sessions weekly to focus on drinking reduction strategies, include her partner in setting weekly drinking reduction goals, and attend conjoint sessions to discuss with her partner how she felt therapy was progressing. N.J. and her partner also agreed that, should N.J. not be able to achieve her drinking reduction goals or should arguments and tensions about drinking continue, N.J. would then work toward a trial of abstinence.

One of the first treatment "strategies" was to unite N.J. and her partner on a treatment goal. Conjoint sessions and a behavioral contract were necessary to clearly outline expectations for both N.J. and her partner and to state the primary goal of drinking reduction and a contingency goal of abstinence. If the early conjoint sessions had been omitted, N.J.'s efforts might have been undermined by the conflict and tension in the relationship regarding her continued drinking. Instead, a treatment plan was outlined from which both N.J. and her partner could benefit.

Individual Sessions.   Individual sessions included discussion of specific drinking reduction strategies, goal setting, problem solving, and relaxation training. N.J. engaged in daily monitoring of her alcohol use and incorporated several drinking reduction strategies each week. Specific drinking strategies included drinking more slowly, alternating nonalcoholic and alcoholic beverages, setting specific limits, preplanning drinking, and using self-talk and self-rewards. N.J. included her partner in setting weekly drinking goals concerning the number of abstinent days each week and the maximum number of standard drinks allowed in a day.

Relaxation training focused on deep breathing exercises and more extensive progressive muscle relaxation to help N.J. cope with panicky and anxious feelings. Problem-solving techniques were incorporated to assist with alcohol-related and general situations.

Contingency Plan.   N.J. stated at intake that she was interested only in reducing her drinking. As a result of the conjoint sessions, she agreed to work toward abstinence if the 2-month trial of drinking moderation training was nonproductive. To this end, a contingency plan for abstinence was developed by the therapist and N.J. to be put into use if N.J. or her partner felt that N.J.'s drinking continued to be problematic.

Outcome and Termination

N.J. first reduced drinking to no more than four beers per day with 2 abstinent days per week. By the end of the 2-month period, N.J. had reduced her drinking to no more than two beers on Friday and Saturday, and one beer on no more than 3 weekdays. During the 2-month trial, N.J. reported no slips or relapses.

Treatment culminated with several sessions on relapse prevention training. N.J. and the therapist (and her partner when present) discussed a variety of relapse prevention strategies. N.J. defined a "slip" as having five standard drinks in one day. She felt that her high-risk situations for a slip were periods of anxiety and frustration about her life (e.g., school, employment opportunities, relationship issues), and she had turned to alcohol in the past in response to such feelings. Techniques focusing on problem solving and relaxation were discussed to cope with these high-risk situations. In addition, N.J. made plans of how to cope with a slip should it occur, including contacting the clinic.

At the end of the course of treatment, N.J.'s outcome was judged as good. She had maintained several consecutive weeks of moderated drinking, and both N.J. and her partner were satisfied with the decrease in tension in their relationship regarding drinking. Three months of treatment, however, is a relative short period, and the therapist and N.J. contracted to maintain monthly and then bimonthly contact over the following 12 months.

Follow-Up and Maintenance

In the year following treatment, N.J. attended most of her scheduled follow-up appointments. Because N.J.'s drinking was no longer an issue, these sessions focused on other short- and long-term goals, including finishing an associate's degree, maintaining a good relationship with her partner, and finding employment in her new field. The therapist continued to encourage the use of problem-solving skills and relaxation techniques to help cope with several school and relationship difficulties. The therapist's role in these follow-up contacts was to help N.J. continue to improve her satisfaction with her life and help to provide methods of coping other than alcohol.

Summary

The assessment and treatment of psychoactive substance use disorders is a complex and often arduous process. There is great heterogeneity among persons presenting with substance use disorders, including variations in severity, symptoms, etiological factors, contributing factors, negative consequences experienced, and resources for treatment (including motivation). There is a range of interventions available for treating substance abusers. Selection of a particular treatment strategy or cluster of strategies will depend on the findings in a comprehensive assessment of the individual client. In addition, it often will be necessary to supplement these specific treatment strategies with other forms of intervention, such as vocational, recreational, financial, and educational counseling. Treatment effectiveness will be enhanced by an ongoing evaluation of the client's progress in treatment so that particular strategies are continually tailored to the current needs of the client and evaluated for their efficacy.

ACKNOWLEDGMENT.   Preparation of this manuscript was supported in part by Grant AA08076 from the National Institute on Alcohol Abuse and Alcoholism.

References

Agosti, V., Nunes, E., Stewart, J. W., & Quitkin, F. M. (1991). Patient factors related to early attrition from an outpatient cocaine research clinic: A preliminary report. *International Journal of the Addictions, 26,* 327–334.

American Psychiatric Association (1980). *Diagnostic and statistical manual of mental disorders* (3rd ed.). Washington, DC: Author.

American Psychiatric Association (1987). *Diagnostic and statistical manual of mental disorders* (3rd ed., rev.). Washington, DC: Author.

Azrin, N. H. (1976). Improvements in the community-reinforcement approach to alcoholism. *Behaviour Research and Therapy, 14,* 339–348.

Carroll, K. M., Rounsaville, B. J., & Keller, S. D. (1991). Relapse prevention strategies for the treatment of cocaine abuse. *American Journal of Drug and Alcohol Abuse, 17,* 249–265.

Collins, R. L. (1990). Family treatment of alcohol abuse: Behavioral and systems perspectives. In R. L. Collins, K. E. Leonard, & J. S. Searles (Eds.), *Alcohol and the family: Research and clinical perspectives* (pp. 285–308). New York: Guilford.

Corder, B. F., Corder, R. F., & Laidlaw, N. D. (1972). An intensive treatment program for alcoholics and their wives. *Quarterly Journal of Studies on Alcohol, 33,* 1144–1146.

Cotton, N. S. (1979). The familial incidence of alcoholism: A review. *Journal of Studies on Alcohol, 40,* 89–116.

Cronkite, R. C., & Moos, R. (1978). Evaluating alcoholism treatment programs: An integrated approach. *Journal of Consulting and Clinical Psychology, 46,* 1105–1119.

Glantz, M., & Pickens, R. (Eds.). (1992). *Vulnerability to drug abuse.* Washington, DC: American Psychological Association.

Goodwin, D. W. (1985). Alcoholism and genetics: The sins of the fathers. *Archives of General Psychiatry, 42,* 171–174.

Helzer, J. E., & Pryzbeck, T. R. (1988). The co-occurrence of alcoholism with other psychiatric disorders in the general population and its impact on treatment. *Journal of Studies on Alcohol, 49,* 219–224.

Hendriks, V. M., Steer, R. A., Platt, J. J., & Metzgar, D. S. (1990). Psychopathology in Dutch and American heroin addicts. *International Journal of the Addictions, 25,* 1051–1063.

Herz, L. R., Volicer, L., D'Angelo, N., & Gadish, D. (1990). Additional psychiatric illness by diagnostic interview schedule in male alcoholics. *Comprehensive Psychiatry, 30,* 72–79.

Hesselbrock, M. N., Meyer, R. E., & Keener, J. J. (1985). Psychopathology in hospitalized alcoholics. *Archives of General Psychiatry, 42,* 1050–1055.

Hilton, M. E. (1987). Drinking patterns and drinking problems in 1984: Results from a general population survey. *Alcoholism: Clinical and Experimental Research, 11,* 167–175.

Hunt, G. M., & Azrin, N. H. (1973). A community-reinforcement approach to alcoholism. *Behaviour Research and Therapy, 11,* 91–104.

Hunt, W. A., Barnett, L. W., & Branch, L. G. (1971). Relapse rates in addiction programs. *Journal of Clinical Psychology, 27,* 455–456.

Institute of Medicine (1990). *Treating drug problems* (Vol. 1). Washington, DC: National Academy Press.

Maisto, S. A., McKay, J. R., & Connors, G. J. (1990). Self-report issues in substance abuse: State of the art and future directions. *Behavioral Assessment, 12,* 117–134.

Marlatt, G. A., & Gordon, J. R. (Eds.). (1985). *Relapse prevention: Maintenance strategies in the treatment of addictive behaviors.* New York: Guilford.

McCrady, B. S. (1989a). Extending relapse prevention models to couples. *Addictive Behaviors, 14,* 69–74.

McCrady, B. S. (1989b). Outcomes of family-involved alcoholism treatment. In M. Galanter (Ed.), *Recent developments in alcoholism: Treatment research* (Vol. 7, pp. 165–182). New York: Plenum.

McCrady, B. S., Stout, R., Noel, N., Abrams, D., & Nelson, H. F. (1991). Effectiveness of three types of spouse-involved behavioral alcoholism treatment. *British Journal of Addiction, 86,* 1415–1424.

Miller, N. S., Gold, M. S., & Millman, R. B. (1989). The prevalence of alcohol dependence in cocaine dependence in an inpatient population. *Annals of Clinical Psychiatry, 1,* 93–97.

Miller, P. M. (1975). A behavioral intervention program for chronic public drunkenness offenders. *Archives of General Psychiatry, 32,* 915–918.

Miller, W. R., & Hester, R. K. (1980). Treating the problem drinker: Modern approaches. In W. R. Miller (Ed.), *The addictive behaviors: Treatment of alcoholism, drug abuse, smoking, and obesity* (pp. 11–141). New York: Pergamon.

Miller, W. R., & Munoz, R. F. (1982). *How to control your drinking* (rev. ed.). Albuquerque: University of New Mexico Press.

Miller, W. R., & Rollnick, S. (1991). *Motivational interviewing: Preparing people to change addictive behavior.* New York: Guilford.

Nathan, P. E. (1991). Substance use disorders in the DSM-IV. *Journal of Abnormal Psychology, 100,* 356–361.

National Institute on Drug Abuse (1988). *National household survey on drug abuse: Main findings, 1985.* Rockville, MD: Author.

Oei, T. P. S., & Jackson, P. R. (1980). Long-term effects of group and individual social skills training with alcoholics. *Addictive Behaviors, 5,* 129–136.

Oei, T. P., & Jackson, P. R. (1982). Social skills and cognitive behavioral approaches to the treatment of problem drinking. *Journal of Studies on Alcohol, 43,* 532–547.

O'Farrell, T. J., Cutter, H. S. G., Choquette, K. A., Floyd, F. J., & Bayog, R. D. (1992). Behavioral marital therapy for male alcoholics: Marital and drinking adjustment during the two years after treatment. *Behavior Therapy, 23,* 529–549.

O'Farrell, T. J., Cutter, H. S. G., & Floyd, J. J. (1985). Evaluating behavioral marital therapy for male alcoholics: Effects on marital adjustment and communication from before to after treatment. *Behavior Therapy, 16,* 147–167.

Ojehagen, A., Berglund, M., Appel, C.-P., Nilsson, B., & Skjaerris, A. (1991). Psychiatric symptoms in alcoholics attending outpatient treatment. *Alcoholism: Clinical and Experimental Research, 15,* 640–646.

O'Leary, D. E., O'Leary, M. R., & Donovan, D. M. (1976). Social skill acquisition and psychosocial development of alcoholics: A review. *Addictive Behaviors, 1,* 111–120.

Powell, B. J., Penick, E. C., Othmer, E., Bingham, S. F., & Rice, A. S. (1982). Prevalence of additional psychiatric syndromes among male alcoholics. *Journal of Clinical Psychiatry, 43,* 404–407.

Prochaska, J. O., DiClemente, C. C., & Norcross, J. C. (1992). In search of how people change: Applications to addictive behaviors. *American Psychologist, 47,* 1102–1114.

Regier, D. A., Farmer, M. E., Rae, D. S., Locke, B. Z., Keith, S. J., Judd, L. L., & Goodwin, F. K. (1990). Comorbidity of mental disorders with alcohol and other drug abuse. *Journal of the American Medical Association, 264,* 2511–2518.

Rohsenow, D. J., Monti, P. M., Binkoff, J. A., Liepman, M. R., & Nirenberg, T. D. (1991). Patient-treatment matching for alcoholic men in communication skills versus cognitive-behavioral mood management training. *Addictive Behaviors, 16,* 63–69.

Rosenberg, H. (1993). Prediction of controlled drinking by alcoholics and problem drinkers. *Psychological Bulletin, 113,* 129–139.

Sanchez-Craig, M., Annis, H. M., Bornet, A. R., & MacDonald, K. R. (1984). Random assignment to abstinence and controlled drinking: Evaluation of a cognitive-behavioral program for problem drinkers. *Journal of Consulting and Clinical Psychology, 52,* 390–403.

Sobell, L. C., & Sobell, M. B. (1990). Self-report issues in alcohol abuse: State of the art and future directions. *Behavioral Assessment, 12,* 77–90.

Sher, K. J. (1991). *Children of alcoholics: A critical appraisal of theory and research.* Chicago, IL: The University of Chicago Press.

Sternberg, D. (1991). Suicide in drug and alcohol addiction. In N. S. Miller (Ed.), *Comprehensive handbook of drug and alcohol addiction* (pp. 663–679). New York: Marcel Dekker.

4

Schizophrenia

Stewart A. Anderson, Petronilla Vaulx-Smith, and Matcheri S. Keshavan

Description of the Disorder

Clinical Features

Schizophrenia is a severe mental disorder characterized by disturbances of thought, perception, emotion, and behavior leading to considerable suffering and social deterioration. Widely believed to have multiple etiologies, schizophrenia is a syndrome with much variability in age at onset, symptomatology, course of illness, and response to treatment. Symptom development may be insidious or abrupt, with peak age at onset for males occurring in late adolescence or early adulthood. Females show a broader and later peak age at onset, with a second, smaller rise in new cases in the fourth decade.

A variety of criterion systems have been utilized to describe the constellation of mental and behavioral disturbances seen in schizophrenia. Schneider (1959) considered the following symptoms to be pathognomonic for schizophrenia in the absence of identifiable brain disease: passivity experiences, in which one's thoughts, feelings, or actions are perceived to be controlled by outside forces; auditory hallucinations of non-self voices anticipating, commenting upon, or repeating one's thoughts; audible thoughts and thought broadcasting, in which one's thoughts are perceived to be readable by others; and primary delusions, composed of false beliefs held with full conviction, arising de novo from normal perceptions and not shared by others from similar cultural backgrounds.

Subsequent research has shown that these "positive" symptoms are not uncommon in affective psychosis (Carpenter, Strauss, & Bartko, 1974) but are particularly

Stewart A. Anderson, **Petronilla Vaulx-Smith**, and **Matcheri S. Keshavan** • Department of Psychiatry, Western Psychiatric Institute and Clinic, Pittsburgh, Pennsylvania 15213.

Handbook of Prescriptive Treatments for Adults, edited by Michel Hersen and Robert T. Ammerman. Plenum Press, New York, 1994.

indicative of schizophrenia when present in conjunction with "negative" symptoms. Negative symptoms include poverty of speech and thought, flat affect, attention impairment, anhedonia, anergia, and social withdrawal. The diagnosis of schizophrenia, per the DSM-III-R (American Psychiatric Association, 1987) is based on the cross-sectional presence of both positive and negative symptoms, a duration of at least 6 months, evidence of deterioration, and absence of either organicity or a mood disturbance primary to the disorder.

Although both positive and negative features of schizophrenia are generally present simultaneously, they may fluctuate together or independently with respect to time and treatment. Accordingly, the clinical course varies considerably among individuals with schizophrenia. Such variability is thought to stem from: (a) the etiologic heterogeneity of the disorder; (b) the diverse effect of environmental factors on both symptom severity and the patient's willingness to engage in treatment; and (c) the apparent diagnostic overlap with psychotic variants of affective disorders, which have a different natural course.

Although cases of marked deterioration from exemplary functioning do occur, careful inspection reveals that disturbances of neurological maturation, cognition, emotional capacity, and social competency hinder the premorbid development of many, if not most, schizophrenic patients (Beitchman, 1985). After onset of symptoms meeting diagnostic criteria, most patients fluctuate between periods of relatively better or worse functioning, punctuated by psychotic relapse, as they regress from their pre-illness baseline. This pattern can be greatly ameliorated, but rarely cured, with antipsychotic medication. Eventually, the spectrum of symptoms often shifts from more positive to more negative, leading to the "burned out" presentation of those affected for many years.

Roughly 20 to 30% of patients with schizophrenia recover sufficiently to lead relatively normal lives, 20 to 30% continue to suffer from moderate symptoms, and 40 to 60% suffer severe, permanent impairment. Factors predicting a better outcome include good premorbid functioning, obvious precipitating factors, acute onset, later age at onset, and the relative predominance of affective, positive, or catatonic symptoms. Higher premorbid intelligence and well-preserved personality are also associated with a better prognosis. Women tend to have a better outcome than men. Schizophrenia in developing countries appears to have a less dismal prognosis.

In the 1950s and 1960s it was recognized that an understimulating hospital environment is associated with a worsening of negative symptoms (the so-called deficit state, or clinical poverty syndrome). On the other hand, an overstimulating environment can trigger relapse of psychotic symptoms. Vaughn and Leff (1976) have reported an association between levels of expressed emotion in the home and the likelihood of relapse. The treatment implications of this finding will be discussed later.

Associated Features

Depressive symptoms are common in schizophrenia, especially following complete or partial recovery from an acute psychotic episode. Approximately 50% of all schizophrenics attempt suicide, and about 10% succeed. Completed suicide is associated with coexistent depression, younger age, male sex, single status, unemployment, and poor response to treatment (Roy, 1986). It is most common soon after discharge from the hospital. Schizophrenics also have greater mortality from accidents and medical illnesses than is found in the general population.

Polydipsia is another common complication, particularly in patients with a longer duration of illness. In severe cases it can result in hyponatremia, delirium, seizures, and even death. Unfortunately, polydipsia responds poorly to antipsychotics, even when symptoms improve.

Epidemiology

Prevalence of schizophrenia is about 1% worldwide. Estimates vary, largely because of differing diagnostic criteria and the subjective nature of the criteria themselves. There appears to be no difference in lifetime prevalence between males and females.

Schizophrenia occurs more commonly in poorer economic classes, especially those inhabiting the inner city. This finding has been ascribed to the "downward drift" of affected individuals and their families (Dunham, 1965). Stressful surroundings and life events are associated with an increased risk of psychotic relapse, but stress appears to play no more than a modest role in the pathogenesis of the disorder.

Family, twin, and adoption studies have indicated that schizophrenia can be transmitted genetically. The offspring of an affected parent, regardless of whether raised by that parent, has roughly a 10% likelihood of developing the disorder. This risk rises to 30% when both parents are affected. Concordance among dizygotic and monozygotic twins is about 20% and 50%, respectively. Lack of perfect concordance in identical twins, and the fact that only about 15% of patients have a first- or second-degree relative with schizophrenia, indicates that the etiology of this illness is not solely genetic.

Etiology

Like its clinical picture, the etiology of schizophrenia appears to be heterogeneous. Many theories have been presented. Those involving the neurotransmitter dopamine have received the most attention, because of the discovery that the clinical potency of most antipsychotics correlates well with their ability to block the D2 dopamine receptor (Creese, Burt, & Snyder, 1975). However, antipsychotic efficacy is not limited to psychosis associated with schizophrenia, and specific pathology within the dopaminergic systems of untreated patients has not been consistently demonstrated. Glutamate neurotransmission (Javitt & Zukin, 1991), developmentally or virally induced structural abnormalities (Murray, O'Callaghan, Castle, & Lewis, 1992), and autoimmunity (Ganguli, Rabin, & Kelly, 1989) are some of the other putative sources of the neuropathology of this disorder. It is likely that discovery of etiologies for schizophrenia, at the molecular and neuronal levels, must await the deeper exploration of neuronal circuitry and its development in other primates and normal humans.

Differential Diagnosis and Assessment

DSM-III-R and DSM-IV Categorization

DSM-III-R provides criteria for making a diagnosis of schizophrenia. First, there must be psychotic symptoms lasting at least one week. These symptoms generally include hallucinations, delusions, or both, but the diagnosis can be made in their absence when severely disorganized thinking and a markedly flat or inappropriate affect are present. Second, there must have been a deterioration in the afflicted person's ability to work, socialize, and care for himself. Third, there must be no concurrent diagnosis of a mood disorder or of schizoaffective disorder, and no known organic cause of the psychotic symptoms. Fourth, some evidence of mental disturbance must have been present for at least 6 months (this requirement may be reduced to 1 month in DSM-IV).

Schizophrenia has been classified into a variety of subtypes throughout the years. The traditional classifications of subtypes presented here continues to be incorporated in DSM-III-R. *Catatonic Type* is characterized by marked psychomotor disturbance involving stupor, negativism, rigidity, excitement, and posturing. *Disorganized Type* is associated with marked loosening of associations, incoherence, grossly inappropriate affect, fragmented delusions, and hallucinations lacking a coherent theme. *Paranoid Type* is characterized by preoccupation with one or more systematized delusions or the presence of frequent hallucinations related to a single theme, in the absence of disorganized or catatonic features. *Undifferentiated Type* blends prominent psychotic symptoms that do not meet criteria for the other subtypes. *Residual Type* is diagnosed by the prior occurrence of at least one episode of schizophrenia with a current clinical picture of mild abnormalities without prominent psychotic symptoms.

Differential Diagnosis

Even with the relatively specific criteria for schizophrenia in DSM-III-R and DSM-IV, clinical practice does not always allow access to historical and collaborating information required to establish this diagnosis. Particularly in the absence of such information, a variety of illnesses, both psychiatric and medical, can present with recent-onset psychosis similar to that seen in new or relapsing cases of schizophrenia. In the acute setting, differentiating among psychiatric causes of psychosis is not necessarily crucial, because antipsychotic agents are likely to be part of the initial treatment in any case. For the long run, however, risk of serious and perhaps irreversible untoward effects associated with antipsychotics makes it imperative to correctly diagnose psychiatric conditions that may not require such agents to sustain remission.

Probably the most difficult psychiatric condition to distinguish from schizophrenia is bipolar disorder when it presents with hallucinations, disorganized thoughts, and bizarre behaviors. The diagnostic challenge is compounded in adolescents, who often present with a mixture of manic, depressive, and psychotic symptoms and may not begin the characteristic bipolar cycling until early adulthood. Werry, McClellan, and Chard (1991) found that about half of subjects diagnosed with bipolar disorder had been termed schizophrenic during adolescence. Factors associated with a persistent schizophrenia diagnosis included "odd personality, poor premorbid adaptive functioning, a history or evidence of major brain dysfunction, a family history of schizophrenia, insidious onset, psychosis lasting over three months, incomplete recovery and poor outcome." Patients who have had a complete recovery from a psychotic episode, particularly those with no negative symptoms, a family history of affective disorders, and good premorbid functioning, probably deserve a trial of lithium or other mood stabilizer followed by gradual withdrawal of antipsychotic agents. Some cases of bipolar disorder with psychotic features will continue to require antipsychotic medication to avoid relapse.

Other psychiatric conditions that must be differentiated from schizophrenia include major depression with psychotic features, personality disorders, and obsessive-compulsive disorder (OCD). The presence of prominent affective symptoms, such as sadness, guilt, and hopelessness in the case of depression; guilt, repulsion, and frustration in the case of OCD; and mood lability in the case of borderline personality, can be helpful in distinguishing these disorders from the classically flat or inappropriate affect of schizophrenics. A pattern of crises in adolescence that may be suggestive of the borderline personality is distinct from the withdrawn, peculiar premorbid behavior of many schizophrenics. Paranoid, schizoid, and schizotypal personalities, however, can resemble pre-schizophrenia and can be especially difficult to distinguish from schizophrenia occurring in patients who are highly guarded and not overtly psychotic. At these diagnostic borders, the treatment of clearly recognizable symptoms should take precedence over attempts to force symptomatology into current diagnostic schema.

A complete discussion of medical conditions that can produce schizophrenia-like symptoms is beyond the scope of this chapter and has been provided elsewhere (see Nasrallah, 1986). Many medications can produce psychotic symptoms. Common offenders include stimulants, medications with prominent anticholinergic effects such as tricyclic antidepressants, and glucocorticoids (see Keshavan & Keshavan, 1992). Psychosis persisting more than 2 weeks after the use of illicit drugs such as LSD, PCP, and amphetamines appears to be quite rare and may well represent true schizophrenia that was unmasked by the drug psychosis (Kane & Selzer, 1991). Toxic psychosis can also result from the chronic ingestion of lead (McCracken, 1987).

Schizophrenia-like states can be produced by systemic disorders (e.g., hyperthyroidism, hypothyroidism, pheochromocytoma), metabolic disturbances (hypercalcemia, hyponatremia), neurologic disorders (central nervous system infections, brain tumors, temporal lobe epilepsy, lupus cerebritis, multiple sclerosis), and genetic disorders (Wilson's disease, acute intermittent porphyria, Huntington's disease) (Nasrallah, 1986).

Assessment Strategies

The assessment of psychosis requires careful attention both to the quality of current symptoms and to their duration, variation, and influencing factors. It is vital to obtain corroborating history from family or friends whenever possible. Although they are rare, the potential reversibility of many "organic" causes of schizophrenia-like illnesses mandates that patients for whom a new diagnosis of schizophrenia is being entertained receive a thorough medical history taking and physical examination. Laboratory studies will vary depending on the history and physical findings, but all "first-episode" psychotic patients should probably receive brain imaging by computed tomographic scan or magnetic resonance imaging (which in addition to space-occupying lesions may also indicate cerebritis due to lupus or multiple sclerosis). Other routine studies include sleep-deprived EEG, complete blood count, electrolyte levels (including calcium), and thyroid function tests.

Treatment

The clinical management of schizophrenia involves the judicious use of antipsychotic medication to reduce acute symptoms, maintenance medication to sustain the period of recovery, and psychoeducation of both patient and family to ameliorate factors related to relapse. There also appears to be a role for supportive and cognitive behavioral psychotherapies for many patients. This section briefly reviews current approaches to the behavioral and pharmacological treatment of schizophrenia.

Behavior Therapy

The awareness that antipsychotic medications generally improve, but rarely eliminate, the symptoms of schizophrenia has encouraged continued efforts to develop psychosocial strategies to aid in the treatment of this disorder. Testing the efficacy of such strategies has proven methodologically difficult, particularly in controlling for compliance with the medication regimen and providing an adequate psychosocial placebo group. Despite these difficulties, data supporting the benefit of several psychosocial treatment approaches has been accumulating (see Schooler & Hogarty, 1987, for review).

Social skills training (SST) is one such approach. Patients participate in classes which use behavioral education aids, such as videotaping, modeling, role playing, and homework. SST has been shown to help some schizophrenic patients learn to interact more appropriately with their social environment (Wallace & Liberman, 1985), although many patients have difficulty generalizing their lessons and tend to regress after courses are completed.

Group therapy focusing on communication and coping skills may be a useful addition to SST and antipsychotic medication (Malm, 1982). Older, less psychotic, and higher functioning patients may also benefit from the social support obtainable in group therapy (Profita, Carrey, & Klein, 1989).

Family therapy also plays an important part in the treatment of schizophrenia. Goldstein, Rodrick, Evans, May, and Steinberg (1978) studied the effect of a 6-week course of therapy designed to help family members accept the presence of a psychotic illness, and to develop their ability to identify and cope with stressors. One hundred and four acutely ill schizophrenic inpatients were randomized and given high- or low-dosage antipsychotic medication, and presence or absence of the six-session therapy. Follow-up at completion of the course and 6 months later revealed less social withdrawal and fewer psychotic relapses in patients whose families had received the therapy, compared to a control group who received the same medications. Subjects who had received standard (25 mg) instead of low-dose (6.25 mg) prolixin decanoate injections every 2 weeks appeared best overall.

Combined SST and family therapy may further improve the schizophrenic patient's ability to function. Hogarty, Anderson, Reiss, Kornblith, and Greenwald (1986) gave 108 subjects either SST, psychoeducational family therapy, both, or neither, and found that the group who received both interventions had less tendency to relapse by the end of one year than those who received either treatment alone (see Anderson, Reiss, & Hogarty, 1986, for details on family psychoeducational workshops). All subjects were given long-acting antipsychotics to ensure compliance, but a control group of patients given neither psychosocial intervention fared worse overall (40% relapse versus about 20% of subjects who received one of the interventions, and none of those who received both psychosocial treatments).

Controlled studies on the efficacy of individual treatment modalities for schizophrenia have been few. Insight-oriented psychotherapy does not appear to be beneficial for most patients (Stanton et al., 1984). It may even have a detrimental effect by pressuring the patient's psychological defenses against his or her biologically driven psychosis.

Recently, efforts have been made to use cognitive behavioral therapy (CBT) in the attempt to (a) help patients differentiate between reality and psychosis, (b) help them identify and avoid aspects of their subjective and objective environment that exacerbate their psychotic thinking, and (c) teach them to steer their attention toward the reality aspect of their moment-to-moment experience. In addition to case reports claiming the utility of cognitive-behavioral approaches in the treatment of schizophrenic delusions (Alford, 1986; Allen & Bass, 1992), Kingdon and Turkington (1992) report that CBT allowed significant reductions in antipsychotic dosage in a series of 64 patients. Despite these reports, efficacy of CBT in schizophrenia will not be established until studies using standardized medication regimens, and non-CBT supportive psychotherapy control groups, have been completed.

As a whole, the studies just discussed suggest that psychosocial interventions can be helpful adjuncts to antipsychotic medication in improving the quality of life and forestalling relapse in the schizophrenic patient. Given the variable presentations of this disorder, it remains to be established which psychosocial treatments will be most beneficial to a particular patient. Individual characteristics such as gender, intelligence, and level of sociality play an important but as yet undetermined role (Schooler & Hogarty, 1987).

Characteristics of the family or social group with which the schizophrenic patient resides also appear to affect illness course. Households that tend to be high in expressed emotion (i.e., argumentative, loud, overinvolved, and highly critical) may dispose the patient to earlier relapse (Vaughn & Leff, 1976), and poorer social adjustment (Hogarty et al., 1988). Psychoeducational approaches designed to reduce the levels of expressed emotion (EE) in families have been shown to decrease relapse rates (Leff, Kuipers, Berkowitz, & Sturgeon, 1985), particularly for young males living with high EE parents (Hogarty et al., 1986).

Thus, while antipsychotic medications remain the mainstay of treatment for schizophrenia, psychosocial interventions can be of considerable benefit to many of those affected. Such interventions include: (a) individual therapy to provide support for, and monitoring of, day-to-day functioning (CBT may also be helpful for some higher-functioning patients); (b) group therapy to provide support, social skills training, and illness education; and (c) family therapy to address blame, teach coping strategies (e.g., avoid arguing against their loved one's delusional thinking), and, when appropriate, decrease levels of EE.

Pharmacotherapy

Evidence has been accumulating for over 30 years that antipsychotic medication, sometimes referred to as "neuroleptics" because of their propensity for causing neurologic side effects, are helpful in the treatment of schizophrenia. They have been shown to reduce symptoms of acute exacerbations (Cole, 1964), shorten hospital stay (May, Tuma, Yale, Potepan, & Dixon, 1976), and decrease rate of relapse (Davis, 1975). More recently it has been suggested that, either by their direct effects or by reducing the intensity and duration of psychotic episodes, antipsychotics positively influence the chronic course of schizophrenia (Crow, MacMillan, Johnson, & Johnstone, 1986; Wyatt, 1991).

Table 4.1 shows commonly used antipsychotic medications. Therapeutically equivalent doses are generally estimated from studies comparing two or more drugs in which doses are blindly titrated to clinical effectiveness. Potencies are often described relative to chlorpromazine (CPZ). For example, haloperidol and CPZ have relative values of 2 and 100, respectively. Five milligrams of haloperidol is therefore estimated to have therapeutic efficacy similar to that of 250 mg of CPZ, or 250 "CPZ equivalents." Methodological difficulties of the studies behind such comparisons are many, but the CPZ equivalent concept remains central to efforts to determine minimum dosage requirements (Kane, 1989).

Problems in Carrying Out Interventions: Side Effects. Clinical potency differentiates the tendency of neuroleptics to cause certain side effects. Low-potency agents generally produce more antiadrenergic (e.g., hypotension) and anticholinergic (e.g., sedation, dry mouth, blurred vision) effects. High-potency antipsychotics more frequently result in extrapyramidal symptoms.

Dystonia. Dystonia refers to sustained muscular spasms that are frightening, painful, and occasionally even life threatening when the pharyngeal musculature is involved. The spasms usually occur while drug levels are in rising and can be quickly reversed with intramuscular or intravenous introduction of anticholinergic medications, such as benztropine or diphenhydramine. Young males appear to be at greatest risk. As might be expected, the experience of an acute dystonia can negatively affect a patient's future compliance (Van Putten, 1974), leading some clinicians to prophylac-

TABLE 4.1. Selected Antipsychotic Drugs[a]

Drug: Generic (trade name)	Class	CPZ equivalent,[b] oral dose	Side effects			
			Extra-pyramidal symptoms	Sedation	Hypotension	Anticho-linergic action
Clozapine (Clozaril)	Dibenzoxazepine	160	X	XXX	XXX	XXX
Chlorpromazine (Thorazine)	Phenothiazine (aliphatic)	100	X	XXX	XXX	XX
Thioridazine (Mellaril)	Phenothiazine (piperidine)	100	X	XXX	XXX	XXX
Loxapine[c] (Loxitane)	Dibenzoxazepine	15	XX	XX	XX	XX
Perphenazine (Trilafon)	Phenothiazine (piperazine)	10	XX	XX	X	X
Trifluoroperazine (Stelazine)	Phenothiazine (piperazine)	5	XXX	X	X	X
Thiothixene (Navane)	Thioxanthene	5	XXX	X	X	X
Fluphenazine (Prolixin)	Phenothiazine (piperazine)	2	XXX	X	X	X
Haloperidol (Haldol)	Butyrophenone	2	XXX	X	X	X

[a]For further details see: Teicher and Glod (1991) and Baldessarini (1990).
[b]Estimates for therapeutically equivalent doses/vary considerably among sources.
[c]Not approved for use under age 16.
CPZ = chlorpromazine.

tically medicate certain patients with anticholinergics, especially those with a previous history of this reaction.

Akathisia. This syndrome of subjective and objective restlessness occurs frequently during treatment with neuroleptics. Symptoms range from a subjective urge to move in an otherwise relaxed appearing patient to pacing, rocking, or other behaviors that reflect severe discomfort associated with remaining motionless. Timing of onset varies but often coincides with the first or second week of steady-state plasma levels. Akathisia can be quite difficult to diagnose, particularly when it coexists with, and probably exacerbates, agitation and anxiety associated with psychosis, incarceration, or both. Anticholinergic medications, benzodiazepines, and beta-adrenergic blockers can be helpful in reducing akathisia. Next to lowering the dosage of the neuroleptic, propanolol administration may present the best risk/benefit profile of these options (Adler et al., 1986).

Parkinsonism. The cardinal features of this syndrome include muscular rigidity, masked facies, tremors, and bradykinesia (slowness of movement). It can develop from days to months into treatment. Although cogwheel rigidity is easy to identify, more subtle parkinsonian-like extrapyramidal symptoms (EPS) can be difficult to diagnose. Bradykinesia can be mistaken for improvement in the previously agitated patient who slows down and becomes easier to manage (Van Putten, Marder, & Mintz, 1990). After acute psychotic symptoms have subsided, psychomotor retardation and blunted affect can be misdiagnosed as postpsychotic depression (Becker, 1988). Antiparkinsonian medications, such as benztropine, biperiden, or amantadine, are effective in reducing this form of EPS. Because, with the exception of amantadine (which can exacerbate psychosis), these agents produce disturbing anticholinergic side effects, they are most useful during the acute phase of treatment and should probably be avoided after several months. Dosage reduction remains the mainstay of treatment for long-term EPS (Kane & Lieberman, 1987).

Tardive Dyskinesia. Tardive dyskinesia (TD) is a potentially debilitating problem caused by chronic exposure to neuroleptics. In young adults, one study has estimated that over the first 5 years of treatment about 4% of patients per year will develop the repetitive, involuntary lip, jaw, and tongue movements characteristic of TD (Kane et al., 1984). In addition to years of treatment, advancing age is also a risk factor (Baldessarini, 1990), although children and adolescents are susceptible (Campbell, Green, & Deutch, 1985). Anticholinergic medications tend to exacerbate symptoms, whereas increasing the dosage of neuroleptic may, paradoxically, suppress them. Although decreasing or withdrawing neuroleptics may initially "unmask" TD, it is the only established treatment. Symptoms may improve very slowly or occasionally not at all. As with EPS, the occurrence of TD highlights the necessity of employing the minimum effective antipsychotic dosage.

Other Side Effects. The neuroleptic malignant syndrome, characterized by severe rigidity, autonomic dysfunction, and delirium, is a rare, potentially fatal side effect that usually develops within 2 weeks of neuroleptic initiation or increase. Treatment involves supportive care and possibly the administration of dantrolene or bromocriptine (Baldessarini, 1990). Other side effects of neuroleptic drugs include leukopenia, hepatitis, and seizures.

With the exception of the "atypical" agent clozapine, the antipsychotics available at the time of this writing, regardless of their potency, appear to have an equal likelihood of causing TD and neuroleptic malignant syndrome. It is hoped that a new generation of more selective antipsychotics will be clinically effective without producing the uncomfortable, problematic, or even devastating side effects of current neuroleptics.

Guidelines for Acute Management

Apart from the limited data suggesting that schizophrenic adolescents, because of their sensitivity to sedation, may better tolerate high-potency neuroleptics (Realmuto, Erickson, Yellin, Hopwood, & Greenberg, 1984), no evidence favors the initial use of one antipsychotic over any other. However, data supporting several guiding principles to neuroleptic use have been accumulating.

1. There appears to be no advantage to a high-dosage, "rapid neuroleptization" approach. Rifkin, Seshagiri, Basawaraj, Borenstein, and Wachpress (1991) studied 87 newly admitted schizophrenic patients who were randomized to receive 10, 30, or 80 mg of haloperidol orally per day and treated for 6 weeks in a double-blind trial. Substantial improvement was noted in all three groups, but no additional benefit was found for those receiving more than 10 mg per day.

2. Significant overlap exists between the therapeutic and untoward effects of a neuroleptic. Van Putten et al. (1990) compared 80 newly hospitalized schizophrenic males randomized to a 4-week trial of 5, 10, or 20 mg of haloperidol daily. Only those patients (28%) with a history of severe dystonic reactions were premedicated with benztropine. As a group, those who received the 20 mg dose improved more quickly, and those who continued to tolerate the higher dose showed greatest improvement throughout the trial. However, this group also scored significantly worse on ratings of blunted affect, social withdrawal, akathisia, and akinesia. In addition, they had a far greater rate of leaving the hospital against medical advice (35% versus only 4% of the subjects receiving 5 or 10 mg). This study highlights the importance of paying close attention to the concurrent development of symptomatic improvement and side effects, and suggests that an individualized, flexible approach to dosing will be most beneficial to the patient.

3. The majority of studies suggest that most acutely ill schizophrenic patients will obtain maximal antipsychotic benefit when receiving between 300 and 700 CPZ equivalents per day (Baldessarini, Cohen, & Teicher, 1988). One recent study has reported that many patients will respond to lower doses given adequate trial length (McEvoy, Hogarty, & Steingard, 1991). One hundred and six acutely ill schizophrenic or schizoaffective inpatients were placed on the minimum dose of haloperidol that produced stiffness or cogwheel rigidity. After two weeks the 95 remaining patients were randomized to either continue their "neuroleptic threshold" dose (averaging 3.4 mg) or to receive a larger dose (averaging 11.6 mg). Double-blind ratings of patient conditions after 4 weeks of treatment at the neuroleptic threshold showed that 72% of the subjects had responded. By comparison, the larger dose group had greater improvement on measures of hostility, but not psychosis, and experienced significantly worse side effects. This study suggests that many patients may be treatable at a substantially smaller dose than is commonly employed, and recommends a systematic approach for establishing this dose.

4. There is no clear evidence that certain symptoms of schizophrenia respond

better to specific antipsychotics. This point becomes particularly relevant with the highly agitated patient, with whom there may be a temptation to utilize a low-potency neuroleptic, or akinesia-inducing doses of high-potency drugs, for combined antipsychotic and sedative purposes. In such cases the side effects will remain after an antipsychotic effect has been achieved, placing the clinician in the uncomfortable position of backing away from a proven effective dose. An alternative is to use benzodiazepines, which have been shown to be useful in treating agitation associated with psychosis (Salzman, 1989), to temporarily sedate the patient while an antipsychotic response to a standard dose is awaited.

5. Given an adequate dose, at least 4 to 6 weeks is necessary to establish the efficacy of an antipsychotic trial (Rifkin & Siris, 1987). Despite pressures from family, hospital administration, and other sources, raising the neuroleptic dosage to unusually high levels (i.e., above 700 CPZ equivalents), changing neuroleptics, or adding adjunctive medications prior to a several week trial is unwarranted.

Long-Acting Injectable Antipsychotics. Both fluphenazine and haloperidol are available in the United States in decanoate preparations, allowing intramuscular administration on a weekly to monthly basis. In addition to assuring compliance, parenterally administered neuroleptics seem to produce fewer EPS at effective doses than do the same drugs taken orally (Deberdt et al., 1980). The half-life of haloperidol decanoate appears to be approximately 3 weeks, allowing monthly injections to maintain adequate plasma levels. Because steady state will not be achieved for at least 3 months, oral doses should be initially maintained and then gradually tapered over this period. A more rapid but risky method for reaching steady state is to load patients by, for example, giving half the expected monthly dose in two divided doses one week apart followed 2 weeks later by monthly dosing.

Fluphenazine decanoate (Flu-D) has been thought to have roughly a 10-day half life, allowing injections every 2 weeks (Jann, Ereshefsky, & Saklad, 1985), although a recent estimation based on a more sensitive assay technique suggest that the half life of Flu-D may actually exceed one month (Simpson et al., 1990). Therefore, patients receiving Flu-D should be carefully monitored for signs of rising neuroleptic levels several months into the trial.

Formulas for converting patients from oral to decanoate preparations vary, but most patients can be maintained on 5 to 25 mg prolixin decanoate every 2 weeks (Yadalam & Simpson, 1988). Haloperidol requires higher dosages, generally between 100 and 200 mg monthly, or 10 to 20 times the oral dose (Jann et al., 1985; Nayak, Doose, & Nair, 1987).

Drug Interactions with Antipsychotics. A variety of medications and substances can affect dosage requirements of neuroleptics. Haloperidol has been best studied, because of fairly reliable detection capabilities and the lack of known active metabolites for this drug. Cigarette smoking and carbamazepine can significantly lower haloperidol levels, whereas buspirone and fluoxetine can raise them (see Goff & Baldessarini, 1993, for a recent review).

Alternative Treatments

Approximately 70% of adult schizophrenics respond adequately to antipsychotics. When symptoms do not improve with standard regimens, prior to considering alternative treatments one should consider several points. First, the agitated or anxious-appearing patient may be suffering from akathisia and thus may improve with a reduced dosage or addition of propanolol. For partially treated or moderately symptomatic patients, the best approach may simply be to continue treatment, since some individuals require 6 weeks or even longer to respond fully (McEvoy et al., 1991). Occasionally, when no EPS are present despite routine dosage (up to 700 CPZ equivalents), serum drug levels might be determined to help identify "rapid metabolizers" who require unusually high antipsychotic doses (Baldessarini et al., 1988). Increasing the haloperidol dosage of nonresponders after 3 weeks at the "neuroleptic threshold" dosage did not produce additional improvement at 5 weeks (relative to those who remained at the lower level), and resulted in significantly increased side effects, in the only controlled study of this issue (McEvoy et al., 1991).

Once a given antipsychotic has proven ineffective, clinicians often begin by switching to a different chemical class, although there are few data to support this approach. Adjunctive therapy with non-neuroleptic medication is frequently tried next. A recent review found that lithium, carbamazepine, reserpine, benzodiazepines, and propanolol have been shown in double-blind trials to have some efficacy as adjunctive agents (Christison, Kirch, & Wyatt, 1991). Because lithium has been by far the best studied, and bipolar disorder with psychotic features can sometimes be difficult to distinguish from schizophrenia, lithium should probably be added first.

Clozapine, considered "atypical" because its side effects and neurochemistry differ from those of other antipsychotics, appears to help at least 30% of patients who did not improve with trials of other agents (Lieberman, Kane, & Johns, 1989). Clozapine has the added advantage of producing no EPS and little or no TD (Kane, 1989). Agranulocytosis, which can be fatal if unrecognized, occurs in about 1.3% of adults who receive this compound but is reversible upon discontinuation of the drug. Although it usually develops 6 weeks to 6 months into treatment, agranulocytosis has been reported over 1 year later, necessitating weekly blood counts for the duration of treatment (Lieberman et al., 1989). Sedation, hypotension, and increased salivation are other side effects of clozapine. Despite these problems, clozapine's potential for improving otherwise refractory symptoms makes it an important option in the treatment of schizophrenia, particularly when at least two classes of conventional neuroleptics, and adjunctive lithium therapy, have proven ineffective.

Unfortunately, some patients remain severely symptomatic despite all mentioned pharmacological interventions, and others are unable to tolerate the side effects of antipsychotics. There are also occasions when the severity of behavioral disturbances associated with schizophrenia necessitates life-saving interventions sooner than an antipsychotic medication response can be expected. In such cases electroconvulsive therapy can be an effective treatment for acute exacerbations of schizophrenia.

Relapse Prevention

Continuing pharmacotherapy for schizophrenia after maximal reduction of acute symptoms has been achieved reduces the likelihood of relapse (Davis, 1975). One review of studies in which patients in the maintenance phase of treatment were given depot neuroleptics found that 0 to 40% of medicated patients relapsed within 1 year, compared to 30 to 80% of those receiving placebo (Kane & Lieberman, 1987). However, despite the proven efficacy of maintenance medication, it appears that even with appropriate pharmacotherapy most patients will relapse within 2 to 3 years

(Crow et al., 1986; Hogarty et al., 1988). At the same time, the potential drawbacks of long-term neuroleptic administration, such as chronic EPS and TD, are well recognized.

Given the substantial risks and important, but noncurative, benefits of these drugs, efforts have been made to establish the minimum effective dose for maintenance pharmacotherapy (see Schooler, 1991, for review). Not surprisingly, studies have demonstrated a risk/benefit trade-off. Low dosages are associated with higher relapse rates than standard dosages (i.e., 5 mg versus 20 mg of Flu-D every 2 weeks) but result in measurably better psychosocial functioning between symptom exacerbations (Kane et al., 1987; Hogarty et al., 1988). Furthermore, patients who begin to relapse on low dosages can in many cases be stabilized without hospitalization by temporarily increasing their medication.

An alternate strategy to reduce the cumulative neuroleptic exposure involves withdrawing neuroleptics several months after symptoms have improved, then targeting the readministration of pharmacotherapy to the earliest signs of relapse (Carpenter et al., 1990). Whereas some patients may benefit from targeted treatment, the increased risk of serious relapse with this method makes it less appropriate for most patients (Schooler, 1991).

In summary, maintenance pharmacotherapy for schizophrenia, like that of acute exacerbations, requires flexible, individualized attention both to its benefits and to its limitations.

Psychopharmacological Education of Patient and Family

The pharmacological treatment of schizophrenia involves both the appropriate use of antipsychotics and the development of a working relationship with the patient and his or her family. Ideally, both should be trained to recognize the symptom and side effect trends pertinent to the given stage of illness and treatment. Initial discussions of EPS, TD, and other common side effects are necessary to obtain informed consent, but time lag before response (2 to 4 weeks), risk of nonresponse (roughly 30%), and likelihood of eventual relapse should also be discussed. During the relatively symptom-free maintenance phase, the patient and family should understand the relationship between antipsychotic dosage, the potential for symptom recurrence, and the appearance of side effects. Prior to the reemergence of clinically apparent psychosis, many patients experience mood and behavioral changes noticeable to themselves and their families (Herz & Melville, 1980). By enlisting their help in recognizing prodromal states, the clinician can attempt to intervene with pharmacological or psychosocial adjustments, or both, before more damaging symptoms have become apparent or inevitable.

Compliance with medication regimens frequently becomes a major issue during maintenance treatment. Seeing the patient alone, while having frequent contact with concerned others, can help develop a therapeutic alliance in which family members feel involved while the affected individual feels appropriately empowered. When relapse does occur, it is important for both the clinician and the family to avoid blaming the noncompliant patient. Relapse frequently occurs despite assured compliance with depot administration (Schooler & Hogarty, 1987), and noncompliance itself may be a result rather than a cause of recurring illness (Schooler, 1991).

One goal of the therapeutic alliance is for the patient to trust his or her clinician to the point where an intention to stop medications can be openly explored. The patient then needs to know that although he or she may experience higher baseline symptoms, and is more vulnerable to serious relapse, symptoms may not recur for many months after antipsychotics have been discontinued. Allowing the patient to participate openly in treatment decisions can also improve his or her willingness to participate in follow-up visits and psychosocial interventions whether or not medication is being used.

Case Illustration

Case Description

R.T., a 19-year-old man, was forcibly brought to the psychiatric emergency room after an altercation at home. His parents had called the police after he responded with verbal abuse, screaming, and throwing furniture to their repeated attempts to enter his room. They reported that R.T. had gradually become more isolative and bizarre since shortly before graduation from high school, some 8 months previously. In the month prior to hospitalization he was noticed frequently to be awake all night, pacing in his room and listening to stereo headphones at loud volume. He became religiously preoccupied, decorating his increasingly disorganized and unclean room with crudely painted or constructed crosses. One evening during dinner he screamed, "Can't you hear them?" and thereafter ate alone between family meals. Efforts to bring him to the family physician were unsuccessful.

R.T. had no prior history of mental illness. He was the third of four children and had had no known birth complications, developmental delays, serious illnesses, or injuries. In school he tended to receive average marks. Socially, he was described as shy and quiet, but he had maintained a few friends throughout childhood. He had not started dating previous to onset of symptoms. Family history was noncontributory.

Mental status examination at initial presentation revealed an unkempt, guarded, frightened, and at times explosive young man. He was fully oriented and hypervigilant, and had a limited attention span. Speech was clear but tended to be both loose and tangential, so that only rarely were his responses perceptibly related to the questions. He seemed to believe he was "at the vortex of the final battle" between good and evil, and admitted to hearing the commands of both sides, speaking to him as well as to each other, on a virtually continuous basis.

The initial interview was concluded when R.T. became assaultive. He was sedated with 5 mg of droperidol administered intramuscularly and was admitted involuntarily to the hospital.

Differential Diagnosis and Assessment

Differential diagnosis included schizophreniform disorder, bipolar disorder with psychotic features, and any of the many identifiably organic causes of psychosis. The history of a gradual onset from a somewhat withdrawn baseline, an illness duration of less than 6 months, the lack of racing thoughts, pressured speech, or prominent affective symptoms, and normal findings in a medical workup that included drug screen, blood count, electrolyte levels, thyroid function tests, EEG, and magnetic resonance imaging, suggested schizophreniform disorder.

R.T. initially required frequent seclusion for assaultive behavior. Lorezepam, eventually 2 mg by mouth or intramuscularly every 6 hours as needed, lessened his agitation and anxiety. On hospital day five R.T., with the urging of his family, agreed to a trial of haloperidol. The initial dosage was 2 mg orally at bedtime, and this was gradually raised to 6 mg over the ensuing week. At this dosage R.T. developed a moderate amount of cogwheel rigidity, which was treated with benztropine, 1 mg twice daily (Figure 4.1).

Treatment Selection

With the exception of clozapine for treatment-resistant cases, there is no evidence that any one antipsychotic is more efficacious than any other. Choice of drug depends on the patient's medication history, the clinician's experience, and the patient's individual needs (i.e., low-potency neuroleptics might be avoided in patients sensitive to sedation or hypotension). We prefer to begin treatment with high-potency neuroleptics, titrating the dosage to onset of EPS, while treating agitation with benzodiazepines as needed. One advantage of haloperidol is the ability to obtain fairly reliable drug levels, which can be helpful when either noncompliance, or non-response at relatively high dosages, is at issue. Both haloperidol and fluphenazine, another high-potency neuroleptic, are available in long-acting injectable preparations which can aid in outpatient compliance.

In addition to medications, R.T. received individual and group therapy. Efforts were made to inform him about the medication's therapeutic and untoward effects (including tardive dyskinesia), to help him cope with symptoms, and to develop insight about the medical nature of his difficulties. Initial family sessions focused on the same topics, and on defusing parental guilt.

Approximately 10 days after reaching a dosage of 6 mg of haloperidol, R.T. began

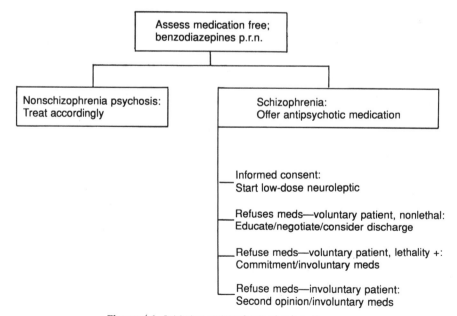

Figure 4.1. Initiating antipsychotic pharmacotherapy.

to report that the voices seemed more distant and less disturbing than usual. However, even as his psychotic symptoms abated, he began to appear more restless, pacing about the unit and tolerating groups less well than the week before. A regimen of propranolol, 10 mg three times daily, was begun. His behavior improved and complaints of nervousness lessened (Figure 4.2).

Treatment Course and Problems in Carrying Out Interventions

The antipsychotic effect of medications generally requires 2 to 4 weeks to develop. Once a therapeutic range (400 to 700 CPZ equivalents) or minimal rigidity (implying adequate blood levels) has been achieved, there are few indications for changing the antipsychotic regimen prior to several weeks into treatment. Extremely violent patients, or those who develop severe side effects, are exceptions.

Akathisia may occur days or weeks after steady-state blood levels have been reached. Lowering the neuroleptic dose, changing to a lower-potency drug, as well as the use of beta-blockers, anticholinergics, and benzodiazepines, can be effective treatments. Failure to recognize and address this highly uncomfortable condition promptly can lead to patient agitation, noncompliance, and requests to leave the hospital against medical advice.

Outcome and Termination

R.T. was discharged 27 days after admission. At that time he denied auditory hallucinations and was reasonably calm but continued to be religiously preoccupied. Discharge medications included haloperidol, 6 mg nightly; propanolol, 20 mg twice daily; and benztropine (Cogentin), 1 mg twice daily. In addition to seeing a nurse-therapist weekly, and a psychiatrist monthly, he was encouraged to attend a day

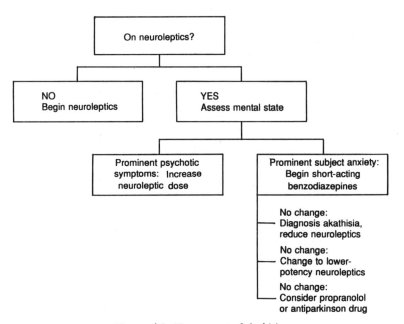

Figure 4.2. Management of akathisia.

treatment program with an educational, social skills emphasis. His parents attended several sessions of a family workshop designed to educate families about the outpatient aspects of schizophrenia, such as the possible prodromal signs of relapse and the importance of adjusting their long-term expectations.

After several weeks of clinical improvement, R.T.'s benztropine dose was adjusted to 0.5 mg twice daily. The return of significant rigidity prompted a decrease of his haloperidol dose to 4 mg. Over the next month benztropine and propanolol were discontinued, leaving a slightly detectable level of rigidity and no visible signs of akathisia.

Follow-Up and Maintenance

The goal of the maintenance phase of pharmacotherapy for schizophrenia is to find the lowest effective antipsychotic dose. Initially, this requires lowering the dose to the level of minimal side effects, preferably discontinuing anticholinergic medications—such as benzotripine, which has its own problematic side effects.

Several months into the maintenance phase of treatment, R.T. stopped attending outpatient appointments and discontinued his haloperidol, saying he did not need "doctors or drugs" and that he desired "to get on with my life." He returned to work in a local fast food restaurant. Approximately 6 months later he was again brought to the hospital by his parents. His condition was similar to that on his first admission, except that he was hospitalized voluntarily in a less agitated state. Psychotic symptoms again responded to 6 mg of haloperidol daily, permitting discharge after several weeks. However, R.T. became withdrawn, apathetic, and complained to his therapist, "It feels like I'm dead." He was treated with benztropine, 2 mg twice daily, which resulted in some improvement in his apparent listlessness. Unfortunately, he had to be readmitted soon after discharge, following a suicide attempt by an overdose of haloperidol, benztropine, and acetaminophen.

Management of Apathy. The differential diagnosis of flattened affect, apathy, and decreased movements in a schizophrenic patient receiving neuroleptic medication includes: (a) akinesis, an extrapyramidal symptom that usually responds to anticholinergic medication or to reduction in the dosage of neuroleptic; (b) depression, which may respond to antidepressant medication; and (c) negative symptoms, which can be treatment resistant but may respond on increase in the dosage of antipsychotic medication or the addition of a serotonin reuptake inhibitor (Figure 4.3).

In this case the problem appeared to be a combination of akinesia and postpsychotic depression. Closer attention to R.T.'s perception of his illness may have revealed the anguish he was experiencing in coming to terms with the chronicity of his disability.

R.T. recovered from his overdose and was treated for depression with fluoxetine, 20 mg daily. Because of compliance problems he was converted from 6 mg of haloperidol by mouth to 75 mg of haloperidol decanoate, administered monthly. Oral doses were continued for 3 months, then tapered over 1 month, with no recurrence of psychotic symptoms. Fluoxetine was eventually discontinued because of patient noncompliance and the improvement of depressive symptoms.

For the next 4 years R.T. was maintained on haloperidol decanoate. He was able to work part-time, had only one hospitalization (precipitated largely by his father's coronary bypass surgery), but continued to have limited socialization. Gradually, despite compliance with appointments and adequate medication blood levels, R.T. again began to deteriorate. He became more paranoid, isolative, and preoccupied with the forces of evil affecting both personal and global circumstances.

Management of Treatment Resistance. Unfortunately, it is not unusual for schizophrenic patients to develop treatment resistance after years of acceptable response to antipsychotics. Once the maintenance medication has become ineffective or intolerable at maintenance and upwardly adjusted doses, there remain several options for pharmacotherapy, including changing the class of antipsychotic, adding a mood stabilizing "adjunctive" agent, or changing to the atypical antipsychotic clozapine (Figure 4.4).

R.T. was placed on 25 mg of fluphenazine decanoate every 2 weeks, which resulted in modest improvement. The addition of lithium carbonate, 900 mg nightly, further reduced R.T.'s paranoia and subjective distress.

Management of Tardive Dyskinesia. Within several years R.T. suffered the gradual onset of involuntary and generally unnoticed tongue movements. These worsened over 6 months until his tongue extruded from his mouth every few seconds. Decreasing the dose of fluphenazine to 12.5 mg initially resulted in worsened tongue movements, which several months later began to slowly improve (Figure 4.5). At the same time, R.T. suffered a recurrence of psychotic symptoms. He was placed on clozapine, eventually 450 mg daily in divided doses, which lessened his psychosis and mildly reduced his tardive dyskinesia. After 2 years on clozapine, R.T. has had problems with oversedation and urinary retention, and some difficulties with compliance. He has, however, remained out of the hospital.

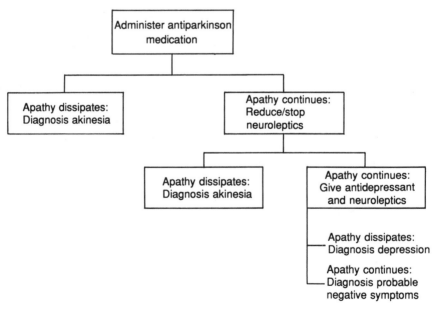

Figure 4.3. Management of apathy.

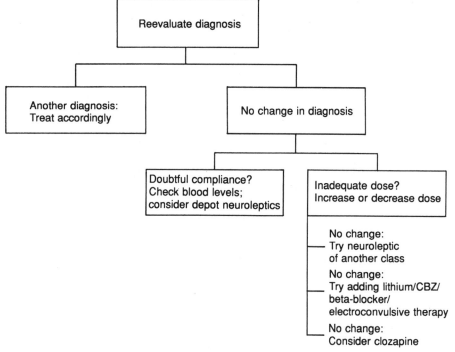

Figure 4.4. Management of treatment resistance.

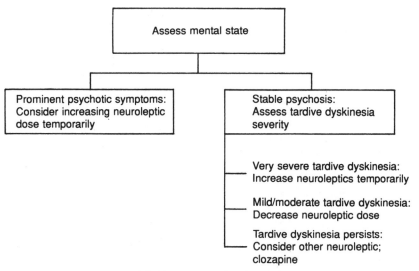

Figure 4.5. Management of tardive dyskinesia.

Summary

Schizophrenia is a severe mental disorder characterized by psychotic symptoms, deterioration in functioning, and considerable residual impairment in most cases. Depression and suicide are frequently associated. The best available treatment involves several modalities: individual therapy, utilizing supportive and cognitive-behavioral approaches to help the patient live with the illness, family psychoeducation to inform them about schizophrenia and teach them ways to minimize stressors at home, and pharmacotherapy with the minimum effective antipsychotic dosage.

Continued research is likely to result in safer and more effective antipsychotic medications, in addition to improving our understanding of etiological factors and thereby helping to prevent this highly debilitating mental illness.

References

Adler, L., Angrist, B., Peselow, E., Corwin, J., Maslansky, R., & Rotrosen, J. (1986). A controlled assessment of propranolol in the treatment of neuroleptic-induced akathisia. *British Journal of Psychiatry, 149*, 42–45.

Alford, G. (1986). Behavioral treatment of schizophrenic delusions: A single-case experimental analysis. *Behavior Therapy, 17*(5), 636–644.

Allen, H., & Bass, C. (1992). Coping tactics and the management of acutely distressed schizophrenic patients. *Behavioral Psychotherapy, 20*(1), 61–72.

American Psychiatric Association (1987). *Diagnostic and statistical manual of mental disorders* (3rd ed., rev.). Washington, DC: Author.

Anderson, C. M., Reiss, D. J., & Hogarty, G. E. (1986). *Schizophrenia in the family*. New York: Guilford.

Baldessarini, R. (1990). Drugs and the treatment of psychiatric disorders. In G. A. Gilman, T. W. Roll, A. S. Nies, & T. Palmer (Eds.), *The pharmacological basis of therapeutics* (pp. 383–435). New York: Pergamon.

Baldessarini, R. J., Cohen, B. M., & Teicher, M. H. (1988). Significance of neuroleptic dose and plasma level in the pharmacological treatment of psychosis. *Archives of General Psychiatry, 45*, 79–91.

Becker, R. B. (1988). Depression in schizophrenia. *Hospital and Community Psychiatry, 39*, 1269–1275.

Beitchman, J. H. (1985). Childhood schizophrenia: A review and comparison with adult-onset schizophrenia. *Psychiatric Clinics of North America, 8*, 793–814.

Campbell, M., Green, W. H., & Deutch, S. I. (1985). *Child and adolescent psychopharmacology*. Beverly Hills, California: Sage.

Carpenter, W. T., Jr., Strauss, J. S., & Bartko, J. J. (1974). Use of signs and symptoms for the identification of schizophrenic patients. *Schizophrenia Bulletin, 11*, 37–49.

Carpenter, W. T., Hanlon, T. E., Heinrichs, D. W., Summerfelt, A. T., Kirkpatrick, B., Levine, J., & Buchanan, R. W. (1990). Continuous vs. targeted medication in schizophrenic outpatients: Outcome results. *American Journal of Psychiatry, 147*, 1138–1148.

Christison, G. W., Kirch, D. G., & Wyatt, R. J. (1991). When symptoms persist: Choosing among alternative treatments for schizophrenia. *Schizophrenia Bulletin, 17*, 217–245.

Cole, J. O. (1964). NIMH-Psychopharmacology Service Center Collaborative Study Group. Phenothiazine treatment in acute schizophrenia: Effectiveness. *Archives of General Psychiatry, 10*, 246–261.

Creese, I., Burt, D. R., & Snyder, S. H. (1975). Dopamine receptor binding predicts clinical and pharmacological potencies of antischizophrenic drugs. *Science, 192*, 481–483.

Crow, T. J., MacMillan, J. F., Johnson, A. L., & Johnstone, E. C. (1986). The Northwick Park study of first episodes of schizophrenia. II. A randomized controlled study of prophylactic neuroleptic treatment. *British Journal of Psychiatry, 148*, 115–120.

Davis, J. M. (1975). Overview: Maintenance therapy in psychiatry. I. Schizophrenia. *American Journal of Psychiatry, 132*, 1237–1245.

Deberdt, R., Elens, P., Berghmans, J., Heykants, R., Woestenborghs, F., Reyntjiens, A., & Van Wungaarden, I. (1980). Intramuscular haloperidol decanoate for neuroleptic maintenance therapy. *Acta Psychiatrica Scandinavica, 62*, 356–363.

Dunham, H. W. (1965). *Community and schizophrenia: An epidemiological analysis.* Detroit: Wayne State University Press.

Ganguli, R., Rabin, B. S., & Kelly, R. H. (1989). Multiple autoantibodies and autoimmune process in schizophrenic patients: Evidence for an autoimmune pathogenesis. In Hadden, J. W., Masek, K., & Nistico, G. (Eds.), *Interaction among CNS, neuroendocrine and immune systems* (pp. 365–383). Rome-Milan: Pythagora.

Goff, C. G., & Baldessarini, R. J. (1993). Drug interactions with antipsychotic agents. *Journal of Clinical Psychopharmacology, 13*(1), 57–67.

Goldstein, M. J., Rodrick, E. H., Evans, J. R., May, P. R. A., & Steinberg, M. R. (1978). Drug and family therapy in the aftercare of acute schizophrenics. *Archives of General Psychiatry, 35,* 1169–1177.

Herz, M. I., & Melville, C. (1980). Relapse in schizophrenia. *American Journal of Psychiatry, 137,* 801–805.

Hogarty, G. E., Anderson, C. M., Reiss, D. T., Kornblith, S. T., & Greenwald, D. P. (1986). Family psychoeducation, social skills training, and maintenance chemotherapy in the aftercare of schizophrenia. *Archives of General Psychiatry, 43,* 633–642.

Hogarty, G. E., McEvoy, J. P., Munetz, M., Dibarry, A. L., Bartone, P., & Cather, R. (1988). Environmental/personal indicators in the course of schizophrenia research group: Dose of fluphenazine, familial expressed emotion, and outcome in schizophrenia. *Archives of General Psychiatry, 45,* 797–805.

Jann, M. W., Ereshefsky, L., & Saklad, S. R. (1985). Clinical pharmacokinetics of the depot antipsychotics. *Clinical Pharmacokinetics, 10,* 315–333.

Javitt, D. C., & Zukin, S. R. (1991). Recent advances in the phencyclidine model of schizophrenia. *American Journal of Psychiatry, 148,* 1301–1308.

Kane, J. M. (1989). The current status of neuroleptic therapy. *Journal of Clinical Psychiatry, 50,* 322–328.

Kane, J. M., & Lieberman, J. A. (1987). Maintenance pharmacotherapy in schizophrenia. In H. Y. Meltzer (Ed.), *Psychopharmacology: The third generation of progress.* New York: Raven.

Kane, J. M., & Selzer, J. (1991). Consideration of "organic" exclusion criteria for schizophrenia. *Schizophrenia Bulletin, 17,* 69–73.

Kane, J. M., Woerner, M., Weinhold, P., Wegner, J., Kinon, B., & Borenstein, M. (1984). Incidence of tardive dyskinesia: Five-year data from a prospective study. *Psychopharmacology Bulletin, 20,* 387–389.

Keshavan, M. S., & Keshavan, A. (1992). Drug induced psychotic disorders. In Keshavan, M. S., & Kennedy, J. S. (Eds.), *Drug-induced dysfunction in psychiatry* (pp. 202–207). New York: Hemisphere.

Kingdon, D. G., & Turkington, D. (1992). The use of cognitive behavioral therapy with a normalizing rationale in schizophrenia: Preliminary report. *Journal of Nervous and Mental Disease, 179*(4), 207–211.

Leff, J., Kuipers, L., Berkowitz, R., & Sturgeon, D. (1985). A controlled trial of social intervention in the families of schizophrenic patients: Two year follow up. *British Journal of Psychiatry, 146,* 594–600.

Lieberman, J. A., Kane, J. M., & Johns, C. A. (1989). Clozapine: Guidelines for clinical management. *Journal of Clinical Psychiatry, 50,* 329–338.

Malm, U. (1982). The influence of group therapy on schizophrenia. *Acta Psychiatrica Scandinavica, 297*(Suppl.), 1–65.

May, P. R., Tuma, A. H., Yale, C., Potepan, P., & Dixon, W. J. (1976). Schizophrenia—A follow-up study of results of treatment. II: Hospital stay over two to five years. *Archives of General Psychiatry, 33,* 481–506.

McCracken, J. T. (1987). Lead intoxication psychosis in an adolescent. *Journal of the American Academy of Child and Adolescent Psychiatry, 26,* 274–276.

McEvoy, J. P., Hogarty, G. E., & Steingard, S. (1991). Optimal dose of neuroleptic in acute schizophrenia. *Archives of General Psychiatry, 48,* 739–745.

Murray, R. M., O'Callaghan, E., Castle, D. J., & Lewis, S. (1992). A neurodevelopmental approach to the classification of schizophrenia. *Schizophrenia Bulletin, 18*(2), 319–332.

Nasrallah, H. A. (1986). The differential diagnosis of schizophrenia: Genetic, perinatal, neurological, pharmacological and psychiatric factors. In H. A. Nasrallah & D. R. Weinberger (Eds.), *Handbook of schizophrenia* (pp. 49–64). New York: Elsevier.

Nayak, R. K., Doose, D. R., & Nair, N. P. V. (1987). The bioavailability and pharmacokinetics of oral and intramuscular haloperidol in schizophrenic patients. *Journal of Clinical Psychopharmacology, 27,* 144–150.

Profita, J., Carrey, N., & Klein, F. (1989). Sustained, multimodal outpatient group therapy for chronic psychotic patients. *Hospital and Community Psychiatry, 40*(9), 943–946.

Realmuto, G. M., Erickson, W. D., Yellin, A. M., Hopwood, J. H., & Greenberg, L. M. (1984). Clinical comparison of thiothixene and thioridazine in schizophrenic adolescents. *American Journal of Psychiatry, 141,* 440–442.

Rifkin, A., Seshagiri, D., Basawaraj, K., Borenstein, M., & Wachpress, W. (1991). Dosage of haloperidol for schizophrenia. *Archives of General Psychiatry, 48,* 166–170.

Rifkin, A., & Siris, S. (1987). Drug treatment of acute schizophrenia. In H. Y. Meltzer (Ed.), *Psychopharmacology: The third generation of progress* (pp. 1095–1102). New York: Raven.

Roy, A. (1986). Suicide in schizophrenia. In A. Roy (Ed.), *Suicide* (pp. 95–112). Baltimore: Williams & Wilkins.

Salzman, C. (1989). Use of benzodiazepines to control disruptive behavior in inpatients. *Journal of Clinical Psychiatry, 49*(Suppl): 13–15.

Schneider, K. (1959). *Clinical psychopathology.* New York: Grune & Stratton.

Schooler, N. (1991). Maintenance medication for schizophrenia: Strategies for dose reduction. *Schizophrenia Bulletin, 17,* 311–324.

Schooler, N., & Hogarty, G. (1987). Medication and psychosocial strategies in the treatment of schizophrenia. In H. Y. Meltzer (Ed.), *Psychopharmacology: The third generation of progress* (pp. 1111–1120). New York: Raven.

Simpson, G. E., Yadalam, K. G., Levinson, D. F., Stephanos, M. J., Lo, E. S., & Cooper, T. B. (1990). Single-dose pharmacokinetics of fluphenazine after fluphenazine decanoate administration. *Journal of Clinical Psychopharmacology, 10*(6), 417–421.

Stanton, A. H., Gunderson, J. G., Knapp, P. H., Frank, A. F., Vanicelli, M. L., Schnitzer, R., & Rosenthal, R. (1984). Effects of psychotherapy in schizophrenia. *Schizophrenia Bulletin, 10,* 520–563.

VanPutten, T. (1974). Why do schizophrenic patients refuse to take their drugs? *Archives of General Psychiatry, 31,* 67–72.

VanPutten, T., Marder, S., & Mintz, J. (1990). A controlled dose comparison of haloperidol in newly admitted schizophrenic patients. *Archives of General Psychiatry, 47,* 754–758.

Vaughn, C. E., & Leff, J. P. (1976). The influence of family and social factors on the course of psychiatric illness. *British Journal of Psychiatry, 129,* 125–137.

Wallace, C. J., & Liberman, R. P. (1985). Social skills training for patients with schizophrenia: A controlled clinical trial. *Psychiatry Research, 15,* 239–247.

Werry, J., McClellan, J., & Chard, L. (1991). Childhood and adolescent schizophrenia, bipolar, and schizoaffective disorders: A clinical and outcome study. *Journal of the American Academy of Child and Adolescent Psychiatry, 30,* 457–465.

Wyatt, R. J. (1991). Neuroleptics and the natural course of schizophrenia. *Schizophrenia Bulletin, 17,* 325–351.

Yadalam, K. G., & Simpson, G. M. (1988). Changing from oral to depot fluphenazine. *Journal of Clinical Psychiatry, 49*(9), 346–348.

5

Unipolar Depression

Lynn P. Rehm, James P. LePage, and Susanne Bailey

Description of the Disorder

Clinical Features

This chapter will discuss unipolar depression excluding bipolar depression entirely. Although the approach may be based on a questionable assumption, most psychological research has focused on unipolar depression, excluding those with bipolar conditions, who are thought to have a more biological dysfunction. Unipolar depression is thought of as a syndrome made up of a constellation of associated clinical symptoms and features. DSM-III-R (American Psychiatric Association, 1987) criteria for depression are shown in Table 5.1. Although depression is referred to as an affective syndrome, sad affect is not necessary for the disorder. Lack of affective responsivity (anhedonia), anxiety, or irritable hostility may typify the affective state of depressed people.

The predominant clinical features of depression can be described in the overlapping areas of somatic, cognitive, and behavioral symptoms. The somatic symptoms of depression involve problems in basic functions of living. Eating is disturbed, as demonstrated by lack of appetite and weight loss; sleep is disrupted by bedtime, middle of the night, or early morning insomnia; and sexual interest may be lacking as well. Weight gain and increased sleep occur in some people and characterize what is referred to as atypical depression. Fatigue and general physical complaints are also common in depression.

In the cognitive realm DSM-III-R lists difficulties in concentration and memory, suicidal thoughts, and feelings of guilt as symptoms. The generalized loss of interest in previously enjoyable activities can also be thought of as a cognitive component of

Lynn P. Rehm, **James P. LePage**, and **Susanne Bailey** • Department of Psychology, University of Houston, Houston, Texas 77204-5341.

Handbook of Prescriptive Treatments for Adults, edited by Michel Hersen and Robert T. Ammerman. Plenum Press, New York, 1994.

many of the DSM symptoms. Low self-esteem and self-depreciation are typically included in standard assessment instruments.

The cognitive indications of depression are complex and may be divided in many ways. Beck (1963, 1967; Beck, Rush, Shaw, & Emery, 1979) defined depression as the cognitive triad of symptoms: a negative view of self, world, and the future. The first of these consists of depressed individuals' views of themselves as defective, inadequate, and worthless. They feel helpless and unable to achieve happiness in life. The second aspect of the triad is the individual's view of the world as filled with negative events and dangers at every turn. Every event is seen in the most pessimistic light. The third symptom is a negative view of the future, in which affected individuals see no improvement ahead and feel hopeless about the possibility of bettering their life circumstances. The depressive processes involved in these views will be discussed later.

Many behaviors are associated with depression. Psychomotor agitation or retardation is noted in the DSM criteria. Sad appearance, lack of eye contact, and drooping posture are sometimes assessed as well. The interpersonal relationships of depressed individuals may be characterized by withdrawal, clinging dependency, or irritability. Research on more specific features of depressive behavior will be noted below.

TABLE 5.1. DSM-III-R Criteria for Major Depressive Episode

A. At least five of the following symptoms have been present during the same two-week period and represent a change from previous functioning; at least one of the symptoms is either (1) depressed mood, or (2) loss of interest or pleasure. (Do not include symptoms that are clearly due to a physical condition, mood-incongruent delusions or hallucinations, incoherence, or marked loosening of associations.)
   (1) depressed mood (or can be irritable mood in children and adolescents) most of the day, nearly every day, as indicated either by subjective account or observation by others
   (2) markedly diminished interest or pleasure nearly every day (as indicated either by subjective account or observation by others)
   (3) significant weight loss or weight gain when not dieting (e.g., more than 5% of body weight in a month), or decrease or increase in appetite nearly every day (in children, consider failure to make expected weight gains)
   (4) insomnia or hypersomnia nearly every day
   (5) psychomotor agitation or retardation nearly every day (observable by others, not merely subjective feelings of restlessness or being slowed down)
   (6) fatigue or loss of energy nearly every day
   (7) feelings of worthlessness or excessive or inappropriate guilt (which may be delusional) nearly every day (not merely self-reproach or guilt about being sick)
   (8) diminished ability to think or concentrate, or indecisiveness, nearly every day (either by subjective account or as observed by others)
   (9) recurrent thoughts of death (not just fear of dying), recurrent suicidal ideation without a specific plan, or a suicide attempt or a specific plan for committing suicide
B. (1) It cannot be established that an organic factor initiated and maintained the disturbance
   (2) The disturbance is not a normal reaction to the death of a loved one (Uncomplicated Bereavement)
C. At no time during the disturbance have there been delusions or hallucinations for as long as two weeks in the absence of prominent mood symptoms (i.e., before the mood symptoms developed or after they have remitted)
D. Not superimposed on Schizophrenia, Schizophreniform Disorder, Delusional Disorder, or Psychotic Disorder NOS.

Table 5.1 is reprinted from the American Psychiatric Association (1987) *Diagnostic and statistical manual of mental disorders, third edition, revised.* Washington, DC: Author. Reprinted with the permission of the American Psychiatric Association.

Recent research from biological, cognitive, and social/behavioral perspectives indicates a number of characteristics associated with depression. Many variables have been investigated in search of a biological marker of depression (see Thase & Howland, 1989, for a thorough review). The metabolites of central nervous system monoamines have been assessed in blood, urine, and spinal fluid as indicators of the status of neurotransmitters associated with depression. Endocrine function has also been explored, and dexamethasone suppression test findings have been found to be correlated with, but not a marker for, severe depression. The most promising attempts to locate a biological marker have come from studies of sleep EEG in depressed persons. Latency to REM sleep is greatly reduced in some depressed individuals and returns to normal with clinical improvement. In recent years brain imaging techniques have begun to explore possible hemispheric activity correlates of depression.

Cognitive processes of distortion have been the focus of Beck's cognitive theory of depression (Beck, 1963, 1967; Beck et al., 1979). Depressive interpretations of information cause the individual to distort objectively neutral or even positive information to fit the individual's negative assumptions. It is the distortion that is then acted upon, not the objective event, leading to continued negative beliefs even when information and events are positive. Beck postulates specific information processing errors that individuals use to validate their beliefs in themselves and the world. These errors include: (a) arbitrary inferences that involve taking blame for externally caused events; (b) selective abstraction, which causes the individual to focus on negative details out of context; (c) overgeneralization of negative events; (d) magnification of failure and minimization of successes; and (e) personalization of negative events that have no clear connection to the individual.

Studies of cognitions and memory in depression also reveal interesting features. Depressed individuals are able to retrieve negatively toned memories more quickly and with greater frequency than positive memories (e.g., Teasdale & Fogarty, 1979; Teasdale, Taylor, & Fogarty, 1980). They also have difficulty suppressing negative thoughts and use negative thoughts as distractions when attempting to avoid thinking of other negative events (Wenzlaff, Wegner, & Roper, 1988).

From a social-psychological point of view a number of interesting behavioral and social-cognitive features of depression have been identified. Wills (1981) described the process of downward social comparison, in which depressed individuals prefer hearing negative information from others so as to compare themselves favorably with that individual. Depressed individuals will often seek negative information about others (Gibbons, 1986; Wenzlaff & Prohaska, 1989; Wood, Taylor, & Lichtman, 1985), often feel worse after learning about positive events from others, and often feel better after learning of negative events from others (Gibbons, 1986; Hammen & Peters, 1978; Wenzlaff & Prohaska, 1989).

Depressed individuals tend to discuss negative events in conversations (Coyne, 1976a; Hokanson, Sacco, Blumberg, & Landrum, 1980), exhibit poorer social skills (Blumberg & Hokanson, 1983), and make frequent self-devaluating comments (Blumberg & Hokanson, 1983; Hokanson, Sacco, Blumberg, & Landrum, 1980).

Epidemiology

Depression is one of the most prevalent psychiatric disorders, with an estimated 2.2% prevalence in the United States population in any given month; lifetime prevalence is estimated at 5.8% (Regier et al., 1988). Gender findings suggest that unipolar depression occurs more often in females than males, with a 3 : 1 ratio (Regier et al., 1988). NIMH data indicate that the average age at onset of the first episode of depression is 25 years (Regier et al., 1988). Recent research suggests, however, that the incidence of depression in adolescents and children is increasing (Robins et al., 1984).

Etiology

The causal theories of depression are as complicated as they are numerous. Hypothesized causes range from interpersonal interactions (e.g., Coyne, 1976b) to cognitive distortions (e.g., Abramson, Seligman, & Teasdale, 1978; Beck, 1967; Seligman, 1975) to behavioral deficits (e.g., Lewinsohn, 1974; Liberman & Raskin, 1971; Rehm, 1977) to biological factors (see Golden & Janowsky, 1990). From a biopsychosocial perspective, factors of biology, psychology, and environment may all contribute and interact to precipitate an episode of depression.

Biological Approaches. Existing biological evidence shows a genetic link in the causes of depression. The NIMH Collaborative Study of the Psychobiology of Depression reports that depression is common in first-degree relatives of depressed patients (Andreasen et al., 1987). Adoption studies suggest that depression in a proband is more likely to be associated with depression in the biological parents than in the adoptive parents. Twin studies suggest that concordance rates for monozygotic twins are approximately 40%, whereas those for dizygotic twins are about 11% (Allen, 1976).

While such evidence suggests a strong genetic role in the causes of depression, lack of 100% concordance between monozygotic twins, who share 100% of their genetic makeup, and the evidence of depression without a family history, suggest that genetic contributions are neither necessary nor sufficient to cause depression. Genetic factors should be thought of as a biological diathesis interacting with stress and psychological coping mechanisms to produce clinical depression.

Psychological Approaches. Several psychological theories suggest cognitive or behavioral conditions or predispositions that contribute to depression. *Reinforcement approaches*, most associated with Lewinsohn (1974), suggest that depression is caused by a disruption in the reinforcers that maintain the individual's normal functioning. When behavior decreases due to a lack of available reinforcers, the symptoms of depression (withdrawal, fatigue, feelings of hopelessness, etc.) will follow. Lewinsohn describes three processes by which the loss or lack of response-contingent reinforcement can occur: (a) reinforcement is no longer available in the environment, as a consequence of loss of employment or divorce; (b) reinforcement is not forthcoming because the person lacks the social skills to obtain it; and (c) reinforcement is available but the individual is unable to enjoy it, as when anxiety interferes with the enjoyment of social interaction.

Interpersonal theorists, such as Beach and O'Leary (1986), Coyne (1976a,b), and Gotlib and Colby (1987), view depression as the result of deficits in the individual's social skills. With his interpersonal model, Coyne (1976b) discusses a process by which depressed people attempt to elicit support and reassurance of their place in their environment through statements of hopelessness and helplessness. The depressed person's social others give the support required, but the depressed person often is unsure of whether the other is being honest and attempts to gain more reassurance. Such continued requests for reassurance alienate important others. This alienation is conveyed through nonverbal communication and through avoidance of the depressed individual, leading to further depression and a vicious cycle of more need for reassurance.

Beach and O'Leary (1986) focus on depression in the interpersonal context of marriage, and they have used marital communication skill treatment strategies for depression. A more recent view by Nezu, Nezu, and Perri (1989) suggests that depression is caused by deficits in problem-solving skills, leading to inefficient attempts to resolve difficulties and to negative outcomes.

The basic tenet of *learned helplessness* theory is that depressed individuals acquire the belief that they are incapable of controlling events in their lives (Seligman, 1975). After several revisions (Abramson, Seligman, & Teasdale, 1978; Alloy, Clements, & Kolden, 1985), the concept of a depressogenic attributional style has emerged that describes the depressed individual's causal attributions for success and failure. Depressed individuals make internal, stable, and global attributions for failures but make external, unstable, and specific attributions about successes. Having such a depressive attribution style makes a person vulnerable to depression when adverse life events do occur. The most recent revision of this theory (Alloy, Clements, & Kolden, 1985) holds that helplessness leads to hopelessness about the future, which then produces depression.

Beck's (1963, 1967) cognitive approach to depression is sometimes referred to as *schema theory*. Schema are structures of information in long-term memory. Schemas affect selection of information for encoding as well as abstraction, interpretation, integration, and reproduction of memory (Alba & Hasher, 1983). Beck believes that depressed people employ negatively biased schemas in processing information. When encoding and retrieving information, depressed individuals select negative aspects of the event to be processed. The depressive schemas also facilitate recalling previously encoded negative information (e.g., Clark & Teasdale, 1982; Teasdale, Taylor, & Fogarty, 1980).

Rehm (1977) defined depression as being characterized by one or more of six deficits in *self-control*. Self-control refers to the way in which individuals influence their own behavior toward long-term goals in the face of immediate external rewards and punishments for alternative behavior. Depression is seen as a deficiency in strategies to direct behavior to long-term goals. The first deficit is selective attention to negative events to the exclusion of positive events. The second is selective attention to the immediate consequences of behavior to the exclusion of delayed consequences. The third is a negative attributional style affecting self-evaluation. Setting of stringent and unreachable standards for one's achievement is a fourth deficit. The last two deficits concern maladaptive strategies to influence one's behavior: excessive self-punishment and insufficient contingent self-reward to maintain behavior.

Environmental Approaches. Negative life events and life stressors seem to precede and often precipitate episodes of depression. Depressed persons are often found to have accumulated a number of stressful life events in the months preceding depression onset. Losses, such as the death of a spouse or child, the loss of a job, or divorce, can readily be seen as precipitating an episode of depression. Even stressful positive events, such as childbirth, can trigger depression. Environments can be protective against depression as well. Good networks of social support and social resources, and confiding relationships help people handle losses and stress without depression (Brown & Harris, 1978).

Interactional Approaches. Though many presumed causes of depression exist, present thinking suggests an integrated theory in which no one condition is necessary and sufficient to cause depression and several conditions working in combination may be necessary for an episode of depression to occur. Life stressors, ability to cope with stressors, biological factors, and cognitive structures may interact to create or avoid an episode of depression (Alloy, Clements, & Kolden, 1985; Lewinsohn, Hoberman, Teri, & Hautzinger, 1985). These models tend to emphasize environmental stressors as the eliciting event of depressive episodes, with biological, interpersonal, and demographic factors seen as contributory causes or predisposing characteristics eliciting or preventing depression. These models suggest that an individual has a set of vulnerabilities and strengths that work together to determine an individual's response to a stressful event.

Differential Diagnosis and Assessment

DSM-III-R and DSM-IV Categorization

DSM-III-R (American Psychiatric Association, 1987) divides mood disorders into depressive disorders and bipolar disorders. Only the unipolar depressive disorders, major depression and dysthymia, will be discussed here. The diagnostic criteria for a major depressive episode were presented in Table 5.1. To diagnose major depressive disorder, a major depressive episode must have occurred and bipolar disorder must be ruled out by the lack of a history of manic or hypomanic episodes. The essential feature of dysthymia is a chronic disturbance of mood (depressed) for at least 2 years that is never absent for more than 2 months at a time. In addition, at least two of the following symptoms must be concurrently present: poor appetite or overeating, insomnia or hypersomnia, low energy, low self-esteem, poor concentration or difficulty making decisions, and feelings of hopelessness. An additional diagnostic category, "depressive disorder not otherwise specified [NOS]," includes disorders with depressive features that do not meet criteria for major depression or dysthymia.

A major depressive episode can further be specified as melancholic or chronic depending on the nature and duration of symptoms. The melancholic type is thought to be more endogenous or biologically based. For a major depressive episode to be labeled chronic, it must have lasted for 2 years without a period of 2 months or longer free of significant depressive symptoms. recurrent major depression can also be specified as exhibiting a seasonal pattern. In this type of depression, a regular temporal relationship between onset of an episode and a particular 60-day period of the year has been identified.

The changes that are to take place in DSM-IV (American Psychiatric Association, 1994) are to be based heavily on a review of current empirical data (First, Frances, Widiger, Pincus, & Davis, 1992). Some changes regarding depressive disorders are proposed for DSM-IV including adding the diagnosis of minor depressive disorder and recurrent brief depressive disorder. Minor depressive disorder is defined as a mood disturbance with at least one of the symptoms listed under major depressive episode.

One of those symptoms must be depressed mood or loss of interest. In recurrent brief depressive disorder, the condition meets the criteria for a major depressive episode, except for its duration. The episode should last for at least 2 days but less than 2 weeks. The depressive periods should occur at least once a month for 12 months and not be associated with the menstrual cycle.

Included among the mood disorders in DSM-IV are secondary mood disorder due to a general medical condition and substance-induced mood disorder. These two disorders were subsumed under organic mood syndrome in the organic mental syndromes and disorders section of DSM-III-R. Finally, a mixed anxiety and depressive disorder (MAD) has been proposed. One reason for including this category in DSM-IV is to increase compatibility with ICD-10 (World Health Organization, 1992; First et al., 1992). Another is that many patients presenting with anxious-depressive symptoms do not easily fit in any of the DSM-III-R depression or anxiety categories but, rather, seem to present with subthreshold symptoms of either one (Boulenger & Lavallee, 1993). The DSM-III-R and the proposed DSM-IV categories are compared in Table 5.2.

Differential Diagnosis

A diagnosis of major depressive episode is given only when it can be established that the episode is not caused by an organic factor, such as influenza or hypothyroidism. If an organic factor can be identified, the diagnosis of organic mood syndrome with depression should be given.

Because disorientation, apathy, difficulty concentrating, and memory loss in elderly patients are often assumed to be symptoms of primary degenerative dementia of the alzheimer type or multi-infarct dementia, depression may be underdiagnosed in older people. Treatment for depression will often result in the disappearance of the symptoms suggesting dementia, which indicates that the diagnosis should have been major depression.

TABLE 5.2.   Categorization of Mood Disorders in DSM-III-R and DSM-IV

Disorder	DSM-III-R	DSM-IV
Mood disorders	Major depression 　Melancholic type 　Chronic type 　With seasonal pattern	Major depression 　Melancholic type 　With atypical features 　With catatonia 　With seasonal pattern 　Postpartum onset
	Dysthymia	Dysthymic disorder
	Depressive disorder not 　otherwise specified	Depressive disorder unspecified
		Minor depressive disorder
		Recurrent brief depressive disorder
		Secondary mood disorder due to a 　general medical condition
		Substance-induced mood disorder
Anxiety disorders		Mixed anxiety and depressive 　disorder (MAD)
Organic mental syndromes and 　disorders	Organic mood syndrome 　with depression	

Patients who have a primary diagnosis of schizophrenia often develop depressive symptoms as well. When these symptoms are superimposed on the residual phase of schizophrenia, or occur briefly during the active phase, a diagnosis of either depressive disorder NOS or adjustment disorder with depressed mood may be made, but not major depression. In the case of schizophrenia, catatonic type, a distinction can be very difficult and can be made only through careful assessment of family history. If there is a family history of mood disorders and the patient's premorbid functioning was good, a diagnosis of major depression is the best choice.

Mood disorder with psychotic features is often hard to distinguish from schizoaffective disorder. To be diagnosed with schizoaffective disorder, the patient must have had periods of at least 2 weeks during which he experienced delusions or hallucinations without prominent mood symptoms.

A diagnosis of uncomplicated bereavement is given when the depressive symptoms are a reaction to the death of a loved one. However, preoccupation with worthlessness, prolonged and marked functional impairment, and marked psychomotor retardation may be an indication that the bereavement is complicated by the development of major depression.

Adjustment disorder with depressed mood is the diagnosis given when the disturbances do not meet full criteria for major depression. Some of the symptoms often seen in this disorder are depressed mood, tearfulness, and feelings of hopelessness. If the disorder has lasted for more than 6 months, a different diagnosis will have to be given (i.e., major depression, dysthymia, or depressive disorder NOS).

Dysthymia is particularly difficult to distinguish from major depression, the main difference being that major depressive episodes usually are separated by periods of normal functioning. With dysthymia, which is often thought of as a depressive personality disorder, there are no apparent acute changes in the person's behavior. In addition, the number and severity of depressive symptoms are usually less in dysthymia. In order to make an accurate differential diagnosis between the two disorders, an assessment of the patient's history is essential.

Assessment Strategies

Assessment can be thought of as a two-stage procedure in which diagnosis based on DSM criteria is involved in the first stage, and a more detailed behavioral assessment that may be undertaken for specific purposes, such as treatment planning and research, is part of the second stage. This section will therefore be divided into two parts: the first will deal with assessment strategies designed to provide the clinician with a diagnosis and a measure of severity of depression; the second will address various instruments designed for identifying cognitive and behavioral deficits judged to be crucial in maintaining the patient's depressive symptoms. The second type of assessment is often developed along with a specific treatment program and is therefore useful when measuring the patient's progress regarding targeted dysfunctional cognitions and behaviors.

Assessment for Diagnosis and Severity of Depression.   Most of the instruments designed for the diagnosis and measurement of depression are either clinician ratings based on interviews of varying degree of structure or paper-and-pencil self-report scales. Some, mostly semistructured interviews, are used predominantly for diagnosis, whereas others, including most of the self-report instruments, are primarily designed to measure severity of depression.

The Schedule for Affective Disorders and Schizophrenia (SADS; Endicott & Spitzer, 1978) is a semistructured interview that allows the clinician to quantify symptoms related to mood and thought disorders. This information enables the interviewer to determine a diagnosis as well as providing a detailed description of the patient's symptomatology.

The Structured Clinical Interview for DSM-III-R (SCID; Spitzer, Williams, Gibbon, & First, 1988) is a semistructured instrument designed to enable a clinically trained interviewer to make DSM-III-R diagnoses. Each major diagnostic class is a separate module of the SCID, which makes it particularly well suited for research, since modules of no interest can be omitted.

The Hamilton Rating Scale for Depression (HRSD) is a widely used clinician-rated scale for estimating severity of depression (Hamilton, 1960). The original HRSD has 17 items, each of which is rated on either a 3-point or 4-point scale. An individual can obtain a score ranging from 0 to 50. The items represent cognitive, behavioral, and somatic symptoms of depression, with emphasis on behavioral and somatic symptoms. In order to represent all three areas equally, items designed to measure cognition have been added to a newer version, resulting in 26 items.

The Zung Self-Rating Depression Scale (SDS) consists of 20 statements rated by the patient (Zung, 1965). The items cover three areas: affective, biological, and psychological. Each statement is evaluated by the individual on a scale from 1 to 4 (i.e., from "Never" to "All the time").

The Beck Depression Inventory (BDI) consists of 21 self-rating items representing the range of depressive symptoms (Beck, Ward, Mendelson, Mock, & Erbaugh, 1961). Each item consists of four statements concerning one symptom listed in order of symptom severity. They are assigned values from 0 to 3. The BDI is the instrument most often used in research as a periodic measure of the severity of depression.

The Inventory to Diagnose Depression (IDD) is a 22-item scale self-report scale specifically designed to diagnose Major Depressive Disorder as well as to quantify severity (Zimmerman, Coryell, Corenthal, & Wilson, 1986). Because the IDD is easily administered, and because the patient has to spend only 15 to 20 minutes to complete it, the instrument is particularly useful when conducting research.

The Minnesota Multiphasic Personality Inventory—Depression Scale (MMPI-D; Hathaway & McKinley, 1940) is composed of 60 true/false questions. The scale was developed empirically and measures symptoms of depression such as poor morale, lack of hope for the future, and general dissatisfaction with one's own life situation. This scale is often used for both research and clinical purposes. The MMPI has been revised as the MMPI-2 with a number of improvements (Butcher, Dahlstrom, Graham, Tellegen, & Kaemmer, 1989).

Instruments Targeted for Specific Cognitive and Behavioral Deficits. This group of instruments is used primarily in research settings. They are often developed by research teams for the purpose of testing theoretical conceptualizations of depression, and to monitor patients' progress during and after intervention aimed at changing targeted behaviors identified to be related to the depression. The instruments might also be used to help decide whether a therapy approach targeting a particular deficit is appropriate.

The Pleasant Events Schedule (PES) is a 320-item questionnaire consisting of a list of pleasant events (MacPhillamy & Lewinsohn, 1982). The individual rates each item for both frequency and enjoyment. The questionnaire attempts to assess reinforcement in the patient's life and is often used in conjunction with reinforcement-oriented therapy approaches to depression.

The Interpersonal Events Schedule (IES) is a 160-item questionnaire developed by Youngren, Zeiss, and Lewinsohn (1976). The IES provide scores on eight scales: Social Activity, Assertion, Give Positive, Receive Positive, Give Negative, Receive Negative, Cognitions, and Conflicts. It can be used in conjunction with reinforcement-oriented treatment to plan interventions and assess outcome in specific domains.

The Problem-Solving Inventory (PSI) provides information about the individual's attitudes toward social problem solving and perceptions of their problem-solving styles (Heppner, 1986). The PSI consists of 35 Likert-type items representing five problem-solving stages. It is a measure of both self-appraised problem-solving ability and problem-solving style and has been used in conjunction with therapy aimed at building problem-solving skills.

The Attributional Style Questionnaire (ASQ) consists of 12 hypothetical situations, 6 with an achievement orientation and 6 with an interpersonal orientation (Peterson et al., 1982). Six are considered to be of a positive nature and six of a negative nature. Each situation is rated on a 7-point Likert scale along three attributional dimensions: internality, stability, and globality.

The Automatic Thoughts Questionnaire (ATQ; Hollon & Kendall, 1980) is a 30-item questionnaire designed to measure the frequency of common negative momentary thoughts associated with depression. Each thought is rated on a 5-point scale, which yields total scores of 30 to 150.

The Dysfunctional Attitude Scale (DAS; Weissman, 1979) consists of two 40-item parallel forms: A and B. The items, which are rated on a 7-point scale, measure the individual's dysfunctional thoughts, such as perfectionism, rigidity, and concern about judgment of others. Whereas the ATQ assesses the symptomatic product of negative distortion, the DAS is intended to assess underlying depressive belief systems or schemas.

The Self-Control Schedule (SCS; Rosenbaum, 1980) is a 36-item instrument developed to assess the individual's tendencies to apply self-control methods to the solution of behavioral problems. These include the use of cognitions and self-statements to control emotional and physiological responses, the use of problem-solving strategies, the ability to delay gratification, and perceived self-efficacy.

The Self-Control Questionnaire (SCQ; Rehm et al., 1981) is a 36-item questionnaire designed to assess attitudes and beliefs associated specifically with the self-control model of depression.

Treatment

Evidence for Prescriptive Treatments

Behavior Therapy. A behavioral approach to therapy for depression was first developed by Lewinsohn in the late 1960s (Lewinsohn, Weinstein, & Shaw, 1969). Based on the assumption that different conditions lead to a lack of response-contingent reinforcement, different treatment strategies have been developed for each condition. Problems caused by loss or lack of reinforcement due to environmental change are treated by various strategies designed to increase pleasant (reinforcing) events in the person's daily life. Pleasant events, identified specifically for the client using the Pleasant Events Schedule, are planned and actual increases in events are reinforced with various contingencies.

Lack of reinforcement due to social skill deficits is dealt with by social skill training. This training may be aimed at general skills in interpersonal interaction, or the patient may be referred for specialized training (e.g., for increasing job skills). If anxiety is etiological, relaxation and systematic desensitization techniques are used. In its most recent version, Lewinsohn's program has been developed into a sequence of modules in a psychoeducational format, consisting of classes that cover topics including activity increase, relaxation, cognitive constructive thinking, social skills, and principles of self-change (Lewinsohn, Antonuccio, Steinmetz, & Teri, 1984).

Social Skill Approaches. Social skill training covers a variety of theories and therapeutic strategies that focus on the goal of improving the client's adaptive interpersonal skills and coping. Many different skills have been the focus of training. McLean (McLean & Hakstian, 1979; McLean, Ogston, & Grauer, 1973) emphasized marital communication and assertion to decrease environmental stressors in the home environment. A more traditional social skill training approach was taken by Bellack, Hersen, and Himmelhoch (1981), who trained depressed patients, for example, to establish better eye contact, improve the modulation of voice, and make more direct statements of their feelings and wishes in social situations with family, co-workers, friends, and strangers. Other examples include the Zeiss, Lewinsohn, and Munoz (1979) focus on identifying problem areas, modeling appropriate responses, and role playing with feedback. Nezu, Nezu, and Perri (1989) focused on problem-solving skills such as problem identification and definition, generating alternative solutions, assessing solutions, and trying an appropriate solution and evaluating its success.

Cognitive Therapy. Cognitive therapy for depression has been developed primarily by Beck (Beck, Rush, Shaw, & Emery, 1979) and is used as a one-to-one psychotherapy technique. Beck focuses on the depressive cognitive triad, the negative schemas maintained by the individual, and the errors in information processing associated with depression. Typically, cognitive therapy follows a general sequence of sessions. Initially, behavioral techniques may be used to mobilize the patient. Graded task assignments and activity scheduling may also be used.

The next focus is on monitoring of automatic thoughts. The patient keeps records of situations in which depressive affect is experienced or worsened. The situation and emotion are recorded, along with any thoughts that may have been associated with the feelings. If the patient has difficulty identifying specific cognitions or avoids situations that would elicit negative cognitions, the therapist can attempt to confront her with an upsetting situation in order to arouse negative cognitions, which are then recorded. Thoughts are then discussed with the patient to determine their evidential basis in addition to possible alternative interpretations of the situation.

As specific automatic thoughts are identified, basic underlying assumptions are revealed. For example, the patient who feels sad and rejected when he sees his friend angry may have the automatic thought "I must have done something to annoy him," but the underlying assumption is "I am responsible if anything goes wrong in my interpersonal relationships." As these assumptions are identified they may be examined for their rationality, tested with homework assignments, and replaced with more reality-based assumptions.

Self-Management Therapy. Self-management therapy was derived from Rehm's self-control model of depression (Rehm, 1977) and targets six areas of possible deficits in self-control. The program is carried out in a psychoeducational group format. Sessions include homework review, discussion of the week's experiences, presentation of self-management concepts about depression, in-session exercises to teach the concept, and subsequent homework assignments to use the concept. Segments of the program focus on monitoring and increasing positive activities, identifying and increasing activities with delayed positive consequences, identifying and replacing inappropriate and unrealistic attributions for success and failure, defining goals and subgoals, and rewarding progress toward goals with self-administered contingent reinforcement and more positive self-talk.

Pharmacotherapy

There are four major classes of psychotropic drugs used in the treatment of unipolar depression. The oldest class of medications are the tricyclic antidepressants, such as imipramine (Tofranil), amitriptyline (Elavil), and doxepin (Sinequan). A newer class of chemically related compounds is the heterocyclic antidepressants, such as bupropion (Wellbutrin) and amoxapine (Asendin). Among the newest antidepressants are the selective serotonin reuptake inhibitors, such as fluoxetine (Prozac) and sertraline (Zoloft). The last class is the monoamine oxidase inhibitors (MAOIs), such as tranylcypromine (Parnate) and isocarboxazid (Marplan).

Tricyclic compounds usually take effect in 1 to 2 weeks, with maximum effectiveness occurring in the 3rd to 6th week. Dosage levels are gradually increased until the desired therapeutic responses are attained. Blood levels of the drugs can be monitored to establish when a therapeutic dose has been achieved. Duration of treatment with tricyclic compounds during an acute episode of depression last from 4 to 6 months.

Side effects with antidepressants include anticholinergic symptoms, such as dry mouth and blurred vision; central nervous system symptoms, such as drowsiness, insomnia, and agitation; cardiovascular symptoms, such as orthostatic hypotension, and cardiac arrhythmia; gastrointestinal distress; and other symptoms such as weight gain. In general, the newer heterocyclics and selective serotonin reuptake inhibitors have fewer side effect than the original tricyclics or MAOIs. Discontinuation of tricyclic medication should be gradual to avoid withdrawal effects, such as nausea, vomiting, and muscle pains. There is also some evidence that manic episodes can be precipitated when bipolar depressions are treated with tricyclics (Prein, Klett, & Caffey, 1973).

The MAOIs have demonstrated efficacy in "atypical" depressions (i.e., those showing hypersomnia and weight gain) (White & Simpson, 1985). However, they are often considered only after tricyclics have been demonstrated to be ineffective. There are more adverse reactions to MAOIs than to tricyclic compounds. The typical side effects can occur, and foods containing tyramine, such as yeasts, certain dairy products, chocolate, some wines, and some beans, are prohibited to avoid the most serious side effect: hypertensive encephalopathy. Also, the combination of MAOIs and tricyclics must be strictly avoided because of the possibility of severe blood pressure effects, and even coma and death.

107

Unipolar Depression

Selecting Optimal Treatment Strategies

The choice of treatments for depression is a complex issue, and in most cases the evidence for choosing one treatment over another is weak at best. Among the psychotherapies, each of the major treatment programs has been studied numerous times and each has been found to be effective. Most studies that have compared one psychotherapy with another have generally found no significant differences (Rehm, in press). For example, studies have found cognitive therapy to be as effective as self-management therapy (e.g., Fleming & Thornton, 1980), behavior therapy (e.g., McNamara & Horan, 1986), and social skills therapy (e.g., Taylor & Marshall, 1977). Behavior therapy has been found to be as effective as social skill training (e.g., Zeiss, Lewinsohn, & Munoz, 1979). Self-management therapy has been broken down into a version targeting cognitive components of depression and a version targeting behavioral components. Results for the two were equivalent for depression and for cognitive and behavioral symptoms (Rehm, Kaslow, & Rabin, 1987).

Within the pharmacotherapies, although no antidepressant has been shown to be more effective than another, there is some consensus about guidelines for treatment. Drug interactions and other psychiatric or medical conditions must be taken into account in selecting medication. History of a positive response to a particular medication is a good predictor of future response. As already mentioned, MAOIs may be more effective with atypical symptom patterns (Depression Guideline Panel, 1993).

In choosing between medication and psychotherapy, there is consensus that medication is more appropriate for the most severe, melancholic/endogenous, or psychotic depressions (Rush et al., 1985). The melancholic/endogenous depressions have been viewed as more biological, with evidence of disturbances in neuroendocrine regulation and neurochemical profiles and reduced REM latency, and were assumed to be resistant to psychotherapies. However, Thase, Simons, Cahalane, and McGeary (1991) found that patients responded more quickly to cognitive therapy when they exhibited biological markers, suggesting that biological depression may simply be more responsive to treatment generally. Medications are clearly called for when patients are unable to utilize or participate actively in psychotherapy. Logic dictates that when psychosocial factors, such as severe life stressors, interpersonal conflict, loss, chronic adjustment problems, or skill deficits, are present, psychotherapy is indicated.

The empirical evidence for the efficacy of pharmacotherapy versus psychotherapy fails to produce a clear program of choice. Psychotherapies have been found to be at least as effective as medication. This finding holds for cognitive therapy (e.g., Murphy, Simons, Wetzel, & Lustman, 1984), behavior therapy (Wilson, 1982), and social skills training (e.g., Hersen, Bellack, Himmelhoch, & Thase, 1984). Some evidence suggests that the combination of medication and psychotherapy is superior to either alone, but the differences are small. Moreover, some studies have found no differences (e.g., Roth, Bielski, Jones, Parker, & Osborn, 1982).

Rude and Rehm (1990) reviewed the evidence for matching patients to psychological treatment based on an assessment of their psychosocial deficits. It is usually assumed that therapy will be most effective when the skill trained matches the patient's skill deficit. Studies that assessed cognitive or behavioral deficits targeted by the therapy programs found no evidence for the compensation effect—that is, in no case did subjects who scored low on the skill factor do better in the therapy. There was some evidence that subjects who scored *higher* in skill (e.g., had more self-control skills or fewer dysfunctional attitudes) on some measures did better in any therapy program. It may be that the active, cognitive-behavioral orientation of most of these programs matched the therapy expectations and beliefs of patients with more self-control skills or fewer dysfunctional beliefs. Matching may prove useful in that it selects a treatment that is seen as helpful or as having face validity by the patient, because it matches the patient's view either of his deficits or of what skills are important to use to produce change.

Although outcome efficacy may vary little among the available treatments, the choice of therapy should also take into account long-term effects and relapse rates. Evans et al. (1992) found that clients in cognitive therapy or a combined treatment program of cognitive therapy and tricyclic medication had significantly fewer relapses over a 24-month follow-up than clients given tricyclic medication alone (50% relapse rate with medication alone; 21% with cognitive therapy alone; 15% with combined therapy). Termination of tricyclic medication after 12 weeks was also associated with significantly more relapses than were found among the patients in a one-year drug maintenance program during the 24-month follow-up. These findings, and others like them (e.g., Blackburn, Eunson, & Bishop, 1986; Simons, Murphy, Levine, & Wetzel, 1986), suggest that cognitive-behavioral therapies may have a prophylactic effect, helping to prevent or delay subsequent episodes. Medication maintenance, and psychotherapy maintenance with monthly sessions, are also useful in enhancing the long-term effectiveness of therapy.

Choosing the proper therapy program is a complex issue that should involve an evaluation of the client's ability to tolerate medication, the intellectual functioning of the client, the resources available to the client, the client's strengths and weaknesses, and the specific areas of difficulty and distress. Because of the relatively quick relief from the depressive features given by medication and the potential long-lasting relief provided by cognitive-behavioral therapies, a sequencing of medication followed by psychotherapy should also be considered.

Problems in Carrying Out Interventions

By far the most important problem in carrying out therapy is the rate of premature termination. Dropout rates for cognitive-behavioral programs have ranged from 5% (McLean & Hakstian, 1979) to 32% (Elkin et al., 1989). A review of some important studies and the dropout rates associated with them are presented in Table 5.3. Factors identified as associated with high levels of dropping out are fewer years of education (Blackburn, Bishop, Glen, Whalley, & Christie, 1981; Rabin, Kaslow, & Rehm, 1985), higher levels of depression (Elkin et al., 1989; Murphy et al., 1984; Rabin et al., 1985), and lower income levels (Rabin et al., 1985). Severity of symptoms may affect dropout rates differently for pharmacotherapy and psychotherapy treatments. It is a clinical observation that more severely depressed patients have higher dropout rates in psychotherapy, and mild to moderately depressed patients have higher dropout rates with pharmacotherapy.

Compliance is also a problem with both medication and psychological treatments. Patients may not comply well with medication regimens because of side effects, lack of rapid relief, or preference for nondrug treatment. Compliance is enhanced by full information as to expected therapeutic effects and side effects, and by good clinical management generally. Most of the effective psychotherapy programs involve extensive homework assignments, and compliance with assignments is difficult for many patients. It is important that the patient understand and agree with the purpose and value of the assignment. The psychotherapy literature reveals little research on compliance in depression programs.

Relapse Prevention

Belsher and Costello (1988) found relapse rates after treatment for depression to be 20% after 2 months, 30% after 6 months, and 40% after 12 months, and then to level off at 50% by 2 years following recovery. With such high levels, it behooves therapists to identify factors leading to relapse as well as ways to prevent it.

The number of previous depressive episodes has been found to be positively correlated with relapse (Keller, Shapiro, Lavori, & Wolfe, 1982; Lewinsohn et al., 1988). At-risk individuals should receive special attention for relapse prevention.

Relapse chances are negatively related to the time that has passed since the last episode of depression. Relapse is related to the level of residual clinical symptoms present after the episode has ended (Faravelli, Ambronetti, Pallanti, & Pazzagli, 1986), and new episodes may be precipitated by periods of life stress (Lloyd, 1980). Continuation of treatment until full recovery, or the use of maintenance therapy, may be useful to bring the patient through the highest risk periods. As has been discussed, there is some evidence of a prophylactic effect from the use of cognitive-behavioral therapies. With these psychological techniques enhancing cognitive, behavioral, and self-control skills, it follows that those so treated should be more resistant to stress and future relapse.

Recent research has shown family levels of expressed emotion (EE) to be related to relapse. Expressed emotion has to do with the open expression of hostile and critical feelings toward the patient in any environment. Hooley, Orley and Teasdale (1986) found that higher percentages of patients from high EE families had relapses, as did those with higher levels of overall marital discord (Hooley & Teasdale, 1989). Marital or family support skills training may also be useful in relapse prevention.

TABLE 5.3. Dropout Rates by Treatment Style

Study	Dropout rates (%s)			
	Drug	PT	Combined	SST
Beck, Hollon, Young, Bedrosian, & Budenz (1985)	26.7	22	—	—
Bellack, Hersen, & Himmelhoch (1981)	55.6	23.5	—	15
Cooper (1989)	50	—	—	—
DiMascio et al. (1979)	50	20	29	
Elkin et al. (1989)	33	32	—	23
McLean & Hakstian (1979)	36	5	—	—
Murphy et al. (1984)	33	20.8	18	—
Roth et al. (1982)	—	23	23	—

Drug = drug condition, usually tricyclic; PT = psychotherapy, usually cognitive-behavioral; combined = combined drug and psychotherapy; SST = social skills training.

Case Illustration   •

Case Description

Mary, 30 years old, was referred to an outpatient clinic for treatment of depression. Two months earlier a female co-worker had suggested to her that she might need to see a physician because she appeared to always "feel bad." At first Mary did not want to follow the advice, but when she started to stay home from work because she could not get out of bed, she decided that her problems were worse than she wanted to admit to herself. When Mary saw her physician, she complained of frequent headaches, fatigue, and inability to sleep. She also told her that she had gained about 20 pounds over the last year, even though she had tried to lose weight. To her relief her physician could find nothing physically wrong with her, and referred her to an outpatient clinic for a psychological evaluation and treatment. She told Mary that she thought she was depressed. After one month of thinking it over, Mary decided to follow the advice, despite her embarrassment at perhaps needing psychological treatment. Her life seemed to have gotten so out control she feared it might cause her to lose her job if she did not do something.

Mary was seen by a psychologist at an outpatient clinic. She appeared fragile and listless, and told him that she was tired because she had slept for only 4 hours the previous night. While talking Mary started to cry and stated that she could not understand what was wrong with her, and that she did not used to be like this.

Mary told the psychologist that she had been divorced for a year, but that she and her husband had not lived together for the last 2 years. She had two children from her marriage: a boy, 6 years old, and a girl, 3 years old. Mary had married at age 19 a man 11 years older than she. At the time of her marriage she was attending college, planning to major in business. Her husband, Dan, who was a lawyer, told her that she would never have to work, and that it therefore was a waste of time for her to go to school. Mary and he decided that it would be better if she spent her time helping him promote his career. They also decided to wait a few years to have children. Early in the marriage Mary went on business trips with her husband and often entertained potential clients in their home. Until the birth of their first child they had what Mary called a "perfect marriage." However, when their son, John, was born, Dan started to go on business trips alone. Mary did leave the baby and accompany Dan a few times, but she felt so guilty about being a "bad mother" that she decided not to go on any more trips. John was a difficult child who required a great deal of attention and who often cried for hours, making it difficult for Mary to keep entertaining Dan's clients. Mary started to feel angry at Dan for not helping her with the baby, but Dan told her that John was her responsibility and that he did not know anything about taking care of babies. When their second child, Ann, was born, their relationship deteriorated even further. Dan stayed away more often and came home late most nights. He said he could not deal with the chaotic situation in the house and indicated to Mary that he did not think she was a very effective disciplinarian, as evidenced by the lack of control she had over the children.

Mary started to suspect that he was seeing other women, which upset her greatly. When Ann was 1 year old, Mary overheard a telephone conversation Dan was having which clearly indicated that her suspicion was right. When she confronted Dan, he admitted that he had been seeing another woman for the past year and that he wanted a divorce. He proceeded to move out of the house.

Mary felt totally overwhelmed by this development. She had no skills that would enable her to get a good job, and Dan was not consistent with his financial support. Mary had to move into an apartment because she no longer could afford house payments. She viewed this as a loss of status which she had little hope of regaining. She felt that she was reduced to nothing, and she was embarrassed about inviting her friends over. Gradually she lost contact with all her friends because she could not tolerate the idea that they might feel sorry for her.

Mary was able to find work as a sales clerk in a department store but after 2 months was laid off because of financial cutbacks. After 3 months without work, she found a job as a checker at a 24-hour food store. She had to agree to some night hours, which made it difficult for her to find someone to take care of the children.

At this point she reported she felt so overwhelmed that she often thought she would be better off dead. The only thing that kept her from committing suicide was the thought of what would happen to her children. The future seemed hopeless to her, because she was just barely making ends meet with her current salary and she was so exhausted that going to school to increase her chances for a better job was totally impossible. Because she felt she had nothing in common with the other residents of the apartment complex where she lived, she kept to herself and did not interact with other adults besides those she met at work.

Mary felt totally helpless and saw no way out of her situation. She felt that she was a failure as a mother and wife, and felt humiliated because she had such a low-paying job. She found herself thinking more and more about all the mistakes she had made in the past and blamed herself for not being able to provide a better life for her children.

Differential Diagnosis and Assessment

A careful diagnostic interview indicated that Mary met the criteria for major depressive episode. She had no history or previous episodes of depression or mania, and no other Axis I or II diagnoses. A 2-7-4 profile on the MMPI-2 was consistent with an anxious, reactive depression. The D-scale score of 82 was consistent with the Beck Depression Inventory score of 31 in indicating a moderate level of depression. The BDI was planned to be used as a weekly index of progress in therapy.

Treatment Selection

Given her physical symptoms and low energy level, it was decided that she should be started on pharmacotherapy and psychotherapy concurrently. After consultation between the psychologist and her family physician, she was begun on a regimen of sertraline, one of the serotonin selective reuptake inhibitors. This relatively new antidepressant is effective, with few side effects. In some instances weight loss is one of the side effects of sertraline, which would be an added benefit in the atypical features of Mary's case.

In discussing Mary's situation with her, the therapist identified three primary areas of difficulty: low rates of reinforcing activity, problem-solving deficits, and cognitive distortion. To facilitate the treatment planning process, Mary was asked to complete some of the self-report questionnaires targeted for these specific cognitive and behavioral deficits. The answers provided the therapist with specific baseline information about the nature and severity of her symptoms. A treatment plan was developed that targeted these deficits roughly in sequence.

1. Over the course of her depressive episode, which seemed to have increased in severity, Mary had clearly lost many of her outside activities and reinforcing events. To assist in the clarification of this particular problem, Mary was asked to complete the Pleasant Events Schedule (PES). Scores on the PES verified a low level of activity, and the potentially reinforcing events that were identified were useful in developing a daily checklist of possible events. For 2 weeks Mary was instructed to collect baseline information about her activities. During this time she became more aware that reinforcing events were occurring in her life, though it looked bleak overall. Next the therapist worked with her to develop plans to increase her pleasant events and to schedule some specific events each day. The therapist asked her to rate her mood on a scale from 1 to 10 in her daily logs at the end of every day, so that Mary could see the correlation between the number of positive events and her mood. As therapy progressed, the event self-monitoring assignment remained and was used to schedule events related to other aspects of therapy.

2. As Mary became more active (a result of both the medication and the activity scheduling), the therapist focused on her sense of diminished control over the environment, and her inability to see her situation as a series of individual problems that could be solved. To assess deficits in this areas, Mary was asked to fill out a Problem Solving Inventory (PSI). Mary's sense of helplessness was addressed through problem-solving techniques (Nezu, Nezu, & Perri, 1989). The major purposes of this approach were to: (a) increase her sensitivity to the fact that problems are part of normal living, (b) minimize the influence of immediate emotional states and self-statements that were likely to interfere with her future ability to solve problems, (c) increase her motivation to engage in future problem-solving attempts, and (d) enable her to learn to focus on successful problem-solving strategies and positive self-statements that were likely to facilitate effective problem-solving behavior in the future. Part of Mary's problem was that without adequate schooling she would be unlikely to find a more fulfilling and better paying job. In order for her to change this situation she and the therapist over a number of sessions employed a problem-solving approach to finding child care on weekends and evenings, identifying a college where she could take night classes, and developing a plan to finance her education.

3. Scores on the Automatic Thoughts Questionnaire (ATQ) and the Dysfunctional Attitude Scale (DAS) both supported the observation that Mary made negative interpretations of her experiences. Mary viewed each daily task as evidence of her inadequacy. That her apartment was not neat was evidence to her that she was inadequate as a housekeeper and mother. Any expression of sympathy or offer of help from her friends was taken as pity and an indication that they thought she was incompetent to help herself. Over the course of therapy and in the context of the event-monitoring and problem-solving strategies, the therapist helped Mary to note when she felt bad in a situation and to attempt to identify and examine what she was saying to herself. She was helped to consider alternative explanations and to dispute negative interpretations. For example, with two small children and a job, keeping the apartment neat at all times is not possible and some degree of clutter is an inevitable part of living. She was helped to test the assumption that her friends looked down on her for living in an apartment and for holding a low-status job.

Treatment Course and Problems in Carrying Out Interventions

Overall, Mary was reasonably compliant with treatment. Initially she had a hard time increasing her reinforcing activities, which she felt would no longer be enjoyable if she did try them. This changed after a couple of weeks with encouragement from the therapist. She found that more positive activities occurred in her life than she had imagined and that many formerly enjoyable activities were indeed rewarding when she engaged in them again. After 5 weeks of treatment she was able to see clearly the correlation between positive events and mood. With such progress and the effects of the antidepressant, BDI scores decreased to the 15 to 20 range. These changes motivated her to work very hard in therapy on the problem-solving strategies, which she now viewed as more likely to be successful. Three months later Mary was attending evening classes at the community college. One of her neighbors was looking after her children in exchange for Mary's looking after the neighbor's children on weekends. Mary became more accepting of her situation and recognized that several of her friends were genuinely interested in seeing her through some difficult times.

Outcome and Termination

After about 8 months of therapy, Mary and her therapist began to discuss termination. Her BDI scores at this point had dropped to the 8 to 10 range. She was pleased with the results of therapy but was concerned that she would not be able to deal with difficulties once therapy had stopped. Mary and her therapist decided to taper off treatment slowly and to discontinue pharmacotherapy. During this tapering-off period the therapist reviewed earlier therapy rationales and strategies and introduced some self-management concepts concerning goal setting and self-reinforcement.

Follow-Up and Maintenance

After six monthly sessions, Mary met with her therapist every 3 months for a year. After the year, they decided she no longer was in need of the maintenance therapy. She was told that if she had a problem she could come back, but that she had developed skills that were likely to sustain her through most future difficulties.

Summary

Depression is a complex phenomenon with somatic, cognitive, and behavioral symptoms and features. It is best viewed as a product of biological predisposition, environmental stress, and psychological coping processes. Genetics, biological and physiological correlates, life events, interpersonal skill deficits, and psychological information processing styles are implicated in depression. The DSM system attempts to deal with the multidimensional nature of depression by a categorization scheme that is based largely on severity and course of symptoms. Depression is often episodic, but especially in its milder forms it may also follow a chronic course. Many self-report and clinician interview instruments have been developed to assess depression severity and diagnostic symptomatology. Additional instruments have been developed to assess specific cognitive and behavioral symptoms and risk factors for depression.

Several treatments have been demonstrated to be effective, including several classes of medications. A number of psychotherapy programs with different theoretical underpinnings have proven equally effective in treating depression. All of these programs provide: (a) a clear rationale for viewing depression, (b) structured techniques that follow from the rationale, (c) homework assignments to enact the program in daily life, and (d) detailed progress feedback to the patients.

There are few clear guidelines for selecting among treatment options. Medication may be most effective for severe depressions, but some combinations of medication and psychotherapy may have a slight advantage over either alone. Psychotherapy seems to be superior in reducing the risk of future episodes. While research evidence does not support the idea of matching psychological treatment method to psychometrically assessed deficits, assessment of those deficits may enhance the acceptability of treatment and provide an index of progress. Lack of motivation in depression decreases compliance with both the pharmacotherapeutic regimens and psychotherapy. Therapists must attend to the patient's understanding and acceptance of treatment strategies. Maintenance therapy appears to be useful to reduce rates of relapse in depression.

References

Abramson, L. Y., Seligman, M. E. P., & Teasdale, J. D. (1978). Learned helplessness in humans: Critique and reformulation. *Journal of Abnormal Psychology, 87*, 32–48.

Alba, J. W., & Hasher, L. (1983). Is memory schematic? *Psychological Bulletin, 93*, 203–231.

Allen, M. G. (1976). Twin studies of affective illness. *Archives of General Psychiatry, 33*, 1476–1478.

Alloy, L. B., Clements, C., & Kolden, G. (1985). The cognitive diathesis-stress theories of depression: Therapeutic implications. In S. Reiss & R. R. Bootzin (Eds.), *Theoretical issues in behavior therapy* (pp. 379–410). Orlando, FL: Academic.

American Psychiatric Association (1987). *Diagnostic and statistical manual of mental disorders*, (3rd ed., rev.). Washington, DC: Author.

American Psychiatric Association (1994). *Diagnostic and statistical manual of mental disorders* (4th ed.). Washington, DC: Author.

Andreasen, N. C., Rice, J., Endicott, J., Coryell, W., Grove, W. M., & Reich, T. (1987). Familial rates of affective disorder: A report from the National Institute of Mental Health Collaborative Study. *Archives of General Psychiatry, 44*, 461–469.

Beach, S. R. H., & O'Leary, K. D. (1986). The treatment of depression occurring in the context of marital discord. *Behavior Therapy, 17*, 43–49.

Beck, A. T. (1963). Thinking and depression: I. Idiosyncratic content and cognitive distortions. *Archives of General Psychiatry, 9*, 324–333.

Beck, A. T. (1967). *Depression: Clinical, experimental, and theoretical aspects*. New York: Harper & Row.

Beck, A. T., Hollon, S. D., Young, J. E., Bedrosian, R. C., & Budenz, D. (1985). Treatment of depression with cognitive therapy and amitriptyline. *Archives of General Psychiatry, 42*, 142–152.

Beck, A. T., Rush, A. J., Shaw, B. F., & Emery, G. (1979). *Cognitive therapy of depression*. New York: Guilford.

Beck, A. T., Ward, C. H., Mendelson, M., Mock, J., & Erbaugh, J. (1961). An inventory for measuring depression. *Archives of General Psychiatry, 5*, 462–467.

Bellack, A. S., Hersen, M., & Himmelhoch, J. M. (1981). Social skill training, pharmacotherapy, and psychotherapy for unipolar depression. *American Journal of Psychiatry, 138*, 1562–1566.

Belsher, G., & Costello, C. G. (1988). Relapse after recovery from unipolar depression: A critical review. *Psychological Bulletin, 104*, 84–96.

Blackburn, I. M., Bishop, S., Glen, A. I. M., Whalley, L. J., & Christie, J. E. (1981). The efficacy of cognitive therapy in depression: A treatment trial using cognitive therapy and pharmacotherapy, each alone and in combination. *British Journal of Psychiatry, 139*, 181–189.

Blackburn, I. M., Eunson, K. M., & Bishop, S. (1986). A two-year naturalistic follow-up of depressed patients treated with cognitive therapy, pharmacotherapy, and a combination of both. *Journal of Affective Disorders, 10*, 67–75.

Blumberg, S. R., & Hokanson, J. E. (1983). The effects of another person's response style on interpersonal behavior in depression. *Journal of Abnormal Psychology, 92*, 196–209.

Boulenger, J. P., & Lavallee, Y. J. (1993). Mixed anxiety and depression: Diagnostic issues. *Journal of Clinical Psychiatry, 54*(1, Suppl.), 3–8.

Brown, R. A., & Harris, T. (1978). *Social origins of depression: A study of psychiatric disorders in women.* New York: Macmillan.

Butcher, J. N., Dahlstrom, W. G., Graham, J. R., Tellegen, A. M., & Kaemmer, B. (1989). *MMPI-2 manual for administration and scoring.* Minneapolis: University of Minnesota Press.

Clark, D. M., & Teasdale, J. D. (1982). Diurnal variation in clinical depression and accessibility of memories of positive and negative experiences. *Journal of Abnormal Psychology, 91,* 87–95.

Coyne, J. (1976a). Depression and the responses of others. *Journal of Abnormal Psychology, 85,* 186–193.

Coyne, J. (1976b). Toward an interactional description of depression. *Psychiatry, 39,* 28–40.

Depression Guideline Panel (1993). *Depression in primary care: Volume 2. Treatment of major depression. Clinical practice guideline, Number 5.* Rockville, MD: U.S. Department of Health and Human Services, Public Health Service, Agency for Health Care Policy and Research, AHCPR Publication No. 93-0551.

DiMascio, A., Weissman, M. M., Prusoff, B. A., Neu, C., Zwilling, M., & Klerman, G. L. (1979). Differential symptom reduction by drugs and psychotherapy in acute depression. *Archives of General Psychiatry, 36,* 1450–1456.

Elkin, I., Shea, T., Watkins, J. T., Imber, S. D., Sotsky, S. M., Collins, J. F., Glass, D. R., Pilkonis, P. A., Leber, W. R., Docherty, J. P., Fiester, S. J., & Parloff, M. B. (1989). National Institute of Mental Health treatment of depression collaborative research program. *Archives of General Psychiatry, 46,* 971–982.

Endicott, J., & Spitzer, R. L. (1978). A diagnostic interview: The Schedule for Affective Disorders and Schizophrenia. *Archives of General Psychiatry, 35,* 837–844.

Evans, M. D., Hollon, S. D., DeRubeis, R. J., Piasecki, J. M., Grove, W. M., Garvey, M. J., & Tuason, V. B. (1992). Differential relapse following cognitive therapy and pharmacotherapy for depression. *Archives of General Psychiatry, 49,* 802–808.

Faravelli, C., Ambronetti, A., Pallanti, S., & Pazzagli, A. (1986). Depressive relapses and incomplete recovery from index episode. *American Journal of Psychiatry, 143,* 461–469.

First, M. B., Frances, A., Widiger, T. A., Pincus, H. A., & Davis, W. W. (1992). DSM-IV and behavioral assessment. *Behavioral Assessment, 14,* 297–306.

Fleming, B. M., & Thornton, D. W. (1980). Coping skills training as a component in the short-term treatment of depression. *Journal of Consulting and Clinical Psychology, 48,* 652–655.

Gibbons, F. X. (1986). Social comparison and depression: Company's effect on misery. *Journal of Personality and Social Psychology, 51,* 140–148.

Golden, R. N., & Janowsky, D. S. (1990). Biological theories of depression. In B. B. Wolman & G. Stricker (Eds.), *Depressive disorders: Facts, theories, and treatment methods* (pp. 3–21). New York: Wiley.

Gotlib, I. H., & Colby, C. A. (1987). *Treatment of depression and interpersonal systems approach.* New York: Pergamon.

Hamilton, M. (1960). A rating scale for depression. *Journal of Neurology, Neurosurgery and Psychiatry, 23,* 56–62.

Hammen, O. L., & Peters, S. D. (1978). Interpersonal consequences of depression: Responses to men and women enacting a depressed role. *Journal of Abnormal Psychology, 87,* 322–332.

Hathaway, S. R., & McKinley, J. C. (1940). A multiphasic personality schedule (Minnesota). I: Construction of the schedule. *Journal of Psychology, 10,* 249–254.

Heppner, P. P. (1986, August). *Manual for the Problem-Solving Inventory.* Paper presented at the 84th annual meeting of the American Psychological Association, Washington, DC.

Hersen, M., Bellack, A. S., Himmelhoch, J. M., & Thase, M. E. (1984). Effects of social skill training, amitriptyline, and psychotherapy in unipolar depressed women. *Behavior Therapy, 15,* 21–40.

Hokanson, J. E., Sacco, W. P., Blumberg, S. R., & Landrum, G. C. (1980). Interpersonal behavior of depressive individuals in a mixed-motive game. *Journal of Abnormal Psychology, 89,* 320–332.

Hollon, S. D., & Kendall, P. C. (1980). Cognitive self-statements in depression: Development of an automatic thoughts questionnaire. *Cognitive Therapy and Research, 4,* 383–395.

Hooley, J. M., Orley, J., & Teasdale, J. D. (1986). Levels of expressed emotion and relapse in depressed patients. *British Journal of Psychiatry, 148,* 642–647.

Hooley, J. M., & Teasdale, J. D. (1989). Predictors of relapse in unipolar depressives: Expressed emotion, marital distress, and perceived criticism. *Journal of Abnormal Psychology, 98,* 229–235.

Keller, M. D., Shapiro, R. W., Lavori, P. W., & Wolfe, N. (1982). Relapse in major depressive disorder. *Archives of General Psychiatry, 39,* 911–915.

Lewinsohn, P. M. (1974). A behavioral approach to depression. In R. M. Friedman & M. M. Katz (Eds.), *The Psychology of depression: Contemporary theory and research* (pp. 157–185). Washington, DC: Winston & Sons.

Lewinsohn, P. M, Antonuccio, D. O., Steinmetz, J. L., & Teri, L. (1984). *The coping with depression course.* Eugene, OR: Castalia Press.

Lewinsohn, P. M., Hoberman, H., Teri, L., & Hautzinger, M. (1985). An integrative theory of depression. In S. Reiss & R. Bootzin (Eds.), *Theoretical issues in behavior therapy* (pp 331–359). New York: Academic.

Lewinsohn, P. M., Weinstein, M., & Shaw, D. (1969). Depression: A clinical-research approach. In R. D. Rubin & C. M. Frank (Eds.), *Advances in behavior therapy.* New York: Academic.

Liberman, P. R., & Raskin, D. E. (1971). Depression: A behavioral formulation. *Archives of General Psychiatry, 24,* 515–523.

Lloyd, C. (1980). Life events and depressive disorder reviewed. II: Events as precipitating factors. *Archives of General Psychiatry, 37,* 541–548.

MacPhillamy, D. J., & Lewinsohn, P. M. (1982). The Pleasant Events Schedule: Studies of reliability, validity, and scale intercorrelation. *Journal of Consulting and Clinical Psychology, 50,* 363–380.

McLean, P. D., & Hakstian, A. R. (1979). Clinical depression: Comparative efficacy of outpatient treatments. *Journal of Consulting and Clinical Psychology, 47,* 818–836.

McLean, P. D., Ogston, K., & Grauer, L. (1973). A behavioral approach to treatment of depression. *Journal of Behavior Therapy and Experimental Psychiatry, 4,* 323–330.

McNamara, K., & Horan, J. J. (1986). Experimental construct validity in the evaluation of cognitive and behavioral treatments for depression. *Journal of Counseling Psychology, 33,* 23–30.

Murphy, G. E., Simons, A. D., Wetzel, R. D., & Lustman, P. J. (1984). Cognitive therapy and pharmacotherapy. *Archives of General Psychiatry, 41,* 33–41.

Nezu, A. M., Nezu, C. M., & Perri, M. G. (1989). *Problem-solving therapy for depression: Theory, research, and clinical guidelines.* New York: Wiley.

Peterson, C., Semmel, A., von Baeyer, C., Abramson, L. Y., Metalsky, G. I., & Seligman, M. E. P. (1982). The Attributional Style Questionnaire. *Cognitive Therapy and Research, 6,* 287–300.

Prein, R. F., Klett, C. J., & Caffey, E. M., Jr. (1973). Lithium carbonate and imipramine in prevention of affective episodes. *Archives of General Psychiatry, 29,* 420–425.

Rabin, A. S., Kaslow, N. J., & Rehm, L. P. (1985). Factors influencing continuation in a behavior therapy. *Behaviour Research and Therapy, 23,* 695–698.

Regier, D. A., Boyd, J. H., Burke, J. D., Jr., Rae, D. S., Myers, J. K., Kramer, M., Robins, L. N., George, L. K., Karno, M., & Locke, B. Z. (1988). One-month prevalence of mental disorders in the United States: Based on five Epidemiological Catchment Area sites. *Archives of General Psychiatry, 45,* 977–986.

Rehm, L. P. (1977). A self-control model of depression. *Behavior Therapy, 8,* 787–804.

Rehm, L. P. (in press). Psychotherapies for depression. In K. S. Dobson & K. D. Craig (Eds.), *Anxiety and depression in adults and children.* New York: Sage.

Rehm, L. P., Kaslow, N. J., & Rabin, A. S. (1987). Cognitive and behavioral targets in a self-control behavior therapy program for depression. *Journal of Consulting and Clinical Psychology, 55,* 60–67.

Rehm, L. P., Kornblith, S. J., O'Hara, M. W., Lamparski, D. M., Romano, J. M., & Volkin, J. (1981). An evaluation of major components in a self-control behavior therapy program for depression. *Behavior Modification, 5,* 459–490.

Robins, L. N., Helzer, J. E., Weissman, M. M., Orvaschel, H., Gruenberg, E., Burke, J. D., Jr., & Regier, D. A. (1984). Lifetime prevalence of specific psychiatric disorders in three sites. *Archives of General Psychiatry, 41,* 949–958.

Rosenbaum, M. (1980). A schedule for assessing self-control behaviors: Preliminary findings. *Behavior Therapy, 11,* 109–121.

Roth, D., Bielski, R., Jones, M., Parker, W., & Osborn, G. (1982). A comparison of self-control therapy and combined self-control therapy and anti-depressant medication in the treatment of depression. *Behavior Therapy, 13,* 133–144.

Rude, S. S., & Rehm, L. P. (1990). Cognitive and behavioral predictors of response to treatments for depression. *Clinical Psychology Review, 11,* 493–514.

Rush, A. J., Erman, M. K., Schlesser, M. A., Roffwarg, H. P., Vasanda, N., Khatami, M., Fairchild, C., & Giles, D. E. (1985). Alprazolam vs. amitriptyline in depressions with reduced REM latencies. *Archives of General Psychiatry, 42,* 1154–1159.

Seligman, M. E. P. (1975). *Helplessness: On depression, development, and death.* San Francisco: Freeman.

Simons, A. D., Murphy, G. E., Levine, J. L., & Wetzel, R. D. (1986). Cognitive therapy and pharmacotherapy for depression. *Archives of General Psychiatry, 43,* 43–48.

Spitzer, R. L., Williams, J. B. W., Gibbon, M., & First, M. B. (1988). *Instruction manual for the structured clinical interview for DSM-III-R.* New York: Biometric Research Department, New York State Psychiatric Institute.

Taylor, F. G., & Marshall, W. L. (1977). Experimental analysis of a cognitive-behavioral therapy for depression. *Cognitive Therapy and Research, 1,* 59–72.

Teasdale, J. D., & Fogarty, S. J. (1979). Differential effects of induced mood on retrieval of pleasant and unpleasant events. *Journal of Abnormal Psychology, 88,* 248–257.

Teasdale, J. D., Taylor, R., & Fogarty, S. J. (1980). Effects of induced elation–depression on the accessibility of happy and unhappy experiences. *Behaviour Research and Therapy, 18,* 339–346.

Thase, M. E., & Howland, R. (1989, April). *The biology of depression.* Paper presented at the First Boulder Symposium on Clinical Psychology: Depression, Boulder, CO.

Thase, M. E., Simons, A. D., Cahalane, J. F., & McGeary, J. (1991). Cognitive behavior therapy of endogenous depression. I: An outpatient clinical replication series. *Behavior Therapy, 22,* 457–467.

Weissman, A. (1979). The Dysfunctional Attitude Scale: A validation study. *Dissertation Abstracts International, 40,* 1389–1390B. (University Microfilm No. 79–19, 533).

Wenzlaff, R. M., & Prohaska, M. L. (1989). When misery prefers company: Depression, attribution, and responses to other's moods. *Journal of Experimental Social Psychology, 25,* 220–233.

Wenzlaff, R. M., Wegner, D. M., & Roper, D. W. (1988). Depression and mental control: The resurgence of unwanted negative thoughts. *Journal of Personality and Social Psychology, 55,* 882–892.

White, K., & Simpson, G. (1985). Should the use of MAO inhibitors be abandoned? *Integrated Psychiatry, 3,* 34–45.

Wilson, P. H. (1982). Combined pharmacological and behavioral treatment of depression. *Behaviour Research and Therapy, 20,* 173–184.

Wills, T. A. (1981). Downward comparison principles in social psychology. *Psychological Bulletin, 90,* 245–271.

Wood, J. V., Taylor, S. E., & Lichtman, R. R. (1985). Social comparison in adjustment to breast cancer. *Journal of Personality and Social Psychology, 49,* 1169–1183.

Youngren, M. A., Zeiss, A. M., & Lewinsohn, P. M. (1976). *The Interpersonal Events Schedule.* Unpublished manuscript, University of Oregon, Eugene, OR.

Zeiss, A. M., Lewinsohn, P. M., & Munoz, R. (1979). Nonspecific improvement effects in depression using interpersonal, cognitive, and pleasant events focused treatment. *Journal of Consulting and Clinical Psychology, 47,* 427–439.

Zimmerman, M., Coryell, W., Corenthal, C., & Wilson, S. (1986). A self-report scale to diagnose depressive disorder. *Archives of General Psychiatry, 43,* 1076–1081.

Zung, W. W. K. (1965). A self-rating depression scale. *Archives of General Psychiatry, 12,* 328–337.

6

Bipolar Disorder

Robert A. Philibert and George Winokur

Description of the Disorder

Clinical Features

Our current understanding of bipolar affective disorder as a distinct entity dates back to Hippocrates' (450 B.C.) delineation of mania as one of six subtypes of mental illness. Since that time, a number of authors, including Bonet (Sedler, 1983), Falret (1854), and Kahlbaum (1874), have described patients with affective syndromes featuring both depressive and manic phases. Kraepelin (1921), building on this rich European literature, first separated "manico-depression" and "dementia praecox" (schizophrenia) as distinct syndromes and described the symptomatology and natural history of the syndrome we now term bipolar affective disorder. Leonhard (1957) further refined Kraepelin's concept by separating bipolar affective disorder (BPAD) from unipolar depression.

Bipolar affective disorder is characterized by distinct, relatively brief, episodes of mania and usually depression interspersed with asymptomatic periods. The hallmark symptoms of the manic episode are euphoria, hyperactivity, and push of speech. In a study of 31 consecutively admitted affectively ill patients suffering from mania, symptoms such as hyperactivity, euphoria, flight of ideas, distractibility, circumstantiality, push of speech, and insomnia were almost invariably found during the course of illness (Table 6.1). Frequently, periods of euphoria are intermingled with periods of irritability, with up to 8% of patients manifesting only irritability during the course of mania (Winokur & Tsuang, 1975). Alternately, up to 70% of patients may experience marked mood lability, as demonstrated by brief periods of melancholia during their manic episode (Winokur, Clayton, & Reich, 1969). During these microepisodes of

Robert A. Philibert and **George Winokur** • Department of Psychiatry, University of Iowa College of Medicine, Iowa City, Iowa 52242-1057.

Handbook of Prescriptive Treatments for Adults, edited by Michel Hersen and Robert T. Ammerman. Plenum Press, New York, 1994.

depression, patients often display restricted affect, tearfulness, psychomotor retardation, and social withdrawal in addition to low mood or irritability. Generally lasting only minutes but sometimes continuing for several days, these mood shifts usually have an abrupt onset which sometimes can be precipitated by asking the subject to recall a sad experience.

In addition to affective symptoms, up to one-half of patients manifest psychotic symptoms, such as religiosity, grandiosity, hallucinations, delusions, ideas of reference, and passivity, during the course of mania (Clayton, Pitts, & Winokur, 1965; Winokur, Scharfetter, & Angst, 1985). In the majority of cases, these schizophrenia-like symptoms are mood congruent. However, in approximately 16% of cases, they are mood incongruent.

Onset of mania can be relatively acute, with the patient's being able to pinpoint the exact time of onset. Episode length can vary from several days to several years, with untreated initial episodes of mania typically lasting approximately two months (Wertham, 1929). Some evidence suggests that in individuals suffering recurrent illness, subsequent episodes tend to lengthen.

A small proportion of bipolar subjects experiences only manic episodes, with the vast majority of patients also experiencing depressive episodes. These depressive episodes manifest relatively high frequency of anergia, hypersomnia, and catatonia (Abrams & Taylor, 1975; Detre et al., 1972) but are otherwise indistinguishable from those suffered in unipolar depression. The reader is referred to Chapter 5 for a complete description of the phenomenology.

Although a substantial number of patients experience only one affective episode in the course of their illness, the majority relapse. The average patient experiences approximately nine episodes with approximately equal frequency of mania and depression (Angst et al., 1973; Ayuso-Gutierrez & Ramos-Brieva, 1982). Often the depressive phase precedes the onset of the manic phase (Winokur et al., 1969). This observation, coupled with frequent tricyclic treatment of the antecedent depression,

TABLE 6.1. Symptoms of Manic Patients

Symptom	Patients with Sx recorded (N)	Patients with Sx recorded as positive	
		%	N
Hyperactivity	31	100	31
Euphoria	31	97	30
Flight of ideas	29	100	30
Distractibility	30	96	20
Circumstantiality	27	96	29
Push of speech	31	100	31
Increased sexuality	23	74	21
Grandiosity/religiosity	24	79	21
Decreased sleep	31	94	29
Delusions	26	73	19
Ideas of reference	26	77	20
Passivity	15	47	7
Depersonalization/derealization	14	43	6

Adapted from Clayton, Pitts, and Winokur (1965).

led some early authors to conclude that these antidepressants induce mania. Subsequent naturalistic studies have demonstrated that this is a noncausal association (Lewis & Winokur, 1982).

Associated Features

Several studies have examined the relationship between BPAD and other Axis I and II disorders. Using Epidemiological Catchment Area (ECA) data, two groups have found that bipolar probands are at increased risk for alcohol and substance abuse (Helzer & Pryzbeck, 1988; Regier et al., 1990). In light of this finding, it is not surprising that personality studies, though varying widely in their methodologies and exact conclusions, have generally indicated a high prevalence of cluster B personality traits in bipolar subjects (Brady & Lydiard, 1992; O'Connell, Mayo, & Sciutto, 1991; von Zerssen & Possl, 1990).

Epidemiology. Since the separation of BPAD from unipolar depression in 1966, only a few studies have examined its prevalence. Reviewing the literature from a variety of countries, including the United States, New Zealand, England, Iceland, and Denmark, Boyd and Weisman (1981) derived lifetime risk rates of 0.6, 0.24, 0.88, 0.79, and 0.61%, respectively. In the landmark ECA study, rates of 1.1, 0.6, and 1.1% were found for the New Haven, Baltimore, and St. Louis catchment areas, respectively.

Bipolar patients tend to become ill earlier in life than unipolar patients, with more than half having onset of either depression or mania before age 30 (Table 6.2). Only a small proportion of patients had onset of illness after age 60. However, given the increasing longevity of the population and greater clinical recognition of geriatric presentations, these numbers may be changing. Later onset of illness is associated with lower rate of familial affective disorder and increased neuropathology (Young & Klerman, 1992).

Etiology

Adoption, twin, and family studies all demonstrate a strong genetic component to BPAD (for review, see Winokur, 1991). In a study of 27 monozygotic and 36 dizygotic bipolar twin pairs, Bertelsen and co-workers, using strict criteria, demonstrated

TABLE 6.2. Age at Onset of First Illness

Patient age at onset	Bipolar (N = 121) %	Unipolar (N = 202) %
10–19	27	5
20–29	30	27
30–39	16	24
40–49	12	23
50–59	13	18
60–69	1	3

Adapted from Winokur (1985).

concordance of 75% and 17%, respectively (Bertelsen, Harvald, & Hauge, 1977). If one includes those co-twins who manifested only depression at the time of the study, the figures rise to 96% and 36%. In the only adoption study of bipolar adoptees, Mendlewicz and Rainer (1977) demonstrated an incidence of affective disorders three times greater in biological than in adoptive parents.

Since Hellenistic times, a wide variety of individuals have noted an association between season and mood disorders. In the hope of demonstrating a causal link between mood and season, several investigators have reviewed hospital admission records. In Northern Hemisphere countries, including Ireland, Greece, and Great Britain, a late spring or early summer (April through June) peak in admissions for mania has been observed (Carney, Fitzgerald, & Monaghan, 1988; Frangos et al., 1980). Conversely, in the Southern Hemisphere (Australia), admissions for mania peak in September through November (Parker & Walter, 1982).

Secondary (organic) manias have been reported in connection with drug intoxications, metabolic disturbances, and brain lesions (Krauthammer & Klerman, 1978). Given the prevalence of their use, it is not surprising that methamphetamine, cocaine, and corticosteroids are some of the substances most commonly implicated in drug-induced manias. A wide variety of central nervous system (CNS) infections, including that of HIV (Keiburtz, Zettelmaier, Ketonen, Tuite, & Caine, 1991), can also produce syndromes mimicking primary mania. Lesion location in secondary mania has been investigated in the hope of elucidating regions of the CNS crucial to the pathogenesis of affective disorders; both bilateral (Jampala & Abrams, 1983) and right-sided (Starkstein, Fedoroff, Berthier, & Robinson, 1991) specificities have been noted.

Differential Diagnosis and Assessment

DSM-III-R and DSM-IV Categorization. The advent of widely accepted criteria for the diagnosis of BPAD has greatly aided communication in psychiatric research. Currently the criteria delineated in DSM-III-R (American Psychiatric Association, 1987) are the most widely used in the United States and are encoded in the ninth revision of the International Classification of Disease (ICD-9) for worldwide usage.

Unlike many prior diagnostic paradigms, the classification system for bipolar spectrum illness in DSM-III-R is etiologically atheoretical in conceptualization. It divides manic syndromes into subgroups including cyclothymia, BPAD, and BPAD not otherwise specified (BPAD-NOS) based on the presence or absence of a clear manic episode as described in parts A and B of the criteria listed in Table 6.3. Although duration of symptoms is not explicitly specified in this definition, symptom severity must be sufficient to socially impair or necessitate hospitalization. Episodes that meet the A and B criteria but do not result in impairment or hospitalization are termed hypomanic. Psychotic symptoms may occur during the course of the episode. However, if they persist for more than 2 weeks in the absence of prominent A and B criteria or the episode occurs in the overall context of a psychotic illness, the episode is not accepted as belonging in the bipolar spectrum of illness. Finally, episodes thought to stem from organic causes such as stroke, stimulants, or traumatic head injury (but not somatic antidepressant treatments) are not included in the definition of mania.

Using this definition of mania, DSM-III-R divides the bipolar spectrum into three distinct diagnostic entities. The first category, bipolar disorder, includes those cases in which at least one manic episode meeting the above definition has occurred

A. A distinct period of abnormally and persistently elevated, expansive or irritable mood.
B. During the period of mood disturbance, at least three of the following symptoms have been present for a significant period of time (four if the mood is only irritable).
  (1) inflated self-esteem or grandiosity
  (2) decreased need for sleep
  (3) pressure of speech or more talkative than usual
  (4) flight of ideas or subjectively racing thoughts
  (5) distractibility
  (6) increase in goal-directed activity or psychomotor agitation
  (7) excessive involvement in pleasurable activities which are potentially harmful.
C. Mood disturbance sufficiently severe to cause marked impairment in social or occupational functioning, or to necessitate hospitalization to prevent harm to self or others.
D. During the disturbance, hallucinations or delusions have not been present for two weeks in the absence of clear mood symptoms.
E. Not superimposed on Schizophrenia, Schizophreniform Disorder, Delusional Disorder or Psychotic Disorder NOS.
F. It cannot be established that an organic factor(s) initiated and maintained the disturbance.

Adapted from the American Psychiatric Association (1987). *Diagnostic and statistical manual of mental disorders, third edition, revised.* Washington, DC: Author.

regardless of the presence or absence of a history of a depressive or hypomanic episode. The second category, cyclothymia, includes those cases in which numerous hypomanic episodes occur along with depressive episodes that just fail to meet the criteria for a major depression. The final bipolar spectrum diagnostic entity, bipolar NOS, includes those syndromes in which at least one episode of hypomania has occurred alone or in the context of a major depressive episode, delusional disorder, residual schizophrenia, or psychotic disorder NOS. Other manic presentations are classified outside the mood disorders spectrum. For instance, those episodes occurring in the presence of presumed organic causes are classified separately under organic mental disorders, whereas those cases in which distinct manic and psychotic episodes coexist are classified under psychotic disorders as schizoaffective.

Several potential improvements in this diagnostic nosology are currently proposed in DSM-IV. Unlike DSM-III, DSM-III-R does not specify the minimum duration for a manic or hypomanic episode. One proposal is to change back to the DSM-III specification of one week. Another proposal is to create a new diagnostic category, Bipolar II Disorder, that would include those individuals who have experienced at least one hypomanic episode and one major depressive episode but have not experienced mania. Already a distinct syndrome according to Research Diagnostic Criteria (RDC) (Spitzer, Endicott, & Robins 1978), this amendment to the nomenclature would recognize the distinctive clinical phenomenology and family history these individuals have compared to those classified as demonstrating the more traditional bipolar disorder (Coryell et al., 1989).

Differential Diagnosis.   The differential diagnosis of mania is often complex and includes schizophrenia, drug intoxication, and organic illnesses such as multiple sclerosis, brain tumors, and AIDS. Irritable mania is particularly difficult, with the combination of irritability, psychomotor agitation, and psychosis being commonly found in paranoid schizophrenia, drug intoxication, and organic mental illness. In contrast, the triad of euphoria, pressured speech, and hyperactivity is highly predictive of bipolar illness (Young, Abrams, Taylor, & Meltzer, 1983). As with other difficult psychiatric presentations, the key to diagnosis is accurate gathering of the acute, premorbid, and family history. Onset of mania should be relatively acute, with the mood syndrome preceding or co-occurring with any psychosis. Although a significant proportion of manics have prior social disabilities, mania is associated with much better premorbid functioning than is schizophrenia. Family history is the most reliable predictor of mania: over half of manics have a family history of affective disorder, whereas mania is not associated with a greater familial prevalence of schizophrenia. Use of informants other than the patient in obtaining the history is essential. This is of particular importance in the case of hypomania, where it should be clear to impartial observers as well as the patient that a clear, sustained change in mood and behavior has taken place.

Assessment Strategies.   After the history is taken, the next step in assessment is a thorough physical and laboratory examination. Abnormal neurological findings should be followed up with the appropriate testing, including neuroimaging and EEG or consultation. Normally, laboratory examination includes a complete blood count with differential, general chemistry panel, and thyroid function tests. However, given the high incidence of substance abuse in manics and ability of psychoactive drugs to mimic mania, a low threshold should be employed in drug testing. The serum concentration of any relevant prescribed drug also should be ascertained.

While these measures are being carried out, the patient should be under the constant surveillance of a trained observer and protected from injurious behavior. Sleep, psychomotor activity, mood, speech, and thought content should be continuously assessed. If necessary, sedatives should be used to ensure patient safety and optimal assessment.

Treatment

Evidence for Prescriptive Treatments

Pharmacotherapy.   Lithium was first introduced as a treatment for mania in 1949 by Cade. However, because of early reports of substantial toxicity, it was not until the late 1960s that this alkali earth metal lithium came into widespread use in the United States for the treatment of acute mania and subsequent affective episode prophylaxis. Since then, the effectiveness of lithium in the treatment of acute mania has been demonstrated in a wide variety of studies. Schou (1959) reviewed 370 cases reported in the literature through 1958 and found an 82% response rate. In the subsequent 20 years a number of double blind, placebo-controlled trials have demonstrated a response rate of approximately 75% in mild to moderate cases of mania (Goodwin & Zis, 1979).

The exact mechanism through which lithium exerts effects is unclear. Since the initial reports of its effectiveness in mania, hypotheses citing direct lithium interactions at ion channels, neurotransmitter reuptake and storage, and the phosphoinositide second messenger pathway have all been advanced. Recently, exciting new work has implicated lithium—G protein interactions as the site of lithium's therapeutic effects (Manji, 1992). However definitive proof for any of these theories is still lacking.

For the treatment of acute mania, lithium is typically initiated at 300 mg two to three times per day. Subsequently, lithium dosing is adjusted to produce a 12-hour steady-state serum level of 0.8 to 1.2 mmol/L. Although parenteral forms of lithium are not commercially available, lithium is available in both solid and liquid forms to facilitate compliance in the acutely manic patient. Typical side effects include nausea and vomiting, diarrhea, tremor, polydipsia, and polyuria. Improvement is usually noted within 1 week of initiation of treatment, with total hospitalization normally lasting less than 3 weeks.

The lack of efficacy of lithium in a significant proportion of individuals with acute manic episodes led to a search for alternate therapies. In 1971, Takezaki and Hanaoka published the first study of carbamazepine use in mania, reporting a 60% response rate in an open study of 10 acutely manic patients (1971). Elphick (1989) reviewed both open and double blind studies to date and found that overall, 51% of acutely manic patients improved significantly while receiving carbamazepine. Although lithium may be more effective in severely ill manics, double blind trials directly comparing the two agents have consistently shown that carbamazepine is therapeutically equivalent to lithium (Lerer, Moore, Meyendorff, Cho, & Gershon, 1987; Luznat, Murphy, & Nunn, 1988; Small et al., 1991).

The success of carbamazepine led to exploration of other anticonvulsants as possible anti-manic agents. Noting earlier studies by Kubanek and Rowell (1946) and Lambert, Carraz, Berselli, and Carrel (1966) reporting the successful use of phenylhydantoin and valpromide, Emrich and co-workers investigated the GABA-ergic anticonvulsant valproic acid (Emrich, Dose, & von Zerssen, 1985). Since Emrich's initial report in 1980, several studies have been published with overall average treatment response in controlled trials of approximately 72% (Brown, 1989). In a recent trial directly comparing valproate to lithium, Freeman and co-workers found lithium overall to be slightly more effective than valproate (Freeman, Clothier, Pazzaglia, Lesom, & Swann, 1992). However, valproate tended to be more effective in patients with high pretreatment depression scores, suggesting that valproate may be particularly indicated in mixed states, a finding consistent with the reported efficacy of valproate in rapidly cycling patients (McElroy, Keck, Pope, & Hudson, 1988).

Dosing regimens for each of these anticonvulsants for BPAD tends to be similar to that for their initial indication (i.e., epilepsy). Starting with carbamazepine, 200 mg two to three times per day, or valproate, 250 mg two to three times per day, the dosage is increased as tolerated until 12-hour steady-state levels of 6 to 12 µg/ml and 50 to 120 µg/ml, respectively, are obtained. Assuming the usual full medical and laboratory evaluation upon hospitalization, following initiation of treatment, serum liver enzymes and drug levels should be monitored periodically to avoid unnecessarily high levels of anticonvulsant, or hepatotoxicity. Furthermore, in patients using carbamazepine, a white blood cell count should be taken approximately one month after treatment is initiated and any time an unusual fever is noted in order to avert possibly fatal aplastic anemia. Typical side effects for each drug include sedation, gastrointestinal distress, and rash (see Brown, 1989, and Elphick, 1989, for complete prescribing recommendations). As with lithium, initial response is usually seen within a week after starting treatment.

Prior to introduction of lithium and anticonvulsants as specific anti-manic agents, neuroleptics were the mainstay of treatment for acute mania. Recent trials comparing therapy with a variety of neuroleptics to standard lithium or carbamazepine treatment found results to be statistically equivalent, although in some studies a trend favoring standard therapy was noted (Grossi et al., 1984; Stoll et al., 1985). Given the potential for potentially fatal or irreversible side effects, such as neuroleptic malignant syndrome and tardive dyskinesia, with neuroleptics, as well as the more favorable side effect profiles of the newer mood-stabilizing agents, most clinicians tend to favor an adjunctive role for antipsychotics. In this accessory role, neuroleptics are a valuable addition to the pharmacologic armamentarium, and their addition to standard lithium therapy significantly accelerates the recovery of severely agitated or psychotic patients. Also, it is possible that neuroleptics have a specific role in the treatment of those patients who mainly exhibit mania (Ahlfors et al., 1981).

The important role of calcium channels in facilitating neurotransmission has resulted in trials of several calcium channel antagonists, including verapamil, nimo-dipine, and nifedipine, as potential anti-manic agents. Most promising of these agents is the relatively nonspecific calcium antagonist verapamil. In two double blind studies involving a total of 68 patients, verapamil in dosages averaging approximately 300 mg per day was found to be therapeutically equivalent to lithium (Garza-Trevino, Overall, & Hollister, 1992; Heschl & Kozeny, 1989) However, in the study by Garza-Trevino and co-workers, the investigators reported more of the adjunctive medications lorazepam and haloperidol in the patients treated with verapamil than in those treated with lithium. Consistent with prior clinical experience in cardiac patients, verapamil was well tolerated, with only minor side effects being noted.

The benzodiazepine clonazepam has also been examined as a potential mood-stabilizing agent in several small case study series, open trials, and one small double blind trial. In the double blind trial, which involved 12 patients and used an unusual crossover design, clonazepam and lithium were found to be equally effective, with clonazepam having significantly fewer side effects (Chouinard, 1987). In a retrospective study with potentially more clinical implications, Sachs and co-workers report that clonazepam may partially or completely replace adjunctive neuroleptic therapy in a significant proportion of patients using lithium prophylaxis (Sachs, Rosenbaum, & Jones, 1990). However, to date clinical experience with clonazepam in BPAD is limited, with the exact role and optimal dosing regimen of this agent not yet established.

Numerous other agents, including alpha- and beta-blockers, thyroid supplements, tryptophan, acetylcholine precursors, and anticholinesterase drugs have been proposed as anti-manic agents. However, double blind trials demonstrating efficacy of these drugs have not yet been conducted.

The short-term pharmacologic treatment of bipolar depression does not differ largely from that of unipolar depression. The major exception is suggested by a series of studies, using first open and then double blind conditions, in which the monoamine oxidase inhibitor tranylcypromine was demonstrated to be superior to imipramine in the treatment of anergic bipolar depression (Himmelhoch, Thase, Mallinger, & Houch, 1991). Although these studies have not yet been replicated, this observation represents a potentially significant advance and suggests that more clinically relevant discoveries lie ahead as the biology of bipolar depression becomes better understood.

Behavior Therapy. The role of psychotherapy in the short-term care of the bipolar patient has not been established. Psychotherapy during the acute phase of mania is not generally thought to be beneficial. Given the effectiveness of cognitive and interpersonal psychotherapies in unipolar depression (Shea et al., 1992), and the similar clinical presentations of unipolar and bipolar depression, it seems reasonable to conclude that psychotherapy should be effective in depressed bipolar outpatients. However, the appropriate studies involving acutely depressed bipolar patients have not been conducted, with the area remaining fertile for research.

The continuous employment of psychotherapeutic principles may, however, be important in the interepisodic care of the bipolar patient. Patient education and establishment of strong patient–physician alliance improve compliance with medication regimens and decrease morbidity. Furthermore, since bipolar disorder is sometimes accompanied by unfortunate social and financial consequences, various psychotherapeutic modalities, including supportive, cognitive, and group approaches, can be useful in improving global functioning in a select group of patients (Vasile et al., 1987). No clear role for dynamic psychotherapy in the care of the bipolar patient has been demonstrated.

Alternative Treatments. The use of electroconvulsive therapy (ECT) in acute mania has fallen into relative disfavor since the advent of effective pharmacologic agents and adverse coverage in the media. However, in the largest prospective controlled study in recent years, Small and co-workers reported that ECT was more effective than standard therapy in 34 patients followed for up to 8 weeks (Small et al., 1988). Furthermore, in a small prospective study of nonresponders to pharmacotherapy, Mukherjee and colleagues reported that all nine patients responded to either unilateral or bilateral ECT (Mukherjee, Sackeim, Lee, Prohovnik, & Warmflash, 1985). In a naturalistic study involving 438 patients, Black and co-workers concluded that ECT was superior to lithium treatment in the treatment of the acute manic episode (Black, Winokur, & Nasrallah, 1987). However, whereas the first two studies indicate that bilateral seizure induction seems to be more effective than unilateral induction, Black and colleagues found no difference. Overall, the literature and our own clinical experience suggest that ECT may be the treatment of choice in elderly or medically ill patients who are unable to tolerate anti-manic agents or those who do not respond to initial pharmacologic therapy.

Selecting Optimal Treatment Strategies

The consensus among psychiatrists is that pharmacotherapy of drug-naive mania without medical complications should begin with lithium. For those not responding to or tolerating adequate lithium therapy or having a medical complication such as epilepsy or renal disease, carbamazepine is probably the best alternative. For those unfortunate individuals unable to tolerate or benefit from either lithium or carbamazepine monotherapy, reasonable alternatives include dual lithium and carbamazepine treatment, valproate monotherapy, and ECT. Care must be taken in each of these cases to ensure that treatment is instituted in the appropriate manner. Only if other treatment options have been exhausted should verapamil or other less-tested agents be initiated. In cases of severe agitation or psychosis, adjunctive therapy, using neuroleptics or benzodiazepines, should be instituted, with the usual daily dose of antipsychotic agent averaging a chlorpromazine equivalent of 800 to 1400 mg. Following stabilization of mania, these accessory medications should be slowly tapered as tolerated.

Relapse Prevention

Following resolution of the manic or depressive episode, the focus of therapy needs to be shifted to the prevention of relapse through prophylactic treatment. Numerous clinical trials have demonstrated the efficacy of lithium in the prophylaxis of BPAD, and it has been recommended by the NIH/NIMH Consensus Development

Panel (CDP) as the drug of first choice in the prevention of relapse (CDP, 1985). Over the years, consensus on the recommended lithium level for prophylaxis has changed from 0.8 to 1.5 mmol/L in 1975 to 0.6 to 0.8 mmol/L (CDP, 1985). This downward trend was fueled largely by early reports of possible long-term side effects of lithium on the kidney. More recent studies, however, have indicated little or no long-term adverse renal effects (Schou, 1988). The decrease in recommended dosage is unfortunate, given recent reports of both increased rates of relapse and subsyndromal symptoms in patients treated with low dosages (0.4 to 0.6 mmol/L) versus more accepted levels (0.8 to 1.0 mmol/L) (Gelenberg et al., 1989; Keller et al., 1992).

Failure of lithium prophylaxis in a substantial minority of patients (20 to 30%) has led to trials of other agents, including carbamazepine, valproate, and clonazepam, as possible preventative treatments. Of these agents, carbamazepine has the best demonstrated efficacy, with at least four double blind studies showing roughly equal responses to lithium and carbamazepine (Coxhead, Silverstone, & Cookson, 1992; Lerer et al., 1987; Post, Uhde, Roy-Byrne, & Joffe, 1987; Small et al., 1991). Clear therapeutic drug levels for carbamazepine have not been conclusively determined. However, the consensus is that a serum level between 6 and 12 μg/ml seems to be most associated with a favorable clinical response. Although studies demonstrating effectiveness in double blind paradigms have not been conducted, a number of single blind and open trials of valproate indicate that it may be beneficial in prophylaxis as well as in acute treatment of mania (for review see McElroy, Keck, Pope, & Hudson, 1992). As with carbamazepine, exact therapeutic guidelines have not been established; overall clinical experience indicates that serum levels between 50 and 125 μg/ml are most beneficial.

Almost all clinicians tend to use the chemotherapeutic agent(s) used in the successful treatment of acute mania in a given patient as that patient's prophylactic agent. During the transition period from acute to chronic treatment, adjunctive agents, such as neuroleptics or benzodiazepines, are tapered as tolerated. For those patients receiving ECT or a regimen without demonstrated prophylactic efficacy, the usual treatment approach begins with lithium prophylaxis. Serum lithium levels are usually checked every 3 to 4 months, and renal and thyroid function are monitored yearly. For the minority of patients not responding to lithium therapy, carbamazepine therapy is the best alternative. Although routine serum level and liver function tests, and white blood cell counts are not mandatory after the first few months of therapy, most clinicians periodically assess serum carbamazepine and liver enzyme concentrations to ensure optimal drug levels and to minimize possible complications and side effects. For those patients unsuccessful with both lithium and carbamazepine monotherapy, either dual therapy or the initiation of valproate therapy is a reasonable option. If all these are unsuccessful, maintenance ECT (Abrams, 1988) and neuroleptic therapy are both possibilities.

Case Report

Case Description

N.B. is a 24-year-old single man, an art student with a 5-year history of bipolar illness and alcohol abuse. Initial onset of the patient's illness occurred near the end of his first semester of college. At that time, the patient's roommates noted an increase in his school-related productivity. This was soon followed by a decreasing need for sleep, with the patient keeping his housemates awake by conducting loud, grandiose phone conversations until 3:00 A.M. After one week of steadily increasing abnormal behavior, the patient stopped going to classes, stating that he already knew more about painting than his instructors. He began drinking heavily at local bars and initiated an affair with a 45-year-old woman. At this point his housemates suggested strongly that he consider seeing a doctor at the local student clinic, but the patient declined, stating, "I feel great." Two days later, N.B. began to experience religious auditory hallucinations and was found by campus police in the college's physics building, naked and lecturing incoherently to students. Upon presentation at the emergency room, the patient was found to be well oriented with labile mood and affect. Thought form was tangential, with delusional religious content. He could not elaborate on whether he was homicidal or suicidal.

Review of the patient's psychiatric/developmental history with his parents revealed him to be bright and slightly introverted but otherwise normal. N.B. and his parents denied a personal history of alcohol or substance abuse. Medical history was normal except for a remote history of febrile seizures. Family psychiatric history revealed a history of BPAD and alcoholism in the patient's biological father and depression in his brother. Social history demonstrated the patient to have been active in band and chorus in high school. His biological parents had divorced when he was 3 years old. Since then, the patient's mother had remarried and N.B. and his older brother had had little contact with their biological father.

Differential Diagnosis and Assessment

On first admission the patient was given the temporary diagnosis of psychosis NOS, with the differential diagnosis including Schizophrenia, BPAD, and psychoactive substance induced mood disorder. Following a physical examination revealing no abnormalities, N.B. was admitted to the seclusion room of the psychiatric unit and observed. While in seclusion overnight, the patient demonstrated marked psychomotor activity elevation and an occasionally irritable mood. Speech was very loud and slightly pressured. The patient's speech content was overtly hypersexual, with efforts to keep the patient clothed repeatedly failing. Overnight, he slept only 1 hour. His overall level of agitation necessitated administration of 2 mg of lorezepam, which he took voluntarily. Routine laboratory tests, including a general chemistry screen and complete blood count with differential, yielded normal results. A urine drug screen was trace positive for marijuana. Phone interviews with the patient's parents and roommates conducted the next morning confirmed the above case history.

Treatment Selection

Since this was the patient's first presentation and renal impairment was not evident in his laboratory screen, following assessment he was started on a regimen of orally administered lithium (600 mg in divided doses), and haloperidol therapy (5 mg orally) was added to control N.B.'s psychosis and agitation. Over the next 3 days, lithium was increased to 1500 mg per day, with the intent of producing a steady-state serum level of 0.9 mmol/L. In addition to the scheduled 5 mg dose of haloperidol, lorazepam (1 mg) or haloperidol (5 mg) was given as needed to control agitation. N.B. quickly responded to therapy, and by hospital day 3 he was released from protective isolation. During his time in isolation, strong therapeutic alliances were established between the ward care team and the patient. Consequently, noncompliance with treatment was not an issue during his hospitalization. On hospital day 8, the patient was enrolled in group and activity therapies. Serial steady-state serum lithium levels confirmed prior predictions that adequate serum levels would be reached using 1500 mg per day. Since by hospital day 10 N.B.'s sleep pattern, psychomotor activity, and thought content had returned to normal, neuroleptic therapy was discontinued. On hospital day 13, a predischarge family meeting was held, and on day 14, the patient was discharged. A routine follow-up clinic visit was scheduled for one week after discharge.

Treatment Course and Problems in Carrying Out Interventions

Six months after discharge, despite therapeutic lithium levels, N.B. began to experience difficulty in completing course work and complained of increased sleep and decreased energy. Two weeks after onset of these changes, a full depressive spectrum of symptoms was noted and concurrent fluoxetine therapy was begun. Four weeks after initiation of antidepressant therapy, clear therapeutic response was noted. By week 8 of antidepressant therapy, onset of hypomania was noted and fluoxetine was discontinued. With cooperation of N.B., a plan was made to initiate dual lithium-carbamazepine therapy, with the overall goal of switching to carbamazepine monotherapy over an extended period on an outpatient basis. Unfortunately, one week into this plan, N.B. became more ill and discontinued all medications.

Three days later, the patient was brought to the emergency room by his parents and housemates. They reported a panoply of manic symptoms accompanied by increased caffeine and alcohol use. On presentation N.B. was euphoric and delusional. He agreed to hospitalization and treatment with the proviso that he be allowed to "go to Jerusalem" in one week. Routine physical and laboratory assessments showed no abnormalities except for a trace of tetrahydrocannabinol (marijuana). Because of the patient's hyperactivity and intrusiveness, he was placed in precautionary seclusion, being assigned the same primary care team as in his first hospitalization. Given the apparent failure of lithium, carbamazepine (400 mg in divided doses) along with haloperidol (5 mg) was initiated. Over the next 3 days, the dosage of carbamazepine was increased to 1000 mg per day. The patient complained of marked sedation secondary to carbamazepine therapy, and perhaps as a consequence did not require any medications for agitation. Such decreased agitation was a key factor in releasing N.B. from seclusion on hospital day 2. On hospital day 4 increases in the patient's sleep and concentration as well as absence of delusionary thought content were noted. On hospital day 6, after a low serum level of carbamazepine was noted, the patient's dosage was increased to 1200 mg per day. On hospital day 7 the patient began group and activity therapy. On hospital day 13 N.B. attended and was enrolled in an outpatient support group; he was discharged in good condition on hospital day 14. Routine white blood cell counts and liver enzyme and serum carbamazepine levels were acceptable at one-week follow-up.

Although readjustment to school was difficult, N.B. did relatively well until 9 months after discharge, when onset of hypomania was noted. Outpatient lithium/carbamazepine therapy was reinitiated, but the patient rapidly decompensated. Two weeks after onset of hypomania, the patient became totally unable to care for himself and was hospitalized. On admission, distinct periods of euphoria interspersed with episodes of irritability were noted. Laboratory evaluation revealed an adequate serum carbamazepine concentration but a low serum level of lithium. The patient was placed under the usual precautions but was not placed in seclusion or prescribed antipsychotics because of the absence of extreme psychomotor agitation or psychosis. During the next week the patient's serum drug levels were optimized but he failed to respond. After further consultation with the patient and his family, consent for ECT was obtained. Two days after a rapid tapering of lithium and carbamazepine administration was begun, bilateral ECT was initiated. A course of seven treatments resulted in a full therapeutic response. After completion of ECT, valproic acid prophylaxis was instituted, and the patient was discharged four days later. Although valproate levels were not therapeutic by the time of discharge, they were quickly optimized on a series of short return visits.

Outcome and Maintenence

In the 3 years since his last discharge, the patient has done well and remained in both medical and supportive treatment, although unfortunately not at this center. Because of his concerns about negative academic and social effects of his illness, N.B. transferred to another university. As he reports in brief follow-up phone calls, his treatment consists of quarterly office visits for medication management and brief supportive therapy. He remains interested in art and plans to finish his degree in the next year.

Summary

The past 30 years have brought great progress in our understanding of manic-depressive illness. Originally conceptualized as a single illness, it now appears that mania and hypomania can occur in several distinct syndromes along the bipolar spectrum. These syndromes have different clinical characteristics and distinct family histories, suggesting separate etiological mechanisms. Unfortunately, at this time the genetic causes and the environmental cues leading to their expression remain mysteries. It is hoped that clinical and basic research will soon resolve some of these issues and lead to more specific therapies with fewer side effects.

Despite progress in our understanding of the etiology and therapy of this disorder, the patient remains the focus of treatment. In each case, an accurate diagnosis must be made before successful treatment can begin. Patient education and establishment of a strong patient–physician alliance still are and will remain the keys to the successful initiation and continuation of therapy.

References

Abrams, R. (1988). *Electroconvulsive therapy*. New York: Oxford University Press.

Abrams, R., and Taylor, M. A. (1975). Catatonia: A prospective clinical study. *Archives of General Psychiatry, 33*, 579–581.

Ahlfors, U. G., Baastrup, P. C., Dencker, S. J., Elgen, K., Lingjaerde, O., Pedersen, V., Schou, M., & Aaskoven, O. (1981). Flupenthixol decanoate in recurrent manic depressive illness: A comparison with lithium. *Acta Psychiatrica Scandinavica, 64*, 236–237.

American Psychiatric Association (1987). *Diagnostic and statistical manual of mental disorders*, (3rd ed., rev.). Washington, DC: Author.

Angst, J., Baastrup, P., Grof, P., Hippius, H., Poldenger, W., & Weis, P. (1973). The course of monopolar depression and bipolar psychoses. *Psychiatria, Neurologia and Neurochirurgia, 76,* 489–500.

Ayuso-Gutierrez, J., & Ramos-Brieva, J. (1982). The course of manic depressive illness. *Journal of Affective Disorders, 4,* 9–14.

Bertelsen, A., Harvald, B., & Hauge, M. (1977). A Danish twin study of manic-depressive disorders. *British Journal of Psychiatry, 130,* 330–351.

Black, D. W. , Winokur, G., & Nasrallah, A. (1987). Treatment of mania: A naturalistic study of electroconvulsive therapy versus lithium in 438 patients. *Journal of Clinical Psychiatry, 48,* 132–139.

Boyd, J., & Weisman, M. (1981). Epidemiology of affective disorders. *Archives of General Psychiatry, 38,* 1039–1046.

Brady, K. T, & Lydiard, R. B. (1992). Bipolar affective disorder and substance abuse. *Journal of Clinical Psychopharmacology, 12,* 17S–22S.

Brown, R. (1989). U.S. experience with valproate in manic-depressive illness: A multicenter trial. *Journal of Clinical Psychiatry, 50* (3, Suppl.), 13–16.

Cade, J. F. T. (1949). Lithium salts in the treatment of psychotic excitement. *Medical Journal of Australia, 2,* 349–352.

Carney, P., Fitzgerald, C., & Monaghan, C. (1988). Influence of climate on the prevalence of mania. *British Journal of Psychiatry, 152,* 820–823.

Chouinard, G. (1987). Clonazepam in acute and maintenance treatment of bipolar affective disorder. *Journal of Clinical Psychiatry, 48*(10, Suppl.), 29–36.

Clayton, P., Pitts, F., & Winokur, G. (1965). Affective disorders. IV: Mania. *Comprehensive Psychiatry, 9,* 31–49.

Consensus Development Panel (1985). Mood disorders: Pharmacological prevention of recurrences. *American Journal of Psychiatry, 142,* 469–475.

Coryell, W., Keller, M., Endicott, J., Andreasen, A., Clayton, P., & Hirshfield, P. (1989). Bipolar II illness: Course and outcome over a five year period. *Psychological Medicine, 19,* 129–141.

Coxhead, N., Silverstone, T., & Cookson, J. (1992). Carbamazepine versus lithium in the prophylaxis of bipolar affective disorder. *Acta Psychiatrica Scandinavica, 85,* 114–118.

Detre, T., Himmelhoch, J., Schwartzburg, M., Anderson, C., Bych, R., & Kupfer, D. (1972). Hypersomnia and manic-depressive disease. *American Journal of Psychiatry, 12,* 1303–1305.

Elphick, M. (1989). Clinical issues in the use of carbamazepine in psychiatry: A review. *Psychological Medicine, 19,* 591–604.

Emrich, H. M., Dose, M., & von Zerssen, D. (1985). The use of valproate, carbamazepine and oxcarbazepine in patients with affective disorders. *Journal of Affective Disorders, 8,* 243–250.

Falret, J. P., (1854). Mémoire sur la folie circulaire, forme de maladie mentale caractérisée par la reproduction successive et réguliére de l'état maniaque, de l'état mélancolique, et d'un intervalle lucide plus ou moins prolongé. *Bulletin de l'Académie de Médecine, 19,* 382–415.

Frangos, E., Althanassenas, G., Tsitourides, S., Psilolignos, P., Robos, A., Katsanou, N., & Bulgaris, C. (1980). Seasonality of episodes of recurrent affective psychoses. *Journal of Affective Disorders, 2,* 239–247.

Freeman, T. W., Clothier, J. L., Pazzaglia, P., Lesom, M. D., & Swann, A. C. (1992). A double-blind comparison of valproate and lithium in the treatment of acute mania. *American Journal of Psychiatry, 149,* 108–111.

Garza-Trevino, E. S., Overall, J. E., & Hollister, L. E. (1992). Verapamil versus lithium in acute mania. *American Journal of Psychiatry, 149,* 121–122.

Gelenberg, A. J., Kane, J. M., Keller, M. B., Lavori, P., Rosenbaum, J. F., Cole, K., & Lavelle, J. (1989). Comparison of standard and low serum levels of lithium for maintenance of bipolar affective disorder. *New England Journal of Medicine, 1989,* 1489–1493.

Goodwin, F. K., & Zis, A. P. (1979). Lithium in the treatment of mania: Comparison with neuroleptics. *Archives of General Psychiatry, 36,* 840–844.

Grossi, E., Sacchetti, E., Vita, A., Conte, G., Faravelli, C., Hautman, G., Zerbi, D., Mesina, A. M., Drago, F., & Motta, A. (1984). Chlorpromazine in mania: A double blind trial. In H. M. Emrich, T. Okuma, & A. A. Muller (Eds.), *Anticonvulsants in affective disorders* (pp. 177–187). Princeton, NJ: Excerpta Medica.

Helzer, J. E., & Pryzbeck, T. R. (1988). The co-occurrence of alcoholism with other psychiatric disorders in the general population and its impact on treatment. *Journal of Studies in Alcoholism, 49,* 219–224.

Heschl, C., & Kozeny, J. (1989). Verapamil in affective disorders: A controlled, double-blind study. *Biological Psychiatry, 25,* 128–140.

Himmelhoch, J. M., Thase, M. E., Mallinger, A. G., & Houch, P. H. (1991). Tranylcypromine versus imipramine in anergic bipolar depression. *American Journal of Psychiatry, 148*, 910–916.

Hirschfield, R. M. A. (1981). Situational depression: Validity of the concept. *British Journal of Psychiatry, 139*, 297–305.

Jampala, V. C., & Abrams, R. (1983). Mania secondary to left and right hemisphere damage. *American Journal of Psychiatry, 140*, 1197–1199.

Kahlbaum, K. (1874). *Die katatonie oder das spannugsirresein*. Berlin.

Keller, M. B., Lavori, P. W., Kane, J. M., Gelenberg, A. J., Rosenbaum, J. F., Walzer, E. A., & Baker, L. A. (1992). Subsyndromal symptoms in bipolar disorder: A comparison of standard and low serum levels of lithium. *Archives of General Psychiatry, 49*, 371–376.

Kieburtz, K., Zettelmaier, A. E., Ketonen, L., Tuite, M., & Caine, E. (1991). Manic syndrome in AIDS. *American Journal of Psychiatry, 148*, 1068–1070.

Kraepelin, E., (1921). *Manic-depressive insanity and paranoia*. Edinburgh: E & S Livingstone.

Krauthammer, C., & Klerman, G. L. (1978). Secondary mania: Manic syndromes associated with antecedent physical illness or drugs. *Archives of General Psychiatry, 35*, 1333–1339.

Kubanek, J. L., & Rowell, R. C. (1946). The use of dilantin in the treatment of psychotic patients unresponsive to other treatments. *Diseases of the Nervous System, 7*, 1–4.

Lambert, P. A., Carraz, G., Borselli, S., & Carrel, S. (1966). Action neuro-psychotrope d'un nouvel anti-epileptique: le depamide. *Annales Medico-Psycologiques, 1*, 707–710.

Leonhard, K. (1979). *The classification of endogenous psychoses* (5th ed., E. Robins, Ed., R. Berman, Trans.). New York: Irvington. (Original work published 1957)

Lerer, B., Moore, N., Meyendorff, E., Cho, S-R., & Gershon, S. (1987). Carbamazepine versus lithium: A double blind study. *Journal of Clinical Psychiatry, 48*, 89–93.

Lewis, J., & Winokur, G. (1982). The induction of mania: A natural history study with controls. *Archives of General Psychiatry, 39*, 303–309.

Luznat, R. M., Murphy, D. P., & Nunn, C. M. H. (1988). Carbamazepine versus lithium in the treatment and prophylaxis of mania. *British Journal of Psychiatry, 153*, 198–204.

Manji, K. K. (1992). G proteins: Implications for psychiatry. *American Journal of Psychiatry, 149*, 746–760.

McElroy, S. L., Keck, P. E., Jr., Pope, H. G., Jr., & Hudson, J. I. (1988). Valproate in the treatment of rapid cycling bipolar disorder. *Journal of Psychopharmacology, 8*, 275–279.

McElroy, S. L., Keck, P. E., Pope, H. G., & Hudson, J. I. (1992). Valproate in the treatment of bipolar disorder: Literature review and clinical guidelines. *Journal of Clinical Psychopharmacology, 12*, 42S–52S.

Mendelwicz, J., & Rainer, J. (1977). Adoption study supporting genetic transmission in manic-depressive illness. *Nature, 268*, 327–329.

Mukherjee, S., Sackeim, H. A., Lee, C., Prohovnik, I., & Warmflash, V. (1985). ECT in treatment resistant mania. In C. Shagass, R. C. Josiasson, W. H. Bridger, K. J. Weiss, P. Stoff, & G. M. Simpson (Eds.), *Biological Psychiatry* (pp. 732–734). New York: Elsevier.

O'Connell, R. A., Mayo, J. A., & Sciutto, M. S. (1991). PDQ-R personality disorder in bipolar patients. *Journal of Affective Disorders, 23*, 217–221.

Parker, G., & Walter, S. (1982). Season variation in depressive disorders and suicide deaths in New South Wales. *British Journal of Psychiatry, 140*, 626–632.

Post, R. M., Uhde, T. W., Roy-Byrne, P. P., & Joffe, R. T. (1987). Correlates of antimanic responses to carbamazepine. *Psychiatric Research, 21*, 71–83.

Regier, D. A., Farmer, M. E., Rae, D. S., Locke, B. S., Keith, S. J., Judd, L. L., & Goodwin, F. K. (1990). Comorbidity of mental disorders with alcohol and drug abuse: Results from the Epidemiology Catchment Area (ECA) study. *Journal of the American Medical Association, 264*, 2511–2518.

Sachs, G. S., Rosenbaum, J. F., & Jones, L. (1990). Adjunctive clonazepam for maintenance treatment of bipolar affective disorder. *Journal of Clinical Psychopharmacology, 10*, 42–47.

Schou, M. (1959). Lithium in psychiatric therapy: Stock-taking after ten years. *Psychopharmacologia, 1*, 65–78.

Schou, M. (1988). Effects of long-term lithium treatment on kidney function: An overview. *Journal of Psychiatric Research, 22*, 287–296.

Sedler, M. J. (1983). Falret's discovery: The origin of the concept of bipolar affective illness. *American Journal of Psychiatry, 140*, 1127–1133.

Shea, T. M., Elkin, I., Imber, S. D., Sotsky, S. M., Watkins, J. T., Collins, J. F., Pilkonis, P. A., Beckham, E., Glass, D. R., Dolan, R. T., & Parloff, M. B. (1992). Course of depressive symptoms over follow-up: Findings from the National Institute of Mental Health treatment of depression collaborative research program. *Archives of General Psychiatry, 49*, 782–787.

Small, J. G., Klapper, M. H., Kellams, J. J., Miller, M. J., Milstein, V., Sharpley, P. H., & Small, I. F. (1988). Electroconvulsive treatment compared with lithium in the management of manic states. *Archives of General Psychiatry, 45,* 727–732.

Small, J. G., Klapper, M. H., Metstein, W., Kellams, J. J., Miller, M. J., Mashenke, J. D., & Small, I. F. (1991). Carbamazepine compared with lithium in the treatment of mania. *Archives of General Psychiatry, 48,* 915–921.

Spitzer, R., Endicott, J., & Robins, E. (1978). *Research Diagnostic Criteria* (3rd ed). New York: Biometrics Research, New York State Department of Mental Hygiene.

Starkstein, S. E., Fedoroff, P., Berthier, M. L., & Robinson, R. G. (1991). Manic-depressive and pure manic states after brain lesions. *Biological Psychiatry, 29,* 149–158.

Stoll, K. D., Bisson, H. E., Fischer, E., Gammel, G., Goncalves, N., Krober, H. L., Moldner, H., Nadler, A., & Troyke, P. (1985). Carbamazepine versus haloperidol in manic syndromes: First report of a multi-centric study in Germany. In C. Shagass, R. C. Josiasson, W. H. Bridger, K. J. Weiss, P. Stoff, & G. M. Simpson (Eds.), *Biological Psychiatry* (pp. 332–334). New York: Elsevier.

Takezeki, H., & Hanaoka, M. (1971). The use of carbamazepine (Tegretol) in the control of manic-depressive psychosis and other manic-depressive states. *Seishinigaku, 13,* 173–183.

Vasile, R. G., Samson, J. A., Bemporad, J., Bloomingdale, K. L., Creasey, D., Fenton, B. T., Gudeman, J. E., & Schildkraut, J. J. (1987). A biopsychosocial approach to treating patients with affective disorders. *American Journal of Psychiatry, 44,* 341–344.

von Zerssen, D., & Possl, J. (1990). The premorbid personality of patients with different subtypes of an affective illness. *Journal of Affective Disorders, 18,* 39–50.

Wertham, F. (1929). A group of benign chronic psychoses: Prolonged manic excitement. *American Journal of Psychiatry, 9,* 17–18.

Winokur, G. (1985). Comparative studies of familial psychopathology in affective disorder. In T. Sakai & T. Tsuboi (Eds.), *Genetic aspects of human behavior* (pp. 87–96). Tokyo: Igaku-Shoin.

Winokur, G. (1991). *Mania and depression: A classification of syndrome and disease.* Baltimore: Johns Hopkins University Press.

Winokur, G., Clayton, P., & Reich, T. (1969). *Manic depressive illness.* St. Louis: Mosby.

Winokur, G., Scharfetter, C., & Angst, J. (1985). A family study of psychotic symptomatology in schizophrenia, schizoaffective disorder, unipolar depression and bipolar depression. *European Archives of Psychiatry and Neurological Sciences, 234,* 295–298.

Winokur, G., & Tsuang, M. (1975). Elation versus irritability in mania. *Comprehensive Psychiatry, 16,* 435–436.

Young, M. A., Abrams, R., Taylor, M. A., & Meltzer, H. Y. (1983). Establishing diagnostic criteria for mania. *Journal of Nervous and Mental Disease, 171,* 676–682.

Young, R. C., & Klerman, G. L. (1992). Mania in late life: Focus on age at onset. *American Journal of Psychiatry, 149,* 867–876.

7

Panic Disorder

Michelle G. Craske and Sachin V. Waikar

Description of the Disorder

Clinical Features

Panic attacks are discrete episodes of intense fear or dread, accompanied by a cluster of physical and cognitive symptoms; these include heart palpitations, dizziness, chest discomfort, paresthesias, depersonalization, and fears of loss of control and death (DSM-III-R, American Psychiatric Association, 1987). Rather than gradually mounting anxious arousal, panic attacks are characterized by suddenness or abruptness of onset. Sometimes the episodes occur unexpectedly, and although the concept of "unexpectedness" is somewhat elusive in the diagnostic criteria, it refers to occurrences of panic *in situations* or *at times* that were not expected. Panic attacks evolve into panic disorder when they occur at least four times within 4 weeks, or the individual is pervasively apprehensive about their recurrence, or both.

Panic Disorder occurs with or without the presence of agoraphobia (PDA and PD, respectively). Agoraphobic avoidance refers to avoidance, or endurance with dread, of situations from which escape might be difficult or in which help might be unavailable in the event of a panic attack or symptoms that could be incapacitating or embarrassing, such as loss of bowel control or vomiting. Agoraphobic situations and places include shopping malls, waiting in line, movie theaters, traveling by car or bus, crowded restaurants, and being alone. Avoidance is rated in terms of degree of impairment in functioning, ranging from mild to moderate to severe. For example, a mildly agoraphobic person hesitates about driving long distances alone but manages to drive to and from work, prefers to sit on the aisle at movie theaters, and feels uncomfortable in crowded places. Moderate agoraphobia is exhibited by a person

Michelle G. Craske and **Sachin V. Waikar** • Department of Psychology, University of California, Los Angeles, Los Angeles, California 90024-1563.

Handbook of Prescriptive Treatments for Adults, edited by Michel Hersen and Robert T. Ammerman. Plenum Press, New York, 1994.

who drives within a 5-mile radius of home and only if accompanied, shops at off-peak times and avoids large supermarkets, and avoids traveling by train. Severe agoraphobia refers to the truly housebound individual.

Associated Features

Rarely does the diagnosis of Panic Disorder occur in isolation. Comorbid Axis I conditions include Simple Phobia, Social Phobia, and Dysthymia (Sanderson, DiNardo, Rapee, & Barlow, 1990). Additionally, several independent investigations have shown that 25 to 60% of individuals with PD, and PDA in particular, meet criteria for an Axis II personality disorder. Most often, these are Avoidant and Dependent Personality Disorders (Chambless & Renneberg, 1988; Mavissakalian & Hamman, 1986; Reich, Noyes, & Troughton, 1987). However, the nature of the relationship between PD/PDA and personality disorders remains unclear. For example, comorbidity rates are highly dependent on the method used to determine the Axis II diagnosis, as well as the co-occurrence of depressed mood (Alneas & Torgersen, 1990; Chambless & Renneberg, 1988) and some "personality disorders" remit after successful treatment of PDA (Mavissakalian & Hamman, 1987; Noyes, Reich, Suelzer, & Christiansen; 1991).

Epidemiology

Several independent investigations have shown that approximately 10 to 12% of the general population has experienced at least one unexpected panic attack in the last year (e.g., Norton, Dorward, & Cox, 1986; Telch, Lucas, & Nelson, 1989). However, only 2 to 6% of the population meet criteria for PD/PDA (Myers et al., 1984). Furthermore, panic attacks occur across a variety of anxiety and mood disorders (Barlow et al., 1985) and are not limited to PD/PDA

Treatment for PD/PDA is usually sought around the age of 34 years, although the mean age at onset ranges from 23 to 29 years (Breier, Charney, & Heininger, 1986; Craske, Miller, Rotunda, & Barlow, 1990; Noyes et al., 1986). A large proportion of these individuals, approximately 72% (Craske et al., 1990), reported identifiable stressors such as marital conflict, bereavement, and negative drug experiences around the time of their first panic attack. However, the number of stressors does not differ from the number experienced prior to the onset of other types of anxiety disorders (Pollard, Pollard, & Corn, 1989; Rapee, Litwin, & Barlow, 1990; Roy-Byrne, Geraci, & Uhde, 1986). Panic disorder is characterized by a fluctuating and often chronic course (Breier et al., 1986), and it (especially PDA) is more common among women than men. Approximately 75% of agoraphobics are female (Bourdon et al., 1988; Weissman, 1986). It has been conjectured that the gender difference can be explained in part by sex-role stereotypes and societal expectations (Barlow; 1988): females may tend to deal with anticipatory/panic anxiety by avoiding situations, whereas males may deal with the same degree of anticipation by forcing themselves to confront situations, particularly with the aid of alcohol or drugs.

Etiology

Biological, psychological, and diathesis-stress models have been proposed to account for the origins of PD/PDA, and it appears increasingly clear that a biopsycho-social approach will be necessary to accommodate all the empirical phenomena

(Barlow, 1988). Biological theories suggest that panic disorder is the manifestation of an inherited neurochemical disease (e.g., Carr & Sheehan, 1984). Used to support this claim is the finding that the tricyclic antidepressant imipramine blocks panic attacks without reducing anticipatory anxiety (Klein, 1964), suggesting that panic is a function of a very specific neurochemical dysregulation. However, subsequent research has demonstrated that imipramine and other anti-panic drugs may have a more general anxiety-reducing effect (Telch, 1988). Other support for biological theories of PD/PDA stems from "challenge tests" of panic, in which physiologic alterations (e.g., infusions of norepinephrine or sodium lactate, or inhalations of carbon dioxide) are used to provoke panic attacks. However, as we will discuss, these procedures may also be accommodated by psychological formulations. Finally, family and twin studies demonstrate that panic disorder is familial, with a concordance rate of approximately 15 to 20% among first-degree relatives (see review in Crowe, 1985).

Beck (1988) and Clark (1988) have proposed cognitive models for PD/PDA. According to these authors, PD/PDA arises from catastrophic misinterpretation of the physical symptoms of anxiety. In other words, normal anxiety responses are misconstrued as signals of threat or immediate danger. For example, chest pains or heart palpitations may signify an impending heart attack, or shakiness and dizziness may indicate imminent loss of control. Although these sensations are internal, external situations may also serve as triggering stimuli for the "flight response"; for instance, mall settings may become endowed with threatening imagery for agoraphobic individuals.

Misappraisal of bodily sensations as threatening leads to increased fearful arousal, increased physiologic symptoms, and, subsequently, intensified perception of threat or danger. Thus, cognitions regarding the setting and symptoms of the first attack are of great importance in the model, as these are responsible for the fixation of attention on the symptoms associated with panic in the future (Barlow, 1988; Wolpe & Rowan, 1988). A growing body of empirical findings supports the ideational components involved in PD/PDA versus other disorders. These include the reported fearfulness of certain bodily sensations by persons with PD/PDA (e.g., Reiss, Peterson, Gursky, & McNally, 1986). In addition, attention seems to be selectively attuned to representation of bodily sensations and death or to loss of control (e.g., Clark et al., 1988; Ehlers & Breuer, 1992). Finally, reappraisal significantly influences fear experienced during panic-provocation challenges (e.g., Rapee, Mattick, & Murrell, 1986).

The biopsychosocial, diathesis-stress approach to PD/PDA proposed by Barlow (1988) is a more comprehensive model. In this approach, the initial panic attack is conceptualized as a misfiring of the fear system under stressful life circumstances in physiologically and psychologically vulnerable individuals. The nature of the physiological vulnerability is under question, but it may be construed, at the very least, as an overly reactive or labile autonomic nervous system. Also, a psychological vulnerability is consistent with the existing familial data for PD/PDA. The psychological vulnerability is conceptualized as a set of danger-laden beliefs about bodily sensations (e.g., "A racing heart could mean a heart attack" or "I'm too weak to control my emotions") and about the world in general (e.g., "Events often proceed uncontrollably"). The concepts of uncontrollability (Barlow, 1988) and anxiety sensitivity (Reiss et al., 1986) seem central to the cognitive schemata of individuals with PD/PDA. Life experience relevant to the development of such schemata may include warnings from significant others about the physical and mental dangers of bodily sensations (e.g., an overly protective parent) and significant negative life events that are unpredictable and uncontrollable (e.g., the loss of a parent). Thus, in Barlow's model, a predisposition, or vulnerability, to anxiety is coupled with negative life stress and cognitive schemata to result in PD/PDA.

Differential Diagnosis and Assessment

DSM-III-R and DSM-IV Categorization

Panic Disorder was first recognized as a specific anxiety problem in DSM-III (American Psychiatric Association, 1980), and its criteria were further refined in DSM-III-R (American Psychiatric Association, 1987). The proposed criteria for DSM-IV differ in several ways. First, the definition of "panic attack" remains the same, but it will be relocated to the beginning of the section on anxiety disorders. This change was made in recognition of the nearly ubiquitous nature of panic, its being observed in almost all the anxiety disorders. In turn, the defining features of PD/PDA emphasize apprehension about the recurrence of panic and its unexpected or uncued quality, at times.

As in DSM-III-R, agoraphobia will be listed as a subtype of Panic Disorder (Panic Disorder with Agoraphobia), given the strong evidence that agoraphobia follows the onset of panic attacks. Nevertheless, for those individuals who never experience a true panic attack (e.g., fears of vomiting or losing bowel control), the category of agoraphobia without a history of panic is likely to remain.

Differential Diagnosis

Though panic attacks occur in numerous DSM-III-R anxiety disorders, they must be the central focus of an individual's concerns for a diagnosis of PD/PDA to be made (Craske, Curtis, McNally, Ost, & Salkovskis, 1992). For example, an individual who worries about financial and educational matters to the point of experiencing panic attacks would be more likely to be suffering from generalized anxiety disorder, so long as the central focus of the worry was not the occurrence of another panic. Similarly, persons with social phobia frequently experience panic, but only when faced with a social situation. Individuals with simple phobias often panic in the presence of the circumscribed phobic object (e.g., a snake) or situation (e.g., a high place). Obsessive compulsive disorder may involve panic attacks provoked by the inability to suppress obsessions or to carry out compulsive rituals. It is important to consider a dual diagnosis of PD/PDA with one of the anxiety disorders described only if panic attacks occur unexpectedly or if a significant level of concern over the next panic attack is present.

Another important area of differential diagnosis involves medical conditions. A full medical evaluation is recommended before a diagnosis of PD/PDA is made. Medical conditions that must be ruled out before making a PD/PDA diagnosis include thyroid abnormalities, caffeine/amphetamine intoxication, drug withdrawal, and pheochromocytoma. Additionally, certain medical syndromes exacerbate PD/PDA by producing bodily sensations that are feared. These include mitral valve prolapse, asthma, and hypoglycemia. However, these conditions do not rule out the diagnosis of PD/PDA.

Although PD/PDA may be superimposed on Axis II personality disorders, it is important not to confuse a general avoidant personality style with the agoraphobia concomitant with PD/PDA. For example, individuals with dependent or avoidant personality disorder demonstrate agoraphobic avoidance, but unexpected panic attacks or significant concern over such attacks must be evident in order for a diagnosis of PD/PDA to be given (Reich et al., 1987). In other words, personality disorders may exist in the absence of panic, even though they may involve avoidance of agoraphobic-type situations.

Assessment Strategies

A thorough assessment is necessary for adequate differential diagnosis and treatment selection. Structured interviews, self-monitoring records, standardized self-report inventories, and behavioral tests have been developed for the assessment of PD/PDA.

One of the most extensively used clinical interviews designed for the assessment of anxiety disorders is the Anxiety Disorders Interview Schedule—Revised (ADIS-R, DiNardo & Barlow, 1988). This instrument contains specific questions concerning DSM-III-R criteria for anxiety disorders, along with Hamilton Rating Scales for Anxiety and Depression (Hamilton, 1959, 1960). The interview takes approximately $1\frac{1}{2}$ to $2\frac{1}{2}$ hours to administer, depending on the experience of the interviewer and the severity of symptoms.

Other, more general diagnostic interviews include the Structured Clinical Interview for DSM-III-R (SCID; Spitzer, Williams, & Gibbon, 1987) and the Schedule for Affective Disorders and Schizophrenia (SADS; Spitzer & Endicott, 1979). These instruments include questions specific to PD/PDA in their protocols. The primary value of structured and semistructured interviews is that they enable diagnoses to be made more reliably, which is important given the issues of differential diagnosis discussed earlier.

Ongoing self-monitoring is another important part of the assessment and treatment of PD/PDA. Retrospective recall tends to inflate estimates of panic frequency and intensity (Margraf, Taylor, Ehlers, Roth, & Agras, 1987; Rapee, Craske, & Barlow, 1990), whereas self-monitoring allows for more objective self-awareness. Panic attack frequency, duration, context, and symptoms may be recorded as soon as possible after an attack occurs, using a form similar to the one depicted in Figure 7.1. Daily levels of anxiety, depression, and medication use can be monitored using the Weekly Record of Anxiety and Depression shown in Figure 7.2. This record is completed at the end of each day. Activities may be recorded by logging daily excursions in a diary, or by checking off activities completed from an agoraphobic checklist.

Several standardized self-report inventories provide information useful for treatment planning, as well as being sensitive markers of therapeutic change. The Mobility Inventory (Chambless, Caputo, Gracely, Jasin, & Williams, 1985) lists common agoraphobic situations, which are rated in terms of degree of avoidance, both when alone and when accompanied. This instrument is especially useful for establishing in vivo exposure hierarchies. The Anxiety Sensitivity Index (Reiss et al., 1986) has received wide acceptance as a trait measure of threatening beliefs about bodily sensations, and it tends to discriminate PD/PDA from other types of anxiety disorders (Telch, Sherman, & Lucas, 1989). More specific information about which bodily sensations are most feared may be obtained from the Body Sensations and Agoraphobia Cognitions Questionnaires (Chambless, Caputo, Bright, & Gallagher, 1984).

Measures of trait anxiety include the State-Trait Anxiety Inventory (Spielberger, Gorsuch, Lushene, Vagg, & Jacobs, 1983) and the Beck Anxiety Inventory (Beck, Epstein, Brown, & Steer, 1991). Measures of interpersonal context include the Dyadic Adjustment Scale (Spanier, 1976) and the Marital Happiness Scale (Azrin, Naster, & Jones, 1973).

Behavioral tests objectively measure avoidance of specific situations. Such measurements may be standardized or individually tailored. The standardized behavioral test usually involves walking or driving a particular route, such as a one-mile loop around the clinic setting. Anxiety levels are rated at regular intervals, and the actual distance walked or driven is measured. Individually tailored behavioral tests entail having the individual attempt three to five situational tasks that the client has identified as being anywhere from somewhat to extremely difficult. These might include driving a distance on the highway, waiting in a bank line, or shopping at a crowded mall. Maximum levels of anxiety and degree of approach (i.e., refused task, attempted but escaped task, or completed task) are recorded for each situation. The advantage of standardized behavioral tests is the relative ease of administration. The disadvantage is that the specific task may not be relevant to all clients; for example, some clients may find a one-mile walk to be only mildly anxiety provoking. Therein lies the value of individually tailored tasks.

PANIC ATTACK RECORD

Name _____

Date _____   Time: _____   Duration: _____ (mins)

With: Spouse _____   Friend _____   Stranger _____   Alone _____

Stressful situation: yes/no   Expected: yes/no

Maximum anxiety (circle):

0	1	2	3	4	5	6	7	8
None				Moderate				Extreme

Sensations (check):

Pounding heart	____	Sweating	____	Hot/cold flash	____
Tight/painful chest	____	Choking	____	Fear of dying	____
Breathlessness	____	Nausea	____	Fear of going crazy	____
Dizziness	____	Unreality	____	Fear of losing	
Trembling	____	Numbness/		control	____
		tingling	____		

Figure 7.1. Panic attack record form and checklist. (Adapted from the Center for Stress and Anxiety Disorders, Albany, New York.)

WEEKLY RECORD OF ANXIETY AND DEPRESSION

Name _____   Date _____

Each evening before you go to bed, please rate your *average* level of anxiety (taking all things into consideration) throughout the day, the *maximum* level of anxiety which you experienced that day, your *average* level of depression throughout the day and your *average* feeling of pleasantness throughout the day. Use the scale below. Next, please list the dosages and amounts of any medication you took. Finally, please rate, using the scale below, how worried or frightened you were on average about the possibility of having a panic attack throughout the day.

Level of anxiety/depression/pleasant feelings

0	1	2	3	4	5	6	7	8
None		Slight		Moderate		A lot		As much as you can imagine

Date	Average anxiety	Maximum anxiety	Average depression	Average pleasantness	Medication: type, dose, number (mg)	Fear of panic

Figure 7.2. Weekly record of anxiety and depression. (Adapted from the Center for Stress and Anxiety Disorders, Albany, New York.)

Michelle G. Craske
and Sachin V.
Waikar

Treatment

Evidence for Prescriptive Treatments

Major developments have occurred in psychological treatments of panic disorder. These treatments fall within the domain of behavioral and cognitive-behavioral therapy. Several independent investigators have converged on a set of very effective procedures for panic attacks that combine cognitive restructuring, breathing retraining or relaxation, exposure to feared bodily sensations, and exposure to feared bodily sensations, and exposure to feared and avoided situations. However, these approaches are recent developments. In contrast, agoraphobia has been targeted specifically by behavioral treatments since the 1970s.

Behavior Therapy

Cognitive-Behavioral Treatment of Agoraphobia. The treatment of choice for agoraphobic avoidance is termed "in vivo situational exposure." In vivo situational exposure refers to repeated confrontation with or approach to an object or situation that is feared and avoided. Typical agoraphobic situations and locations include shopping malls, crowded places, public transportation, and others from which escape might be difficult or help might be unavailable in the event of a panic attack. When dropouts are excluded, approximately 60 to 70% of agoraphobics show substantial clinical improvement with this type of exposure-based therapy. Furthermore, the success rate is generally maintained for an average of 4 years or more (Jansson & Ost, 1982). However, 30 to 40% fail to benefit, and the treatment attrition rate is about 12 to 20%. Furthermore, fewer than half achieve high end-state functioning (a "symptom-free" status) (Burns, Thorpe, & Cavallaro, 1986; Cohen, Monteiro, & Marks, 1984; Hafner, 1976; Jacobson, Wilson, & Tupper, 1988; Jansson, Jerremalm, & Ost, 1986; Marks, 1971; Munby & Johnston, 1980). Jacobson et al. (1988) concluded from their review that whereas 50% showed statistically reliable improvement, only 25% on average were no longer agoraphobic by the end of treatment. Finally, as many as 50% who have benefitted clinically may relapse, although the relapse tends to be transient and is followed by return to levels of therapeutic gain (Munby & Johnston, 1980).

Attempts to decrease these qualifications to the efficacy of exposure treatments for agoraphobia have been ongoing. For example, attention has been given to formats such as massed versus spaced exposure. At its most intensive, exposure therapy may be conducted for 3 to 4 hours a day, 5 days a week. Long, continuous sessions are generally considered more effective than are shorter or interrupted sessions (Chaplin & Levine, 1981; Marshall, 1985; Stern & Marks, 1973). The optimal rate for repeating exposure is unclear. Some have found massed sessions on a daily basis to be superior to spaced sessions on a weekly basis, at least on a short-term basis (Foa, Jameson, Turner, & Payne, 1980). However, others have argued against massed aproaches, because they are likely to lead to higher rates of attrition and relapse (Barlow, 1988; Emmelkamp & Ultee, 1974). Chambless (1989), however, recently found spaced and massed exposure to be equally effective in short-term and long-term treatment, as well as comparable in attrition and relapse rates. As Chambless notes, however, unlike those in the usual protocol for spaced exposure, clients in this condition were prevented from conducting between-session practices. Homework assignments are likely to enhance the efficacy of spaced exposure.

A second issue concerns whether exposure should be conducted in a progressive hierarchy or in an intense flooding fashion. Usually, exposure proceeds from least to most difficult items. However, Feigenbaum (1988) recently reported very successful short-term and long-term results from an intense exposure approach.

Other procedural variations concern whether clients should be encouraged to endure high levels of distress during exposure, or to discontinue an exposure trial upon feeling unduly high levels of distress. There is some reason to believe that effective exposure requires the experience of intense anxiety and subsequent anxiety reduction during a single exposure session (Marks, 1971). However, several studies show that equally effective results are obtained when exposure trials are repeatedly terminated as anxiety reaches a certain ("strong") level (e.g., Rachman, Craske, Tallman, & Solyom, 1986). Similarly, the mastery approach developed by Williams and Zane (1989) is effective even though "mastery" subjects tend to report the least anxiety during the exposure. (In this approach, individuals are taught to correct defensive behaviors that interfere with the attribution of performance to personal capabilities.) Nevertheless, some degree of anxiety seems necessary (Foa & Kozak, 1986).

Another consideration is the role of distraction. Exposure is believed to be most functional when attention is directed fully toward the phobic object and internal and external sources of distraction are minimized (Foa & Kozak, 1986). Preliminary evidence suggests that distraction during exposure tends to limit improvement following treatment completion (Craske, Street, & Barlow, 1989).

Finally, several studies have examined the efficacy of including significant others in the treatment of agoraphobia. Significant others are important for several reasons, including the change in roles that can occur as a function of agoraphobic disability. The assumption of tasks and activities by a significant other may inadvertently reinforce agoraphobic behavior. Also, miscommunication or stressful, conflictual relationships may impede clients' progress. Barlow, O'Brien, and Last (1984) found very beneficial effects from involving the spouse as a "coach" who attended each treatment session and aided the client in between-session exposure practices. Even more significant, however, were the much stronger trends for continuing improvement over the 2 years following treatment completion for patients whose spouses were involved versus those whose spouses did not participate (Cerny, Barlow, Craske, & Himadi, 1987).

Cognitive-Behavioral Treatment of Panic.   The cognitive-behavioral treatment for panic has developed mostly during the late 1980s and early 1990s. The approach entails several components, including cognitive restructuring, breathing retraining, and interoceptive exposure. It is not yet known which of these components are necessary, sufficient, or both. Cognitive restructuring targets misappraisals of bodily sensations as being threatening. It involves the provision of a rationale for the role of cognitions in anxiety and panic, identification of aberrant cognitive structures, and the challenging of misinterpretations and biases through reasoning and experience. In an uncontrolled study, Sokol and Beck (Beck, 1988) treated 25 patients with cognitive techniques in combination with behavioral strategies for an average of 17 sessions. Panic attacks were eliminated at the end of treatment and 12 months later in the 17 patients who did not have additional diagnoses of personality disorder. Certainly it is difficult to attribute the outcome specifically to cognitive strategies, because they were combined with behavioral strategies. However, preliminary reports from Margraf (1989) and a series of single case designs (Salkovskis, Clark, & Hackmann, 1991) suggest that cognitive strategies used without exposure are highly effective means of controlling panic attacks.

Breathing retraining is another important component to treatment, because 50 to 60% of panic patients describe hyperventilatory symptoms as being very similar to their panic attack symptoms. In the conception that emphasizes hyperventilation, panic attacks are viewed as stress-induced respiratory changes that either provoke fear because they are perceived as frightening, or augment fear already elicited by other phobic stimuli (Clark, Salkovskis, & Chalkley, 1985). Two case reports have described successful application of breathing retraining in the context of cognitive reattribution of panic symptoms (Rapee, 1985; Salkovskis, Warwick, Clark, & Wessels, 1986). Clark et al. (1985) reported a larger-scale—although uncontrolled—study in which 18 patients received two weekly sessions of respiratory control and cognitive reattribution training. Panic attacks were reduced markedly. Salkovskis et al. (1986) provided further confirmation of the effectiveness of breathing retraining in combination with cognitive strategies. Because cognitive strategies are typically included with breathing retraining, it is difficult to attribute the results specifically to breathing retraining. In an extensive review of therapeutic mechanisms, Garssen, de Ruiter, and van Dyck (1992) conclude that breathing retraining effects change through cognitive mechanisms of distraction and enhancement of a sense of control. Others have used progressive muscle relaxation techniques instead of breathing retraining. In particular, Ost (1988) reported very favorable results from applied progressive muscle relaxation in comparison to nonapplied progressive muscle relaxation.

Interoceptive exposure is emphasized particularly in the treatment protocol developed at the Center for Stress and Anxiety Disorders (Barlow & Craske, 1988). The purpose of interoceptive exposure (as in the case of exposure to external phobic stimuli) is to disrupt or weaken associations between specific bodily cues and panic reactions. Such exposure is brought about through procedures that reliably induce panic-type sensations, such as cardiovascular exercise, inhalations of carbon dioxide, spinning in a swivel chair, and hyperventilation. In the first controlled study, Barlow, Craske, Cerny, and Klosko (1989) compared the following four conditions: applied progressive muscle relaxation, interoceptive exposure plus breathing retraining and cognitive restructuring, their combination, and a wait-list control. The two conditions involving interoceptive exposure and cognitive restructuring were significantly superior to applied progressive muscle relaxation and wait-list conditions. Eighty-seven percent of the two former groups were free of panic after treatment. The results were maintained at follow-up up to 24 months following treatment completion for the group receiving interoceptive exposure and cognitive restructuring without progressive muscle relaxation, whereas the group receiving combined treatment tended to deteriorate over time (Craske, Brown, & Barlow, 1991). Nevertheless, progressive muscle relaxation was particularly effective for general anxiety reduction.

This high level of success has been replicated in several studies using similar approaches (Margraf, 1989; Michelson et al., 1990; Ost, 1988). Furthermore, the results are obtained within relatively short periods, with an average of ten sessions. However, almost all the outcome studies just described involved patients with panic disorder with minimal or no agoraphobic avoidance. An important question that awaits investigation is the extent to which panic control treatments enhance the well-established situational exposure approaches for agoraphobia at moderate or severe levels.

Pharmacotherapy. The pharmacological treatment of panic disorder has an extensive empirical base, following research conducted by Klein in 1964. Several studies have established the efficacy of the tricylic antidepressant imipramine, with 50 to 90% of patients showing moderate to marked overall improvement in panic symptoms. The dosage of imipramine has been shown to be an important variable. For example, Mavissakalian and Michelson (1986) found that 75% of patients receiving 150 mg or more per day had no or minimal symptoms at the end of treatment, compared to 25% of patients receiving 125 mg or less per day. Other tricyclic antidepressants have anti-panic effects as well. These include clomipramine and desipramine (Lydiard, 1985).

Monoamine oxidase inhibitors (MAOIs) are also effective anti-panic agents. The most commonly used drug of this class is phenelzine. However, the negative side effects of MAOIs often prohibit their use. The high-potency benzodiazepine alprazolam has been shown to be quite effective also. However, the frequent and severe withdrawal symptoms during discontinuation, and relapse after discontinuation, of alprazolam present serious problems (Fyer, Sandberg, & Klein, 1991).

It seems that drugs from a variety of classes control or reduce panic for 70% of patients, on average. The main differences among the various medical regimens appear to be side effects and patient susceptibility. However, data on drug discontinuation and follow-up are lacking or contradictory. Relapse rates have been reported to be as high as 90% in patients withdrawing from alprazolam. Follow-up studies of imipramine treatment suggest that relapse is less frequent, but further investigation is needed. Also, further investigation is needed on specific target effects of anxiolytics. Some studies suggest that medications block panic, while others suggest that the primary effect of all classes of drugs is to lessen anticipatory anxiety (Barlow, 1988).

Another issue is the combination of drug treatments with behavioral and cognitive-behavioral therapy. Even in a select sample of persons seeking help from a psychology clinic, approximately 50% reportedly use prescription anxiolytic medications (Barlow et al., 1989). The results of controlled investigations suggest that imipramine enhances the efficacy of in vivo exposure therapy for agoraphobia, and vice versa (e.g., Marks et al., 1983; Telch, Agras, Taylor, Roth, & Gallen, 1985). A recent study confirms these findings (Agras, Telch, Taylor, Roth , & Brouillard, in press). Agras et al. (in press) present some preliminary evidence to suggest that the therapeutic effect of imipramine is not on panic attacks but, rather, on phobic avoidance. To date, there are no published studies concerning the interactive effects of medications and cognitive-behavioral treatments for panic attacks.

Clinically, it is important to note the potential for interference from medications with cognitive-behavioral treatments. For example, because some medications lessen physical symptoms, behavioral treatments that emphasize exposure to feared physical sensations may be detrimentally affected. Also, clients may attribute their success to medications. The resultant lack of perceived self-efficacy may increase relapse potential when medication is withdrawn or alternately, contribute to maintenance of a medication regimen because of the client's belief that he or she cannot function without it. The soothing and sometimes sedating effects of medication may also lower levels of motivation and thereby reduce the effort and time devoted to behavioral practices. Also, side effects such as sedation may interfere with learning processes. State dependency of learning has been cited as another possible cause of increased return of fear when medication is withdrawn (Bouton & Swartzentruber, 1991).

Alternative Treatments.   Various other forms of treatment have been implemented for panic and agoraphobia. These include hypnosis, general psychotherapy, and psychoanalytic approaches (Michels, Frances, & Shear, 1985). Unfortunately, very little controlled investigation has been conducted to examine the effectiveness of these alternate treatment approaches. For this reason, and because of the established efficacy of short-term cognitive-behavioral treatments (80% rate of significant improvement, on average), a consensus statement from the National Institute of Health (1991) recommended that referrals should be made to cognitive-behavioral or medication treatments if changes are not observed within the first 6 to 8 weeks of alternative treatment. Nevertheless, continued investigation of alternate approaches is encouraged, given that not all individuals will respond well to either medication or to cognitive-behavioral treatments.

The presence of coexisting personality disturbances is not a contraindication for cognitive-behavioral therapy. Several studies have shown that patients suffering Axis II conditions still benefit from cognitive-behavioral treatments for panic, although possibly at a slower rate (e.g., Beck, 1988). In addition, sometimes the personality disturbances remit after the panic and agoraphobia have been successfully controlled (e.g., Mavissakalian & Hamman, 1987).

Selecting Optimal Treatment Strategies

Very little research has examined predictors of response to behavioral versus medication treatments. It is commonly suggested that individuals experiencing more severe symptoms would benefit most from immediate medication. However, this suggestion has not been empirically validated. A related question is whether persons seeking help from medical centers are necessarily experiencing more severe distress than are individuals seeking help from psychological centers. Again, empirical data are lacking.

Medications are possibly more appropriate for persons seeking immediate relief because of external demands. A common example is the business executive who is required to travel within the next few weeks and is particularly fearful of experiencing panic in the plane. In this case, the almost immediate sedating effects of the benzodiazepines seems to be particularly appropriate. Usually, the behavioral treatments take effect within 5 to 6 weeks, although Clark and colleagues (Hackman, Clark, Salkovskis, Wells, & Gelder, 1992) have recently shown cognitive treatment for panic to be effective within four sessions.

The presence of complicating medical factors may be an important consideration. Those who are at risk due to, for example, high blood pressure or arrhythmias may benefit from more rapid alleviation of panic symptoms through the use of benzodiazepine medications.

Problems in Carrying Out Interventions

Compliance tends to be the greatest problem with both medical and psychological interventions. The side effects of medications, particularly tricyclic antidepressants and MAOIs, frequently lead to noncompliance with medication regimens. Furthermore, individuals who are fearful of medication (which is not uncommon in panic disorder) may be less likely to comply with prescribed dosages or schedules of medication. Finally, some individuals may prefer to use medications (particularly the fast-acting benzodiazepines) on an "as needed" basis. However, some evidence suggests that "as needed" use of medication is particularly counteractive to the relearning that takes place during behavioral exposure treatments (e.g., Gray, 1987).

Noncompliance with behavioral treatment procedures arises for several reasons. First, individuals who remain intensely fearful may be less compliant. In this case the exposure practices should be designed in a graduated fashion, and more discussion of cognitive principles is likely to be helpful. The second reason for noncompliance is lack of perceived credibility of the treatment. For example, individuals may hold onto the misconception that they are different from other persons with panic disorder because of a certain symptom they experience. Third, a lack of social support may minimize motivation and compliance with the treatment. Finally, concomitant levels of depression may reduce motivation for behavioral treatment compliance.

Relapse Prevention

Unlike addiction, there has been very little work on relapse prevention with anxiety disorders. Relapse prevention is a much more important issue with medication treatments than with behavioral therapy. Long-term follow-up evaluations conducted 2 to 5 years after a behavioral treatment for agoraphobia showed very little relapse (e.g., Feigenbaum, 1988). As noted earlier, the inclusion of significant others facilitates continuing improvement after the end of treatment for agoraphobia (Cerny et al., 1987). The percentage of panic disorder patients who were panic free after receiving cognitive restructuring, interoceptive exposure, and breathing retraining was almost identical to the proportion who were panic free 2 years later in the Albany study (Craske, Brown, & Barlow, 1991). Similarly, Beck (1988) has found maintenance of therapeutic gains 1 year after treatment completion. As mentioned earlier, however, relapse after medication treatments has been a significant problem, particularly with the benzodiazepines. For that reason, several investigators are currently focusing on methods of minimizing relapse by conducting behavioral treatment procedures during discontinuation of medications. Bruce, Spiegel, Falkin, and Nuzzarello (1992) found that behavioral treatments significantly reduced withdrawal symptoms and relapse rates following the use of alprazolam.

Case Illustration

Case Description

History and Symptomatology.   Mark was a 45-year-old married man who was working as an electrician. He had experienced his first panic attack 2 years prior to treatment while working inside an elevator shaft at a library. At that time, Mark's symptoms included shortness of breath, rapid heart rate, increased sweating, dizziness, hot flashes, and a fear of dying. He was taken to the emergency room by his co-workers, where he was given a sedative to ease these symptoms, after being told that he had experienced a "common anxiety attack."

Since his first panic attack, Mark had experienced an average of one full-blown and four to six limited symptom attacks each month. Most of these episodes began with his noticing shortness of breath. The panics were most likely to occur when Mark was driving on the highway, shopping at crowded malls, or speaking to authority figures (e.g., his boss). He noted that he felt most panicky in "hot places" (e.g., elevators and small rooms). The attacks were interfering significantly with his life, as he was unable to travel far from home or to be in strange surroundings. Mark expressed considerable worry over his "next" attack (i.e., the idea of experiencing another attack was always on his mind, and he was unable to plan activities without considering how to cope with or escape from an attack). During the panic episodes, he noted that he would tell himself, "It's all right; this will be over soon." Mark usually escaped the situation and returned home, where he would listen to a relaxation tape. After his first attack, Mark had been prescribed imipramine. He was taking this drug (125 mg a day) at the time that he entered cognitive-behavioral treatment for panic. Nevertheless, Mark continued to panic, worry about panic, and avoid situations because of anticipation of panic.

Distal and Proximal Precipitating Events. Mark reported that stressful circumstances had existed at work at the time of his first attack. He felt pressured to perform at a superior level under the constant scrutiny of his boss. He noted that he was competing for a "performance award," and that he was often preoccupied with the idea of winning this prize. Additionally, around the time of his first panic, Mark was experiencing marital difficulties related to his wife's recent miscarriage.

More distally, Mark had had school phobia as a child. His fear of attending school was followed by general shyness through his elementary school years. Additionally, Mark reported that his father had been a "nervous" man who never seemed comfortable in social situations and had numerous fears (e.g., flying in airplanes) that Mark had never understood.

Differential Diagnosis and Assessment

Before beginning cognitive-behavioral treatment for panic, Mark underwent assessment procedures including a structured interview, a number of self-report instruments, and a behavioral assessment. Some of the measures included were the Anxiety Sensitivity Index (ASI) and the Mobility Inventory (see Assessment Strategies section).

Based on findings on the ADIS-R, Mark was given a diagnosis of Panic Disorder (moderate) with agoraphobia (mild). The severity of this diagnosis was 5 (on a 0–8 scale), representing a moderate level of severity. Mark's Hamilton Anxiety Scale score was 15, also reflecting moderate anxiety. Additionally, Mark's individualized Fear and Avoidance Hierarchy revealed that he was most fearful of entering crowded department stores, moderately avoidant of driving on the highway, and least fearful of being in smaller, empty stores. Items were chosen from that hierarchy for a behavioral test. First, Mark was asked to drive a short loop (i.e., one mile) around campus. Mark completed this task, during which he experienced a moderate level of anxiety. However, Mark experienced severe anxiety when he was asked to enter a crowded department store and wait in line to ask a salesperson a question. He was unable to complete the task and left the store prematurely.

Treatment Selection

Mark received a 12-session group treatment for panic disorder and agoraphobia. The therapy entailed (a) cognitive restructuring, (b) breathing and relaxation training, (c) interoceptive exposure, and (d) in vivo exposure. A brief description of each of these components of Mark's treatment follows.

Cognitive Restructuring.   After education regarding the nature of panic and the basis for anxiety symptoms, Mark learned to conceptualize the way in which his interpretations of a given event, internal or external, determined his emotional response, which in turn might confirm or disconfirm the original interpretation. Then, Mark became able to classify his own experiences in terms of the two primary cognitive errors of overestimation and catastrophization. The tendency to "jump to conclusions" regarding the meaning of panic symptoms and to magnify the negative reactions of others to his own panic attacks was explored. He realized that he usually regarded his panic symptoms as precursors to a heart attack, and that he was fearful of the potential embarrassment that he faced when experiencing an attack in public. To increase Mark's awareness of such cognitions, he was asked to keep a record of instances of overestimation or catastrophization. He recorded the situation in which his cognitions occurred, the probability that an event (e.g., heart attack) would occur as he saw it at that time, counter-cognitions based on an examination of the evidence and a search for alternatives, and a re-rating of the probability of the event. By keeping such a record, Mark was able over time to effectively combat his cognitive distortions. However, he had some difficulty accepting the idea that he could survive some level of embarrassment after experiencing an attack in public. Mark was aided toward this end by the notion that he could ask himself, "So what?" if such an event occurred, revealing to him that he was amplifying the meaning of others' reactions. Additionally, he was asked to engage in hypothesis testing by telling other people how he felt and then observing their reactions. In every case he learned that he was able to cope with their responses, which were usually more positive than he had predicted.

Breathing and Relaxation Training.   During this portion of treatment, Mark was taught to be more aware of his breathing patterns and to breathe using the muscles of his diaphragm, rather than the breathing apparatus of the upper chest. He was given a complete explanation of the physiology of overbreathing so that he would understand its purpose and effects and realize that its symptoms are rarely dangerous. To further develop this skill, he was asked to visualize a long tube running from his mouth through his chest to a chamber (i.e., the diaphragmatic cavity) at the end, and to imagine himself filling this chamber with air and then releasing it. With the help of modeling and corrective feedback from the therapist, Mark learned to breathe in and out steadily, using a 3-count (i.e., a 6-second cycle for inhalation-exhalation). To make this style of breathing more natural, Mark practiced it outside of the session, at home and at work. Although he initially felt uncomfortable focusing on his breathing, repeated practice in "safe," relaxing environments eventually enabled Mark to control his breathing effectively. Then he was able to implement this strategy when he felt anxious or experienced symptoms of anxiety.

Interoceptive Exposure.   In addition to breathing retraining, Mark was taught to be less fearful of the physiological sensations of anxiety by repeated interoceptive exposure methods. Through hyperventilating, spinning, and tube breathing (i.e, respirating through a small, narrow tube), Mark purposely brought on the shortness of breath, dizziness, and other symptoms that he associated with anxiety and panic. This procedure was repeated enough times for Mark to learn to be less fearful of the sensations aroused by the exercises and to allow for generalization to other anxiety-provoking exercises. Mark practiced inducing sensations outside of therapy as well, in order to enhance generalization away from the safety of the clinic setting. Although his overall response to this portion of treatment was good, Mark had some difficulty with the dizziness created by spinning, perhaps because he found it the most similar to his own experience of panic. With repeated practice during treatment sessions and at home, he was eventually able to experience this symptom with minimal fear.

In Vivo Exposure.   The interoceptive exposure component of Mark's treatment dealt with his fear of bodily sensations regardless of their context. The next step was to deal with the feared contexts or agoraphobic situations in which he anticipated the occurrence of panic attacks. Mark was instructed to approach the situations that he feared, as listed on his Fear and Avoidance Hierarchy, progressively. During exposures, Mark applied his cognitive restructuring and breathing retraining strategies. In addition, he was instructed to expect bodily sensations and to be objectively aware of them, rather than attempting to distract himself from his internal experiences.

On one occasion at a mall, he experienced hot flashes and the anticipation of having a panic attack. Mark escaped from this situation by retreating to his car, where he felt safer. After this experience Mark was asked to review the cognitions that intensified his fearfulness and motivated his escape behavior, and to challenge them, if possible. He noted that he was most fearful of suffering a heart attack and then being embarrassed by his condition. The "stuffiness" and heat in the mall were unexpected, inducing him to fall into his "old" cognitive style of misinterpretation. Mark was able to successfully challenge these cognitions by reviewing the probability of his having a heart attack and by asking himself, "So what if other people notice me?" Following this session he was more successful in his in vivo practice. For example, he was able to view a movie in its entirety in a crowded theater. By the end of treatment, Mark had much greater confidence in his ability to enter previously anxiety-provoking situations, and he had given up many of the "safety signals" (e.g., a paper bag for breathing) that he had carried earlier. However, he reported that he had not been able to relinquish his use of a relaxation tape that he carried with him into arousing situations. As medications can be, the relaxation tape was a source of reassurance for Mark that he had a "tool" on hand should he become anxious.

Outcome and Termination

After the twelve sessions Mark felt that he had been "cured" of his panic disorder. He was able to enter formerly anxiety-provoking places and situations (e.g., malls, elevators, and highway driving) with little anxiety, and he was using cognitive techniques regularly when faced with anxiety symptoms (e.g., he no longer felt that anxiety was a signal of an impending heart attack).

A posttreatment ADIS-R assessment revealed that in the month following treatment, Mark experienced one limited-symptom panic attack involving hot flashes and dizziness, and no full-blown attacks (Figure 7.3). Additionally, he had a very mild level of worry concerning his next attack; he thought about panic attacks only "in passing." Similarly, Figure 7.3 depicts Mark's Anxiety Sensitivity Index and Mobility Inventory scores; as demonstrated by the graph, they were significantly reduced from pre-

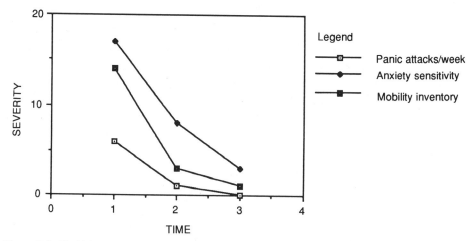

Figure 7.3. Mark's improvement on three measures of panic disorder over time (Time 1 = Prettreatment, Time 2 = Posttreatment, Time 3 = 6-month follow-up).

treatment ratings, reflecting Mark's decreased agoraphobia and interoceptive sensitivity.

Mark was assigned a posttreatment diagnosis of "Panic Disorder in Remission." However, he continued to take medication (a reduced dosage of imipramine) and to use his relaxation tape during the posttreatment period. Additionally, he noted that he desired to maintain contact with his therapist, "just in case" he suffered any additional attacks. In other words, a mild level of apprehension was still present.

Follow-Up and Maintenance

A follow-up assessment revealed that Mark continued to improve over the 6 months following treatment. As demonstrated in Figure 7.3, Mark was panic free; he had experienced no limited-symptom or full-blown attacks during the 3 months prior to the follow-up. Similarly, Mark's scores on the other measures were lower than his posttreatment ratings (see Figure 7.3). He was able to attend movies and shop at crowded malls and markets regularly, and he had taken a 6-hour drive during a recent vacation. Additionally, Mark rarely worried about experiencing a panic attack, and he had discontinued his medication and the use of the relaxation tape. Mark felt secure about his future experience of anxiety, and he was able to discontinue comfortably his contact with the therapist.

Summary

The cognitive-behavioral treatments for agoraphobia, and more recently for panic attacks, are impressively effective. A series of independent investigations has shown that an average of 70 to 90% of panic sufferers stop panicking after cognitive-behavioral treatment. Similarly, agoraphobic avoidance significantly diminishes for 70 to 80% of persons who complete treatment. Several areas are in need of further exploration: the combination of cognitive-behavioral and medication approaches; the combination of cognitive-behavioral approaches for panic and for agoraphobia; and generalization of cognitive-behavioral approaches to individuals with other problems in addition to panic disorder and agoraphobia (these include personality disorders, substance abuse, and complicating medical conditions). Treatment of panic disorder is one of the most exciting areas of psychotherapy, given the success being demonstrated for treatment of this very common and severely debilitating condition.

References

Agras, W. S., Telch, M. J., Taylor, C. B., Roth, W. T., & Brouillard, M. (in press). Imipramine and exposure therapy in agoraphobia: The type of exposure may matter. *Behavior Therapy*.

Alneas, R., & Torgersen, S. (1990). DSM-III personality disorders among patients with major depression, anxiety disorders, and mixed conditions. *Journal of Nervous and Mental Disease, 178*, 693–698.

American Psychiatric Association (1980). *Diagnostic and statistical manual of mental disorders* (3rd ed.). Washington, DC: Author.

American Psychiatric Association (1987). *Diagnostic and statistical manual of mental disorders* (3rd ed., rev.). Washington, DC: Author.

Azrin, N., Naster, B., & Jones, R. (1973). Reciprocity counselling: A rapid learning-based procedure for marital counselling. *Behaviour Research and Therapy, 11*, 365–382.

Barlow, D. H. (1988). *Anxiety and its disorders: The nature and treatment of anxiety and panic*. New York: Guilford.

Barlow, D. H. & Craske, M. G. (1988). *Mastery of your anxiety and panic*. Albany, NY: Graywind.

Barlow, D. H., Craske, M. G., Cerny, J. A., & Klosko, J. S. (1989). Behavioral treatment of panic disorder. *Behavior Therapy, 20*, 261–282.

Barlow, D. H., O'Brien, G. T., & Last, C. G. (1984). Couples treatment of agoraphobia. *Behavior Therapy, 15*, 41–58.

Barlow, D. H., Vermilyea, J., Blanchard, E., Vermilyea, B., DiNardo, P., & Cerny, J. (1985). Phenomenon of panic. *Journal of Abnormal Psychology, 94*, 320–328.

Beck, A. T. (1988). Cognitive approaches to panic disorder: Theory and therapy. In S. J. Rachman & J. D. Maser (Eds.), *Panic: Psychological perspectives* (pp. 91–110). Hillsdale, NJ: Erlbaum.

Beck, A. T., Epstein, N., Brown, G., & Steer, R. A. (1991). An inventory for measuring clinical anxiety; the Beck Anxiety Inventory. *Journal of Consulting and Clinical Psychology, 56*, 893–897.

Bourdon, K. H., Boyd, J. H., Rae, D. S., Burns, B. J., Thompson, J. W., & Locke, B. Z. (1988). Gender differences in phobias: Results of the ECA community survey. *Journal of Anxiety Disorders, 2*, 227–241.

Bouton, M., & Swartzentruber, D. (1991). Sources of relapse after extinction in Pavlovian conditioning and instrumental conditioning. *Behavioral Neuroscience, 104*, 44–55.

Breier, A., Charney, D. S., & Heninger, G. R. (1986). Agoraphobia with panic attacks. *Archives of General Psychiatry, 43*, 1029–1036.

Bruce, T. J., Spiegel, D. A., Falkin, S. M., & Nuzzarello, A. (1992, March). *Does cognitive behavioral therapy assist slow-taper alprazolam discontinuation in panic disorder?* Poster presented at the conference of the National Anxiety Disorders Association of America, Houston.

Burns, L. E., Thorpe, G. L., & Cavallaro, L. A. (1986). Agoraphobia eight years after behavioral treatment: A follow-up study with interview, self-report, and behavioral data. *Behavior Therapy, 17*, 580–591.

Carr, D. B., & Sheehan, D. V. (1984). Panic anxiety: A new biological model. *Journal of Clinical Psychiatry, 45*, 323–330.

Cerny, J. A., Barlow, D. H., Craske, M. G., & Himadi, W. G. (1987). Couples treatment of agoraphobia: A two-year follow-up. *Behavior Therapy, 18*, 401–415.

Chambless, D. L. (1989, November). *Spacing of exposure sessions in the treatment of phobia.* Poster presented at the convention of the Annual Association for the Advancement of Behavior Therapy, New York.

Chambless, D. L., Caputo, G., Bright, P., & Gallagher, R. (1984). Assessment of fear in agoraphobics: The Body Sensations Questionnaire and the Agoraphobic Cognitions Questionnaire. *Journal of Consulting and Clinical Psychology, 52*, 1090–1097.

Chambless, D. L., Caputo, G., Gracely, S., Jasin, E., & Williams, C. (1985). The Mobility Inventory for agoraphobia. *Behaviour Research and Therapy, 23*, 35–44.

Chambless, D., & Renneberg, B. (1988, September). *Personality disorders of agoraphobics*. Paper presented at World Congress of Behavior Therapy, Edinburgh, Scotland.

Chaplin, E. W., & Levine, B. A. (1981). The effects of total exposure duration and interrupted versus continued exposure in flooding therapy. *Behavior Therapy, 12*, 360–368.

Clark, D. M. (1988). A cognitive model of panic attacks. In S. Rachman & J. D. Maser (Eds.), *Panic: Psychological perspectives* (pp. 71–89). Hillsdale, NJ: Erlbaum.

Clark, D., Salkovskis, P., & Chalkley, A. (1985). Respiratory control as a treatment for panic attacks. *Journal of Behavior Therapy and Experimental Psychiatry, 16*, 23–30.

Clark, D. M., Salkovskis, P., Gelder, M., Koehler, C., Martin, M., Anastasiades, P., Hackmann, A., Middleton, H., & Jeavons, A. (1988). Tests of a cognitive theory of panic. In I. Hand & H. Wittchen (Eds.), *Panic and phobias II* (pp. 71–90). Berlin: Springer-Verlag.

Cohen, S. D., Monteiro, W., & Marks, I. M. (1984). Two-year follow-up of agoraphobics after exposure and imipramine. *British Journal of Psychiatry, 144*, 276–281.

Craske, M. G., Brown, T. A., & Barlow, D. H. (1991). Behavioral treatment of panic disorder: A two-year follow-up. *Behavior Therapy, 22*, 289–304.

Craske, M. G., Curtis, G. C., McNally, R. J., Ost, L. G., & Salkovskis, P. (1992). An integrative review of issues related to the diagnosis of Simple Phobia. *DSM-IV Source Book*. Washington, DC: American Psychiatric Press.

Craske, M. G., Miller, P. P., Rotunda, R., & Barlow, D. H. (1990). A descriptive report of features of initial unexpected panic attacks in minimal and extensive avoiders. *Behaviour Research and Therapy, 28*, 395–400.

Craske, M. G., Street, L., & Barlow, D. H. (1989). Instructions to focus upon or distract from internal cues during exposure treatment for agoraphobic avoidance. *Behaviour Research and Therapy, 27*, 663–672.

Crowe, R. R. (1985). The genetics of panic disorder and agoraphobia. *Psychiatric Developments, 2*, 171–186.

DiNardo, P., & Barlow, D. H. (1988). *Anxiety Disorders Interview Schedule—Revised (ADIS-R)*. Albany, NY: Phobia and Anxiety Disorders Clinic, The University of Albany, State University of New York.

Ehlers, A., & Breuer, P. (1992). Increased cardiac awareness in panic disorder. *Journal of Abnormal Psychology, 101*, 371–382.

Emmelkamp, P. M. G., & Ultee, K. A. (1974). A comparison of "successive approximation" and "self-observation" in the treatment of agoraphobia. *Behavior Therapy, 5*, 606–613.

Feigenbaum, W. (1988). Long-term efficacy of ungraded versus graded massed exposure in agoraphobics. In I. Hand & H. Wittchen (Eds.), *Panic and phobias: Treatments and variables affecting course and outcome* (pp. 149–158). Berlin: Springer-Verlag.

Foa, E. B., Jameson, J. S., Turner, R. M., & Payne, L. L. (1980). Massed vs. spaced exposure sessions in the treatment of agoraphobia. *Behaviour Research and Therapy, 18*, 333–338.

Foa, E. B., & Kozak, M. S. (1986). Emotional processing of fear: Exposure to corrective information. *Psychological Bulletin, 99*, 20–35.

Fyer, A. J., Sandberg, D., & Klein, D. F. (1991). The pharmacological treatment of panic disorder and agoraphobia. In J. R. Walker, G. R. Norton, and C. A. Ross (Eds.), *Panic disorder and agoraphobia: A comprehensive guide for the practitioner* (pp. 211–251). Belmont, CA: Brooks/Cole.

Garssen, B., de Ruiter, C., & van Dyck, R. (1992). Breathing retraining. A rational placebo? *Clinical Psychology Review, 12*, 141–153.

Gray, J.A. (1987). *The psychology of fear and stress*. Cambridge, UK: Cambridge University Press.

Hackmann, A., Clark, D., Salkovskis, P., Wells, A., & Gelder, M. (1992, June). *Making cognitive therapy for panic more efficient: Preliminary results with a four session version of treatment*. Paper presented at the World Congress of Cognitive Therapy, Toronto, Canada.

Hafner, R. J. (1976). Fresh symptom emergence after intensive behavior therapy. *British Journal of Psychiatry, 129*, 378–383.

Hamilton, M. (1959). A rating scale for depression. *British Journal of Medical Psychology, 32*, 50–55.

Hamilton, M. (1960). The assessment of anxiety states by rating. *Journal of Neurology, Neurosurgery, & Psychiatry, 23*, 56–62.

Jacobson, N. S., Wilson, L., & Tupper, C. (1988). The clinical significance of treatment gains resulting from exposure-based interventions for agoraphobia: A re-analysis of outcome data. *Behavior Therapy, 19*, 539–554.

Jansson, L., Jerremalm, A., & Ost, L.-G. (1986). Follow-up of agoraphobic patients treated with exposure in-vivo or applied relaxation. *British Journal of Psychiatry, 149*, 486–490.

Jansson, L., & Ost, L.-G. (1982). Behavioral treatments for agoraphobia: An evaluative review. *Clinical Psychology Review, 2*, 311–336.

Klein, D. F. (1964). Dissection of two drug-responsive anxiety syndromes. *Psychopharmacologia, 5*, 397–408.

Lydiard, B. (1985, October) *Desipramine in panic disorder: An open fixed-dose study*. Paper presented at the meeting of the American Academy of Clinical Psychiatry, San Francisco.

Margraf, J. (1989, June). *Comparative efficacy of cognitive, exposure, and combined treatments for panic disorder*. Paper presented at the annual meeting of the European Association for Behavior Therapy, Vienna.

Margraf, J., Taylor, C. B., Ehlers, A., Roth, W. T., & Agras, W. S. (1987). Panic attacks in the natural environment. *Journal of Nervous and Mental Disease, 175*, 558–565.

Marks, I. M. (1971). Phobic disorders four years after treatment: A prospective follow-up. *British Journal of Psychiatry, 118*, 683–686.

Marks, I., Grey, S., Cohen, S. D., Hill, R., Mawson, D., Ramm, E., & Stern, R. (1983). Imipramine and brief therapist-aided exposure in agoraphobics having self-exposure homework: A controlled trial. *Archives of General Psychiatry, 40*, 153–162.

Marshall, W. L. (1985). The effects of variable exposure in flooding therapy. *Behavior Therapy, 16*, 117–135.

Mavissakalian, M., & Hamman, M. (1986). DSM-III personality disorder in agoraphobia. *Comprehensive Psychiatry, 27*, 471–479.

Mavissakalian, M., & Hamman, M. (1987). DSM-III personality disorder in agoraphobia: II. Changes with treatment. *Comprehensive Psychiatry, 28*, 356–361.

Mavissakalian, M., & Michelson, L. (1986). Two-year follow-up of exposure and imipramine treatment of agoraphobia. *American Journal of Psychiatry, 143*, 1106–1112.

Michels, R., Frances, A. J., & Shear, M. K. (1985). Psychodynamic models of anxiety. In A. H. Tuma & J. D. Maser (Eds.), *Anxiety and the anxiety disorders* (pp. 595–618). Hillsdale, NJ: Erlbaum.

Michelson, L., Mavissakalian, M., Marchione, K., Ulrich, R., Marchione, N., & Testa, S. (1990). Psycho-physiological outcome of cognitive, behavioral, and psychophysiologically-based treatments of agoraphobia. *Behaviour Research and Therapy, 28*, 127–139.

Munby, J., & Johnston, D. W. (1980). Agoraphobia: The long-term follow-up of behavioural treatment. *British Journal of Psychiatry, 137*, 418–427.

Myers, J., Weissman, M., Tischler, C., Holzer, C., Orvaschel, H., Anthony, J., Boyd, J., Burke, J., Kramer, M., & Stoltzam, R. (1984). Six-month prevalence of psychiatric disorders in three communities. *Archives of General Psychiatry, 41*, 959–967.

National Institute of Health. (1991, September 25–27). *NIH Consensus Development Conference on Panic, 9*, No. 2.

Norton, G., Dorward, J., & Cox, B. (1986). Factors associated with panic attacks in nonclinical subjects. *Behavior Therapy, 17*, 239–252.

Noyes, R., Crowe, R. R., Harris, E. L., Hamra, B. J., McChesney, C. M., & Chaudhry, D. R. (1986). Relationship between panic disorder and agoraphobia: A family study. *Archives of General Psychiatry, 43*, 227–232.

Noyes, R., Reich, J., Suelzer, M., & Christiansen, J. (1991). Personality traits associated with panic disorder: Change associated with treatment. *Comprehensive Psychiatry, 32*, 282–294.

Ost, L.-G. (1988). Applied relaxation vs. progressive relaxation in the treatment of panic disorder. *Behaviour Research and Therapy, 26*, 13–22.

Pollard, C. A., Pollard, H. J., & Corn, K. J. (1989). Panic onset and major events in the lives of agoraphobics: A test of contiguity. *Journal of Abnormal Psychology, 98*, 318–321.

Rachman, S. J., Craske, M. G., Tallman, K., & Solyom, C. (1986). Does escape behavior strengthen agoraphobic avoidance? A replication. *Behavior Therapy, 17*, 366-384.

Rapee, R. M. (1985). A case of panic disorder treated with breathing retraining. *Behavior Therapy and Experimental Psychiatry, 16*, 63–65.

Rapee, R. M, Craske, M. G., & Barlow, D. H. (1990). Subject described features of panic attacks using a new self-monitoring form. *Journal of Anxiety Disorders, 4*, 171–181.

Rapee, R. M., Litwin, E. M., & Barlow, D. H. (1990). Impact of life events on subjects with panic disorder and on comparison subjects. *American Journal of Psychiatry, 147*, 640–644.

Rapee, R. M., Mattick, R., & Murrell, E. (1986). Cognitive mediation in the affective component of spontaneous panic attacks. *Journal of Behavior Therapy and Experimental Psychiatry, 17*, 245–253.

Reich, J., Noyes, R., & Troughton, E. (1987). Dependent personality disorder associated with phobic avoidance in patients with panic disorder. *American Journal of Psychiatry, 144*, 323–326.

Reiss, S., Peterson, R., Gursky, D., & McNally, R. (1986). Anxiety sensitivity, anxiety frequency, and the prediction of fearfulness. *Behaviour Research and Therapy, 24*, 1–8.

Roy-Byrne, P. P., Geraci, M., & Uhde, T. W. (1986). Life events and the onset of panic disorder. *American Journal of Psychiatry, 143*, 1424–1427.

Salkovskis, P., Clark, D., & Hackmann, A. (1991). Treatment of panic attacks using cognitive therapy without exposure or breathing retraining. *Behavior Research and Therapy, 29*, 161–166.

Salkovskis, P., Warwick, H., Clark, D., & Wessels, D. (1986). A demonstration of acute hyperventilation during naturally occurring panic attacks. *Behaviour Research and Therapy, 24*, 91–94.

Sanderson, W. C., DiNardo, P. A., Rapee, R. M., & Barlow, D. H. (1990). Syndrome comorbidity in patients diagnosed with a DSM-III-R anxiety disorder. *Journal of Abnormal Psychology, 99*, 308–312.

Spanier, G. (1976). Measuring dyadic adjustment: New scales for assessing the quality of marriage and similar dyads. *Journal of Marriage and the Family, 38*, 15–38.

Spielberger, C., Gorsuch, R., Lushene, R., Vagg, P., & Jacobs, G. (1983). *Manual for the State-Trait Anxiety Inventory*. Palo Alto, CA: Consulting Psychologists Press.

Spitzer, R. L., & Endicott, J. (1979). *The Schedule for Affective Disorders and Schizophrenia—Lifetime Version* (3rd ed.). New York: New York State Psychiatric Institute, Biometrics Research.

Spitzer, R. L., Williams, J. B. W., & Gibbon, M. (1987). *Structural Clinical Interview for DSM-III-R (SCID)*. New York: New York State Psychiatric Institute, Biometrics Research.

Stern, R. S., & Marks, I. M. (1973). Brief and prolonged flooding: A comparison of agoraphobic patients. *Archives of General Psychiatry, 28*, 270–276.

Telch, M. J. (1988). Combined pharmacological and psychological treatments for panic sufferers. In S. Rachman & J. D. Maser (Eds.), *Panic: Psychological perspectives* (pp. 167–187). Hillsdale, NJ: Erlbaum.

Telch, M. J., Agras, W. S., Taylor, C. B., Roth, W. T., & Gallen, C. (1985). Combined pharmacological and behavioral treatment for agoraphobia. *Behaviour Research and Therapy, 21*, 505–527.

Telch, M. J., Lucas, J. A., & Nelson, P. (1989). Nonclinical panic in college students: An investigation of prevalence and symptomatology. *Journal of Abnormal Psychology, 98*, 300–306.

Telch, M. J., Sherman, M., & Lucas, J. (1989). Anxiety sensitivity: Unitary personality trait or domain specific appraisals? *Journal of Anxiety Disorders, 3*, 25–32.

Weissman, M. M. (1986). The relationship between panic disorder and agoraphobia: An epidemiologic perspective. *Psychopharmacology Bulletin, 22*, 787–791.

Williams, S. L., & Zane G. (1989). Guided mastery and stimulus exposure treatments for severe performance anxiety in agoraphobics. *Behaviour Research and Therapy, 27*, 237–245.

Wolpe, J., & Rowan, V. (1988). Panic disorder: A product of classical conditioning. *Behaviour Research and Therapy, 26*, 441–450.

8

Social Phobia

Richard P. Mattick and Gavin Andrews

Description of the Disorder

Clinical Features

Social phobia was first delineated from other anxiety disorders in the 1960s, being described by Taylor (1966), in a classic summary, as affecting patients who

> . . . avoid all competitive activities, such as examinations or games; . . . are unable to talk to superiors, to appear in front of an audience, to eat in a restaurant or even at home when another person is present, to sit opposite others on a bus or in a tube, to have people walk behind them, to walk past a queue of people, to look at themselves in a mirror. They may be unable to write, or to carry on any routine activity, when they feel themselves under observation. Some can only leave their house when it is so dark or foggy that they cannot easily be seen. Some have a fear of blushing or of attracting attention by behaving awkwardly or fainting (p. 160).

Marks (1969) noted that these patients are able to engage in certain activities "only as long as nobody's eyes are upon them. A glance from another person will precipitate the phobia concerned" (p. 153). In these early descriptions the emphasis was on circumscribed *scrutiny fears*. Yet there is often a more pervasive fear of criticism and an avoidance of social interaction—but more of that later.

DSM-III (American Psychiatric Association, 1980) suggested that social phobia was a relatively circumscribed disorder, and although it was noted to be chronic and unremitting, it was said to be rarely incapacitating. Liebowitz, Gorman, Fyer, and Klein (1985), contrary to this view, reported that socially phobic individuals are often markedly impaired in occupational, educational, and social functioning. This report

Richard P. Mattick • National Drug and Alcohol Research Centre and Clinical Research Unit for Anxiety Disorders, University of New South Wales, Sydney 2033 Australia.   **Gavin Andrews** • Clinical Research Unit for Anxiety Disorders, University of New South Wales, Sydney 2010 Australia.

Handbook of Prescriptive Treatments for Adults, edited by Michel Hersen and Robert T. Ammerman. Plenum Press, New York, 1994.

has been confirmed by Turner, Beidel, Dancu, and Keys (1986) and others (Cappe & Alden, 1986), who have presented findings that indicate that for the majority of sufferers in their clinic, the disorder had a significant impact on life functioning, and although there was no "report of complete incapacitation, significant impairment was highly prevalent" (Turner et al., 1986, p. 391).

Not only is significant impairment frequent, but social phobia can be a complex disorder. Contrary to early suggestions (American Psychiatric Association, 1980), it is frequently multiphobic, with fears of specific situations where one may be observed undertaking everyday activities (e.g., eating, drinking, writing, signing documents, speaking in front of a group, simply appearing in public places, using public toilets) often coexisting; as noted earlier, there may also be a pervasive anxiety about social interactions (Mattick & Peters, 1988; Mattick, Peters, & Clarke, 1989; Turner et al., 1986). DSM-III-R (American Psychiatric Association, 1987) has made this point by specifying two aspects of disturbance in social phobia: the circumscribed fears of scrutiny mentioned above, and the more "general fears of [social interactions, including] saying foolish things or not being able to answer questions" (p. 241). Two-thirds of a clinical sample suffer this generalized disorder, in addition to fears of multiple specific situations (Mattick et al., 1989). It is apparent that we can no longer consider social phobia a monosymptomatic phobia with minimal impact on the sufferer.

Associated Features

DSM-III-R suggests that, if there is generalized avoidance of most social situations, the additional diagnosis of avoidant personality disorder should be considered. Inspection of the criteria for this disorder indicates that the avoidant personality is likely to show a "pattern of social discomfort, fear of negative evaluation, and timidity, beginning in early adulthood, and present in a variety of contexts" (p. 352). Whereas some socially phobic individuals may show fear and avoidance of only a relatively circumscribed set of social situations, and otherwise function reasonably well in social interactions, others will display a generalized inability to make and maintain interpersonal relationships resulting from fear of rejection, of acting foolish, or of being embarrassed by showing signs of anxiety in front of others. The description in DSM-III-R does not do full justice to the potential extent and nature of the underlying pathology in the avoidant personality based on clinical impression and the descriptions of Millon (1969).

Millon (1969) has provided an insightful summary of the Avoidant Personality, not available in the bland descriptions found in the taxonomies:

> Anxiety-ridden, denied encouragement and belittled and disparaged in childhood, the avoidant personality has a deep mistrust of others and a markedly deflated image of his own self-worth. He has learned through bitter experience that the world is unfriendly, cold and humiliating, and that he himself has few personal skills and talents. . . . He expects to be slighted and demeaned wherever he turns; he has learned to be watchful, to be on guard against the ridicule and contempt he anticipates from others. He must be ever-alert, exquisitely sensitive to [often imagined] signs of censure and derision. And looking inward offers him no solace since he finds none of the attributes he admires in others (p. 237).

These patients are characterized by long-standing, pervasive, and active withdrawal from social relationships, they are utterly devastated by perceived disapproval, and they are constantly vigilant for any signs of ridicule (Millon, 1981). Nichols (1974) has catalogued a similar list of traits as typical of "severe social anxiety," suggesting an overlap (rather than a discontinuity) between the phobia and more pervasive maladaptive personality traits (cf. Kendell, 1975). Findings of recent studies have been largely consistent in this regard, suggesting that generalized social phobia and avoidant personality disorder are overlapping problems that have only minor differences in terms of the severity of the dysfunction and symptoms present (Herbert, Hope, & Bellack, 1992; Holt, Heimberg, & Hope, 1992; Turner, Beidel, & Townsley, 1992). This result is also consistent with clinical experience, and it is noteworthy that the introduction of the diagnosis of avoidant personality into DSM-III-R was not based on any empirical studies demonstrating a discontinuity (Kendell, 1975) between social phobia and the personality disorder.

Several other problems are associated with social phobia. Research has indicated that self-medication using alcohol or prescribed anxiolytic medications is frequent, and that it is not unusual for this self-medication to escalate into significant substance abuse (Liebowitz et al., 1985; Mattick & Peters, 1988; Mattick et al., 1989; Stockwell, Smail, Hodgson, & Canter, 1984). Significant depressive symptoms are reported to be quite common, being found in half the patients in one study (Amies, Gelder, & Shaw, 1983), one in eight of this large sample having a history of "parasuicidal" acts. It has also been reported that there are frequently clinically significant levels of generalized anxiety (Liebowitz et al., 1985). Most recently, Schneier, Jonson, Hornig, Leibowitz, and Weissman (1992) reported that clinical social phobia shows substantial comorbidity, especially with other anxiety disorders and depressive disorders. Only 31% of those with social phobia had no other lifetime disorder. This study also confirmed the presence of alcohol and drug abuse, as well as suicidal ideation and suicide attempts.

Epidemiology

The 1-month, 6-month, and lifetime prevalence of social phobia has been estimated at 1.3, 1.5, and 2.8%, respectively (Regier et al., 1990). Overall, based on this study, social phobia appears to be present in one-third of the instances of "clinical phobias" (social and agoraphobia combined). However, the figures reported are likely to overestimate the prevalence of "pure" social phobia: agoraphobic patients may also suffer social phobia symptoms (Marks, 1987), and the Myers et al. (1984) study did not report clearly on the co-occurrence of social phobia with an agoraphobia diagnosis.

Etiology

There is a consensus that an excessive fear of negative evaluation by others underlies the disorder. Butler (1985, 1989), among others, has argued that reduction of this fear is an important mediator of improvement, and that the disorder may be resistant to treatment that does not include a "cognitive element." In support of this view, others have been able to show that the extent to which the fear of negative evaluation is reduced within treatment is predictive of long-term functioning (e.g., Mattick & Peters, 1988; Mattick et al., 1989).

Similarly, the importance of social skills deficits and their role in maintaining the disorder has received some attention, with early workers focusing on attempting to teach appropriate skills to sufferers on the assumption that their difficulties were due in large part to a lack of appropriate social skills. According to this argument the disorder may occur from faulty socialization (such as inadequate parental models or simply a lack of social experience). Certainly an apparent lack of social skills may be secondary to some other pathology, but in practice an apparent lack of appropriate skills seems here to be taken at face value without any presumption of an underlying disturbance. In those cases in which a lack of social skill is secondary, sufferers may have their normally adequate (and intact) social repertoire inhibited or disrupted by anxiety. Marks (1985) has argued for a distinction between social phobia and social skills deficit in terms of descriptive factors and treatment response, asserting that the presence of apparent skills deficits suggests the diagnosis of avoidant personality disorder. In support of this assertion, Turner et al. (1986) have reported that patients with the avoidant personality disorder diagnosis do exhibit significantly poorer social skills than do socially phobic individuals without that diagnosis, although as noted elsewhere in this chapter the disorders appear to be continuous. Others have developed sociological interpretations, suggesting that there is a crucial period for learning social fearfulness, and that a social hierarchy exists that affects some individuals by making them anxious and withdrawn (Ohman, 1986).

Viewed critically, the majority of these explanations of the etiology of social phobia are speculative, circular, or without any solid supporting evidence. More recently, sophisticated statistical modeling procedures have been used to demonstrate an important genetic component in the genesis of the anxiety disorders (Andrews, Stewart, Allen, & Henderson, 1990; Kendler, Neale, Kessler, Heath, & Eaves, 1992), although it remains a matter of debate whether there is a general contribution to "neurotic" symptoms or specific heritability of distinct anxiety disorders (Andrews et al., 1990). Kendler et al. (1992) have reported an impressive twin study in which it was found that the familial co-occurrence of *any* phobia appears to result from genetic but not from familial-environmental factors (a result that does not eliminate environmental influences from having an important role). Consistent with the genetic twin study research findings are the intriguing results reported by Kagan, Reznick, and Snidman (1988), who studied shyness in children in two longitudinal studies and found evidence of a biological basis of social restraint and avoidance. The role of environmental influences has also been attested to by this research into genetic factors, although the environmental factors responsible have yet to be identified. These important etiological issues are addressed in more detail elsewhere (Mattick, Page, & Lampe, in press).

Differential Diagnosis and Assessment

DSM-III-R and DSM-IV Categorization

If the essence of social phobia (as discussed earlier in this chapter) is the fear and avoidance of situations in which one might be exposed to scrutiny while undertaking routine activities and then become anxious, possibly perform poorly, and thereafter be judged negatively, then it is of interest how well the classifications describe this syndrome. A summary of the diagnostic criteria of three classification systems is presented in Table 8.1. The DSM-III-R criteria are published, the DSM-IV criteria were still in draft form but essentially final (Taskforce on DSM-IV, 1993), and the ICD-10 Diagnostic Criteria for Research are published (World Health Organization, 1993).

ICD-10 is included because it is the lingua franca for recording health information throughout the world, although with the adoption in DSM-IV of the ICD-10 numerical system, it will become the de facto standard in North America without the need for the cross coding necessary with DSM-III and ICD-9 CM.

Given that all three descriptions were the result of committee deliberations, it is surprising how similar they are in broad terms. DSM-IV has changed the diagnostic criteria very little from DSM-III-R, and this seems to be fully appropriate given the small amount that has been learned about the disorder over the past 6 years. Much more work is necessary in determining the nature of the disorder, and studying the pattern of symptoms will be required before we can usefully alter the criteria. Alteration without such information would be based on personal opinions, and that is not a suitable basis for the development of an international taxonomy.

There will be discussion over the clinical significance of the detailed wording of the various criteria, but in broad terms, whereas DSM-III-R and DSM-IV are very similar, ICD-10 contains two important differences. The first is that in order for one to make the diagnosis, the person must have had, in a feared situation, either blushing, or fear of vomiting, or urgency or fear of micturition or defecation. There is no mention of sweating, shaking, trembling, or similar common symptoms of the disorder. Clinically, this ICD-10 requirement is too narrow. It may well be that all social phobics

TABLE 8.1. Comparison of the DSM-III-R, ICD-10, and DSM-IV Diagnostic Criteria for Social Phobia

DSM-III-R 300.23 Social phobia	ICD-10 F40.1 Social phobias	DSM-IV F40.1 Social phobia
A. Fear of scrutiny in case of humiliation (e.g., speaking poorly, trembling, unable to eat, unable to urinate in the presence of others)	A. Marked fear and avoidance of being the focus of attention or embarrassment or humiliation occurring in such social situations	A. Marked fear of social or performance situations in case of actions or anxiety that will be humiliating or embarrassing
C. Exposure to feared situation provokes anxiety	B. Exposure to feared situation provokes anxiety; required is a fear of vomiting, micturition, defecation, or blushing	B. Exposure to feared situation provokes anxiety
	E. Symptoms linked to feared situations	
F. Person recognizes that the fear is excessive or unreasonable	D. Person recognizes that the fear or avoidance is excessive or unreasonable	C. Person recognizes that the fear is excessive or unreasonable
D. Phobic situation is avoided or endured with anxiety	A. (Avoidance is included in criterion A.)	D. Phobic situation is avoided or endured with anxiety
E. Disorder distresses or handicaps	C. Disorder produces significant distress	E. Disorder distresses and handicaps
B. Not due to other mental disorder	F. Not due to organic mental disorders, depression, schizophrenia, or obsessive compulsive disorder	F. Not substance induced, not secondary to panic disorder or schizoid personality disorder
B. Not due to physical disorder	No equivalent criterion present, although ICD-10 criterion D makes DSM-IV criterion G redundant	G. Not an expected reaction to stuttering, Parkinson's disease, or other nonanxiety disorder

Source: World Health Organization (1993), Taskforce on DSM-IV (1993).

do have such symptoms or concerns, in which case this diagnostic restriction is not important, but if research shows that a significant number of individuals complaining of fear and distress in social situations do not experience such symptoms but do meet the other criteria, then wise clinicians using ICD-10 will ignore this proviso. Clinically, our experience tells us that the application of this criterion would exclude many patients from the diagnosis, and because of this problem we strongly question the use of this system for diagnosing this disorder. The other difference between the DSM-III-R and ICD systems is that ICD-10 mentions the very real possibility that some persons with psychotic disorders, or with obsessive-compulsive disorder, will fear and avoid social situations. Further enquiry will make it clear that neither anxiety nor fear of humiliation or embarrassment is the driving force behind these behaviors.

Differential Diagnosis

In all phobias the clinician should avoid making a quick diagnosis based on the situation that is feared and avoided, at least until the reason for this behavior is clarified. For instance, in the ICD-10 caveats listed in Table 8.1, psychotic patients when asked will explain their delusional beliefs and persons with obsessive-compulsive disorder explain the obsession that is driving the avoidance.

The principal differential diagnostic problem will be distinguishing social phobia from panic disorder with agoraphobia. Both groups of patients can avoid crowded places like shopping centers, movie theaters, concert halls, and formal social occasions; both groups commonly avoid public transportation; but because the cognitions associated with each disorder differ considerably, patients respond differently when asked the reason. Agoraphobics are concerned about the physical consequences of panic and reply, "In case I panic, collapse, and die." Social phobics, on the other hand, are concerned about social evaluation and reply, "In case others present notice I am anxious." Often the disorders coexist and patients exhibit both types of cognitions, but when symptoms of both are present, one set of cognitions usually is perceived as secondary to the other. The agoraphobic who primarily fears the panic outcome may also think that it would be embarrassing to collapse or lose control. The social phobic who avoids primarily because of fear of negative evaluation may also find the severity of the panic aversive and at times will also avoid for fear of panic. In both cases only the criteria for the primary diagnosis are satisfied even though elements of both syndromes are present. If the clinician is in doubt the question "Could you perform/cope in front of an audience of blind persons?" often produces clarification. Social phobics understand the intend of the question and answer that they could, or, more rarely, explain why the blind would still be able to detect the anxiety in their voice. Agoraphobics who are afraid for their own physical safety should they panic, psychotic persons who are preoccupied with their delusions, and persons with obsessive-compulsive disorder who are reacting to the obsessional fear will be mystified at what they consider a dumb question, and eager to clarify the reason behind their fear and avoidance.

Schizoid personality disorder (characterized by coldness, aloofness, and indifference to others) is a cause of people's not establishing friendships and not attending social functions, but the motivation is clearly different. The sufferer does not fear or avoid the situation; he or she simply does not see why ordinary humans value the personal interactions that occur in such situations. This disorder should seldom cause confusion with social phobia. Avoidant personality disorder is quite different. A majority of persons who meet criteria for either 301.82 DSM-III-R or F60.6 ICD-10 avoidant personality disorder will also meet criteria for social phobia. Conversely, some proportion (in our clinical material about one-third) of persons presenting for treatment for social phobia will also meet criteria for the more severe and disabling personality disorder. We have already mentioned the relationship between the two syndromes and find that, in clinical practice, they are best considered to be two aspects of the same or very closely related disorders. One important reason to identify whether a patient meets criteria for avoidant personality disorder is that treatment is considerably more difficult. At the conclusion of our 80-hour cognitive-behavioral program for social phobia, persons with social phobia without personality disorder are mastering their fears and their avoidances, whereas persons with avoidant personality disorder as well are only just beginning to do so. We have doubled the length of the program, we have emphasized social skills training and conducted special programs for persons with avoidant personality disorder, and we are still unconvinced that we have an effective remedy for this condition. It is severe, chronic, and unresponsive. Therefore, the importance of differentiation is in regard to prognosis: one can expect to cure a narrow social phobia, but one cannot expect to do the same with avoidant personality disorder. Where the phobia ends and the personality disorder picks up is unclear, and this issue and treatment response should remain a focus for research.

Avoidance of public places also occurs in persons with physical illnesses such as epilepsy, episodic cardiac arrhythmias, and severe diabetes, and in persons withdrawing from psychoactive substances. Again the reason behind the avoidance will differentiate these conditions from social phobia. Although the phenomenon is mentioned in DSM-IV, persons with stuttering, Parkinson's disease, or eating disorders—or any disfiguring disorder—rarely shrink from public scrutiny. We have experience with chronic and severe adult stutterers. We are constantly amazed at the normalcy of their social and work relationships, for unlike persons with social phobia, they do not perceive their disorder to lessen their intrinsic worth to others. Persons with parkinsonism or eating disorders seem to perceive themselves no differently than do the rest of us. The inclusion of stuttering, Parkinsonism, and eating disorder as special conditions in DSM-IV may have been related more to the concerns of members of the committee over careful diagnosis than to realities of clinical presentation.

Assessment Strategies

The purpose of conducting an assessment is to ensure that the correct diagnosis is made, to identify any serious comorbid conditions, to identify personality and coping strengths and weaknesses, and to explore the detailed ramifications of the disorder in the patient. The purpose of conducting the assessment in a standardized fashion is to ensure that opinions on which treatment is to be based will be in accord with standard and accepted criteria. Clinical judgment is a necessary, but no longer sufficient, basis for constructing a treatment plan.

The instruments used for assessment will vary from clinic to clinic. The procedures adopted in our clinic are as follows. When patients first attend, having been referred for treatment of a putative anxiety disorder, they complete a questionnaire battery before seeing the clinician. The intake battery consists of the Eysenck Personality Inventory (Eysenck & Eysenck, 1964), the Locus of Control of Behavior Scale (Craig, Franklin, & Andrews, 1984), the Defense Style Questionnaire (Andrews, Pollock, & Stewart, 1989), the Hopkins Symptom Checklist-90R (SCL-90R; Derogatis, 1977), and a questionnaire designed to tap panic attacks, phobic avoidance, and related cognitions. Each patient is then seen by a clinician, who takes a diagnostic history and makes a formulation based on the letter from the referring agency, the computer-scored results of the intake battery, and the results of the clinical interview. Additionally, a formal diagnosis is made.

Given a patient with uncomplicated social phobia, by the end of the first interview, the clinician would expect to have elicited symptoms consistent with that diagnosis, clarified the extent of current prescription medication and any self-medication with drugs or alcohol, and discussed a treatment plan. The clinician would expect that Eysenck Neuroticism and Introversion scores would be more than one standard deviation above the population mean, as would scores on the Locus of Control of Behavior Scale and the Immature factor of the Defense Style Questionnaire. Likewise, the panic, phobia, and cognitions questionnaire results should support the clinical picture, as should the scores on the Anxiety, Phobia, and Interpersonnel Sensitivity Scales on the SCL-90R. When the questionnaire results are not in accord with expectations, then the clinician should consider alternative diagnoses along the lines discussed earlier, or consider whether current substance use or dependence are clouding the current presentation. If, however, the picture is consistent, we make an offer of treatment conditional on a further assessment. The clinician, then, with the patient's help, encapsulates the patient's principal complaint. Fear of scrutiny is often identified as the principal complaint in social phobia, and the patient rates the extent to which this fear now interferes with his or her "life and activities" and the extent to which it did 12 months earlier.

On a second assessment day each patient completes the Anxiety, Depression, and Substance Use sections of the computerized Composite International Diagnostic Interview (World Health Organization, 1990) and further questionnaires, including the Fear of Negative Evaluation and Social Avoidance and Distress Scales (Watson & Friend, 1969), and then the patient is interviewed by an independent clinician, who administers the Personality Disorder Examination (Loranger, Susman, Oldham, & Russakoff, 1987). Given that all the information is consistent with the diagnosis of social phobia and that there is no drug or alcohol dependence, major depressive episode, or personality disorder other than avoidant personality disorder, the patient will be accepted for treatment.

The intake questionnaire, the Fear of Negative Evaluation scale, and the patient's individualized principal complaint statement are used to assess progress with both symptoms and the underlying vulnerability to social phobia. These questionnaires are readministered immediately prior to treatment, at the end of treatment, and 3 months and 12 months later. Other specific measures of aspects of the disorder are available, and the interested reader is directed to the work of Beidel, Turner, and Cooley (1993) and Heimberg, Mueller, Holt, Hope, and Leibowitz (1992), for information on these newly developed scales.

Treatment

Evidence for Prescriptive Treatments

Given that narrow views of the complexity of social phobia have only recently been superseded, it is unsurprising that treatment approaches reported on have tended toward narrow (and relatively brief) interventions. These interventions have generally derived from unitary models of the disorder. Among the postulated causes of the disorder are the conditioning approaches, irrational and maladaptive thought processes, and social skills deficits. It may not be surprising that just as there has been relatively little empirical research on the nature of this disorder, the treatment outcome literature in this area is limited.

Much of the early research focused on behavioral interventions (skills training and exposure), and only recently have cognitive interventions and pharmaco-therapies been investigated. It is very disappointing that there have been few trials combining pharmacotherapy and psychotherapeutic interventions to address the possibility of synergistic effects, and this is an important area for future research, especially for the more severe cases involving generalized social anxiety or avoidant personality.

Behavior Therapy. Early studies of the effectiveness of exposure therapies using systematic desensitization in imagination suggested that these approaches were of limited value (see review by Marks, 1985). Later work examined the effect of in vivo exposure therapy and found the approach to exert statistically and clinically significant effects on social phobia (e.g., Butler, Cullington, Munby, Amies, & Gelder, 1984; Mattick & Peters, 1988; Mattick et al., 1989). Yet it has been reported that simple exposure to the feared situation does not always produce the cognitive changes that are thought to be required to maximize progress (e.g., Butler et al., 1984; Mattick et al., 1989).

Skills training has been found to be useful for patients suffering from avoidant personality. Two studies have reported skills training to be superior to exposure therapy (Cappe & Alden, 1986; Trower, Yardley, Bryant, & Shaw, 1978). Additionally, skills training has been found effective for social phobia where skills deficits are not present, a result that possibly is due to the systematic and repeated exposure to social stimuli that skills training, by its nature, involves (Trower et al., 1978).

The general clinical impression that social phobia is a disorder that is more "cognitively mediated" than other phobias has given rise to a small number of trials examining the effects of a variety of cognitive therapies. Despite the view that excessive fears of negative evaluation by others is the single most important diagnostic, underlying, and maintaining process in the disorder (cf. Bulter, 1985), the supporting evidence is rather sparse. Similarly, the argument that cognitive restructuring approaches have a unique or specific role in the treatment of the disorder remains tentative: firstly, the research on the role of cognitive interventions for the disorder has not clearly supported the efficacy of these approaches beyond that of more traditional exposure-based and skill-based approaches, and second, even those studies that have supported the role of cognitive interventions (although suggestive) cannot be used to argue that faulty cognitions are an important maintaining factor. Simply classifying therapeutic techniques as cognitive or behavioral on procedural grounds and subsequently implying different mechanisms of action is to confuse process with procedure, and it is well recognized that relying on the results of experiments contrasting such procedures with each other to suggest the nature of the disorder under study is a weak experimental approach. The success (or failure) of a therapeutic procedure that is said to act through a certain mechanism does not necessarily imply that it does in fact act through that mechanism.

Two types of study examining the role of cognitive interventions for this disorder have been conducted: those comparing the effects of cognitive therapy alone (i.e., without concurrent behavioral interventions) with the results with therapy, and those comparing the effects of combined cognitive therapy and behavioral approaches with the outcome of a behavioral intervention alone. In the first case the results are equivocal. Early research suggested that brief cognitive therapy did not have a role in the treatment of the condition (e.g., Biran, Augusto, & Wilson, 1981). More recently, Emmelkamp, Mersch, Vissia, and Van der Helm (1985) reported results showing that both self-instructional training and rational-emotive therapy were essentially equivalent to exposure therapy in their effects on the disorder. Similarly, Mattick et al. (1989) reported data to indicate that cognitive restructuring without additional behavioral treatment could have a significant and lasting impact upon the disorder, although the effects were slow in appearing relative to those of the behavioral (exposure-based) treatments used. Note that the gains obtained in the studies with cognitive component per se, as this approach may act to motivate patients to undertake self-directed exposure. No study to date has adequately addressed this possibility, although there have been attempts (e.g., Mattick et al., 1989).

Four studies have assessed whether cognitive restructuring conferred benefits beyond those achieved by behavioral interventions. The results have been generally positive, with one null finding. One study by Stravinski, Marks, and Yule (1982) reported that brief cognitive therapy did not increase the effects of social skills training for socially dysfunctional patients. Butler et al. (1984), in contrast, reported that exposure was inferior to exposure combined with an anxiety management package involving "rational self-talk." However, the fact that the latter anxiety management package also contained relaxation and distraction techniques makes it impossible to ascribe the superiority of the combined intervention solely to the cognitive component. Two recent studies have indicated that socially phobic patients do improve more with a combination of cognitive restructuring and behavioral therapy (exposure in vivo) than with behavioral therapy alone, although between-group differences were apparent for only some of the outcome variables assessed (Mattick & Peters, 1988; Mattick et al., 1989). Thus, while there are data to support the role of cognitive procedures with this disorder, the evidence is not particularly compelling, and those advantages that have been found for cognitive procedures have been slight. It may be that the cognitive treatments used have been too brief and focused to show their potential (cf. Biran et al., 1981; Stravinski et al., 1982), and that longer and more intensive therapy is required to maximize their effects. This is certainly our clinical experience, and it will be important to study the effectiveness of more intensive psychotherapeutic treatments using these procedures, especially given the limited gains that can accrue from treatment.

Turning away from the relative effects of these treatment approaches to the issue of the mechanisms whereby they might exert their effects, we receive little guidance from the literature. Research has shown that reduction in fear of negative evaluation is predictive of long-term outcome (Mattick & Peters, 1988; Mattick et al., 1989). However, this finding might be critically viewed as trivial and obvious. Put simply, changes in the cardinal symptom of the disorder might reasonably be expected to correlate well with patient status. Even so, the importance of ensuring that excessive concerns over the opinions of others are decreased cannot be overlooked in treatment. It remains for the research community to turn attention to the factors that are responsible for optimal outcome to better allow us to understand the mechanisms that underlie the effects of these treatments.

Little attention has been given to assessing the clinical significance of the changes that treatment achieves. Only a few studies have addressed the issue. Using stringent criteria of end-state functioning, it has been found that only about one-third (37 and 33%, respectively) of patients who receive relatively brief cognitive-behavioral interventions achieve high or very high end-state functioning (Mattick & Peters, 1988; Mattick et al., 1989). Thus, some two-thirds of patients treated with such methods are likely to be left with significant pathology, although the majority do show improvement in symptoms. Some basic efforts have been made to categorize patients as responders or nonresponders to pharmacotherapeutic interventions (Liebowitz et al., 1992). Future studies must routinely assess end-state functioning in this order. It may be that improved outcomes will be achieved through broadening the range of intervention provided, and that greater treatment duration will enhance outcome.

Pharmacotherapy. The research on pharmacotherapy also has not been extensive. It generally favors the effects of the monoamine oxidase inhibitor (MAOI) phenelzine, and has usually failed to address the issue of the return of symptoms after discontinuation of medication. Early clinical trials suggested that both beta-adrenergic blockers and MAOIs might be of benefit. The evidence for the role of the beta-blockers came mostly from studies of performance anxiety in students, musicians, and other groups that were not necessarily socially phobic (see the review by Liebowitz et al., 1985). Open clinical trials with socially phobic patients in research attempting to infer the presence of an underlying pathophysiological state showed positive effects for both MAOIs and beta-blockers (Klein & Leibowitz, 1985), while others found no advantage of beta-blockers over placebo (Falloon, Lloyd, & Harpin, 1981).

Recently, Gelernter and colleagues (1991) compared the effects of cognitive-behavioral treatment without medication, alprazolam plus self-exposure instructions, phenelzine plus self-exposure instructions, and placebo medication plus self-exposure instructions. The treatments were delivered over a 12-week period. Significant changes resulted across the course of treatment for all of the groups involved. The effect of each of the therapies was roughly equivalent, suggesting that cognitive-behavioral intervention without medication is as effective as medication with basic exposure instructions. Unfortunately, the study did not look at the synergistic potential of psychological and pharmacological interventions. To its credit, the study also incorporated a withdrawal phase during which patients receiving pharmacotherapy had their medication tapered and then discontinued. No condition showed consistent superiority over another, but a follow-up conducted some 2 months after a 4-week tapering showed an interesting pattern of results. The phenelzine group continued to show an advantage over placebo, whereas the subjects in the alprazolam group deteriorated to be equivalent in their status to subjects in the placebo group. An arbitrary method of determining whether patients were treatment "responders" or "nonresponders" produced evidence favoring the MAOI: 69% of the phenelzine-treated group were categorized as responders compared with 38%, 24%, and 20% of the alprazolam treated, cognitive-behaviorally treated, and placebo-treated patients, respectively. How these subjects appear in the medium to longer term is not reported in this study, and it would be impressive if the MAOIs maintained their benefits. This would also be a result out of keeping with the typical outcome associated with the removal of medication in the treatment of anxiety disorders, and with clinical expectations given the nature of social phobia; a return of symptoms is usual.

Yet, more recent research has suggested an advantage for MAOIs over other medications and placebo in blind controlled research (Liebowitz et al., 1992). Liebowitz et al. (1992) have reported that MAOI phenelzine to be markedly superior to either a beta-blocker (atenolol) or placebo among 74 patients who met criteria for social phobia. The rationale provided by these authors for the use of an MAOI in the treatment of social phobia was the fact that this class of drugs has previously been found to be efficacious in the treatment of depression, and that depression and social phobia have in common "the feature of interpersonal hypersensitivity (excessive perception of and/or difficulty coping with criticism or rejection from others)" (p. 290). These authors do not mention the fact that MAOIs appear to have a general anxiolytic effect, and that such a general mechanism is the most parsimonious explanation for the effects of these drugs. Nor is there any discussion of the role of tricyclic antidepressants. They found at the end of a 16-week treatment phase that phenelzine was superior to placebo, but that atenolol produced an intermediate effect that did not differ significantly from the effects of either placebo or the MAOI. They also found evidence that patients with generalized social phobia symptoms were preferentially responsive to the MAOI, suggesting that the more severe form of the disorder may be specifically targeted by these more powerful psychotropic drugs.

The conclusion that is drawn from this research is that MAOIs are effective treatments, especially for the more generalized and severe social phobias, but the long-term impact of these drugs, after they have been discontinued, is unclear. Symptomatic relief will also occur with benzodiazepine administration, but relief will tend to disappear when the medication is withdrawn. Discrete or specific social phobias are more likely to respond to beta-blockers, which are not a useful intervention for the more severe and pervasive variants of the disorder. It is likely that other medications, such as the tricyclic antidepressants, will be found to have a role with this disorder, and it would be unfortunate if the neuropsychiatric researchers who test the efficacy of these drugs infer a unique or specific pathophysiology based on a drug response (as has occurred with other anxiety disorders).

Alternative Treatments. There is no published evidence for the efficacy of other treatment approaches for this disorder. Psychodynamic and other interpretative psychotherapies have not been tested, and it remains for proponents of these approaches to provide even the most basic evidence of the power of these interventions. Until such time they must be considered to be unproven procedures for the treatment of this disorder.

Selecting Optimal Treatment Strategies

The optimal treatment strategy will take into account the severity of the problem and prior treatment history. In some cases of very highly circumscribed and infrequently occurring phobic reactions (for occasional speeches, or for musicians who react only when performing), selective intervention with a beta-adrenergic blocker (preferably atenolol) will be useful to reduce the peripheral signs of anxiety, and this should be considered especially if other approaches have been tried without success. More generalized and severe social phobias will respond poorly to beta-blockers alone, and their use is not recommended in such cases.

Relatively circumscribed and specific fears (e.g., of eating, drinking, writing, walking past crowds, being in public places), even when more than one is present in a given patient, will usually respond well to repeated, graduated exposure and cognitive restructuring involving daily homework assignments, along with additional procedures (such as relaxation training, and hyperventilation control) to ameliorate any generalized anxiety symptoms and thereby potentiate the effects of exposure. For more severe cases of social phobia, especially where there is a generalized social anxiety present, more prolonged procedures are advocated, as is an exploration of self-image issues within a cognitive therapy framework. When a diagnosis of avoidant personality disorder is present, there is likely to be a need for longer-term contact. The intention of such longer-term contact and psychological intervention is to maintain and extend the benefits derived from a standard cognitive-behavioral approach. The ability of this longer-term therapy to exert beneficial effects has yet to be established in empirical research. It was noted earlier that interpretative psycho-therapies possess no evidence of efficacy, and given the clear evidence that is available for the effectiveness of cognitive-behavioral approaches in this disorder, there can be no justification for choosing untested and unproven techniques.

Pharmacotherapy is unlikely to provide long-term alteration in symptoms, and cessation of medication will typically result in relapse. It is not recommended that medication be used, except in three circumstances. First, if psychotherapeutic procedures have had no or limited effect, the phobia is deemed to be incapacitating, *and* when the adequacy of the delivery of the nonpharmacologic procedures has been checked (nondrug treatments are not always delivered faithfully or well), medication can be tried Anxiolytic medication (MAOIs or benzodiazepines) is preferable to self-medication with alcohol, which can escalate into significant substance abuse. The second use of medication is in cases in which the feared situation occurs infrequently (e.g., speech giving); medication here is preferable to no treatment, or to failing to offer the sufferer any assistance. The third use of medication is with a patient who is suffering significant distress; medication can be used to provide temporary relief while psychotherapeutic procedures are put in place. Medication has an important role to play, but it cannot be expected to cure a (typically) long-standing disorder like social phobia.

Problems in Carrying Out Interventions

One major problem unique to the social phobias relates to exposure therapy. Clinicians who employed exposure in the United Kingdom in the early days of the use of exposure treatment lamented the failure of unsupervised exposure. Send the phobic alone and unaided into the feared situation and fear the worst result: the maintenance or exacerbation of the fear. For the social phobic, the feared conse-quence is that others will evaluate him negatively. Since the patient cannot easily have this fear disconfirmed through exposure (whereas the fears involved in other phobias are more easily disconfirmed), exposure can prove less effective (cf. Foa & Kozak, 1986). Given that it is unusual for others in fact to be negatively evaluating the patient, it is important to address the feared consequences more directly through cognitive restructuring. Butler (1985) has provided an excellent discussion of this problem and other difficulties in the behavioral treatment for the disorder. She lists four principal difficulties, including the difficulty already discussed. Second, she notes that tasks cannot always be clearly specified, repeated, or graduated because of the unpredict-able nature of social situations. Third, many social interactions are necessarily time limited, and it is difficult to organize the prolonged exposure required for a decline in anxiety to occur. Fourth, many social phobics will avoid relatively few social situa-tions, although they endure those they enter with significant anxiety.

A further problem relates to the conduct of cognitive restructuring treatment. There is a danger that the patient will not believe the alternative explanations and appraisals of the actions and thoughts of other people who observe them. Our experience is that occasionally a patient will dutifully practice rational reappraisals of the imagined feared consequences of behaving awkwardly or appearing anxious, without improvement. Upon careful questioning it becomes clear that the patient does not believe the reappraisals. Thus, it is important to ensure that the interpretations that the patient practices during cognitive restructuring are believed. This can best be achieved by getting the patient to actually ask a friend or another patient (in group programs) whether the feared negative evaluation occurred. Typically the friend will not have noticed the problem that the patient fears has been seen (e.g., shaking). Even if it is noticed, it is generally disregarded, or at worst thought of as a symptom of anxiety. If the patient probes further, it will usually become apparent that the friend does not think of the sufferer as the odd, inferior person that she imagines. Getting patients to "test out" their beliefs is a useful strategy in itself. To skip this procedure is to slow the rate of recovery, or in the worst case stall improvement completely.

Relapse Prevention

Relapse prevention has been little addressed for anxiety disorders generally, and for social phobia specifically. Because social phobia is a chronic disorder, there is little reason to believe that a relatively brief, circumscribed intervention will be sufficient to always ensure success. Research with unassertive persons has shown the value of "booster" sessions, and it is strongly recommended that such sessions be a part of treatment for social phobia. As a guide, these sessions should be scheduled at monthly intervals for 4 months and then spaced 2 months apart for a further 8 months if the patient is progressing adequately. This will allow the patient to receive structured support in practicing skills learned within treatment proper, and will allow the clinician to assist in dealing with new situations as they arise during the patient's new found freedom.

Case Illustration

Case Description

Patient Identification.   Mr. Jones is a 35-year-old married man who works as an accountant for a large company. He was referred by his family doctor for attacks of anxiety, for which the doctor had prescribed diazepam.

Presenting Complaint.   He sought help because he feared, and whenever possible avoided, business meetings, particularly those at which he had to speak. At those meetings, and to a lesser extent in anticipation of such occasions, he became anxious and panicky, and complained that he experienced a pounding heart, trembling, sweating, and blushing. He felt that he was unable to speak clearly or fluently, and tended to minimize the duration of time that he spoke. He feared that others would notice his anxiety and consequently decide that he was unreliable and unsuited for promotion within his organization. He sought help at this time because his fear and avoidance of meetings were jeopardizing his chances of promotion to middle management.

History of Presenting Complaint. He had first noticed being uncomfortable in social situations at high school. At that stage and in the early years of college it was not difficult to remain unnoticed, but in the final year at college, when seminars had to be presented, he took to relieving his anxiety with alcohol prior to his presentations. His early years in the workforce also allowed him to be anonymous but lately, with increasing seniority and responsibility, he found it impossible to avoid all presentations.

He said that the most social situations in which he could possibly be a focus of attention caused him distress. He was not anxious at home with his wife and family or with his own parents, but he found visiting his wife's family stressful. He avoided writing or computing if others were looking over his shoulder, avoided telephoning if others were listening, avoided parties if possible, was uncomfortable traveling by public transportation, especially if he could not get a seat at the back of the bus or train, and was uncomfortable standing in lines. In these situations he was concerned that he might do something foolish or embarrassing—"Like they would see me blush or my hands shake and then they would never respect me again." He said that while he "sort of knew" that these fears were excessive, he could not put them out of his mind. Although he could force himself to endure a stressful presentation, his critical reworking of the experience sensitized him further and made the next presentation no easier.

Previous Psychiatric and Medical History. He had not previously sought help. His local doctor reported that he was in good physical health, although some years previously he had noted that the patient was consuming too much alcohol. The patient had been using alcohol to alleviate his symptoms of anxiety in work and social situations but was able to follow advice and reduce his intake.

Family and Personal History. He described his mother as nervous and his younger sister as shy and a worrier, "a bit like me." Neither had sought help. He was the eldest of three children in a blue collar family. He was the only son, and his mother had placed considerable pressure on him to secure a respectable white collar job. He described himself as having been a normal child, not particularly shy or anxious, in elementary school. In high school he began to feel self-conscious and instead of being overly concerned ("I thought I'd grow out of it," he said), he was able to direct his energies into his studies. He did well, gained a degree in commerce, and had been with the same company since graduation. His social anxieties meant he socialized little and did not have a girlfriend until he met his wife, to whom he was devoted; "She is one of the few people I really trust," he said. She had been a secretary at his workplace but had since retired to care for their two children. He described her as quiet but sociable, and his constant excuses to avoid social interaction distressed her and placed a strain on the marriage.

Mental State at Examination. Mr. Jones was a neatly attired man who appeared ill at ease and initially avoided eye contact. Although nervous, he did not obviously blush, shake, or sweat, even though he apologized for doing so. His speech was fluent and there was no evidence of delusions, hallucinations, or significant depression. At the end of this interview he identified his principal complaint as fear of scrutiny and identified it as interfering with his life and activities almost totally. He was made a provisional offer of treatment and returned for the second assessment interview.

Differential Diagnosis and Assessment

He scored 17/23 on the Eysenck Neuroticism scale and 3/23 on the Extraversion scale, both scores 1.5 standard deviation (SD) units from the population mean. He scored 30 on the locus of control measure, within the normal range, indicating that although the disorder was chronic he had been able to continue his life despite it. He scored 2 SD above the mean on the Immature factor of the Defense Style Questionnaire, endorsing the projection and devaluation items very highly, and scored normally on the Mature factor, which reflected his ability to stoically endure if avoidance was not possible. On the Fear of Negative Evaluation scale, he endorsed 26 of 30 items, a high score typical of this disorder. On the Personality Disorder Examination he met criteria for two items (DSM-III-R 5 and 6, the social phobic items) and was therefore diagnosis negative; he met one criterion for dependent personality disorder, again diagnosis negative. On the SCL-90R he scored high on anxiety, phobias, and interpersonal sensitivity. On the computerized Composite International Diagnostic Interview, his only current diagnosis was social phobia, onset at age 15, although he met criteria for alcohol dependence from age 21 to age 27.

No differential diagnosis was considered to be sufficiently likely to warrant additional investigations. The unreasonable fear of negative evaluation provoked significant anxiety in situations in which he could come under scrutiny. Some of the physiological reactions of anxiety caused further distress in themselves, for he worried that they would proclaim his anxiety to others and thereby attract negative evaluation. Avoidance of social situations was prominent and responsible for marital stress and lost job opportunities. Although there was overlap with agoraphobia in some of the situations avoided, there was a different underlying fear. This fear the patient recognized as excessive, and there were no features to suggest schizophrenia or obsessive-compulsive disorder. He would socialize if it were not for his anxiety, hence schizoid personality disorder was excluded. Avoidant personality disorder, a common comorbid condition, was excluded by the normal findings on the Personality Disorder Examination.

Treatment Selection

This patient had tried self-medication with alcohol. His family doctor had given him prescriptions for diazepam. Although there are drugs reported to help this disorder, we could not assure the patient of their proven long-term efficacy, and he, as might be expected from his scores on the locus of control scale and mature coping factor, was keen to learn to control the disorder himself. As he commented, "I asked around and came to you because of your reputation for nondrug treatment." We recommended the cognitive-behavioral therapy program for social phobia.

Treatment Course and Problems in Carrying Out Interventions

The program is conducted in a small discussion group format, usually with about six people in a group. The treatment is intensive: 9:00 A.M. to 5:00 P.M. Monday through

Friday in week 1, homework assignments for week 2, and then full days again for 5 days in week 3; yielding 80 hours of therapy in all. The compliance rate is high. Treatment follows a 70-page treatment manual (Andrews, 1991) issued to each patient and read and discussed with the therapist during the sessions. There are seven sections to the manual and hence to the program: education about the nature of anxiety and social phobia; control of hyperventilation and panic; relaxation training; graded exposure and the control of situational fears; specific anxieties in social phobia; cognitive restructuring; and assertiveness, included because the person with fear of negative evaluation becomes unassertive and it is helpful to address this specifically. The treatment schedule is iterative, with patients encouraged to work completely through the manual in the first few days, and then as feared tasks are completed to use the anxiety management and cognitive restructuring sections again and again to develop full mastery.

The anxiety management strategies are standard and are taught first, giving patients techniques to control their anxiety as they confront their situational fears. Beginning on day 1 and continuing throughout the 10 days, about half the time is spent in confronting situational fears—beginning with brief, simple impromptu talks in front of the group, soon videotaped and played back, and ending with a formal presentation in an auditorium to a group of strangers. Parallel with this graded hierarchy of speaking tasks, hierarchies of eating, drinking, and writing, or whatever group members identify as tasks that they previously avoided, are developed and carried out. In both weeks of active treatment group members separately and together carry out a variety of tasks in which they perform in public, drawing attention to themselves and challenging the public to think less of them. Associated with each graded exposure task from day 4 of the program onwards, patients are encouraged to identify the associated cognitions, identifying, disputing, challenging, and reframing their irrational beliefs. Cognitive restructuring must address two core distortions: The risk of being negatively evaluated is always exaggerated, as are the unpleasant consequences of negative evaluation. Patients can be helped to confront these issues if asked, "How likely is it that people will notice? How likely are they to evaluate negatively? How much does it matter?"

Teaching the anxiety management package is relatively simple. Supervising graded exposure tasks outside the clinic is more difficult. Patients are tempted to confront the core fear only partially, and the therapist must remain alert to this. The most difficult task is to gradually restructure the cognitions, for they are endemic. It is here that the experience and reasonableness of the therapist and the opinions of the other members of the groups can be important in allowing patients to explore the cognitions, see the irrationality, and finally experiment with the rational thinking patterns that are essential to their long-term recovery. Mr. Jones, like many patients, said it perfectly: "I force myself to confront feared situations but it does not get any easier." It only gets easier when the irrational cognitions are identified and replaced with more accurate and realistic thinking.

During the assessment period we ascertain whether people are using alcohol, benzodiazepines, or other relevant psychoactive substances. If so, we attempt an arrangement with a withdrawal program prior to the social phobia treatment program. We believe, without data, that if consciousness is clouded by such substances, new learning does not occur. Also, occasionally we have found that patients will increase their use of psychotropic substances to cope with exposure rather than using the anxiety management procedures or adjusting the difficulty of the exposure tasks. We therefore exclude from the program persons who use alcohol or drugs to help them confront difficult situations during the treatment program. This exclusion is, of course, contrary to the research evidence that suggests that drug-dependent persons can benefit from psychotherapeutic procedures, both in their drug use and in their psychiatric symptoms (Ward, Mattick, & Hall, 1992), but the exclusion makes the program function more easily, and that is our main aim. Such individuals should be provided assistance in a one-to-one therapeutic intervention.

Outcome and Termination

During the program, Mr. Jones mastered the anxiety management skills quickly and soon ceased to comment on sweating, shaking, or blushing. He gradually mastered the development of task hierarchies, becoming quite adept at dividing tasks into subsets of easier components. During the cognitive restructuring sessions, he learned that he was excessively fearful of negative evaluation, reviewing all comments made about his performance for their critical and aggressive content and devaluing all compliments. He gradually learned to identify these distortions and very slowly began to see things more rationally. His final public presentation was excellent in form and content. In discussion afterward he was able to accept credit and even took home a videotape to show his wife. At the end of treatment his locus of control scale had further internalized, his score on the Immature defense factor had fallen, and the score on the Fear of Negative Evaluation Scale had fallen to 18/30.

Follow-Up and Maintenance

Mr. Jones attended follow-up sessions at 3 and 12 months. At 3 months he reported that he was continuing to look for opportunities to make presentations of gradually increasing difficulty at work and that he had begun to socialize. His relationship with his wife was improving as his social relationships normalized. At the 5-month point he came back for an additional consultation prior to an interview for an important job with a different company, which he obtained. At 12 months he no longer met criteria for social phobia on the Composite International Diagnostic Interview, his Eysenck Neuroticism scale had fallen to 12/23, his locus of control and defense style measures remained low, and his fear of negative evaluation score was now 14/30 (normal). He now rated his principal complaint—fear of scrutiny by others—as affecting his life and activities only a little. His introversion score remained low. He was discharged as cured and his cased closed.

Summary

Social phobia occurs in 1 to 2% of the population and is often a chronic, debilitating, and severe disorder that has tended to be unrecognized in its effects on the sufferer. Fears of scrutiny while undertaking routine activities frequently coexist with a more generalized social anxiety, or avoidant personality disorder. Self-medication by social phobics with alcohol and anxiolytic agents is frequent, as is substance abuse, depression, and other anxiety disorders.

Differential diagnosis of social phobia from agoraphobia, schizoid personality disorder, psychotic disorders, and other anxiety disorders is generally achieved by clarifying the reasons for fear and avoidance. Assessment should take the form of a standardized battery and address the diagnosis, comorbid states, the situations avoided, reasons for avoidance, and personality variables, such as fear of negative evaluation.

Treatment research has attested to the efficacy of cognitive-behavioral therapy for the disorder. It appears that the reduction of excessive concerns about the opinions of others combined with repeated exposure and anxiety management procedures can bring about lasting changes in fear and avoidance, as well as in symptoms that appear to underlie the disorder. Beta-blockers (for reactions in which peripheral signs of anxiety are paramount) and MAOIs (for more generalized reactions) are effective while they are taken, but based on current evidence they are no more effective than cognitive-behavioral approaches. Benzodiazepines also assist by providing symptomatic relief.

References

American Psychiatric Association (1980). *Diagnostic and statistical manual of mental disorders* (3rd ed.). Washington, DC: Author.

American Psychiatric Association (1987). *Diagnostic and statistical manual of mental disorders* (3rd ed., rev.). Washington, DC: Author.

Amies, P. L., Gelder, M. G., & Shaw, P. M. (1983). Social phobia: A comparative clinical study. *British Journal of Psychiatry, 142*, 174–179.

Andrews, G. (1991). *Social phobia treatment manual*. Darlinghurst, Sydney: Clinical Research Unit for Anxiety Disorders, St. Vincent's Hospital.

Andrews, G., Pollock, C., & Stewart, G. (1989). The determination of defense style by questionnaires. *Archives of General Psychiatry, 46*, 455–460.

Andrews, G., Stewart, G., Allen, R., & Henderson, A. S. (1990). The genetics of six neurotic disorders: A twin study. *Journal of Affective Disorders, 19*, 23–29.

Beidel, D. C., Turner, A. M., & Cooley, M. R. (1993). Assessing reliable and clinically significant change in social phobia: Validity of the Social Phobia and Anxiety Inventory. *Behaviour Research and Therapy, 31*, 331–337.

Biran, M., Augusto, F., & Wilson, G. T. (1981). In vivo exposure vs. cognitive restructuring in the treatment of scriptophobia. *Behaviour Research and Therapy, 19*, 525–532.

Butler, G. (1985). Exposure as a treatment for social phobia: Some instructive difficulties. *Behaviour Research and Therapy, 23*, 651–657.

Butler, G., (1989). Issues in the application of cognitive and behavioral strategies to the treatment of social phobia. *Clinical Psychology Review, 9*, 91–106.

Butler, G., Cullington, A., Munby, M., Amies, P., & Gelder, M. (1984). Exposure and anxiety management in the treatment of social phobia. *Journal of Consulting and Clinical Psychology, 52*, 642–650.

Cappe, R. F., & Alden, L. E. (1986). A comparison of treatment strategies for clients functionally impaired by extreme shyness and social avoidance. *Journal of Consulting and Clinical Psychology, 54*, 796–801.

Craig, A., Franklin, J., & Andrews, G. (1984). A scale to measure locus of control of behaviour. *British Journal of Medical Psychology, 57*, 173–180.

Derogatis, L. R. (1977). *SCL-90 revised version manual*. Baltimore: Johns Hopkins Hospital School of Medicine.

Emmelkamp, P. M. G., Mersch, P. P., Vissia, E., & Van der Helm, M. (1985). Social phobia: A comparative evaluation of cognitive and behavioral interventions. *Behaviour Research and Therapy, 23*, 365–369.

Eysenck, H. J., & Eysenck, S. B. G. (1964). *Manual of the Eysenck Personality Inventory*. London: University of London Press.

Falloon, I. R. H., Lloyd, G. G., & Harpin, R. E. (1981). Real-life rehearsal with nonprofessional therapists. *Journal of Nervous and Mental Disease, 169*, 180–184.

Foa, E. B., & Kozak, M. J. (1986). Emotional processing of fear: Exposure to corrective information. *Psychological Bulletin, 99*, 20–35.

Gelernter, C. S., Uhde, T. W., Cimbolic, P., Arnkoff, D. B., Vittone, B. J., Tancer, M. E., & Bartko, J. J. (1991).

Cognitive-behavioral and pharmacological treatments of social phobia: A controlled study. *Archives of General Psychiatry*, *48*, 938–945.

Heimberg, R. G., Mueller, G. P., Holt, C. S., Hope, D. A., & Leibowitz, M. R. (1992). Assessment of anxiety in social interaction and being observed by others: The social interaction anxiety scale and social phobia scale. *Behavior Therapy*, *23*, 53–73.

Herbert, J. D., Hope, D. A., & Bellack, A. S. (1992). Validity of the distinction between generalized social phobia and avoidant personality disorder. *Journal of Abnormal Psychology*, *101*, 332–339.

Holt, C. S., Heimberg, R. G., & Hope, D. A. (1992). Avoidant personality disorder and the generalized subtype in social phobia. *Journal of Abnormal Psychology*, *101*, 318–325.

Kagan, J., Reznick, J. S., & Snidman, N. (1988). Biological bases of childhood shyness. *Science*, *240*, 167–171.

Kendell, R. E. (1975). *The role of diagnosis in psychiatry*. Oxford: Blackwell Scientific.

Kendler, K. S., Neale, M. C., Kessler, R. C., Heath, A. C., & Eaves, L. J. (1992). The genetic epidemiology of phobias in women: The interrelationship between agoraphobia, social phobia, situational phobia, and simple phobia. *Archives of General Psychiatry*, *49*, 273–281.

Klein, D. F., & Liebowitz, M. R. (1985). Social phobias: Diagnosis, pathophysiology, and treatment. *Psychopharmacology Bulletin*, *21*, 610–614.

Liebowitz, M. R., Gorman, J. D., Fyer, A. J., & Klein, D. F. (1985). Social phobia: Review of a neglected anxiety disorder. *Archives of General Psychiatry*, *42*, 729–736.

Liebowitz, M. R., Schneier, F., Campeas, R., Hollander, E., Hatterer, J., Fyer, A., Gorman, J., Papp, L., Davies, S., Gully, R., & Klein, D. F. (1992). Phenelzine vs. atenolol in social phobia: A placebo-controlled comparison. *Archives of General Psychiatry*, *49*, 290–300.

Loranger, A. W., Susman, V. L., Oldham, J. M., & Russakoff, L. M. (1987). The personality disorder examination: A preliminary report. *Journal of Personality Disorders*, *1*, 1–13.

Marks, I. M. (1969). *Fears and phobias*. London: Heinemann.

Marks, I. M. (1985). Behavioral treatment of social phobia. *Psychopharmacology*, *21*, 615–618.

Marks, I. M. (1987). *Fears, phobias, and rituals: Panic, anxiety, and their disorders*. Oxford: Oxford University Press.

Mattick, R. P., Page, A., & Lampe, L. (in press). Cognitive and behavioral theories of social phobia. In M. B. Stein (Ed.), *Social phobia: Clinical and research perspectives*. New York: American Psychiatric Press.

Mattick, R. P., & Peters, L. (1988). Treatment of severe social phobia: Effects of guided exposure with and without cognitive restructuring. *Journal of Consulting and Clinical Psychology*, *56*, 251–260.

Mattick, R. P., Peters, L., & Clarke, J. C. (1989). Exposure and cognitive restructuring for social phobia: A controlled study. *Behavior Therapy*, *20*, 3–23.

Millon, T. (1969). *Modern psychopathology: A biosocial approach to maladaptive learning and functioning*. Philadelphia: Saunders.

Millon, T. (1981). The avoidant personality. In J. R. Lion (Ed.), *Personality disorders, diagnosis and treatment: Revised for DSM-III* (2nd ed.) (pp. 103–120). Baltimore: Williams & Wilkins.

Myers, J. K., Weissman, M. M., Tischler, G. L., Holzer, C. E., Leaf, P. J., Orvaschel, H., Anthony, J. C., Boyd, J. H., Burke, J. D., Kramer, M., & Stoltzman, R. (1984). Six-month prevalence of psychiatric disorders in three communities 1980–1982. *Archives of General Psychiatry*, *41*, 959–967.

Nichols, K. A. (1974). Severe social anxiety. *British Journal of Medical Psychology*, *47*, 301–306.

Ohman, A. (1986). Face the beast and fear the face: Animal and social fears as prototypes of evolutionary analyses of emotion. *Psychophysiology*, *23*, 123–145.

Regier, D. A., Farmer, M. E., Rae, D. S., Locke, B. Z., Keith, S. J., Judd, L. L., & Goodwin, F. K. (1990). Comorbidity of mental disorders with alcohol and other drug abuse: Results from the epidemiologic catchment area (ECA) study. *Journal of the American Medical Association*, *264*, 2511–2518.

Schneier, F. R., Johnson, J., Hornig, C. D., Leibowitz, M. R., & Weissman, M. M. (1992). Social phobia: Comorbidity and morbidity in an epidemiologic sample. *Archives of General Psychiatry*, *49*, 282–288.

Stockwell, T., Smail, P., Hodgson, R., & Canter, S. (1984). Alcohol dependence and phobic anxiety states. II: A retrospective study. *British Journal of Psychiatry*, *144*, 58–63.

Stravinski, A., Marks, I., & Yule, W. (1982). Social skills problems in neurotic outpatients: Social skills training with and without cognitive modification. *Archives of General Psychiatry*, *39*, 1378–1385.

Taskforce on DSM-IV (1993). *Work in Progress: DSM-IV draft Criteria—3.1.93*. Washington, DC: American Psychiatric Association.

Taylor, F. K. (1966). *Psychopathology: Its causes and symptoms*. London: Butterworths.

Trower, P., Yardley, K., Bryant, B. M., & Shaw, P. (1978). The treatment of social failure: A comparison of anxiety-reduction and skills-acquisition procedures on two social problems. *Behavior Modification*, *2*, 41–60.

Turner, S. M., Beidel, D. C., Dancu, C. V., & Keys, D. J. (1986). Psychopathology of social phobia and comparison to avoidant personality disorder. *Journal of Abnormal Psychology, 95*, 389–394.

Turner, S. M., Beidel, D. C., & Townsley, R. M. (1992). Social phobia: A comparison of specific and generalized subtypes and avoidant personality disorder. *Journal of Abnormal Psychology, 101*, 326–331.

Ward, J., Mattick, R. P., & Hall, W. (1992). *Key issues in methadone maintenance treatment.* Sydney: University of New South Wales Press.

Watson, D., & Friend, R. (1969). Measurement of social-evaluative anxiety. *Journal of Consulting and Clinical Psychology, 33*, 448–457.

World Health Organization (1990). *Composite International Diagnostic Interview (CIDI): (a) CIDI-interview (version 1.0), (b) CIDI user manual, (c) CIDI training manual, (d) CIDI computer programmes.* Geneva: Author.

World Health Organization (1993). *ICD-10 classification of mental and behavioral disorders: Diagnostic criteria for research.* Geneva: Author.

9

Simple Phobia

F. Dudley McGlynn

Description of the Disorder

Clinical Features

Jane was a 20-year-old college student whose graduation was in doubt because she was too fearful to perform mandatory dissections in a required biology class. When merely thinking about "cutting up animals," Jane experienced palpitations, breathlessness, nausea, and goosebumps. Michael was a 48-year-old journalist whose health was jeopardized because he was intensely fearful when being examined by physicians, dentists, or nurses. Michael avoided medical and dental settings steadfastly, and he experienced intense fear accompanied by lowered heart rate, lowered blood pressure, and fainting when avoidance was not possible. Kathy was a 29-year-old retail saleswoman whose livelihood was threatened by an intense fear of black men. She was too fearful to work alone, and she avoided all places in which black men might be encountered. Jane, Michael, and Kathy all suffered from a specific anxiety disorder called simple phobia.

DSM-III-R (American Psychiatric Association, 1987) considers simple phobia an anxiety disorder characterized by "a persistent fear" of some object or situation. The feared object or situation is avoided habitually, and anxiety behaviors occur when avoidance is precluded. The diagnosis of simple phobia is made when, in addition, the fear behavior interferes with the person's functioning, when the fear is acknowledged as irrational, and when the fear is not a constituent of another anxiety disorder or condition.

Stimulus Control. The major feature that separates simple phobias from other anxiety disorders is the relatively narrow stimulus control over anxious responses.

F. Dudley McGlynn • Department of Psychology, Auburn University, Auburn, Alabama 36849-5214.

Handbook of Prescriptive Treatments for Adults, edited by Michel Hersen and Robert T. Ammerman. Plenum Press, New York, 1994.

Sometimes there is tangible and direct stimulus control, as seen, for example, when the sight of a cockroach instantly cues narrowed attention, cardiac acceleration, breathlessness, goosebumps, and the experience of fear. Sometimes there is tangible stimulus control in which the functional stimulus control is abstract or thematic. Thus, elevators, stairways, theaters, and buses can be tangible venues that are fearfully avoided because, in common, they have the property of constraining one's freedom of movement.

Response Properties.   The anxiety behaviors seen in phobias probably are not different fundamentally from those present in other anxiety disorders. Accordingly, the differential diagnosis of phobias is linked to the conditions under which anxiety behaviors occur, not to differences in the anxiety behaviors themselves (Lipschitz, 1988).

Phobic anxiety behaviors can be described as more or less organized patterns of emotional, cognitive, physiologic, and overt behavioral responses. Emotional anxiety behaviors involve a combination of heightened attention to cues that are phobia relevant, fear-related negative affectivity, and a sense of diminished control over behavioral outcomes. Cognitive anxiety behaviors mainly involve irrational and catastrophic thinking (e.g., overestimating the danger involved in encountering the feared cue stimulus, and underestimating one's ability to cope effectively in its presence). Physiologic anxiety behaviors reflect sympathetic activation (heightened alpha-adrenergic action) as well as recruited metabolic support for cognitive and motor fear behaviors. Response patterning varies across individuals (Lacey, 1967) and can include altered cardiac function, increased blood pressure, increased blood flow to the skeletal muscles, increased respiration rate, and electrodermal lability, among other phenomena (Papillo, Murphy, & Gorman, 1988). Motoric anxiety behaviors can range from headlong flight to "freezing" and can include such diverse decrements in performance quality as speech dysfluencies and clumsiness.

The nature of the connections between emotion, cognition, physiology, and behavior in anxiety is controversial. Different theoretical views posit different sequences and different feedback loops among events in emotion, cognition, arousal, and behavior (Barlow, 1988). The orthodox behavioral view (Wolpe, 1958) for example, holds that autonomic arousal is basic to anxiety; anxious cognition and anxious behavior are driven by sympathetic arousal. The cognitive view, in contrast, holds that events at the level of cognition are basic to anxiety; autonomic arousal and anxious behavior result from catastrophic thinking (Beck & Emery, 1985), from sudden interruption of ongoing thinking (Mandler, 1975), and the like.

When different anxiety behaviors are measured simultaneously, the resulting correlations usually are positive but modest. Similarly, when multiple measures of anxiety behavior are tracked concurrently over time, fluctuations of the measures are not well synchronized (Rachman & Hodgson, 1974). Discordance and desynchrony among measures of anxiety might reflect the true organization of anxiety behaviors but might, instead, be artifactual consequences of actuarial research methodologies.

Associated Features

Simple phobias occur along with other anxiety disorders, with mood disorders, and with various correlates of those conditions. Barlow and coworkers (1985) studied reports of panic among 7 simple phobics in a comorbidity study of 108 consecutive patients at an anxiety disorders clinic. Barlow, DiNardo, Vermilyea, Vermilyea, and Blanchard (1986) included those 7 simple phobics in a report about co-occurring depression and other anxiety disorders. Sanderson, Rapee, and Barlow (1987) diagnosed 17 simple phobics in a subsequent study of comorbidity among 132 anxiety clinic patients. Sanderson and Barlow (1990) included simple phobia in a study of comorbidity among 22 patients with a primary diagnosis of generalized anxiety disorder. These studies were all conducted with demonstrably reliable structured interview formats intended for working with DSM-III-R categories. The results suggest that half of persons diagnosed with simple phobia will receive at least one additional diagnosis, and that additional diagnoses will include panic disorder, social phobia, generalized anxiety disorder, and various depressive syndromes. There is likewise little doubt that simple phobias sometimes overlap with somatoform disorders and with some personality disorders.

Epidemiology

Epidemiologic data on anxiety disorders are being produced by the National Institute of Mental Health Epidemiological Catchment Area program. Myers et al. (1984) described the 6-month prevalence of simple phobia among men and women in New Haven, Baltimore, and St. Louis. Rates among men ranged from 2.3 to 7.3%. Rates among women ranged from 6.0 to 15.7%. Robins and colleagues (1984) described the lifetime prevalence of simple phobia among men and women in those same cities; rates among men ranged from 3.8 to 14.5%, and among women from 8.5 to 25.9%. Data about the prevalence of several subcategories of simple phobia were produced some years ago by Agras, Sylvester, and Oliveau (1969). Blood/illness/injury phobias were the most prevalent (13 per 1000). Also widespread were phobias related to storms (2.3 per 1000) and to animals (1.5 per 1000).

Robins et al. (1984) found differences in phobia prevalence as a function of race and of education: blacks and persons with modest educational achievements reported higher prevalence rates than did whites and college graduates. Reich (1986) reviewed the epidemiologic literature carefully and concluded that 2.5% of United States residents experience simple phobia at some time in their lives.

Etiology

Anxiety behaviors per se are part of normal survival mechanisms that operate when people are faced with signals of danger. Etiological accounts of simple phobias are, therefore, less concerned with the origins of anxiety behaviors than with factors that produce functional connections between anxiety behaviors and their controlling signals.

From the psychodynamic perspective (e.g., Cameron, 1963), phobia-cue stimuli derive their controlling power from a process of repression and subsequent displacement. For example, momentary conscious recognition of a frightening urge to leap through a window to one's death is followed by repressing the incident and projecting and displacing the fearful affect onto tall buildings or other places that present suicidal opportunities.

According to the behavioral perspective, phobia-cue stimuli derive their controlling power from person-environment histories that include one or more of the following: aversive respondent conditioning experiences, vicarious fear experiences, and exposure to information (or misinformation) that an object or event is dangerous (see Rachman, 1977). Once a phobia-cue function has been acquired, behaviors that are instrumental in removing or replacing the phobia-cue stimulus are reinforced (see Delprato & McGlynn, 1984). There are variations on the theme. Thus, arguments have been made that some stimuli become conditioned fear cues more readily than do others (Seligman, 1971), that some persons more readily develop conditioned fears than do others (Barlow, 1988), and so forth. Behavioral, neurobiological, and cognitive theories are available that explain the mechanisms of fear acquisition and maintenance that presumably are imbedded in these histories (e.g., Eysenck, 1976; Gray, 1988; Reiss, 1980).

Rachman (1977) and others have proposed that the pathway by which a phobia develops influences the nature of the resultant anxiety behaviors. Thus, phobias with important cognitive elements develop out of histories that involve information/misinformation; phobias with strong somatovisceral components develop out of aversive respondent conditioning experiences, and so on. Despite the intuitive appeal of such formulations, they are not supported by data (Ost & Hugdahl, 1981).

Differential Diagnosis and Assessment

DSM-III-R and DSM-IV Categorization

In DSM-III-R the diagnosis of simple phobia is listed among other anxiety disorders: panic disorder with agoraphobia, panic disorder without agoraphobia, agoraphobia without history of panic disorder, social phobia, obsessive-compulsive disorder (or obsessive-compulsive neurosis), posttraumatic stress disorder, and generalized anxiety disorder. Diagnostic criteria are provided for each disorder, and there is, in each case, a narrative that summarizes available information about age at onset, course, impairment, complications, predisposing factors, prevalence, sex ratios, and some of the issues in differential diagnosis. In DSM-IV simple phobia is referred to as specific phobia and is subdivided into three categories based on the nature of the phobia stimulus: natural, man-made, and blood-injury-illness.

Differential Diagnosis

Differential diagnosis of simple phobia mainly involves establishing that the focal anxiety behaviors are not constituents of conditions that are sometimes similar, such as panic disorder, social phobia, agoraphobia, and avoidant personality disorder. These discriminations are not always straightforward. For example, fearful avoidance of crowded or enclosed places (apparent claustrophobia) might or might not be motivated by fear of panicking in those places (panic disorder), by fear of behaving foolishly in front of the people in those places (social phobia), or other factors. Within the category of simple phobias, a case can be made for differential diagnosis of animal phobias and of blood/injury phobias (Ost, Sterner, & Lindahl, 1984).

Recent interest in improving the reliability of psychiatric classification has prompted the development and validation of various structured interview formats for use with the DSMs and with subsections of the DSMs. For anxiety disorders, the preferred format is the Anxiety Disorders Interview Schedule—Revised (ADIS-R; DiNardo & Barlow, 1985).

The treatments of choice for phobias are derived from the behavior therapy tradition. A hallmark of that tradition is careful assessment of the to-be-treated behavior: assessment that provides bases for choosing among treatments, for conducting treatments, and for evaluating therapeutic efficacy. Problematically, there are three orientations to the conduct of behavior therapy for phobias, and the details of assessment differ according to each. Assessment in orthodox behavior therapy (Wolpe, 1990) includes very careful study of the stimuli that patients fear, as well as measurement of autonomic, motoric, and private/cognitive fear behaviors during imaginal and in vivo stimuli presentations. Assessment in an exposure technology approach to behavior therapy (e.g., Marks, 1981) is restricted mainly to evaluation of motor performances in the presence in vivo of fear stimuli. Assessment in social-cognitive behavior therapy (e.g., Bandura, 1977) includes procedures such as those above and adds measures of cognitive constructs, such as performance outcome expectations and self-efficacy expectations. The narrative here follows from the orthodox behavior therapy tradition (Wolpe, 1958, 1990).

In order to plan phobia treatment we need to know the specific cue stimuli that control anxious behavior; the exact features, dimensions, or meanings of those stimuli that influence gradations in anxiousness; and the nature of the anxiety behaviors themselves, that is, their cognitive, physiologic, and motoric characteristics. The information is provided by self-report, behavioral, and psychophysiologic assessment methods.

Self-Report Methods

Interviews. Interviews seek information that will guide subsequent assessment and early treatment planning. In general, the diagnostic interview seeks to answer four questions. What is the problem? What is the history of the problem? What are the current maintaining conditions and adverse effects of the problem? What strengths or resources are available that can be brought to bear in dealing with the problem?

As noted earlier, interest in improving the reliability of psychiatric diagnosis has produced various structured interview formats. Initial interviews can be guided by a standard format such as the Diagnostic Interview Scale (Robins, Helzer, Croughan, & Ratcliff, 1981) or the Structured Clinical Interview for DSM-III (Spitzer, Williams, & Gibbon, 1985). Once the area of anxiety disorder has been targeted, more narrow interview structure is afforded by formats such as the ADIS-R (DiNardo & Barlow, 1985), mentioned previously. Many interview structures are available that are still narrower. For example, Vrana, McNeil, and McGlynn (1986) developed a structured interview concerned with pinpointing problems related to fear of dental treatment.

Questionnaires. Omnibus fear inventories such as the Fear Survey Schedule-III (Wolpe & Lang, 1964) can be used routinely in assessing phobic patients, and they sometimes pinpoint difficulties not identified during interviewing. Tests of more general "neuroticism" can assist in conceptualizing how a patient's fear behaviors are related to other problems. The Willoughby Personality Schedule, for example, is reproduced in an appendix of Wolpe's (1990) classic text on the conduct of behavior therapy.

Many specific fears have been of such widespread interest that questionnaires for assessing them in detail have been developed. Ordinarily such instruments are used for research because, by and large, they are insufficiently idiographic for clinical assessment. Nonetheless, many specific-fear questionnaires have demonstrable reliability and discriminant validity, and their use can occasionally help narrow the focus of therapy. For example, Kleinknecht, McGlynn, Thorndike, and Harkavy (1984) factor analyzed a 20-item questionnaire about fear of dentistry so as to provide separate scores for geographic avoidance of dental settings, for perceived autonomic responsivity within dental settings, and for subjective fear intensity vis-à-vis the various cues encountered in dental settings.

Other Self-Reports. When patients self report on questionnaires, the actual stimuli are verbal descriptions of objects or events that are not present when the responses are given. It is preferable to use real objects and situations to occasion self-reports when it is feasible to do so.

The Fear Thermometer (Walk, 1956) is a 10-point rating scale ("completely calm" to "absolute terror") that the patient uses to rate experienced fear levels during encounters with phobia cues. Subjective anxiety scaling, or SUD scaling (e.g., Wolpe, 1990), is a common variation of the format in which a 100-point rating scale ("absolutely calm" to "worst anxiety you can imagine") is used.

Because of the historical influence of methodological behaviorism in behavior therapy, information obtained by self-reports has been viewed with skepticism. There is no reason for skepticism about self-reports per se so long as self-reporting is regarded as behavior and self-report data are used in convergent validation strategies to make clinical decisions.

Behavioral Assessment

Contrived Behavioral Tests. Approach/avoidance of a phobia-cue stimulus can be assessed in both contrived and naturalistic settings. The behavioral avoidance test or behavioral approach test (BAT) refers typically to work done in contrived settings (see McGlynn, 1988). Typically a targeted fear stimulus (e.g., spider, rat, snake) is caged at the end of a 10- to 20-foot walkway along which distances to the cage are indicated at regular intervals. The patient is provided with a behavioral checklist that describes a hierarchical series of discrete activities, and is instructed to perform as many of them as he or she can. The patient might be provided also with various performance aides such as a pointer or gloves.

Contrived behavioral testing is an assessment mode, not a specific test. Hence, there is room for variation in the timing and content of instructions, the activities and locations of therapists or other assessors during the tests, and so forth. Variations are possible also in the exact nature of the assessment data that BATs produce, such as degree of approach, latency to touch the target stimulus, and Fear Thermometer ratings at various points during the test. Use of the BAT strategy is not restricted to stimuli such as snakes and spiders. Claustrophobics can be evaluated when instructed to remain in small, dark, closed areas; acrophobics can be encouraged to climb clinic stairways.

Contrived BATs are inexact. Internal validity is problematic because behavior in a BAT is influenced by contextual and procedural factors unrelated to levels of fear. External validity is a problem because content-valid assessment requires representative fear context sampling that is not possible in contrived settings. For these reasons, and others, contrived BATs should be used as precursors and guides to naturalistic assessment, or used when naturalistic assessment is inconvenient.

Naturalistic Behavioral Assessment. Ideally, assessments of phobic behavior will be made during adaptively significant interactions with problematic objects and events in the patient's environment. Increasingly, therapists are entering problematic environments alongside their patients and recording behavioral observations. Sometimes informants, such as graduate students, interns, or spouses, are used. Naturalistic assessment shares validity problems with behavioral assessment in contrived settings, including reactivity and content validity. Nonetheless, naturalistic behavioral assessment can provide valuable information. Naturalistic contexts afford opportunities for evaluating physiologic, emotional, and cognitive fear behaviors as well as motoric ones. Behavioral assessors working in the natural environment should be provided with checklists or similar documents to structure their observations and recordings.

Naturalistic Self-Monitoring. Self-assessment of fear behavior has proven to be a viable approach to clinical evaluation. Self-assessment became popular as a natural component of self-managed exposure protocols in clinical phobia treatments (Marks, 1978, 1981). Marks (1978) provides standardized formats and instructions for self-assessment of anxiety. In general, they look for the same information that is sought when therapists or informants are used.

Psychophysiologic Assessment. Depending on the general approach to behavioral fear therapy that is followed, assessment of phobic behavior might or might not involve systematic evaluation of physiologic responsivity to phobia signals. Psychophysiologic response measurement can be coupled with actual or imagined (i.e., instructed) fear signals and typically will include heart rate and electrodermal flow as well as special purpose measures (see Papillo, Murphy, & Gorman, 1988).

Psychophysiologic assessment of emotional imaging is basic to traditional phobia therapy (e.g., Wolpe, 1990). First the patient is given some instruction in progressive muscle relaxation. Then instructions to continue relaxing are interspersed with instructions to imagine phobia-related scenarios and, perhaps, other scenarios that do not involve fear but do involve similar activity. For example, a patient being evaluated for dental phobia might sometimes imagine going to a hair salon in which the operator's behaviors correspond closely to those of the dentist (e.g., McGlynn & Vopat, 1994). During these sessions the therapist can observe muscle tremors, grimaces, and the like as the equipment records psychophysiologic events. Of course, heart rate and respiration rate can be recorded manually.

The role of psychophysiologic assessment in behavior therapy for phobias is controversial. Many authorities have expressed doubts about the reliability and clinical relevance of psychophysiologic information (e.g., Arena, Blanchard, Andrasik, Cotch, & Myers, 1983).

Treatment

Evidence for Prescriptive Treatments

Behavior Therapy. One impetus to the behavior therapy movement was the claim (Eysenck, 1952) that psychotherapy does not work. The early behavior therapists attempted to show that approaches based on conditioning concepts are superior to those based on psychodynamic formulations. Indeed, concern with demonstrating beneficial outcomes, and with developing the requisite methodologies, has been a hallmark of behavior therapy since its inception.

As noted earlier, there are three approaches to behavior therapy for phobias and related disorders: orthodox behavior therapy (e.g., Wolpe, 1958, 1990), social-cognitive behavior therapy (e.g., Bandura, 1977; Beck & Emery, 1985), and exposure technology (e.g., Marks, 1978). Recently, it has become standard to assert that exposure to feared objects or events is the crucial component in all successful fear therapies and, in turn, to classify fear therapies according to the way they implement exposure, e.g., slow vs. fast exposure, graded vs. ungraded exposure. For some purposes the exposure-based taxonomy of therapies is acceptable because available data support the basic assertion that exposure is fundamental to success, and because the taxonomy can provide guidance for researchers and clinicians. For other purposes the exposure-based taxonomy is less acceptable because the procedures of some behavior therapies reflect treatment goals other than arranging for exposure, such as producing conditioned inhibition of anxious responding (Wolpe, 1990) or producing increased self-efficacy concerning fear-related performances (Bandura, 1977). The following narrative is organized using traditional categories.

Systematic Desensitization. For many years the treatment of choice for simple phobias was systematic desensitization (Wolpe, 1958, 1990). The list of phobias and anxiety-related conditions for which systematic desensitization has produced beneficial outcomes by clinical criteria includes death, injury, disaster, illness, heart attack, atomic holocaust, water, storms, animals, birds, insects, reptiles, automobiles, airplanes, dissections, injections, hospitals, ambulances, sanitary napkins, childbirth, authority figures, and many others. Clinical evidence for the efficacy of systematic desensitization comes from individual case reports, grouped case reports, and retrospective analyses of treated patient cohorts.

Evidence concerning the efficacy of systematic desensitization is available also from "controlled experiments" in which systematic desensitization was compared with some or all of the following: no treatment, competing treatment(s), and pseudo-treatments designed to estimate the contribution of demand-placebo variance to global indices of therapy outcome (see Kazdin & Wilcoxon, 1976). College students served as subjects in most of the experiments. For that reason, among others, the experiments were criticized on grounds of suspect external validity (e.g., Bernstein & Paul, 1971). However, not all the experiments were equally open to that criticism, and not all criticisms of the early experiments were legitimate (McGlynn, Mealiea, & Landau, 1981). Paul (1969a, 1969b) prepared reviews in painstaking detail of 75 clinical and experimental reports. The reports covered the use of desensitization by more than 90 therapists with nearly 1,000 patients, and the findings were "overwhelmingly positive" (p. 159).

Modeling. The influence of the social learning theory perspective on behavior therapy (Bandura, 1969) caused modeling procedures to be used in early attempts to treat fear-related problems. The bulk of research took the form of comparing modeling with other forms of treatment (e.g., desensitization), and of evaluating modeling outcomes when modeling procedures were varied (e.g., single vs. multiple models; coping vs. mastery models). Rachman (1972) reviewed 17 of the early experiments in which modeling was used to overcome fear and concluded that "modeling produces significant and lasting reduction of fear which generalizes to similar situations and stimuli" (p. 385).

Participant Modeling. Rachman (1972) noted that "other things being equal, participant modeling appears to be more effective than vicarious modeling" (p. 390).

Marks (1975) reviewed 13 experiments that appeared after Rachman's review, and offered the same conclusion. At the same time, participant modeling treatment protocols were developed (e.g., Bandura, Jefferey, & Gajdos, 1975; Bandura, Jefferey, & Wright, 1974) that included several standard procedures for optimizing generalized treatment effects. The literature shows very clearly that the total package of participant modeling procedures is reliably effective (Bandura, 1977).

Exposure-Based Treatment. As noted, systematic desensitization and modeling incorporate exposure to fear signals, but their procedural details are guided by additional goals derived from explicit theories of how the therapies work. Exposure technology, in contrast, is not driven by theories of fear reduction; the goal of exposure technology is to bring about functional exposure to fear signals. Historically there has been an informal connection between exposure technology and the concept of fear habituation. Therefore, some importance has been placed on using exposure times that are sufficiently long for habituation to occur, roughly 2 to 4 hours (Watson, Gaind, & Marks, 1972). Other procedural guidelines for using exposure technology are not easily determined. "Flooding" is a major variant of exposure technology. In flooding, patients are constrained, in any way short of outright force, to confront their phobia-cue stimuli as soon as possible, as intimately as possible, and for as long as possible, or until fear subsides. "Graduated exposure" is a somewhat standard variant of exposure technology in which the patient is exposed to increasing forms of fear stimuli at his or her own, unforced pace. "Self-directed exposure" (Marks, 1978) is a variant in which the patient guides his or her own assessment and exposure with the remote assistance of a therapist.

Exposure technology is currently the most popular approach to treating simple phobias. There has been discussion about optimally matching patients with specific exposure protocols based on differences in phobia histories, differences in phobic response characteristics, and other characteristics. To date, however, there are few data on which to base any matching strategy.

Pharmacotherapy. Most of the literature on pharmacotherapy in phobia cases concerns use of medication as an adjunct to behavior therapy. Usually a benzo-diazepine or a beta-blocker has been the medication, and some variant of exposure technology or of desensitization has been the behavior therapy (e.g., Campos, Solyom, & Koelink, 1984; Sartory, 1983). An early example was reported by Marks, Viswanathan, Lipsedge, and Gardner (1972). They conducted 2-hour flooding sessions for 18 phobics during "peak" periods of diazepam effectiveness, during "waning" periods of diazepam effectiveness, or during placebo periods. Multiple clinical assessments showed that the greatest effects from flooding occurred during "waning" diazepam effectiveness periods, followed by "peak" periods and then by placebo periods.

Barlow (1988) noted that occasional, transitory drug effects have been reported in pharmacotherapy–behavior therapy studies, but that "the firm and consistent conclusion is that drugs do not contribute to therapy and may even hinder the effects of exposure-based therapy" (p. 490). Wardle (1990) concluded a review of benzo-diazepine effects on behavior therapy outcomes somewhat less pessimistically. In general, the effects of behavior therapy on phobias are sufficiently strong that drugs should not be needed. In addition, the issue of state-dependent drug effects (e.g., Sartory, 1983) has not been resolved. Therefore, prudence calls for the use of drugs only in refractory cases.

Alternative Treatments. Sloan, Staples, Cristol, Yorkston, and Whipple (1975) published results from one experiment in which the outcomes of behavior therapy were characterized as not different from those of brief psychoanalytic therapy among mixed psychoneurotic patients. Soon afterward Smith and Glass (1977) reported a meta-analysis of outcomes from 400 studies; the effects of behavior therapy ("systematic desensitization, behavioral modification") were not found to be superior to the effects of other approaches ("Rogerian, psychodynamic, rational-emotive, transactional analysis, etc."). These reports became cornerstones of the argument, in some circles, that outcomes of various forms of psychological therapy for psychoneuroses are equivalent. The fact is, however, that various forms of psychological therapy for anxiety disorders are not equivalent; behavior therapies are superior to all others. The experiment of Sloan et al. (1975) was not well controlled by modern standards, and it used dependent variables that were inappropriate to the evaluation of behavior therapy. In addition, careful scrutiny of their data shows differential support for behavior therapy (Wolpe, 1990). Similarly, the meta-analytic approach used by Smith and Glass (1977) has been criticized (e.g., Searles, 1985; Wilson & Rachman, 1983), and subsequent reports based on improved methods favor behavior therapy outcomes (e.g., Andrews & Harvey, 1981; Giles, 1983). Clearly, there is no legitimate replacement for behavior therapy in the treatment of phobias.

Selecting Optimal Treatment Strategies

Exposure Technology. There are no data that would justify a firm choice of one exposure format over another based on differential outcomes (Linden, 1981). Those data that do exist are interpretively marginal or based on research with nonclinical subjects. Therefore, choice of exposure protocol should rest on matters such as cost, efficiency, and feasibility. Various feasible approaches, including self-directed exposure, should be described to the patient, and the patient should be allowed to choose the format best suited to his or her circumstances. At this level, graduated participant modeling can be presented as a variant of exposure technology.

Behavior Therapy. Behavior therapy for simple phobias is guided, to some extent, by the three-channel conceptualization of anxiety in which fear cognition, fear behavior, and fear physiology are idiosyncratically patterned response modes. The twofold clinical implication of the three-channel perspective is that some channels are more important than others in individual cases, and that behavior therapy can target behaviors in one, two, or all three channels. For example, fear cognition can be approached by correcting misconceptions, fear behavior can be changed by participant modeling, and fear-related autonomic arousal can be reduced by systematic desensitization (Wolpe, 1981). As with exposure technology, there are no data that serve to justify a firm commitment to working in the manner just described. However, there is no compelling argument to do otherwise. It is simply reasonable to apply behavior therapy according to the details of anxiety as they are revealed by assessment of cognitive, motoric, and physiologic phenomena.

Problems in Carrying Out Interventions

There are pitfalls in the use of systematic desensitization. Problems arise when the patient is unable to learn to relax, has problems generating adequate imagery, or has numerous fear cues. Sometimes the course of desensitization is not smooth in one way or another. Within limits the problem of multiple fears can be addressed during the hierarchy construction phase of desensitization. Wolpe's (1990) classic text provides guidance for hierarchy construction in the form of clinical cases that include the hierarchies used. The DSM-III-R and DSM-IV categories provide some guiding schema, as do factor-analytic studies of ratings on omnibus fear questionnaires. Ways to deal with various problems in "the mechanics of desensitization" have been discussed elsewhere (McGlynn, 1978). Sometimes patients experience intense fear or panic episodes during the course of relaxation training, episodes that seemingly are related to fear of losing control (Heide & Borkovec, 1984). Some behavior therapists (e.g., Goldfried & Davison, 1976) routinely prepare patients for perceiving loss of control before relaxation training.

The principal problem with participant modeling is a restricted range of application. Ordinarily, participant modeling uses only those fear stimuli that are easy to locate and transport to the treatment setting. A second problem with participant modeling is that fear reduction in the treatment setting might very well not transfer to adaptively significant encounters with fear stimuli in the natural environment. In such cases, naturalistic exposure is required; participant modeling will have been superfluous.

Exposure technologies carried out in the natural environment also are limited to circumstances that can be located conveniently. In addition, naturalistic exposure can be time consuming. For example, a good part of a day can be absorbed by driving across town, parking, walking to and riding in a particular bank of elevators for 3 or 4 hours, debriefing and rescheduling the patient, and returning to the office. There also are potential problems related to premature termination and relapse. Approximately 12% of patients drop out of exposure-based treatments (Jansson & Ost, 1982), and as many as 50% of patients show some degree of relapse after such treatments (Munby & Johnston, 1980).

Relapse Prevention

Some theoretical accounts of the therapeutic effects of exposure (e.g., habituation, extinction) allow for the prediction that fear levels will increase some time after treatment. Hence, patients should be instructed to expect the return of fear so that it will not be interpreted as an indication of failure. Patients should be instructed also *never* to give in to escape or avoidance dispositions. Finally, the availability of booster treatment sessions should be made known, and patients should be encouraged to schedule such sessions as needed.

Case Illustration

Case Description

The case material that follows in some respects reflects exposure technology; in others it illustrates behavior therapy.

Kelley was a 25-year-old female graduate student. She presented for treatment to the psychology department clinic at a southeastern university. During the initial interview she mentioned unhappiness, uneasiness about being far away from home, self-doubts about her ability to succeed in graduate school and about her matrimonial prospects, insomnia, diminished appetite, and chronic tension. I reassured her that some of her concerns were to be expected, given her circumstances, and that others could probably be addressed in due course. She left after voicing a commitment to return to the clinic, and to share more about her concerns and difficulties at that time.

During the second visit Kelley told of a family history of panic disorder among maternal relatives, and returned to the theme of her increasing uneasiness during the early weeks of graduate school in a new environment. She denied ever having had spontaneous panic experiences, but she reported having seen her mother during numerous panic attacks, and she expressed concern that her own accelerating uneasiness might eventuate in a panic disorder. She alluded also to worry about the health of her parents and of her grandparents, about the emotional adjustment of a college-bound sibling, about the adequacy of her finances and the reliability of her car, about the prospect of failure in school, and about her ability to someday be a good wife and mother. In addition, she described several frightening experiences with stinging insects and cockroaches that had occurred, for the most part, when she was moving into her apartment. The picture that emerged from the two interviews was one of an immature individual who had led a sheltered life, who was in some conflict about her long-term future, and who was doubtful about dealing adequately with various aspects of the novel circumstances in which she found herself.

Differential Diagnosis and Assessment

During the third visit the Anxiety Disorders Interview Schedule—Revised (DiNardo & Barlow, 1985) and the Fear Survey Schedule—III (Wolpe & Lang, 1964) were used. Panic disorder was ruled out despite Kelley's concern. Social phobia was likewise ruled out; her fear of academic failure was specific. (Items on the FSS-III about "Looking foolish," "Meeting someone for the first time," "Speaking before a group," and the like were endorsed as prompting little or no fear.) The anxiety disorder diagnoses suggested were generalized anxiety disorder and simple phobia. The phobic fears contributed to the generalized anxiety by providing themes for needless worry. However, simple phobia was diagnosed separately.

Spiders and stinging insects were endorsed on the FSS-III as causing "very much fear." Interviewing confirmed generalized fear of insects and pinpointed specific fears of spiders, wasps, cockroaches, and millipedes. Kelley had been fearful of insects for as long as she could remember but had resided in locations where insects were encountered infrequently and where someone else had dealt with those around her living quarters. On moving to the South, and into a student apartment at the end of the summer, she had encountered stinging insects nesting close to her door, and cockroaches and spiders inside her apartment. Some of the cockroaches were "large, flying ones" of a sort she had not seen before.

Behavioral Assessment.   Separate behavioral walkway tests with live specimens housed in a 20-gallon aquarium were undertaken using one garden spider plus one Daddy Longlegs, then five cockroaches, and then two millipedes. In each case Kelley approached and stood next to the cage but refused to remove the lid or touch the specimens, even though gloves and a pointer were available. In each case also, Fear Thermometer ratings showed increasing fear with increasing proximity to the specimens. After the tests a behavioral diary was begun in which all encounters with targeted insects were chronicled so as to include the date and time of day, Kelley's location and distance from the insect(s), the movements of the insect(s), her response to the encounter, and how frightened she was, indicated on a 10-point Fear Thermometer scale. Kelley was instructed to bring the diary to all clinic visits.

Various stinging insects were "presented in imagination" and were interspersed with imagery about birds (control) after Kelley had received one session of relaxation training (described below). Imagery scripts were developed around the dimensions of distance to the insect or bird, and movement of the insect or bird. Instructions involving blue wasps and yellowjackets were used. Pulse rates were recorded manually during various wasp, bird, and intervening instructions. Kelley's imagery involving both blue wasps and yellowjackets was associated with pulse acceleration when the wasps were nearby or flying toward her. Her imagery that involved birds, bees, and distant wasps was not associated with pulse rate increases.

Treatment Selection

Fears related to spiders, cockroaches, and millipedes were treated simultaneously using graduated participant modeling. Participant modeling was chosen because it was feasible and has a strong supporting literature. Kelley's fears of wasps were treated with systematic desensitization. Systematic desensitization in imagination was chosen because wasps do not lend themselves conveniently to modeling or exposure methods, and because Kelley showed increased heart rates after insect imagery instructions but not after corresponding bird imagery instructions.

Treatment Course and Problems in Carrying Out Interventions

A 25-step behavioral gradient was developed around the walkway, cage, gloves, pointers, and specimens that were used in the behavioral assessment. The hierarchy of to-be-performed activities began with "Stand next to a closed cage containing spiders, roaches, and millipedes," and ended with three parallel items: "Gently pick up the spider [or roach or millipede], then let it crawl around on the palm or back of your bare hand for 5 minutes." Among the intermediate items were "Touch each millipede with the tip of a pointer held in a bare hand" and "Touch each roach while wearing a glove."

Participant Modeling.   Once the behavioral gradient was developed, we began a series of modeling-with-guided-participation sessions, each of which lasted for 20 to 25 minutes. During each I performed several steps in the series calmly, I pointed out to Kelley that I was not frightened and was not being harmed, and I encouraged Kelley to reproduce my actions.

Sometimes Kelley and I performed the behavioral checklist activity together after my demonstration. Sometimes one or two female graduate students took my place for modeling and conjoint performance trials. After Kelley was able to perform a behavior alongside a model, she and the model performed it several times, then Kelley was encouraged to do it on her own. After Kelley performed the behavior on her own, she was encouraged to do it several times or for several minutes, or both. We then proceeded to the next steps of the behavioral gradient and began the process anew. Each session after the first began and ended with a successful, autonomous performance. During the eighth modeling session Kelley performed the 25th checklist activity with a millipede for 5 minutes. After that a series of three self-directed mastery experiences was undertaken. In each case Kelley was provided opportunity to handle the specimens as she wished for 90 minutes and was observed from a distance occasionally.

Systematic Desensitization. Kelley's fears of wasps were treated with the "orthodox" procedure for systematic desensitization in imagination (Wolpe, 1990). First, a to-be-visualized hierarchy of 17 scenes involving wasps was jointly developed. In brief, 25 scenarios were typed individually on index cards; then Kelley ordered the cards along a 100-point SUDS scale of increasing fearsomeness. She then deleted cards that were too similar in content or in their SUDS ratings. The organizing dimensions of the hierarchy were the numbers and distances of the wasps, and the directions of their flight toward or away from Kelley. By and large, the imagery scripts described scenes around Kelley's apartment and three specific sidewalks on the university campus. Again, blue wasps and yellowjackets were used interchangeably.

As part of the fear assessment, Kelley received one session of relaxation training. The training continued during the visits used for hierarchy construction. Kelley was seated in a large reclining chair and exposed verbatim to muscular relaxation instructions in the manual provided by Bernstein and Borkovec (1973). During the first four sessions the 16-muscle-group transcript was used. During each of the next two sessions the 4-muscle-group transcript was used and was repeated once. During all relaxation training sessions after the first, Kelley was instructed to elevate an index finger if a targeted muscle group was not relaxed after training. Finger elevations prompted repeating of the relevant instructions until no finger elevation was observed.

Orthodox systematic desensitization began with the 4-muscle-group relaxation instructions. Then Kelley was instructed to relax and, simultaneously, to visualize a series of three idyllic scenes in which she pictured herself viewing pastures, streams, red barns, and grazing cattle. After the relaxed imagery practice, Kelley was instructed to begin formal desensitization by remaining relaxed and visualizing the lowest item on the 17-item hierarchy. During nine ensuing 25-minute sessions, Kelley was relaxed and was instructed to visualize each of the scenes on the hierarchy, and to signal the presence of discomfort with a finger elevation as before. Three successive visualizations without a finger elevation were followed by progressing to the next scene on the hierarchy. Each session began and ended with three successful visualizations. Throughout the nine sessions of systematic desensitization Kelley was instructed to rehearse her successfully visualized scenarios in real life, given opportunities to do so. She was told also that real-life practice should lag three or four items behind progress in imagination. Finally, she was instructed to record real-life practice opportunities and their outcomes in her behavioral diary.

Intervention Difficulties. There were no problems with the participant modeling format except that of finding fearless female models to handle the cockroaches. There were, likewise, no unanticipated problems with the conduct of systematic desensitization. Because of Kelley's concern over panic behaviors, she was alerted that she might experience a sense of loss of control during relaxation training and that the experience was not unusual. Repeated finger elevations signaled the continued presence of anxious discomfort at five points along the desensitization hierarchy. For four of these the problem was handled by Kelley's constructing and visualizing new hierarchy items. For one, the problem was handled by having Kelley rehearse the 16-muscle-group relaxation transcript twice, and then visualize the troublesome scene.

Toward the end of treatment Kelley was instructed to contact her apartment manager and request a pest-control visit. She was instructed also to expect to find dead insects for several days after pest-control treatment, and to dispose of them herself after tolerating them for 24 hours.

Outcome and Termination

Kelley returned to the clinic and performed the behavioral test with simultaneous specimens once a week for 3 weeks after the third self-directed mastery trial. On the first and third visits she also received 4-muscle-group relaxation rehearsal, after which her heart rate and skin conductance following insect imagery instructions and bird imagery instructions were evaluated in a psychophysiology laboratory. Kelley's behavioral test performances were calm and competent. There was only a very slight increase in skin conductance during imagery about insects over that found during imagery about birds; no heart rate differences were observed. Treatment for Simple Phobia was considered finished when the posttreatment testing was done.

Kelley encountered a spider unlike those we had dealt with not long after the posttreatment evaluations. While she was cleaning a window behind a curtain in her apartment, the spider seemingly "jumped at her" as she drew the curtain to one side. Kelley retreated from the room and made a tearful call to the psychology clinic. After the episode Kelley was seen for five sessions of stress inoculation training (Meichenbaum, 1977). In addition, she was instructed to videotape and watch two programs about insects on public television. Kelley was instructed to watch both of them several times, to practice 4-muscle-group relaxation during viewing, and to take note of her diminishing fear.

Follow-Up and Maintenance

Three months and 9 months after treatment, the behavioral tests with simultaneous specimens were repeated. Kelley's performances were competent and fearless. After each test she was reminded that her fear of insects might return from time to time with or without incidents such as that of the jumping spider. She was instructed to never give in to her fear of insects, to improvise her own behavioral performances as opportunities arose, and to call the clinic for booster treatment if that became necessary.

Summary

Simple phobias are disorders in which anxiety behaviors such as fearful affect, physiologic arousal, and motoric escape and avoidance are cued by relatively objective stimuli such as thunderstorms, elevators, dentists, and spiders. Simple phobias usually coexist with other anxiety disorders, with mood disorders, or with other correlates of those conditions. These phobias have a lifetime prevalence in the United States of 2.5 to 5%.

The controlling influence of phobia-cue stimuli can derive from aversive respondent conditioning experiences, from vicarious fear experiences, and from exposure to information. Once stimulus control over anxious behavior has been established, behaviors are reinforced that remove or replace the controlling stimulus. The means by which various experiences produce and maintain phobic responses have been explained with behavioral, neurobiological, and cognitive concepts. There are disagreements about exactly how behavioral, physiologic, and cognitive mechanisms combine to produce complex phobic displays, about the sequences or feedback loops that exist among the component processes.

The procedures used for assessing phobias vary according to the allegiance of the therapist; behavior therapists, social-cognitive therapists, and exposure technicians proceed somewhat differently. Self-report assessment is done with interviews, questionnaires, and ratings. Behavioral assessment is carried out during actual performances with feared stimuli in contrived and naturalistic settings. Assessment of fear-related physiology is done manually, with specialized equipment, or both.

Treatments for phobias likewise vary according to the allegiance of the therapist. Exposure-based treatments are used most widely. These have the goal of bringing about prolonged, functional exposure to phobia-cue stimuli. Behavior therapy regimens such as systematic desensitization and modeling are used in some cases. Treatments, such as systematic desensitization and modeling, have goals above and beyond that of prolonged exposure to phobia-cue stimuli. The goals are derived from theories of how fear reduction occurs.

Exposure technology, behavior therapy, and social-cognitive therapy constitute the treatments of choice for phobias. There is no need for pharmacotherapy and no justification for other forms of psychological therapy. Exposure technology is the most common treatment; behavior and social-cognitive therapy are applicable potentially when exposure is not feasible.

References

Agras, W. S., Sylvester, D., & Oliveau, D. (1969). The epidemiology of common fears and phobia. *Comprehensive Psychiatry, 10,* 151–156.

American Psychiatric Association (1987). *Diagnostic and statistical manual of mental disorders* (3rd ed., rev.). Washington, DC: Author.

Andrews, G., & Harvey, R. (1981). Does psychotherapy benefit neurotic patients? *Archives of General Psychiatry, 38,* 1203–1208.

Arena, J. G., Blanchard, E. B., Andrasik, F., Cotch, B. A., & Myers, P. E. (1983). Reliability of psychophysiological assessment. *Behaviour Research and Therapy, 21,* 447–460.

Bandura, A. (1969). *Principles of behavior modification.* New York: Holt, Rinehart & Winston.

Bandura, A. (1977). Self-efficacy: Toward a unifying theory of behavioral change. *Psychological Review, 84,* 191–215.

Bandura, A., Jefferey, R. W., & Gajdos, E. (1975). Generalizing change through self-directed performance. *Behaviour Research and Therapy, 13,* 141–152.

Bandura, A., Jefferey, R. W., & Wright, C. L. (1974). Efficacy of participant modeling as a function of response induction aides. *Journal of Abnormal Psychology, 83,* 56–64.

Barlow, D. H. (1988). *Anxiety and its disorders: The nature and treatment of anxiety and panic.* New York: Guilford.

Barlow, D. H., DiNardo, P. A., Vermilyea, B. B., Vermilyea, J. A., & Blanchard, E. B. (1986). Comorbidity and depression among the anxiety disorders: Issues in diagnosis and classification. *Journal of Nervous and Mental Disease, 174,* 63–72.

Barlow, D. H., Vermilyea, J. A., Blanchard, E. B., Vermilyea, B. B., DiNardo, P. A., & Cerny, J. A. (1985). The phenomenon of panic. *Journal of Abnormal Psychology, 94,* 320–328.

Beck, A. T., & Emery, G. (1985). *Anxiety disorders and phobias: A cognitive perspective*. New York: Basic Books.

Bernstein, D. A., & Borkovec, T. D. (1973). *Progressive relaxation training*. Champaign, IL: Research Press.

Bernstein, D. A., & Paul, G. L. (1971). Some comments on therapy analogue research with small animal "phobias." *Journal of Behavior Therapy and Experimental Psychiatry, 2*, 225–238.

Cameron, N. (1963). *Personality development and psychopathology: A dynamic approach*. Boston: Houghton Mifflin.

Campos, P. E., Solyom, L., & Koelink, A. (1984). The effects of timolol maleate on subjective and physiological components of air travel phobia. *Canadian Journal of Psychiatry, 29*, 570–574.

Delprato, D. J., & McGlynn, F. D. (1984). Behavioral theories of anxiety disorders. In S. M. Turner (Ed.), *Behavioral theories and treatment of anxiety* (pp. 1–49). New York: Plenum.

DiNardo, P. A., & Barlow, D. H. (1985). *Anxiety Disorders Interview Schedule Revised (ADIS-R)*. Albany: Phobia and Anxiety Disorders Clinic, State University of New York at Albany.

Eysenck, H. J. (1952). The effects of psychotherapy: An evaluation. *Journal of Consulting Psychology, 16*, 319–338.

Eysenck, H. J. (1976). The learning theory model of neurosis: A new approach. *Behaviour Research and Therapy, 14*, 251–267.

Giles, T. R. (1983). Probable superiority of behavioral interventions. I: Traditional comparative outcome. *Journal of Behavior Therapy and Experimental Psychiatry, 14*, 29–32.

Goldfried, M. R., & Davison, G. C. (1976). *Clinical behavior therapy*. New York: Holt, Rinehart & Winston.

Gray, J. A. (1988). The neuropsychological basis of anxiety. In C. G. Last & M. Hersen (Eds.), *Handbook of anxiety disorders* (pp. 10–37). New York: Pergamon.

Heide, F. J., & Borkovec, T. D. (1984). Relaxation-induced anxiety: Mechanisms and theoretical implications. *Behaviour Research and Therapy, 22*, 1–12.

Jansson, L., & Ost, L. G. (1982). Behavioral treatments for agoraphobia: An evaluative review. *Clinical Psychology Review, 2*, 311–336.

Kazdin, A. E., & Wilcoxon, L. A. (1976). Systematic desensitization and nonspecific treatment effects: A methodological evaluation. *Psychological Bulletin, 83*, 729–758.

Kleinknecht, R. A., McGlynn, F. D., Thorndike, R. M., & Harkavy, J. (1984). Factor analysis of the Dental Fear Survey with cross validation. *Journal of the American Dental Association, 108*, 59–61.

Lacey, J. I. (1967). Somatic response patterning and stress: Some revisions in activation theory. In M. H. Appley & R. Trumbull (Eds.), *Psychological stress: Issues in research* (pp. 14–37). New York: Appleton-Century-Crofts.

Linden, W. (1981). Exposure treatments for focal phobias. *Archives of General Psychiatry, 38*, 769–775.

Lipschitz, A. (1988). Diagnosis and classification of anxiety disorders. In C. G. Last & M. Hersen (Eds.), *Handbook of anxiety disorders* (pp. 41–65). New York: Pergamon.

Mandler, G. (1975). *Mind and emotion*. New York: Wiley.

Marks, I. (1975). Behavioral treatments of phobic and obsessive-compulsive disorders: A critical appraisal. In M. Hersen, R. M. Eisler, & P. M. Miller (Eds.), *Progress in behavior modification*, Vol. 1 (pp. 65–158). New York: Academic Press.

Marks, I. M. (1978). *Living with fear*. New York: McGraw-Hill.

Marks, I. M. (1981). *Cure and care of neuroses*. New York: Wiley.

Marks, I. M., Viswanathan, R., Lipsedge, M. S., & Gardner, R. (1972). Enhanced relief of phobias by flooding during waning diazepam effect. *British Journal of Psychiatry, 121*, 493–505.

McGlynn, F. D. (1978). Adults with anxiety-based disorders. In M. Hersen & A. S. Bellack (Eds.), *Behavior therapy in the psychiatric setting* (pp. 259–285). Baltimore: Williams & Wilkins.

McGlynn, F. D. (1988). The behavioral avoidance test. In M. Hersen & A. S. Bellack (Eds.), *Dictionary of behavioral assessment techniques* (pp. 59–60). New York: Pergamon.

McGlynn, F. D., Mealiea, W. L., Jr., & Landau, D. L. (1981). The current status of systematic desensitization. *Clinical Psychology Review, 1*, 149–179.

McGlynn, F. D., & Vopat, T. (1994). Simple phobia. In C. G. Last & M. Hersen (Eds.), *Adult behavior therapy casebook* (pp. 139–151). New York: Plenum.

Meichenbaum, D. (1977). *Cognitive-behavior modification: An integrative approach*. New York: Plenum.

Munby, J., & Johnston, D. W. (1980). Agoraphobia: The long-term follow-up of behavioural treatment. *British Journal of Psychiatry, 137*, 418–427.

Myers, J. K., Weissman, M. M., Tischler, C. E., Holzer, C. E., III, Orvaschel, H., Anthony, J. C., Boyd, J. H., Burke, J. D., Jr., Kramer, M., & Stoltzman, R. (1984). Six-month prevalence of psychiatric disorders in three communities. *Archives of General Psychiatry, 41*, 959–967.

Ost, L. G., & Hugdahl, K. (1981). Acquisition of phobias and anxiety response patterns in clinical patients. *Behaviour Research and Therapy, 19,* 439–447.

Ost, L. G., Sterner, U. S., & Lindahl, I. L. (1984). Physiological responses in blood phobics. *Behaviour Research and Therapy, 22,* 109–117.

Papillo, J. F., Murphy, P. M., & Gorman, J. M. (1988). Psychophysiology. In C. G. Last & M. Hersen (Eds.), *Handbook of anxiety disorders* (pp. 217–250). New York: Pergamon.

Paul, G. L. (1969a). Outcome of systematic desensitization. I: Background, procedures, and uncontrolled reports of individual treatment. In C. M. Franks (Ed.), *Behavior therapy: Appraisal and status* (pp. 63–104). New York: McGraw-Hill.

Paul, G. L. (1969b). Outcome of systematic desensitization. II: Controlled investigations of individual treatment, technique variations, and current status. In C. M. Franks (Ed.), *Behavior therapy: Appraisal and status* (pp. 105–159). New York: McGraw-Hill.

Rachman, S. J. (1972). Clinical application of observational learning, imitation, and modeling. *Behavior Therapy, 3,* 379–397.

Rachman, S. J. (1977).The conditioning theory of fear acquisition: A critical examination. *Behaviour Research and Therapy, 15,* 375–387.

Rachman, S. J., & Hodgson, R. S. (1974). Synchrony and desynchrony in fear and avoidance. *Behaviour Research and Therapy, 12,* 311–318.

Reich, J. (1986). The epidemiology of anxiety. *Journal of Nervous and Mental Disease, 174,* 129–136.

Reiss, S. (1980). Pavlovian conditioning and human fear: An expectancy model. *Behavior Therapy, 11,* 380–396.

Robins, L. N., Helzer, J. E., Croughan, J., & Ratcliff, K. S. (1981). National Institute of Mental Health Diagnostic Interview Schedule: Its history, characteristics and validity. *Archives of General Psychiatry, 38,* 381–389.

Robins, L. N., Helzer, J. E., Weissman, M. M., Orvaschel, H., Gruenberg, E., Burke, J. D., & Regier, D. A. (1984). Prevalence of specific psychiatric disorders in three sites. *Archives of General Psychiatry, 41,* 949–958.

Sanderson, W. C., & Barlow, D. H. (1990). A description of patients diagnosed with DSM-III-R Generalized Anxiety Disorder. *Journal of Nervous and Mental Disease, 178,* 588–591.

Sanderson, W. C., Rapee, R. M., & Barlow, D. H. (1987, November). *The DSM-III—Revised Anxiety Disorder Categories: Description and patterns of co-morbidity.* Paper presented at the annual meeting of the Association for Advancement of Behavior Therapy, Boston.

Sartory, G. (1983). Benzodiazepines and behavioural treatment of phobic anxiety. *Behavioural Psychotherapy, 11,* 204–217.

Searles, J. (1985). A methodological critique of psychotherapy outcome meta-analysis. *Behaviour Research and Therapy, 23,* 453–463.

Seligman, M. E. P. (1971). Phobias and preparedness. *Behavior Therapy, 2,* 307–320.

Sloane, R. B., Staples, F. R., Cristol, A. H., Yorkston, N. J., & Whipple, K. (1975). *Psychotherapy versus behavior therapy.* Cambridge, MA: Harvard University Press.

Smith, M. L., & Glass, G. V. (1977). Meta-analysis of psychotherapy outcome studies. *American Psychologist, 32,* 752–760.

Spitzer, R. L., Williams, J. B. W., & Gibbon, M. (1985). *Instruction manual for the Structured Clinical Interview for DSM-III* (SCID; 7/1/85 revision). New York: Biometrics Research Department, New York State Psychiatric Institute.

Vrana, S., McNeil, D. W., & McGlynn, F. D. (1986). A structured interview for assessing dental fear. *Journal of Behavior Therapy and Experimental Psychiatry, 17,* 175–178.

Walk, R. D. (1956). Self ratings of fear in a fear-invoking situation. *Journal of Abnormal and Social Psychology, 52,* 171–178.

Wardle, J. (1990). Behaviour therapy and benzodiazepines: Allies or antagonists? *British Journal of Psychiatry, 156,* 163–168.

Watson, J. P., Gaind, R., & Marks, I. M. (1972). Physiological habituation to continuous phobic stimulation. *Behaviour Research and Therapy, 10,* 269–278.

Wilson, G. T., & Rachman, S. J. (1983). Meta-analysis and the evaluation of psychotherapy outcome: Limitations and liabilities. *Journal of Consulting and Clinical Psychology, 51,* 54–64.

Wolpe, J. (1958). *Psychotherapy by reciprocal inhibition.* Stanford, CA: Stanford University Press.

Wolpe, J. (1981). The dichotomy between classical conditioned and cognitively learned anxiety. *Journal of Behavior Therapy and Experimental Psychiatry, 12,* 35–42.

Wolpe, J. (1990). *The practice of behavior therapy* (4th ed.). New York: Pergamon.

Wolpe, J., & Lang, P. J. (1964). A fear survey schedule for use in behaviour therapy. *Behaviour Research and Therapy, 2,* 27–30.

10

Obsessive-Compulsive Disorder

Conor Duggan

Description of the Disorder

Clinical Features

Obsessive-compulsive disorder (OCD) is one of a series of disorders in which the predominant symptom is anxiety. This anxiety arises either from thoughts (i.e., obsessions) or the need to carry out certain behaviors (i.e., compulsions). Most presentations involve a combination of obsessions and compulsions; single obsessions or compulsions are less common (Marks, 1987). Classifying OCD on the basis of the stimulus is generally not helpful, because this tends to produce an almost endless list. Nevertheless, certain groups of concerns in OCD naturally coalesce and hence are useful in practice. Obsessions, for instance, commonly center around thoughts of contamination, violence, doubting, and worries about sexual or religious prohibitions. Compulsions commonly involve checking, washing, and counting (Rasmussen & Eisen, 1988).

The compulsive behaviors often have the function of undoing the perceived harm from the mentalistic process. For instance, a fear of contamination is commonly associated with compulsive washing, a fear of violence with checking behaviors, and so on. Thus, the behaviors reinforce and maintain the disturbance by temporarily decreasing anxiety. Indeed, Foa, Steketee, and Ozarow (1985) propose that obsessions and compulsions cause and reduce anxiety, respectively. However, the anxiogenic stimulus may itself be a behavior, which then has to be undone by a mental ritual. Thus a simple model to have in mind is that of an anxiogenic stimulus—usually

Conor Duggan • Department of Psychiatry, The University of Nottingham, Nottingham NG3 6AA England.

Handbook of Prescriptive Treatments for Adults, edited by Michel Hersen and Robert T. Ammerman. Plenum Press, New York, 1994.

an obsession—which drives an anxiolytic response. Obsessional slowness refers to the abnormal length of time taken for everyday tasks. Although the emphasis is on the behavior, it is usually secondary to the patient's ruminating on whether a particular act has been carried out properly or being abnormally indecisive (Veale, 1993).

Associated Features

In addition to the basic obsession/compulsion, secondary avoidance is common, with idiosyncratic thinking leading individuals to believe that the slightest contact with the feared object will spell catastrophe. The effect of this avoidance is that the core feature of the disorder (i.e., anxiety) may not be evident. Family members are often forced to offer repeated reassurance and to go to extraordinary lengths to comply with the avoidance behavior. Hence, they may be useful allies in constructing a therapeutic regimen.

The adoption of a nonhierarchical system of classification has led to identification of multiple diagnoses. In the Epidemiological Catchment Area study, individuals with OCD had a 75% chance of having at least one additional diagnosis (Karno & Golding, 1991). Clinically, the most important of these disorders is depression, found in 30% of patients at presentation with OCD (Rasmussen & Eisen, 1988), other anxiety states, and drug abuse (commonly iatrogenic). The long-assumed association between OCD and Tourette's syndrome has recently been questioned (Crino, 1991). In addition, several other psychiatric disorders, including anorexia (Holden, 1990), trichotillomania, hypochondriasis, and body dysmorphic disorder, are regarded by some as representing variants of OCD (Tynes, White, & Steketee, 1990). However, it is probably best to consider these as separate from the core OCD syndrome.

Epidemiology

Recent epidemiologic studies have shown that previously reported rates of OCD were underestimates, with lifetime prevalence rates ranging from 2.2 to 3% (Bland, Newman, & Orn, 1988; Myers et al., 1984; Oakley-Browne, Joyce, Wells, Bushnell, & Hornblow, 1989). This makes OCD the fourth most common psychiatric disorder (after phobias, substance abuse, and major depression). Although the gender ratio is approximately 1:1, the ratio differs among the subtypes of OCD, with females and males predominating among compulsive washers and those with compulsive slowness, respectively (Marks, 1987). OCD typically commences in late adolescence and early adulthood. Females appear to have a later onset than males, and the epidemiologic findings also point to females who develop OCD after age 60.

OCD is often precipitated by an adverse life event (McKeon, Roa, & Mann, 1984), an association shared with many anxiety states (Marks, 1987). In some cases there is an immediate deterioration after onset, while in others the development is much more gradual and insidious. Once OCD is established, spontaneous remissions are unusual, with most individuals having a chronic course, exacerbations often being precipitated by adverse life events (Rasmussen & Eisen, 1992).

Etiology

Current etiological theories focus on an interaction between social learning theory and biological vulnerability. A genetic basis for OCD has not been supported by careful research. For instance, controlled studies (Black, Noyes, Goldstein, & Blum, 1991; McKeon & Murray, 1987) have failed to replicate the familial association in OCD found in uncontrolled studies (Lenane et al., 1990; Swedo, Rapoport, Leonard, Lenane, & Cheslow, 1989), although the prevalence of other anxiety disorders was greater than normal. Again, although an increased monozygotic concordance has been reported for OCD (Marks, 1986b), Andrews, Stewart, Allen, & Henderson (1990) failed to replicate this finding with a large sample of twin pairs.

Inferring causality on the basis of successful pharmacologic treatment is also notoriously unreliable, and the serotonergic deficit explanation for OCD is similarly not straightforward (Barr et al., 1992). However, the association of OCD with several neurological illnesses such as Sydenham's chorea, Postencephalitic parkinsonism, and Tourette's syndrome have lead to neuroimaging studies that are producing interesting findings (Insel, 1992). Attention has focused on the orbitofrontal cortex, cingulate cortex, and caudate nucleus, and it is suggested that these form a circuit that is hyperactive in OCD. Of especial interest is the finding, using positron emission tomographic scanning, that caudate nucleus activity decreased in OCD subjects treated with either fluoxetine or 10 weeks of behavior therapy (Baxter et al., 1992). However, these advances in the identification of the vulnerable biological substrate need to be integrated with the other known psychological factors to develop a comprehensive etiological model of OCD.

Differential Diagnosis and Assessment

DSM-III-R Categorization

DSM-III-R delineates a bipartite classification with (a) definitions of both obsessions and compulsions, and (b) the requirement that these have a significant impact on the individual's life.

Obsessions are defined as existing if: (a) there are recurrent and persistent ideas, thoughts, or impulses that are experienced, at least initially, as intrusive and senseless; (b) an attempt is made to ignore or suppress these thoughts or impulses or to neutralize them with some other thought or action; and (c) the individual recognizes that these thoughts are the product of his or her own mind and are not imposed from outside. Compulsions exist if (a) repetitive, purposeful, and intentional behaviors are performed in response to an obsession or according to certain rules or in a stereotyped fashion; (b) the behavior is designed to neutralize or to prevent discomfort or some dreaded event or situation; and (c) the person recognizes the behavior as excessive or unreasonable.

The obsessions or compulsions cause marked distress, take a significant amount of time (i.e., at least one hour a day), and have an impact on the individual's occupation or leisure or relationships with others (American Psychiatric Association, 1987).

Differential Diagnosis

Obsessional Compulsive Personality Disorder (OCPD) and Other Axis II Diagnoses. Conventionally, OCPD traits are considered ego syntonic (i.e., not distressing or alien), whereas OCD symptoms are ego dystonic. This distinction becomes problematic when the beliefs in OCD become embedded with a degree of secondary avoidance, so that subjective distress becomes minimal and resistance to the intrusion disappears. Research has shown estimates of the co-occurrence of OCPD and OCD varying from 30 to 70%. Recent evidence suggests that this co-occurrence is less common than indicated in earlier studies, while the rate of other personality disorders is considerably more (Crino, 1991). Because the occurrence of an Axis II disorder makes more difficult treatment of the Axis I disorder, whether with medication (Baer et al., 1992; Reich & Green, 1991), with behavior therapy (Turner, 1987), or with self-help methods in general (Tyrer, Seivewright, Ferguson, Murphy, & Johnson, 1993), this finding has important treatment and prognostic implications.

Other Anxiety States.   Clinically, it may be difficult to decide whether an individual has a phobia or OCD (Marks, 1987). In addition, other anxiety states commonly co-occur with OCD, with one study showing that OCD subjects had a 40% likelihood of having a phobic disorder and a 10% probability of panic disorder (Mulder, Sellman, & Joyce, 1991). In addition, longitudinal investigations of anxiety states do not support their separate identity, although OCD appears more stable than other anxiety conditions (Tyrer, 1985).

Depression.   Depression is the most important and common co-occurring condition, with a lifetime prevalence of 70%. Some 25 to 30% of patients with OCD will be depressed at presentation (Rasmussen & Eisen, 1988). This co-occurrence has a number of implications: (a) the individual with long-standing OCD may present for treatment only after developing depression; (b) the depression commonly increases the severity of OCD (Kendell & Discipio, 1970); and (c) the presence of depression worsens the outcome of anxiety disorders in general (Mulder et al., 1991) and the response of OCD to treatment in particular (Foa et al., 1983).

OCD as a Prelude to Psychosis.   It may sometimes be difficult to distinguish OCD from an overvalued idea, especially if the belief has been held for some time and resistance has disappeared. An overvalued idea is considered to be reasonable (vs. futile), natural (vs. intrusive), and not resisted (McKenna, 1984). Another important differential is whether the OCD symptomatology represents a defense against an acute psychotic breakdown or a more gradual deterioration of personality (Rosen, 1957). In an 18-year follow-up study of depressed patients, high scores on the Leyton Obsessional Inventory at index were associated with the subsequent development of schizophrenia or schizoaffective psychosis (Duggan, Lee, & Murray, 1990).

Assessment Strategies

Preassessment Preparation.   If the patient wants a psychotherapeutic approach rather than medication, then it is useful for the patient to have read a self-exposure manual (e.g., *Living with Fear*, I. M. Marks, 1978) before being seen by the therapist. This has the effect of informing the patient what will be required of him or her, and will subtly convey that the patient's active involvement in the treatment will be required.

Clinical Assessment.   The current disturbance must be examined in terms of the anxiogenic stimulus (usually the obsession), the resultant anxiety state, and then the anxiolytic response. The anxiogenic stimulus may occur spontaneously or be cued by a number of other stimuli, which that individual will avoid. The undoing ritual may be overt (i.e., a behavior that is excessive) or covert, in the form of a mental ritual. Because the ritual reduces anxiety, it has an important maintaining, reinforcing, or even preemptive function. What is the impact on the individual's relationships and occupational functioning? One should inquire as to what treatments have been applied in the past. Were they appropriate, and what was the response? One also needs to assess the drug and alcohol intake of the patient. Commonly, other medications have been prescribed, and the consumption of benzodiazepines in particular should be reduced, because these will affect habituation in behavior therapy. At the Maudsley Hospital's Psychological Treatment Unit, the practice has been not to commence treatment until the individual is taking at most 10 mg of diazepam (or equivalent), and preferably less. It is also important to assess the mental state to decide if there is any concomitant depression or any evidence of psychosis. Finally, use of an informant (a close family member) is often very helpful in that (a) the individual with OCD may minimize the level of disability or omit crucial avoidances, and (b) the family member may need guidance in order to avoid offering excessive reassurance.

Another important issue, especially for behavior therapy, is to assess motivation for change. Experience has shown the following to be useful indicators:

1. A desire to obtain therapy and to have read about the rationale for treatment before being assessed. Conversely, an individual whose consultation is arranged by a long-suffering spouse or parent is not likely to be motivated to change behavior.
2. A commitment to homework from the beginning of treatment.
3. A desire to extemporize and develop one's own treatment program so that the therapist can quickly take a back seat. Individuals who do well generally do so early in treatment. By session 4 or 5, the treatment needs to be reviewed if there is no demonstrable progress.

Measurement of Symptoms. At the completion of the assessment, the therapist and the patient should be clear as to the nature of the OCD and the problems that it produces, and together they should determine a list of specific targets that the patient wishes to achieve. These should again be quantified to form a baseline whereby the impact of the therapy may be judged. There are several instruments available to assess OCD symptoms, including the Yale Brown Obsessional Scale (Y-BOCS; Goodman et al., 1989a, 1989b), the Maudsley Obsessive Compulsive Inventory (MOCI; Rachman & Hodgson, 1980), and the Leyton Obsessional Inventory (Cooper, 1970). However, these are most often used in a research setting. As a routine package, I advise using the self-report Compulsions Checklist, a Fear Questionnaire (Marks & Mathews, 1979), and the Beck Depression Inventory (Beck, Ward, Mendelson, Mock, & Erbaugh, 1961; see Marks, 1986a).

Treatment

Evidence for Prescriptive Treatments

Successful treatments should be (a) efficient to deliver, (b) acceptable and accessible to a majority of sufferers, and (c) effective. An additional consideration with OCD is that it often takes patients many years to present for treatment (Duggan, Marks, & Richards, 1993; Pollitt, 1957). In this they are little different from those with other anxiety disorders. Thus there is a considerable unmet need in the community. One of the challenges of the mental health professional is to make sufferers aware that effective treatments are available and how these can be accessed. Controlled evaluative research has identified two methods of treatment as being effective for OCD: behavior therapy and pharmacotherapy.

Behavior Therapy. Meyer (1966) has been credited with establishing the early credentials for behavior therapy for OCD. This procedure involves self-exposure to the anxiogenic stimulus together with response prevention. Treatment time has been reduced so that 15 to 20 treatment sessions is usually adequate to effect a significant improvement. Treatment time has been reduced (increasing treatment availability and making it more successful) by emphasizing the centrality of self-exposure, excluding relaxation training, and omitting therapist-assisted exposure (Marks, 1991).

There is now compelling evidence from several studies that this treatment, if applied by the patient, will be effective in most patients with OCD, even when the condition has been severe and chronic (Cottraux, 1989; Duggan et al., 1993; Marks, 1987; Rachman & Hodgson, 1980). For instance, in a series of 261 patients with OCD treated with behavior therapy at Maudsley Hospital, 70% were in the "much improved" category and only 10% showed no improvement (Duggan et al., 1993). Foa and colleagues drew much the same conclusion in their review of patients treated with behavior therapy in different countries. Foa et al. (1985) concluded that 51% of patients achieved a 70% reduction in symptoms and only 10% showed no improvement. Furthermore, the gains achieved tend to be maintained in follow-up studies running for up to 12 years (see O'Sullivan & Marks, 1990). The message for patients is therefore clear: for those with OCD who commit themselves to an exposure program, there is a 70% chance that their symptoms will be substantially reduced and that, moreover, these gains will persist many years after the completion of treatment.

Pure Obsessional Ruminations. This subset of OCD had a particularly poor response in the past to behavioral techniques of thought stopping and distraction (Emmelkamp, 1982; Rachman, 1983). Conceptualizing obsessive ruminations as both anxiogenic thoughts and anxiolytic or cognitive neutralizing rituals—which have the same maintaining effect as overt compulsive behavior—has improved the success rate with this condition (Salkovskis & Westbrook, 1989). The treatment consists of the patient (again as a part of homework) recording his or her anxiogenic thoughts on a cassette tape and playing these thoughts continually until habituation occurs, while omitting anxiolytic or cognitive neutralizing thoughts.

Inpatient Units. In the past, OCD was thought to be such a serious and refractory disorder that inpatient intensive work was required to effect change. There has been a swing away from such treatment, with the recent emphasis on self-exposure without the aid of the therapist. However, there may be a case for referring a patient if intensive work is indicated and the person has little access to behavior therapy locally. For the gain to be maintained, however, some local support is necessary for the treatment to be continued after the patient has been discharged. Considerations in deciding on referral are the severity of the disorder, concomitant depression, and the need to involve other members of the family in rehearsing not giving reassurance (Thornicroft, Colson, & Marks, 1991). In the main, however, hospitalization is not necessary; it is likely that the gains made in the hospital may well be lost after discharge.

Treatment Failures. Foa, Steketee, Grayson, and Doppelt (1983) have identified the following types of treatment failure in behavior therapy for OCD:

1. Treatment refusal. Here a patient considered suitable for treatment refuses because the treatment is perceived as being too demanding, inappropriate, or too frightening. The rates of treatment refusal for OCD vary from 5 to 25% (see Foa et al., 1983).
2. Treatment dropout. This refers to premature termination of treatment (i.e., by the fourth session) (McDonald, Marks, & Blizzard, 1988). The rates of dropout are lower than those of treatment refusal; from 0 to 12% has been reported from different series (Foa et al., 1983).
3. Treatment failure. Groups in which 10% showed no improvement despite treatment have been reported (Duggan et al., 1993; Foa et al., 1983).
4. Relapse. O'Sullivan and Marks (1990) estimate that there is a relapse rate of 20% in OCD treated with behavior therapy over an extended period of follow-up.

Collapsing these data across studies suggests that about one-quarter to one-third of patients will not get an adequate course of treatment, either because of treatment refusal or because of premature dropout. In addition, 10 to 15% will not respond (true treatment failures) and an additional 10 to 20% will relapse. Thus, some 30 to 50% of OCD patients referred for treatment and believed to be suitable for behavior therapy will make little or no progress.

Foa and colleagues have investigated some of the predictors of failure in OCD. They identified initial severe depression, late age at symptom onset, pretreatment anxiety, and overvalued ideation (Foa, 1979; Foa et al., 1985) as having a negative effect on outcome. Depression prevented habituation from taking place at all, whereas with overvalued ideation, habituation took place within the session but not outside the session. Duration and severity of symptoms did not affect outcome.

Cognitive Therapy. Cognitive therapy has been used infrequently because of the belief that OCD patients are already overly preoccupied with intellectualizing their problems. Where cognitive therapy may be of advantage is in persuading an individual to take the risk of engaging in a behavioral "experiment." This may be especially true when the obsession has the quality of overvalued ideation. Cognitive therapy might then be employed to render the thought more ego dystonic and thereby more amenable to challenge by a behavioral intervention (Salkovskis & Warwick, 1985). Cognitive therapy may also be used to improve compliance, which is a major problem in behavior therapy. One trial has compared a form of cognitive therapy (rational-emotive therapy) with exposure in vivo in OCD, and no differences between the two approaches were found (Emmelkamp & Beens, 1991). Furthermore, there was no additional benefit when cognitive therapy added anything to exposure in vivo.

Pharmacotherapy. In the United States, drugs are the mainstay of treatment for OCD, and recent studies have clarified what types, dosages, and lengths of treatment are effective, in addition to highlighting certain problems. Although there have been individual case reports of successful treatment with a diverse series of drugs, controlled evaluation points to the efficacy of clomipramine and, more recently, several of the specific serotonergic reuptake inhibitors (SSRIs). These drugs achieve a significant symptom reduction in 30 to 60% of cases (White & Cole, 1990). However, even in cases with residual symptomatology, the individual usually regards the reduction as a major benefit (Jenike, 1990).

Clomipramine has been the most extensively studied of any drug prescribed for OCD, and placebo-controlled trials have shown it to be effective. For example, a recently completed large multicenter study showed a 40% reduction in Y-BOCS scores in the actively treated group, as compared to 2 to 5% in the placebo control (Clomipramine Collaborative Study Group, 1991). The findings from this and several other studies can be summarized as follows: (a) improvement with the active drug continues throughout the initial phase of treatment and is generally not apparent until 6 weeks; (b) dosages need to be high (up to 250 mg a day); (c) the side effects are primarily anticholinergic, but sexual difficulties are also common (Monteiro, Noshirvani, & Marks, 1987); (d) the response of OCD symptomatology is independent of baseline depressive symptomatology; and (e) drugs not affecting the serotonergic process are ineffective (Goodman, McDougle, & Price, 1992; Jenike, 1990).

There have been encouraging reports from double blind, placebo-controlled studies for the SSRIs fluvoxamine (Jenike, Baer, & Greist, 1990), fluoxetine (Jenike, 1990), and sertraline (Chouinard, Goodman, & Griest, 1990). Although the side effect profile of these drugs is less severe than that of clomipramine, these drugs are associated with nausea, diarrhea, and motor restlessness. A meta-analysis comparison between clomipramine and fluoxetine showed the former to have the greater effect but also to have more side effects (Jenike et al., 1991).

Although the chances of obtaining symptomatic relief are high, what about relapse once medication is stopped? The evidence is not reassuring for our present drug regimens, with one study showing a 90% relapse rate on abrupt discontinuation of medication (Pato, Zohar-Kadouch, & Zohar, 1988). Since the natural history of OCD points to chronicity, this relapse pattern is not surprising. Thus, although to date there have been no controlled evaluative studies, there may be a case for long-term maintenance treatment of OCD.

Treatment Resistance.   What are the alternatives once a drug of choice has failed? Goodman et al. (1992) recommends first switching the patient to an alternative 5HT blocker. If this fails, then the standard medication could be augmented by a series of drugs, including lithium (10% respond), an MAOI, buspirone, tryptophan, or a neuroleptic, although here again there is no clear data to attest to their effectiveness.

Combining Behavior Therapy with Medication.   Because neither pharmacotherapy nor behavior therapy for OCD is entirely satisfactory when prescribed alone, a logical alternative is to use a combined approach to optimize the response. What is the evidence that combining drugs with behavior therapy for OCD is advantageous? In two studies conducted by Marks and colleagues, clomipramine was added to an exposure regimen and then compared to pure exposure and placebo. Although clomipramine initially enhanced the effect of exposure, this drug effect disappeared at 2-year follow-up (Marks et al., 1988; Marks, Stern, Mawson, Cobb, & McDonald, 1980; Mavissakalian & Jones, 1989). In another combination study, Foa, Kozak, Steketee, and McCarthy (1992) pretreated a group of patients with OCD and depression with an antidepressant prior to treatment with behavior therapy. The study found that: (a) this pretreatment did not enhance the effects of behavior therapy for OCD (as compared to placebo), (b) the antidepressant reduced the depressive but not the OCD symptoms, and (c) behavior therapy reduced the OCD symptoms. Thus, a reasonable summary of the present evidence is that a behavioral approach used as the primary intervention seems a sufficient treatment in itself and does not require adjunctive medication except to treat concomitant depression. However, when medication is used as the primary intervention, it is helpful to complement it with behavior therapy to prevent relapse once the medication has been stopped.

Alternative Treatments. Although rarely used nowadays, psychosurgical techniques such as cingulotomy, anterior capsulotomy, and modified leucotomy have been shown to have some effect when the two conventional treatments have failed. Reviews point to a 30 to 60% improvement in symptoms with psychosurgery for OCD but with the side effects of seizures, transient mania, and memory and intellectual changes (Jenike et al., 1991; O'Sullivan & Marks, 1990). Because surgery may improve the response to conventional treatments, behavior therapy or medication is worth trying again postoperatively even if ineffective previously.

Selecting Optimal Treatment Strategies

Psychotherapy vs. Pharmacotherapy. The advantages of behavior therapy over drugs are that it produces a greater overall improvement, and the improvement, once established, persists. The disadvantages are the difficulties of initial engagement of the patient and the expense and necessity of trained therapists to supervise treatment. Since there is no research to inform us on the indications for either of these treatments, the selection depends on patient preference and the availability of trained behavior therapists. Assessment for co-occurring depression is important, because this condition may necessitate prescribing an antidepressant if behavior therapy is offered as the front-line treatment. Augmentation of behavior therapy with cognitive therapy would appear to be indicated for an overvalued idea. As other diagnoses are documented in addition to OCD, it may be possible to develop a rational policy of management for the overall treatment of the patient. Thus, although certain authors argue that there is no role for relaxation training (e.g., Marks, 1991), it may be of value in a subgroup of patients in whom the anxiety level is so high as to prevent engagement in the exposure exercises or preclude habituation. However, there is little evidence as yet to help us predict which patients are likely to need adjunctive techniques (if indeed there are any needed at all).

Problems in Carrying Out Interventions

Because the problem of drug compliance in OCD is no different than in other conditions, we will concentrate here on some of the difficulties in carrying out behavior therapy.

Failures of Engagement. The behavioral analysis provides essential data and creates a therapeutic alliance in which the patient feels understood. Some individuals will recognize the validity of the behavior analysis, yet not be willing to take a risk with the treatment. To encourage the patient to take this step, one can point to the following: (a) although anxiety is uncomfortable, it may not be as uncomfortable as the patient anticipates; (b) the amplitude and duration of anxiety will diminish over time; and (c) the prediction that something catastrophic will happen may be disconfirmed. One should avoid getting drawn into an intellectual debate about the pros and cons of the individual's behavior; this is likely to be used by the patient to provide reassurance.

Failures to Habituate. Failure to carry out the homework task properly must be considered when habituation does not occur. Patients generally underestimate the amount of homework involvement necessary to overcome their OCD. Typically, the patient needs to spend at least 1 hour every day practicing homework tasks. Records should be made of the homework on a simple diary (Figure 10.1). Taking homework seriously is as important for the therapist as for the patient; hence, a large proportion of every session should be given over to an examination of the homework diary, which usually identifies the reasons for failure in treatment. These include (a) not doing homework at all—which unfortunately is quite common; (b) doing homework but not systematically or regularly enough to be effective (e.g., two days out of seven); (c) and carrying out an inadequate exposure exercise—suggested by a rating of less than 4 in the anxiety scale—either because the task was insufficiently anxiety provoking or was ended prematurely, or because some mode of distraction was used. Thus a typical therapy session focuses initially on how well the patient has carried out the homework exercises, followed by a discussion of any difficulties that may have arisen in their implementation; finally, homework exercises for the next session are set. Because the patient will be setting more and more of the homework tasks in a successful treatment, the length of a session can be short—on the order of 15 to 20 minutes.

Ways of dealing with reasons (a) and (b) have already been discussed; reason (c) refers to a small group of patients ("true nonhabituators")—possibly about 2%—who, despite carrying out homework assignments, nevertheless do not habituate. Unfortunately, they are a group who can be discovered only by default and cannot be predicted.

Relapse Prevention

Since we know that adverse life events and depression are often associated with a recrudescence of OCD, patients need to learn to predict likely times of relapse. This should be made explicit, and the patient can then be coached into introducing the appropriate exposure and response prevention exercises. Short booster courses of therapy (i.e., a few sessions) may be necessary to reestablish the previous program.

Case Illustration

Case Description

A psychiatrist referred a 17-year-old unmarried girl with the core problem of intrusive, persistent distressing thoughts that she would cause harm to others. She believed that this harm would ensue from her carelessness so that she needed to be on constant alert. These thoughts of harm to others occupied about 70% of her day and were alien to her, but she was not capable of suppressing them. They were cued by her

HOMEWORK DIARY

Name _____

Week commencing _____

Goals for the week
1. ____
2. ____
3. ____
4. ____

Level of Anxiety

0	2	4	6	8
No anxiety	Slight anxiety	Definite anxiety	Marked anxiety	Panic

Session			Goal number	Task performed	Anxiety			Comments (including coping tactics)	Co-signed
Date	Began	Ended			Before	During	After		

Figure 10.1. Homework diary.

being in public places, where she might meet babies and other vulnerable individuals; hence these situations were avoided so that she became increasingly housebound. While at home, she avoided the kitchen and food preparation to ensure that she not poison her family. She checked letters for incriminating statements about herself. She spent at least one hour a day seeking reassurance from her parents. These thoughts spoiled her social life and private leisure and affected her ability to concentrate. They had commenced a year previously, when she believed that she had somehow strangled a child, and had gradually become worse. Her past treatment had involved clomipramine, 75 mg (she would not tolerate a larger dose), and also a 1- to 2-week exposure regimen with counseling from a psychologist.

Family History. Her parents were in their forties and had separated 5 years previously. Her mother had subsequently begun living with another man, with whom the patient had a good relationship. She reported that she was very close to her mother. She had one older sister (aged 21). There was a history of anxiety in the family, but no one had sought treatment.

Personal History. She had been born prematurely and spent some time in an incubator. There was no evidence of any developmental delay. She was always somewhat shy and anxious and had been bullied at school. She had left school at age 15 without any qualifications and over the previous two years had had two brief periods of work as a shop assistant. She now lived at home with her family, occupying herself with occasional work for her stepfather. Menarche had been at 12 years of age, and she had regular periods. She was not sexually experienced and was apprehensive about sex but did not want any help with this. There was no history of illicit drug use, and she drank sparingly. She described her premorbid personality as shy, anxious, and a worrier.

At interview, she was well dressed and a clear informant but needed to be encouraged to amplify aspects of her obsessions. She appeared depressed and said that she did not have a future. Specific questioning revealed that she had considered suicide and that she had superficially cut her wrists 6 weeks previously. There was no evidence of psychosis, and she appeared to be of normal intelligence although somewhat immature.

Differential Diagnosis and Assessment

The primary problem was undoubtedly that of obsessional ruminations with a worry that she might harm others. She managed these anxiogenic thoughts with checking rituals and reassurance seeking. There was nothing to suggest that she was psychotic, but in the referral letter it was stated that when her symptoms commenced, she was 90% certain that she had strangled a baby; at that time the phenomenology may have been that of an overvalued idea.

A second problem, however, was her depression, which was probably more severe than she admitted. Here, a Beck Depression Inventory (BDI) might give a more accurate picture than direct questioning. Could it be that this was the primary problem and OCD was secondary? Again, the course of the disorder would likely settle this.

The third issue concerned her personality. There was evidence of long-standing but mild personality disturbance involving dependency and avoidance. There was the additional evidence of her immaturity and the reported closeness with her mother. The latter needed further exploration, because the therapy risked being sabotaged by the mother's failing to withhold reassurance. An additional question was why she had had such inadequate treatment in the past. However, at this stage, she was diagnosed as having OCD (ruminations) with a secondary depression and a dependent personality.

Treatment Selection

It was decided to treat her with a self-exposure program to real-life feared situations with response prevention of her rituals. In addition, she was to be given exposure to her thoughts of harm by audiotape. The medication (clomipramine, 75 mg) was continued for her mood disturbance.

As part of the treatment, she was asked to describe her main problem and three targets with her therapist. She described her main problem as "Constant intrusive thoughts that I will have harmed others through my actions, leading to checking, distracting, and reassurance seeking." Her three targets were: (A1) to go out with friends three times per week for 3 hours without having anxiety or intrusive thoughts; (A2) to go to public places (e.g., shops, cinema) for 2 hours twice a week without having intrusive thoughts; and (A3) to reduce the frequency and discomfort and increase the control over the thoughts by 70%. She also rated the amount of handicap and the effect of the problem on her life, her work, her family, and social interactions and private leisure. Finally, she completed a Fear Questionnaire, a BDI, and a Compulsive Checklist.

Defining and quantifying the main problem, targets, and consequences are important for the following reasons: (a) the specificity of the problem and targets clarifies the problem behavior; (b) the rating introduces the patient to have a dimensional rather than a categorical view of his or her problem; and (c) the patient has an important role in this negotiation process so that from the outset he or she has an active involvement in the treatment.

The initial rating and their change at midtreatment (at 12 weeks) and at treatment completion (24 weeks) are given in Figure 10.2. There are some interesting anomalies. Although she gave the main problem a near maximum rating, the amount of handicap it caused was minimal. This suggests that there was probably a significant amount of covert avoidance, which had the effect of reducing anxiety. If this is the case, then one would predict that the effect of the exposure program would be to increase these ratings, and to a certain extent this is what transpired. This was also the case in some aspects of the fear questionnaire. The clinician's concern about her mood were well founded; her pretreatment BDI score was 27.

Treatment Course and Problems in Carrying Out Interventions

The patient was given 19 sessions of therapy, which involved 10 hours of therapist time (including the assessment). The patient set herself certain tasks (such as not checking that she had filled the kettle properly when she was making tea for her family) and was asked to keep a diary recording the task, the number of times it had been performed, and the resultant anxiety and the amount of time required for this anxiety to diminish. Following are verbatim transcripts from the therapist's notes, which give a flavor of the therapy:

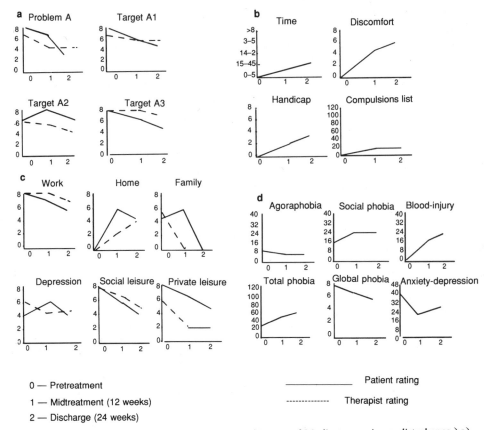

0 — Pretreatment
1 — Midtreatment (12 weeks)
2 — Discharge (24 weeks)

—————————— Patient rating

------------- Therapist rating

Figure 10.2. Initial ratings and change with treatment. (A score of 8 indicates maximum disturbance.) a) Main problems and targets. b) Obsessive-compulsive: Total time, discomfort, handicap. c) Effect of the problem on work, home, family, depression, and social and private leisure. d) Fear questionnaire: Self rating.

Session 3. 30 min. Therapist writes 3 exposure tasks performed, which seemed to have been prescribed by mother. The patient distracts herself when carrying out the task. Patient given antidistraction instruction. Mood—stable. Ruminative belief still 90% but does reduce on challenging. Homework [(H/W)]: To make drinks for family twice every day without refilling kettle.

Session 4. 40 min. Completed (H/W) twice during week but ritualized once before filling kettle. Still using distraction when has anxiogenic thoughts by either carrying out some task very thoroughly or possibly with the use of neutralizing thoughts. Same (H/W) given.

Session 5. 40 min. Made infrequent drinks for family but distracted during carrying out of task. Mood—very low, tearful; therapist to contact mother and treating psychiatrist. (H/W): Drinks for family; to write a script of the original episode when she believed she had strangled the baby so that this might be put on audiotape.

Session 6. 30 min. (H/W) not done consistently, mood low, thoughts of strangling baby prominent, guilty, feels she is being and should be punished. (H/W): Drinks for family, write up script of incident (still not done).

Session 7. 20 min. (H/W): Has made drinks regularly but has not recorded anxiety and says it bothers her very little. Script started but very sparse and needs more detail. Mood better but she feels that there has not been any improvement. (H/W) as for the last session.

Session 8. 45 min. (H/W) written script, but because of anxiety has written little. Consistency stressed in homework practice. Given relaxation tape to try to reduce background anxiety. (H/W): Prepare drinks for family as before. Turn gas fire off daily without checking. Cross roads for 30 min. without undue checking. Make a loop tape of anxiogenic thoughts.

Session 9. 20 min. (H/W) has listened to tape and gets bored and cannot concentrate after 25 minutes. Not doing (H/W) frequently enough. Told friend of problem, which she found useful. (H/W) as for last week.

Session 10. 15 min. Discussed (H/W). Still not consistent and still ritualizing; mother worried that treatment not working; mood OK. (H/W) as for last week.

Session 11. 30 min. (H/W) inconsistent; sustained exposure reiterated. (H/W) as previously.

Session 12. 15 min. Minimal (H/W). Further encouragement given to make loop tape with anxiogenic detail.

Session 13. 30 min. (H/W) increased exposure causes increase in rituals. Spontaneously spoke about the kitchen being anxiety provoking because of the presence of kitchen fluids that she might inadvertently use and thereby poison her family. Three-system model of anxiety discussed again and reiterated need for adequate exposure for anxiety to habituate. Patient feels that she is not dealing with main fear of strangling baby but it was pointed out to her that she must work toward this. (H/W): To spend 1 hr. in kitchen without distraction.

Session 14. 10 min. Still not doing (H/W) regularly. Feels 1 hr. is too long. Told to do exposure for 1 hr. or until anxiety is reduced by 50%, also (H/W) to be done daily.

Session 15. 15 min. Rates 6 on anxiety in kitchen and no reduction within 30 min. but then engages in ritual. Also has magazine, which she glances at. Goes shopping but sees baby, becomes anxious, and returns home. Core belief becomes clearer to therapist (i.e., has to be in control, otherwise may have amnesia when anything could happen). (H/W): 1 hr. in kitchen without distraction.

Session 16. 20 min. Mother contacted unit as daughter has become very distressed. She has been out in a car and believes that she has caused an accident. Mood low and tearful. Therapist asked to call patient. Finally made contact. Patient described how she put head out of the car window and later came to believe that she had caused an accident. Therapist is able to challenge the belief so that it reduces 50%. Encouraged patient to do this herself.

Session 17. 60 min. Parents seen with patient. They describe many rituals that the patient has never disclosed (e.g., spends 4 hours in the bathroom every morning ritualizing). Also has many cognitive (i.e., neutralizing) rituals. Patient does not see connection between program and her thought about harming the baby. (H/W): Time to get ready in the mornings to be reduced to 2 hours before next appointment. Parents given instructions about withholding reassurance, and principles of therapy amplified.

Session 18. 30 min. Therapist has clearer idea of sequence: If anxious will become amnesic and then behave recklessly without knowing it, hence has a certain sequence of allaying anxiety. Encouraged to act spontaneously and obey parents' commands. (H/W): Avoid checking gas taps and doors.

Session 19. 45 min. Patient stated that she could not comply with treatment at present. At discharge 15 to 20% improvement in symptoms. Depression is also slightly better, but there is a question as to whether this is accurate. She is encouraged to adopt a self-help approach, and the door is kept open should she wish to return. Therapy terminated.

Follow-Up

No follow-up data are available, but 9 months post treatment she had not made any contact with the unit.

Although the program for behavior therapy with OCD is straightforward, this case illustrates that the application of the approach in the real world is often complicated and requires considerable skill. With the advantage of hindsight, certain key aspects of the case become apparent: It is clear, for instance, that the patient's commitment to homework was halfhearted. This became very evident during her crisis (Session 16), when she became extremely anxious and wanted reassurance. It appears that the therapist missed an opportunity here and should have persisted with the model. This would have involved the patient's carrying out the same anxiogenic behavior again and again until her anxiety had diminished. Instead, he challenged her thoughts, which was a subtle form of inadvertent collusion and possibly offered her reassurance. This episode also suggests that her mother is actively involved in offering her reassurance and may be sabotaging therapy. At this point, if not before, she should have been involved in treatment. One should also note that despite the thorough initial assessment, certain worries (e.g., about kitchen fluids) and avoidances were not disclosed and her initial ratings were probably misleading. There is the question of whether helping her manage her anxiety initially with anxiety management training might have facilitated greater compliance with the behavior program subsequently, but, as in all cases of this type, this is an issue apparent only in retrospect. Finally, there is the issue of her mood disturbance, which may still be exerting a significant detrimental effect on the behavioral program. It might have been wise to have switched to an SSRI drug, because the amount of clomipramine she was able to tolerate was probably subtherapeutic.

Since this patient never consistently carried out homework, the foremost question is: If the therapist had said that he would refuse to see her after the fourth session unless she agreed to carry out homework tasks properly, would not a great deal of time have been saved? He clearly thought that with time he would be able to increase her compliance, but this was not to be. Questions as to when treatment should be abandoned have not preoccupied us up to now, but with limited health budgets, this will clearly be an important area to examine in the future. When patients are not doing homework, it is not necessarily a time for despair or blaming the patient; rather, it is an invitation to evaluate again the adequacy of the initial formulation. There remain a substantial number of patients with OCD who will not attempt something that is potentially advantageous, and to understand this refusal remains a challenge for the future.

Summary

Obsessive-compulsive disorder (OCD) is a relatively common condition with a lifetime prevalence of 2.5%. The basic neuropathology, centering on the orbitofrontal cortex, is gradually becoming understood. Although OCD was previously thought to be refractory to treatment, behavior therapy or drugs have now been shown to be effective in controlled research. Behavior therapy is successful in up to 70% of cases treated, and these gains persist, as shown in several long-term follow-up studies. Recent advances in conceptualization of obsessional ruminations suggest that this subtype of OCD may also respond well to a behavioral approach. A cognitive component to treatment appears unwarranted except in the treatment of overvalued ideation.

Depression often co-occurs with OCD and requires specific treatment when a behavioral approach is employed. Serotonergic receptor blocking drugs also produce substantial symptom reduction in 30 to 60% of patients; this improvement is not due to pretreatment levels of depression. However, relapse is common once the medication has been stopped. There is no evidence, as yet, to support combining behavior therapy with medication; the effect of the combined treatment is similar to that of either treatment offered alone. However, augmentation of drug therapy with psychological approaches seems sensible to prevent relapse. Future research should focus on making treatment available to those in the community who fail to present as well as improving engagement and compliance in those who do.

ACKNOWLEDGMENT.   I am indebted to Jonathan Ash, Clinical Nurse Specialist at The Maudsley Hospital, for providing details on the case illustration, and to the patient who graciously provided permission to publish the material presented herein.

References

American Psychiatric Association (1987). *Diagnostic and statistical manual of mental disorders* (3rd ed., rev.). Washington, DC: Author.

Andrews, G., Stewart, G., Allen, R., & Henderson, S. (1990). The genetics of six neurotic disorders: A twin study. *Journal of Affective Disorders, 19*, 23–29.

Baer, L., Jenike, M. A., Black, D. W., Treece, C., Rosenfeld, R., & Griest, J. (1992). Effect of Axis II diagnoses on treatment outcome with clomipramine in 55 patients with obsessive compulsive disorder. *Archives of General Psychiatry, 49*, 862–867.

Barr, L. C., Goodman, W. K., Lawrence, M. D., Price, H., McDougle, C. J., & Charney, D. S. (1992). The serotonin hypothesis of obsessive compulsive disorder: Implications of pharmacologic challenge studies. *Journal of Clinical Psychiatry, 53*, 17–28.

Baxter, L. T., Jr., Schwartz, J. M., Bergman, K. S., Szuba, M. P., Guze, B. H., Mazzitotta, J. C., Alazraki, A., Selin, C. E., Ferng, H. K., Munford, P., & Phelps, M. E. (1992). Caudate glucose metabolic rate changes with both drug and behavior therapy for obsessive compulsive disorder. *Archives of General Psychiatry, 49*, 681–689.

Beck, A. T., Ward, C. H., Mendelson, M., Mock, J. E., & Erbaugh, J. K. (1961). An inventory for measuring depression. *Archives of General Psychiatry, 4*, 561–571.

Black, D. W., Noyes, R., Goldstein, R. B., & Blum, N. (1991). A family study of obsessive compulsive disorder. *Archives of General Psychiatry, 49*, 362–371.

Bland, R. C., Newman, S. C., & Orn, H. (1988). Lifetime prevalence of psychiatric disorders in Edmonton. *Acta Psychiatrica Scandinavica, 77*, 24–32.

Chouinard, G., Goodman, W., & Griest, J. (1990). Obsessive-compulsive disorder—treatment with sertraline: A multicenter study. *Psychopharmacological Bulletin, 26*, 279–284.

Clomipramine Collaborative Study Group (1991). Clomipramine in the treatment of patients with obsessive-compulsive disorder. *Archives of General Psychiatry, 48*, 730–738.

Cooper, J. E. (1970). The Leyton Obsessional Inventory. *Psychological Medicine, 1*, 48–64.

Cottraux, J. (1989). Behavioral psychotherapy for obsessive-compulsive disorder. *International Review of Psychiatry, 1*, 227–234.

Crino, R.D. (1991). Obsessive-compulsive disorder. *International Review of Psychiatry, 3*, 189–201.

Duggan, C. F., Lee, A. S., & Murray, R. M. (1990). Does personality predict long-term outcome in depression? *British Journal of Psychiatry, 157*, 19–24.

Duggan, C. F., Marks, I., & Richards, D. (1993). Clinical audit of behavior therapy training of nurses. *Health Trends, 25*, 25–30.

Emmelkamp, P. M. G. (1982). *Phobic and obsessive compulsive disorders*. New York: Plenum.

Emmelkamp, P. M. G., & Beens, H. (1991). Cognitive therapy with obsessive compulsive disorder: A comparative evaluation. *Behaviour Research and Therapy, 29*, 293–300.

Foa, E. B. (1979). Failure in treating obsessive-compulsives. *Behaviour Research and Therapy, 17*, 169–176.

Foa, E. B., Kozak, M. J., Steketee, G. S., & McCarthy, P. R. (1992). Treatment of depressive and obsessive-compulsive symptoms in OCD by imipramine and behaviour therapy. *British Journal of Clinical Psychology, 31*, 279–292.

Foa, E. B., Steketee, G., Grayson, J. B., & Doppelt, H. G. (1983). Treatment of obsessive compulsives: When do we fail? In E. B. Foa (Ed.), *Treatment Failures* (pp. 10–33). New York: Wiley.

Foa, E. B., Steketee, G. S., & Ozarow, B. J. (1985). Behavior therapy with OCD. In M. Mavissakalian (Ed.), *Obsessive compulsive disorder*. New York: Plenum.

Goodman, W. K., McDougle, C. J., & Price, L. H. (1992). Pharmacotherapy of obsessive compulsive disorder. *Journal of Clinical Psychology, 53*, 29–37.

Goodman, W. K., Price, L. H., Rasmussen, S. A., Masure, C., Fleishmann, C., Hill, C., Heninger, G., & Charney, D. (1989a). The Yale Brown Obsessive Compulsive Scale (Y-BOCS) I: Development, use, and reliability. *Archives of General Psychiatry, 46*, 1006–1011.

Goodman, W. K., Price, L. H., Rasmussen, S. A., Masure, C., Fleishmann, C., Hill, C., Heninger, G., & Charney, D. (1989b). The Yale Brown Obsessive Compulsive Scale (Y-BOCS) II: Validity. *Archives of General Psychiatry, 46*, 1012–1016.

Holden, N. (1990). Is anorexia nervosa an obsessive-compulsive disorder? *British Journal of Psychiatry, 157*, 1–5.

Insel, T. R. (1992). Toward a neuroanatomy of obsessive-compulsive disorder. *Archives of General Psychiatry, 49*, 739–744.

Jenike, M. A. (1990). The pharmacological treatment of obsessive-compulsive disorders. *International Review of Psychiatry, 2*, 411–425.

Jenike, M. A., Baer, L., Ballantine, M. D., Martuza, R. L., Tynes, S., Giriunas, I., Buttolph, L., & Cassem, N. H. (1991). Cingulotomy for refractory obsessive compulsive disorder. *Archives of General Psychiatry, 48*, 548–550.

Jenike, M. A., Baer, L. & Greist, J. H. (1990). Clomipramine vs fluoxetine in obsessive-compulsive disorder: A retrospective comparison of side-effects and efficacy. *Journal of Clinical Psychopharmacology, 10*, 122–124.

Karno, M., & Golding, J. M. (1991). Obsessive compulsive disorder. In L. Robins & D. A. Regier (Eds.), *Psychiatric disorders in America: The Epidemiological Catchment Area Study* (pp. 204–219). New York: Free Press.

Kendell, R. E., & Discipio, W. J. (1970). Obsessional symptoms and obsessional personality traits in depressive illness. *Psychological Medicine, 1*, 65–72.

Lenane, M. C., Swedo, S. E., Leonardo, H., Pauls, D. L., Sceery, W., & Rapoport, J. L. (1990). Psychiatric disorders in the first degree relatives of children and adolescents with obsessive compulsive disorder. *Journal of the American Academy of Child and Adolescent Psychiatry, 29*, 407–412.

Marks, I. M. (1978). *Living with Fear*. New York: McGraw-Hill.

Marks, I. M. (1986a). *Behavioural psychotherapy: The Maudsley pocket book of clinical management*. Bristol, UK: Wright.

Marks, I. M. (1986b). Genetics of fear and anxiety disorders. *British Journal of Psychiatry, 149,* 406–418.

Marks, I. M. (1987). *Fears, phobias, and rituals.* Oxford, UK: Oxford University Press.

Marks, I. M. (1991). Self-administered behavioral treatment. *Behavioural Psychotherapy, 19,* 42–46.

Marks, I. M., Lelliot, P., Basoglu, M., Noshirsvani, H., Monteiro, W., Cohen, D., & Kasvikis, Y. (1988). Clomipramine, self-exposure, and therapist-aided exposure for obsessive-compulsive rituals. *British Journal of Psychiatry, 152,* 522–534.

Marks, I. M., & Mathews, A. M. (1979). Brief standard self-rating for phobic patients. *Behaviour Research and Therapy, 17,* 263–267.

Marks, I. M., Stern, R. S., Mawson, D., Cobb, J., & McDonald, R. (1980). Clomipramine and exposure for obsessive compulsive rituals: 1. *British Journal of Psychiatry, 136,* 1–25.

Mavissakalian, M. R., & Jones, B. A. (1989). Antidepressant drugs plus exposure treatment of agoraphobia/panic and obsessive-compulsive disorders. *International Review of Psychiatry, 1,* 275–281.

McDonald, R., Marks, I. M., & Blizzard, R. (1988). Quality assurance of outcome in mental health care: A model for routine use in clinical settings. *Health Trends, 20,* 111–119.

McKenna, P. J. (1984). Disorders with overvalued ideas. *British Journal of Psychiatry, 145,* 579–585.

McKeon, P., & Murray, R. (1987). Familial aspects of obsessive compulsive neurosis. *British Journal of Psychiatry, 151,* 528–534.

McKeon, P., Roa, B., & Mann, A. (1984). Life events and personality traits in obsessive-compulsive neurosis. *British Journal of Psychiatry, 144,* 185–189.

Meyer, V. (1966). Modification of expectations in cases with obsessional rituals. *Behaviour Research and Therapy, 4,* 273–280.

Monteiro, W. O., Noshirvani, H. F., & Marks, I. M. (1987). Anorgasmia from clomipramine in obsessive compulsive disorder: A controlled trial. *British Journal of Psychiatry, 151,* 107–112.

Mulder, R. T., Sellman, D., & Joyce, P. R. (1991). The comorbidity of anxiety disorders with personality, depressive, alcohol and drug disorders. *International Review of Psychiatry, 3,* 253–263.

Myers, J. K., Weissman, M. M., Tischler, G. L., Holzer, C. E., Leaf, P. J., Orvaschel, H., Anthony, J. C., Boyd, J. H., Burke, J. D. T., Kraemer, M., & Stotzman, R. (1984). Six month prevalence of psychiatric disorders in three communities. *Archives of General Psychiatry, 41,* 959–967.

Oakley-Browne, M. A., Joyce, P. R., Wells, J. E., Bushnell, J. A., & Hornblow, A. R. (1989). Christchurch psychiatric epidemiology study, Part 11. Six month and other period prevalences for specific psychiatric disorders. *Australian and New Zealand Journal of Psychiatry, 23,* 327–340.

O'Sullivan, G., & Marks, I. M. (1990). The treatment of anxiety. In M. Roth (Ed.), *Handbook of Anxiety.* New York: Elsevier.

Pato, M. T., Zohar-Kadouch, R., & Zohar, J. (1988). Return of symptoms after discontinuation of clomipramine in patients with obsessive compulsive disorder. *American Journal of Psychiatry, 144,* 1543–1548.

Pollitt, J. (1957). Natural history of obsessional states. *British Medical Journal, 1,* 195–198.

Rachman, S. J. (1983). Obstacles to the successful treatment of obsessions. In E. B. Foa & P. Emmelkamp (Eds.). *Failures in behavior therapy* (pp. 35–57). New York: Wiley.

Rachman, S. J., & Hodgson, R. J. (1980). *Obsessions and compulsions.* Englewood Cliffs, NJ: Prentice Hall.

Rasmussen, S. A., & Eisen, J. L. (1988). Clinical and epidemiological findings of significance to neuro-pharmacologic trials in obsessive compulsive disorder. *Psychopharmacological Bulletin, 24,* 466–470.

Rasmussen, S. A., & Eisen, J. L. (1992). The Epidemiology and differential diagnosis of obsessive compulsive disorder. *Journal of Clinical Psychiatry, 53,* 4–10.

Reich, J. H., & Green, A. I. (1991). Effect of personality disorders on outcome of treatment. *Journal of Nervous and Mental Diseases, 179,* 74–82.

Rosen, I. (1957). The clinical significance of obsessions in schizophrenia. *Journal of Mental Science, 103,* 773–785.

Salkovskis, P. M., & Warwick, H. M. C. (1985). Cognitive therapy of obsessive-compulsive disorder: Treating treatment failures. *Behavioural Psychotherapy, 13,* 243–255.

Salkovskis, P. M., & Westbrook, D. (1989). Behaviour therapy and obsessional ruminations: Can failure be turned into success? *Behaviour Research and Therapy, 27,* 149–160.

Swedo, S. E., Rapoport, J. L., Leonard, H., Lenane, M., & Cheslow, D. (1989). Obsessive compulsive disorder in children and adolescents: Clinical phenomenology of 70 consecutive cases. *Archives of General Psychiatry, 46,* 335–341.

Thornicroft, G., Colson, L., & Marks, I. (1991). An in-patient behavioral psychotherapy unit: Description and audit. *British Journal of Psychiatry, 158,* 362–367.

Turner, R. M. (1987). The effects of personality disorder diagnosis on the outcome of social anxiety symptom reduction. *Journal of Personality Disorders, 1,* 136–143.

Tynes, L. L., White, K., & Steketee, G. S. (1990). Toward a new nosology of obsessive compulsive disorder. *Comprehensive Psychiatry, 31,* 465–480.

Tyrer, P. (1985). Classification of mental disorders—Neurosis divisible. *Lancet, 1,* 685–688.

Tyrer, P., Seivewright, N., Ferguson, B., Murphy, S., & Johnson, A. L. (1993). The Nottingham study of neurotic disorder and effect of personality status on response to drug treatment, cognitive therapy and self help over two years. *British Journal of Psychiatry, 162,* 219–226.

Veale, D. (1993). Classification and treatment of obsessional slowness. *British Journal of Psychiatry, 162,* 198–203.

White, K., & Cole, J. (1990). Pharmacotherapy. In A. S. Bellack & M. Hersen (Eds.), *Handbook of comparative treatments* (pp. 266–284). New York: Wiley.

11

Trichotillomania

Gary Alan-Hue Christenson and Thomas Brooke Mackenzie

Description of the Disorder

Clinical Features

The essential feature of trichotillomania (TM) is the pulling out of one's hair over a prolonged period, resulting in noticeable hair thinning or bald spots. The majority of hair pullers describe the act as an automatic behavior that occurs during sedentary, contemplative activities such as reading, writing, watching television, speaking on the phone, driving, or lying in bed (Christenson, Mackenzie, & Mitchell, 1991).

Many trichotillomanics (TMs) distinguish "focused" hair pulling which has a compulsive quality with patients actively seeking out hairs to pull, from "automatic" hair pulling, which is initially out of awareness; approximately one-fourth describe the majority of their hair pulling as focused (Christenson, Mackenzie, & Mitchell, 1992, unpublished observations). The ratio of focused to automatic pulling may vary with the site being pulled or the chronological progression of the disorder.

Virtually all hair pullers have attempted to resist or control their hair pulling at some time. Self-imposed remedies have included taping fingers together, applying lubricants to fingers or hair, impairing grasp by cutting nails short (or allowing them to grow long), wearing mittens, utilizing head barriers (e.g., wigs, scarves, hats), and avoiding associated activities (e.g., reading).

Any body hair may be targeted in TM; most patients pull from two or more sites. A recent study reported that the following sites are involved in descending order of frequency: scalp (75%), eyelashes (53%), eyebrows (42%), pubus (17%), arm

Gary Alan-Hue Christenson and **Thomas Brooke Mackenzie** • Department of Psychiatry, University of Minnesota, Minneapolis, Minnesota 55455.

Handbook of Prescriptive Treatments for Adults, edited by Michel Hersen and Robert T. Ammerman. Plenum Press, New York, 1994.

(10%), beard/face (10%), moustache (7%), leg (7%), chest (3%), and abdomen (2%) (Christenson et al., 1991a).

Hair pulling can develop at any age, although onset is typically in childhood or adolescence. The mean age at onset is 13 years (Christenson, Mackenzie, & Mitchell, 1991). It has been suggested that childhood-onset TM often resolves spontaneously after a brief course with minimal or no intervention (Friman, Rostain, Parrish, & Carey, 1990). However, this impression appears to be based on anecdotal impressions; long-term studies of the natural course of TM are lacking. One report suggests that if, at the time of presentation in children, hair pulling has been present for less than 6 months, the prognosis for recovery with minimal intervention is good; otherwise a chronic pattern of hair pulling is typical (Chang, Lee, Chiang, & Lü, 1991).

Large clinical studies of TMs indicate that 70 to 90% are female (Christenson, Mackenzie, & Mitchell, 1991; Muller, 1990). However, a recent survey of college freshmen suggests that the lifetime prevalence of DSM-III-R TM may be equal for both sexes (Christenson, Pyle, & Mitchell, 1991).

Associated Features

Oral manipulation of pulled hair is reported in 48% of TMs (Christenson, Mackenzie, & Mitchell, 1991). This may involve rubbing hair along the mouth, chewing the end of the hair, or complete ingestion of hair. The last behavior, which is reported to some degree in 10% of TMs, may on rare occasions lead to the formation of a trichobezoar (a mass of connected hair in the stomach or bowel). The mortality rate for untreated trichobezoars is approximately 70% (DeBakey & Ochsner, 1938). A recent report noted that 6 (25%) of 24 TM patients had a trichobezoar and 3 (12.5%) had a trichophytobezoar (mass of hair and vegetable fiber); 22.2% of these patients were asymptomatic (Bhatia et al., 1991). This observation underscores the importance of always inquiring about hair ingestion in the assessment of TM.

TM, by definition, results in visible hair loss, which may vary from minimal thinning to complete alopecia of the involved area. Patients are typically upset and ashamed about their appearance and attempt to disguise the involved area. For scalp pullers this frequently involves adaptation of their hair style. At times patients apply makeup to the scalp; the wearing of scarves, hats, and wigs is common among severe TMs. Attempts to hide hair loss may lead to avoidance of windy weather, swimming, or situations in which the scalp would be more visible (e.g., sitting in bleachers). Pubic hair pullers may avoid routine physical examinations. Hair pulling from any site may lead to avoidance of intimate relationships.

Hair pulling may result in physical changes including lack of hair regrowth, hair color changes (to gray or white), or hair curling (Rebora, Chiappara, Guarrera, & Parodi, 1990). Textural changes may exacerbate TM; hair pulling often targets "thick," "kinky," "curly," or "coarse" hair (Christenson, Mackenzie, & Mitchell, 1991; Swedo & Leonard, 1992).

TM is frequently associated with psychiatric comorbidity. One large study reported high lifetime prevalences of mood (65%), anxiety (57%), chemical use (22%), and eating (20%) disorders (Christenson, Mackenzie, & Mitchell, 1991). Elevated rates of mood and anxiety disorders have also been noted in children and adolescents with TM (Reeve, Bernstein, & Christenson, 1992).

Personality disorders, particularly borderline and compulsive personality disorders, have also been suggested to be prevalent in TM (Christenson, Chernoff-

Clementz, & Clementz, 1992). A recent report of 48 TMs noted high rates of histrionic (14.6%), avoidant (10.4%), obsessive-compulsive (8.3%), and dependent (8.3%) personality disorders. However, personality disorders were no more common among a group of psychiatric outpatients presenting to the same clinic (Christenson, Chernoff-Clementz, & Clementz, 1992). In light of these observations, all TMs should undergo a thorough psychiatric assessment.

Epidemiology

TM has traditionally been considered a rare disorder. Early accounts suggested a prevalence of 0.05 to 0.6% in clinical psychiatric populations (Christenson, Pyle, & Mitchell, 1991).

In an attempt to better characterize the prevalence of TM, Christenson, Pyle, and Mitchell (1991) surveyed 2,579 college freshmen regarding lifetime history of hair pulling. Of 2,534 respondents, 0.6% of both males and females fulfilled DSM-III-R TM criteria at some time. Additionally, hair pulling resulting in visible hair loss but failing to meet full DSM-III-R criteria was reported by 1.5% of males and 3.4% of females.

Etiology

Although the etiology of TM remains unknown, some theories regarding its origins have been proposed. Early accounts often offered psychoanalytic explanations. For example, Greenberg and Sarner (1965) suggested that TM was multidetermined, with different symbolism at different stages of psychosexual development. Typical family dynamics are reportedly a "hair-pulling symbiosis" characterized by mothers who are double binding and controlling toward hair-pulling daughters in the presence of a passive father (Greenberg & Sarner, 1965).

Several authors note the association of hair-pulling onset with loss or perceived loss or trauma, such as divorce of parents, death of a friend or relative, family move, birth of a sibling, change of schools, illness of patient or family member, or physical abuse (Greenberg & Sarner, 1965; Monroe & Abse, 1963; Oguchi & Miura, 1977; Orange, Peereboom-Wynia, & De Raeymaecker, 1986). Histories of sexual abuse are present in 18.6% of cases and in certain instances may be a contributing factor (Christenson, Mackenzie, & Mitchell, 1992).

More recently, it has been speculated that TM belongs to a spectrum of disorders related to obsessive-compulsive disorder (OCD) (Swedo & Leonard, 1992; Swedo et al., 1989). Supporting such an assertion are observed similarities between TM and OCD regarding phenomenology, neuropsychological test performance, response to serotonin reuptake blockers, and familial association (Swedo & Leonard, 1992). Arguing against this construct are observations of the frequent automatic quality of hair pulling and the lack of obsessions or other compulsions in TM (Christenson, Mackenzie, & Mitchell, 1991). Additionally, TM and OCD differ in baseline positron emission tomography (PET) profiles (Swedo et al., 1991), response to lithium (Christenson, Popkin, Mackenzie, & Realmuto, 1991), age at onset, and clinical sex ratios (Christenson, Mackenzie, & Mitchell, 1991).

Another theory is that TM is the human equivalent of displacement activities, a well-known phenomenon in the ethological literature (Swedo & Rapoport, 1991). In such a model, TM is viewed as an abnormal grooming behavior elicited in response to stress in the context of limited options for motoric behavior and tension release; hair pulling typically occurs in the context of sedentary postures with the patient engaged in heightened concentration (Christenson, Mackenzie, & Mitchell, 1991).

Differential Diagnosis and Assessment

DSM-III-R and DSM-IV Categorization

TM is currently included in DSM-III-R under the Impulse Control Disorders, Not Elsewhere Classified, along with Intermittent Explosive Disorder, Pyromania, Kleptomania, and Pathological Gambling (American Psychiatric Association, 1987). According to DSM-III-R, impulsive behaviors are consistent with the will of the individual at the time they are executed. However, the individual may later object to the behavior or its consequences. Impulse control disorders are additionally characterized by mounting tension preceding the behavior and release of tension or gratification following the behavior. The specific criteria for TM, which go little beyond these minimal descriptors, include: (a) recurrent failure to resist impulses to pull out one's hair, resulting in noticeable hair loss; (b) increasing sense of tension immediately before pulling out the hair; (c) gratification or a sense of relief when pulling out the hair; and (d) no association with a preexisting inflammation of the skin, and not a response to a delusion or hallucination. The utility of criteria (b) and (c) has been challenged, because these qualities are not experienced in 17% of chronic hair pullers (Christenson, Mackenzie, & Mitchell, 1991).

Revisions being considered for DSM-IV will not substantially alter these current criteria (Task Force on DSM-IV, 1991). Some consideration has been given to including TM with disorders usually first diagnosed in infancy, childhood, or adolescence because of the typical age at onset, or under the Anxiety Disorders because of some similarities with OCD (see above); however, both considerations have been rejected. A minor change has been suggested for criterion (d), recognizing that hair pulling is a common feature of other psychiatric and nonpsychiatric conditions. The suggested criterion reads: "Not better accounted for by another mental disorder (e.g., Delusional Disorder) and not due to a nonpsychiatric medical condition (e.g., a dermatological disorder)."

Differential Diagnosis

The diagnosis of TM is rarely difficult, in that the primary sign of the syndrome, alopecia, is generally readily observable on examination and the patient usually admits to her or his hair pulling. Disclosure of the behavior may be somewhat less common in young children or hair pullers of any age who are extremely embarrassed about their TM. In such cases alopecia from TM may be misdiagnosed as another disorder of hair loss, such as alopecia areata. In suspected cases involving the scalp, a skin biopsy will correctly discern TM.

Under the current schema TM should not be diagnosed if hair pulling is due to an inflammatory scalp condition, although we are not in complete agreement with this distinction; the first few individuals with TM described by the French dermatologist Hallopeau (who named the disorder) pulled hair in response to an intense itch, presumably the same reason someone with an inflammatory skin condition would pull out hair (Hallopeau, 1894). As Hallopeau pointed out, responding to pruritus by pulling out hair should be considered additional pathology.

Twisting and pulling at hair with or without occasional hair loss of insufficient severity to produce thinning or alopecia is probably a common behavior and should not be diagnosed as TM. Hair pulling with or without hair loss can be one of many self-stimulating stereotypies of mental retardation or autism. In many cases it can lead to severe hair loss. Because of the difficulty of eliciting the phenomenologic experiences of these individuals necessary for the DSM-III-R diagnosis, and the similarity of hair pulling to other stereotypies in these circumstances, hair pulling in these cases is best diagnosed under the DSM-III-R category Stereotypy/Habit Disorders.

Hair pulling that is in response to obsessions (e.g., need to keep hair symmetrical) and that is ego dystonic, intrusive, resisted, and the cause of significant distress to the individual often will meet criteria for OCD as well as TM. In these cases TM is still the preferred diagnosis. If other obsessions and compulsions (e.g., washing, checking) are present, the diagnosis of OCD may be warranted.

Hair pulling in the presence of a psychotic disorder would not necessarily preclude the diagnosis of TM unless the hair pulling is specifically related to a delusion or in response to a hallucination; in such cases hair pulling should be subsumed under the psychotic disorder.

Hair pulling infrequently has self-abusive intent similar to that encountered in patients who intentionally lacerate themselves and who often manifest personality disorders. However, hair pulling usually does not occur in the context of similar behaviors. Borderline personality disorder, which often has associated self-abusive behavior, is not a frequent comorbid diagnosis, as had been suggested (Christenson, Chernoff-Clementz, & Clementz, 1992). In the case of comorbid personality disorders a separate TM diagnosis is appropriate.

Assessment Strategies

The proper assessment of TM includes both a comprehensive exploration of the individual's hair-pulling behavior and a thorough screening for psychiatric co-morbidity. Hair-pulling onset and duration should be noted. Knowledge of events associated with onset is often intriguing, although in our experience this is unnecessary for successful treatment. More crucial are the patient's current environmental stressors and how they relate to hair pulling. Identification of which "high-risk" circumstances (e.g., watching television, driving, reading, lying in bed) and emotions (anxiety, anger, frustration, depression, boredom) are likely to accompany hair pulling is useful if behavioral treatment will be considered. One should always inquire as to oral manipulation of hair and hair ingestion. If hair ingestion is accompanied by gastrointestinal complaints, appropriate medical referral should be sought so as not to miss a potential trichobezoar.

TM's impact on self-esteem, mood, and avoidant behavior should be noted, because these characteristics may require additional supportive or other psychotherapeutic interventions. The sites of hair pulling should be observed and the amount of hair loss assessed. Occasionally this is deferred until the patient is more comfortable with examination for hair loss. Evidence of a skin disease (skin reddening or scaling) calls for a referral to a dermatologist. In the case of suspected hair pulling in a patient not willing to admit the behavior, a scalp biopsy by a dermatologist may confirm the diagnosis.

The patient's motivation for change should be explored, because some interventions (e.g., behavior therapy) require considerable effort on the part of the patient. This assessment is particularly important in the case of children and adolescents, who may be ambivalent about the desirability of intervention. Family dynamics should always be explored; parents with good intentions may actually exacerbate their child's hair pulling by excessive attention, pressure to change, or both.

Screening for affective disorders, anxiety disorders, substance abuse disorders, and eating disorders is essential in light of the high rates of comorbidity with these disorders and the frequent exacerbation of hair pulling under circumstances of increased psychological discomfort. Although rare, psychotic processes that direct hair pulling should be explored.

Treatment

Evidence for Prescriptive Treatments

Behavior Therapy. The majority of treatment literature on TM pertains to behavior therapy. Unfortunately, although many reports utilize sound experimental methodology, most are confined to case reports or small series of subjects and use such a diversity of techniques that a clear consensus on the best treatment strategy does not emerge. Treatments have included self-monitoring (counting hair pulls), covert desensitization (self-imposed punishment in the form of imagining highly stressful events when hair pulling or urges to pull are experienced), punishment paradigms (snapping a rubber band against the wrist, performing sit-ups, receiving mild electric shock, smelling aromatic ammonia, or hand slaps in response to pulling), token economies (rewards given for periods without hair pulling), attention reflection (providing periods of nonevaluative, noncontingent play for child hair pullers), and habit reversal (see below) among many others (Friman, Finney, & Christophersen, 1984). Techniques vary according to the patient's ability to participate in the treatment plan. For example, mentally handicapped hair pullers may respond to mildly aversive consequences for hair pulling, such as facial screening (which simultaneously produces time out), response prevention, and sensory extinction by covering the patient's head with a soft terrycloth cover whenever hair pulling is observed; children may respond well to token economies, whereas adults with normal intelligence may respond to more complex behavioral programs in which primary responsibility for treatment rests with the patient. The effectiveness of various programs appears to increase with the number of specific behavioral components (Friman et al., 1984). This finding is consistent with the current widespread use of the habit reversal method in the treatment of TM.

In the largest study of behavioral interventions for TM, Azrin, Nunn, and Frantz (1980) treated 34 subjects randomly assigned to two groups, one receiving habit reversal ($N = 19$), the other negative practice (instructed to act out the motion of pulling out hair without doing any damage) ($N = 15$). Training for both therapies was accomplished during a 2-hour session, and follow-up data (recorded number of hair-pulling episodes) was collected through the mail or over the phone for 4 months for both treatments and up to 22 months for habit reversal. Although negative practice was somewhat beneficial, habit reversal was statistically superior. At 4-month follow-up, those using habit reversal ($N = 18$) demonstrated a 91% reduction in hair pulling; an 87% reduction was noted at 22 months for subjects ($N = 12$) for whom data were available.

As utilized in Azrin et al.'s (1980) study, habit reversal comprises 13 components:

1. During *competing response training*, the patient is instructed to grasp or clench her hands for 3 minutes in response to hair pulling or when hair pulling is likely to occur.
2. *Awareness training* teaches the patient to become aware of the detailed movements involved in pulling out hair by observing the behavior in a mirror.
3. Hair pulling *precursor identification* informs the patient of what behaviors (e.g., face touching, hair straightening) precede his pulling.
4. Similarly, *identification of TM prone situations* (e.g., reading, driving, studying, watching T.V.) is emphasized.
5. *Relaxation training* uses deep breathing and postural adjustment exercises to target the commonly associated precursor states of nervousness and tension.
6. During *prevention training*, the patient practices the competing response whenever encountering nervousness, response precursors, or habit-prone situations.
7. Similarly, when hair pulling is encountered, the patient intervenes by immediately executing the competing response (*habit interruption*).
8. *Positive attention (overcorrection)* is the use of appropriate grooming behaviors (e.g., hair combing, hair brushing, applying makeup to lashes or brows) after each hair pulling episode.
9. The subject is additionally instructed in *daily practice of competing response* in front of a mirror to demonstrate inconspicuousness of the act and gain self-confidence.
10. Greater awareness of hair pulling is sought with *self-recording* on a hair-pulling chart of each hair pulling episode and urge to pull; this also provides feedback for progress in relinquishing hair pulling.
11. In *display of improvement*, the patient is encouraged to immediately seek out previously avoided situations, reinforcing his efforts at control.
12. A significant other is instructed during one of the sessions to positively encourage and remind the patient not to pull, thus offering *social support*.
13. Finally, motivation for improvement is increased via *annoyance review*, in which the patient lists and discusses various negative implications of hair pulling.

Since Azrin et al.'s (1980) study, others have also noted success with modifications of this technique, often using fewer behavioral components (De Luca & Holborn, 1984; Rosenbaum & Ayllon, 1981; Tarnowski, Rosén, McGrath, & Drabman, 1987). In general, frequent sessions have been necessary in contrast to the brief intervention originally proposed by Azrin et al. (1980). This often has been due to frustration encountered when patients experience brief exacerbations in hair pulling, and also serves as an aid to consistent application of techniques. In addition, incorporation of cognitive behavioral techniques (Ottens, 1982) is often of benefit.

Pharmacotherapy. Medication trials for TM are limited. Only two controlled studies, both investigating the antitrichotillomanic effects of serotonin reuptake inhibitors, have been reported in the literature.

Swedo et al. (1989), noting phenomenologic similarities of TM and OCD, compared the tricyclic antidepressant, antiobsessional agent clomipramine to the tricyclic antidepressant, non-antiobsessional agent desipramine in a double blind crossover study of 13 women with TM. Subjects received the two drugs consecutively for 5 weeks each with no washout between. Despite this relative small sample size and brief treatment period, clomipramine was demonstrated to be superior to desipramine on investigator assessments of TM impairment and overall improvement. The mean tolerated clomipramine dose was 180 mg a day. Three subjects completely remitted, and another 9 experienced decreased severity of 50% or more. Nine subjects continued clomipramine treatment and maintained clinical response at 6-month follow-up. This study has now been extended to 22 subjects, with similar results (Swedo & Leonard, 1992). An anecdotal report (Pollard et al., 1991) on the experience with 4 patients suggests that clomipramine response may diminish over time; it is further suggested that an initial rapid and dramatic response may prove to be a predictor of eventual relapse. However, Swedo and Leonard (1992) recently reported 2-year follow-up data on the first 16 subjects treated in the clomipramine vs. desipramine study and noted that 7 subjects demonstrated moderate to marked improvement (40 to 100%); 6 remained on serotonin reuptake inhibitors (clomipramine or fluoxetine), although other interventions (psychotherapy, behavior therapy, other medication) had been used also in several cases.

The other controlled study (Christenson, Mackenzie, Mitchell, & Callies, 1991) compared fluoxetine to placebo in a double blind crossover design. Fifteen subjects completed a 6-week course of fluoxetine with a final dosage of 80 mg a day; a 16th subject dropped out after 4 weeks on fluoxetine with a final dosage of 60 mg a day. Fluoxetine was no better than placebo on measures of change in severity of hair pulling, severity of urge to pull, number of hair-pulling episodes, and estimated hair loss. However, several open label trials of fluoxetine suggest that this agent may be effective (Benarroche, 1991; Winchel, Jones, Stanley, Molcho, & Stanley, 1992), although placebo effects cannot be ruled out. For example, Winchel et al. (1992) recently reported on 12 patients treated in an open 16-week trial of fluoxetine at dosages of up to 80 mg daily. Hair pulling was assessed using the Clinician's Trichotillomania Severity Scale (CTSS), a 5-item, 35-point instrument designed by the authors that inquires about the number of hair-pulling sites, daily duration of the behavior, severity of hair loss, ability to resist the behavior, and the severity of distress or functional interference caused by the symptoms. Response was defined as a 20% decrease in the CTSS score from baseline. Among 8 responders thus identified, the mean decrease in severity score was 60%. Benarroche (1991) reported relapse following discontinuation of fluoxetine in all of 10 patients treated for 1 year.

Case reports note improvement in TM using a number of other psychotropic agents. In one of the larger studies (Christenson, Popkin, et al., 1991), diminished hair pulling with mild to marked hair regrowth was observed in 8 of 10 patients treated with lithium; 3 patients experienced relapse upon subsequent discontinuation of lithium. Lithium doses ranged from 990 to 1,500 mg a day, with effective serum levels of 0.5 to 1.2 mEq/L. Carol Pleasants (personal communication, February 1992) has also reported positive responses to lithium, in some cases in individuals unresponsive to serotonin reuptake blockers. Case reports have also supported individual responses to the tricyclic antidepressants imipramine and amitriptyline, and the monoamine oxidase inhibitor (MAOI) isocarboxazid (Krishnan, Davidson, & Miller, 1984; Sachdeva & Sidhu, 1987; Snyder, 1980). Imipramine (Weller, Weller, & Carr, 1989) and clomipramine (Naylor & Grossman, 1991; Wilens, Steingard, & Biederman, 1992) were utilized in the few reported cases of children or adolescents treated successfully with medication. Buspirone was effective at a dosage of 30 mg a day in a patient with TM and several months of paroxysmal episodes of acute anxiety associated with autonomic hyperactivity (Reid, 1992).

Neuroleptics have occasionally been reported as effective; Childers (1958) successfully used chlorpromazine in two cases; however, both patients were psychotic and hair pulling improved with the psychosis, thereby suggesting a causal relationship. Spiegel and Spiegel (1978) reported successful treatment with trifluoperazine, initially alone and later, following discontinuation and relapse, in combination with hypnosis. Haloperidol resolved hair pulling in a boy with autism and mental retardation (Ghaziuddin, Tsai, & Ghaziuddin, 1991). Stein and Hollander (1992), suggesting a similarity between hair pulling and motor tics, used pimozide to augment serotonin reuptake blockers in incomplete responders and nonresponders, and noted that 6 of 7 patients thus treated benefitted. Although neuroleptics may be helpful in individual cases, care should be taken in considering their use for TM because they carry significant long-term risks such as tardive dyskinesia. Pimozide carries an additional risk of cardiac toxicity.

Finally, Black and Blum (1992) noted additional improvement when a topical steroid was added to clomipramine therapy in a patient whose TM was a response to pruritus.

Alternative Treatments. A number of case reports and case series note the successful treatment of TM with hypnosis, often in combination with behavioral or other psychotherapeutic techniques. Controlled studies of hypnosis have yet to be conducted.

The largest report on hypnosis concerns the treatment of 5 patients (Hynes, 1982). In these patients age regression was first used to bring the patient to the time before hair pulling onset, at which point conflicts were explored prior to refocusing the patient on the present. Subjects were instructed while in the hypnotic state to think "stop" when finding themselves hair pulling. Three of 5 were instructed in self-hypnosis. Of the 5 patients, 3 ceased to pull. The 2 failures did not use self-hypnosis and 1 dropped out of treatment; both were described as leading stressful lives.

Barbasz (1987) treated 4 patients with hypnosis, 3 of whom also received brief restricted environmental stimulation (REST). The REST environment consisted of a sound- and light-attenuated chamber with a reclining chair; REST environments have been shown to enhance the hypnotic state. All subjects were instructed during hypnosis to become aware of the hand as it approached the hair; that it was the patient's choice to pull or to control the effort was emphasized. Several patients received ongoing psychotherapy. Three patients responded with complete cessation of hair pulling. A 4th patient had initial improvement but later relapsed.

Hypnotic techniques have varied greatly in the hypnotic suggestions used. Such suggestions have included that the patient's hand warm upon contacting the hair (Hall & McGill, 1986), that pulling would be painful (Galski, 1981; Rodalfa, 1986; Rowen, 1981), that there would be increased awareness of hair pulling or its antecedents (Galski, 1981; Gardner, 1978), that the patient would become relaxed instead of pulling (Galski, 1981; Rodalfa, 1986), that the behavior be replaced with hair stroking (Spiegel & Spiegel, 1978) or by using another area of skin to produce pain (Jonas, 1970); and that the patient exercise good hair grooming (Gardner, 1978). The efficacy of these different hypnotic techniques remains difficult to assess, considering the lack of controlled trials and the confounding nature of incorporating a number of different strategies (relaxation training, assertiveness training, behavior monitoring, supportive and psychodynamic therapies) into the treatment.

Selecting Optimal Treatment Strategies

Treatment selection is hindered by an absence of published studies comparing different treatment modalities (e.g., behavior therapy vs. hypnosis). However, a recent report has suggested that habit reversal may be more effective than the serotonin reuptake inhibitor clomipramine (Rothbaum & Ninan, 1992). Despite these limitations, some general guidelines can be offered.

For patients with uncomplicated TM (e.g., those without psychiatric comorbidity, compulsive ritualized hair pulling, or severe hair loss), nonpharmacologic interventions such as behavior therapy or hypnosis are often appealing to both therapist and patient. Not only are these techniques devoid of medication side effects, but patients often feel greater mastery and self-esteem from the notion that they implement the treatment (autohypnosis, behavioral homework) with the therapist's guidance. Furthermore, there are few data on the required length of treatment with medications, although relapse during and after discontinuation has been reported (Benarroche, 1991; Pollard et al., 1991), and patients often prefer nonpharmacologic treatments because the therapist cannot advise accurately as to how long a patient will need to remain on medication. Nonpharmacologic treatments are not ideal for all patients, however. Habit reversal demands that the patient self-monitor and practice competing response consistently, which may prove difficult for the easily frustrated, busy, or unmotivated patient. The technique requires active patient cooperation and understanding, so it is often inappropriate for the hair-pulling child or the intellectually impaired. Other specialized behavioral techniques should be considered in such cases. Finally, success in hypnosis is affected by the patient's hypnotizability, confidence in the technique, and motivation for change.

Severe TM (i.e., nearly complete scalp denudement) is an indication to consider a medication strategy despite the absence of psychiatric comorbidity. Additionally, medications should be considered when other psychiatric comorbidity would also benefit from pharmacologic intervention. In light of the antidepressant and antiobsessional nature of the serotonin reuptake inhibitors clomipramine and fluoxetine, these should be used when a patient has additional major depression, dysthymia, or obsessions and compulsions. It has been suggested that as depression clears so does TM (Krishnan et al., 1984), indicating that in the presence of clinical depression standard tricyclic antidepressants, MAOIs, or novel antidepressants can be considered, although serotonin reuptake inhibitors remain the agents of choice. Because some TM is clearly more ritualized and reminiscent of a monosymptomatic manifestation of OCD, serotonin reuptake inhibitors should additionally be considered in these cases even if additional psychiatric comorbidity is absent.

For individuals with comorbid bipolar disorder, cyclothymia, frequent fluctuation in mood, or indications of a pattern of impulsivity, lithium should be considered. Comorbid general anxiety disorder would suggest the use of buspirone. Neuroleptics might be considered in situations in which coexisting conditions—such as psychosis, autism, or tics—would also benefit, although, considering the risk of tardive dyskinesia, neuroleptics should be avoided in cases in which such conditions are absent. Although the neuroleptic pimozide has been suggested as an effective adjunct to serotonin reuptake blockers, other strategies (addition of lithium, combination with habit reversal) are probably safer. Topical steroid creams may benefit hair pullers who pull in response to pruritus.

Children and adolescents represent a special consideration. Although there exists one report of a 7-year-old child responding to the tricyclic antidepressant imipramine (Weller et al., 1989), and two cases of adolescents responding to clomipramine (Naylor & Grossman, 1991; Wilens et al., 1992), experience with this population is limited. Additionally, some childhood TM has been considered to be more benign and rarely serious enough to need medication (Friman et al., 1990).

The benefit of combining therapeutic modalities has not been studied. Clinically, we have found that combinations of medication, behavior therapy, and/or hypnosis have resulted in gains beyond those that initially resulted from a single modality, and we would recommend such strategies when successful resolution of TM has not been achieved.

Problems in Carrying Out Interventions

The potential development of side effects may affect treatment choice or tolerance. Clomipramine, although best supported for the treatment of TM, can cause dry mouth, blurred vision, constipation, urinary retention, orthostatic hypotension, weight gain, and drowsiness. Fluoxetine is frequently better tolerated and is therefore often considered first; common side effects include jitteriness (which often resolves), insomnia, and decreased appetite with weight loss. Both fluoxetine and clomipramine can be associated with sweating, myoclonic jerks, and sexual dysfunction. Lithium may cause nausea, diarrhea, polyuria, tremor, sedation, and weight gain; prolonged use has been associated with nephrotic syndrome and hypothyroidism, both of which are usually reversible. Serum blood urea nitrogen, creatinine, and thyroid-stimulating hormone levels should be checked every 6 months when patients receive extended lithium therapy.

Buspirone is usually well tolerated, although dizziness, nausea, headache, nervousness, and lightheadedness are occasionally experienced. Neuroleptics are generally not indicated in TM and have been associated with potentially severe complications including tardive dyskinesia, neuroleptic malignant syndrome, pseudoparkinsonism, and acute dystonic reactions. Pimozide has the additional risk of cardiac toxicity. Women of childbearing age should practice some form of birth control when taking any of the above agents; little is known about fetal effects for many of them, whereas some, such as lithium, have clearly demonstrated teratogenicity.

The development of side effects may limit the dosage used or may necessitate discontinuation or change to a different medication. At times, side effects can be treated with the addition of another agent, such as a small dose of trazodone (e.g., 50 mg at bedtime) for insomnia associated with fluoxetine.

Patients are often eager for change and frustrated if they do not experience an early response. Although there is limited information on treatment response, most studies support changes occurring within 5 to 6 weeks of treatment initiation (Benarroche, 1991; Swedo et al., 1989; Winchel et al., 1992). Considering the theoretical association with OCD and OCD's longer treatment response, it is not unreasonable to attempt medication treatment for up to 10 weeks before considering a particular medication ineffective.

As we have indicated, motivation can have a considerable effect on a patient's response to behavior therapy and hypnosis. Although habit reversal and autohypnosis can be taught in relatively brief periods (e.g., one large study of habit reversal utilized a single training session) (Azrin et al., 1980), the unmotivated patient may require more frequent contact with the therapist in order to benefit from social pressure to complete assigned tasks and support during the treatment effort. Flexibility with all components is advised, with adaptation of treatment to meet the individual patient's needs. For example, the usual competing response recommended for habit reversal, clenching one's fist for 3 minutes, is not suitable for every patient; we have found that many individuals prefer manipulating a malleable substance (e.g., "Silly Putty") as an alternative. Additionally, we have found that incorporation of cognitive restructuring into habit reversal often augments its effect.

Family members can be both allies and hindrances to treatment. They are often concerned and supportive but may put undue pressure on patients to improve. Patients occasionally comment on the nagging quality of a spouse's or parent's intervention and the way this can exacerbate hair pulling; at times hair is pulled to spite the other or to demonstrate to the patient and others that the patient can ultimately do as she pleases. A session with family members is often indicated under such circumstances. In general, family members should remain distant to hair-pulling issues, leaving most aspects of treatment to the patient and therapist.

Relapse Prevention

Most crucial to relapse prevention are maintaining the patient's confidence in his ability to improve and avoiding inappropriate expectations that might discourage eventual treatment response and lead to loss of treatment effect. Patients may have high expectations for rapid improvement with medications, leading to abandonment of any strategy that has not worked in the first few days or weeks. Discontinuation of treatment often occurs or is contemplated when an initial response is followed by a temporary increase in hair pulling. Such fluctuation is to be expected, because hair pulling is often influenced by changes in psychosocial stressors. Reassurance that such lapses (in contrast to relapses) are to be occasionally expected is usually helpful. Some therapists have even suggested planned lapses in certain cases (Cohen, 1990). Review of hair-pulling diaries (useful during any treatment technique) often reveals to the patient that the frequency, duration, or intensity of her hair pulling is, in fact, less than at the beginning of treatment and inconsistent with the negative cognitions often associated with temporary increases in hair pulling.

Case Illustration

To demonstrate how treatment strategies can be applied, the following hypothetical case, a composite of extensive experience with actual patients, is presented.

Case Description

Ms. Jones is a 33-year-old married professional who presented to a general psychiatry outpatient clinic with a chief complaint of hair pulling. She recalled hair pulling developing around age 13, a time notable for increased stress related to moving to a new town and school. Although the patient eventually adjusted to these changes, hair pulling persisted. Pulling involved both the scalp and eyelashes. On presentation the lateral aspect of the upper eyelashes was absent and the scalp was afflicted with a large bald spot over the vertex. Ms. Jones described her hair pulling as usually occurring during times of increased tension while engaged in sedentary activities. These activities included working on her computer at the office, driving between work and home, and lying in bed at night. Typically, the last was associated with ruminations about her work performance and attempts to plan the next day. After some reflection, the patient stated that approximately 30% of her hair pulling occurred while she was fully focused on the behavior and while experiencing ego-dystonic urges to continue pulling. She described mounting tension prior to pulling and release of tension after pulling in some, but not all, instances. Rarely, she felt compelled to pull in a symmetrical fashion. The remaining 70% of hair pulling was described as occurring automatically; the patient claimed that she would literally find piles of hair about her desk without knowledge of having pulled it out. She often bit the ends of pulled hair, but denied hair ingestion.

Psychiatric history revealed that the patient had experienced recurrent bouts of depression associated with insomnia, low appetite and weight loss, poor concentration, fatigue, and occasional thoughts that life wasn't worth living. Episodes lasted from several weeks to 4 months. One such depression had begun approximately 1 month prior to presentation. The patient additionally had received outpatient treatment for alcohol dependency; she had maintained sobriety for the last 3 years. In addition to episodes of depression, the patient described a pattern of mood lability that persisted despite resolution of her depressive episodes.

The patient had been treated for depression and TM one year earlier with 150 mg a day of clomipramine; sedation and orthostatic hypotension had prevented a higher dosage. She achieved modest improvements in hair pulling and complete resolution of depression After 4 months the patient discontinued the medication on her own. In addition the patient had tried several techniques to control TM on her own, such as wearing a cap to bed, taping her fingers together, and sitting on her hands. She was easily frustrated by lack of progress, however, and soon abandoned such attempts. Concern about increasing hair loss and the possible need for a wig had directed the patient to seek additional help. She was assessed to be frustrated but motivated to change.

Differential Diagnosis and Assessment

Ms. Jones met DSM-III-R criteria for Trichotillomania. She pulled out hair to the point of visible hair loss (criterion A), and for at least some hair pulling described mounting tension prior to (criterion B) and release of tension after (criterion C) hair pulling. There was no evidence of scalp inflammation or hair pulling in response to psychosis (criterion D). She also met criteria for recurrent major depression and history of alcohol dependence. There was no evidence of obsessions or compulsions, although at least some of her hair pulling seemed compulsive. Besides her previous alcohol use, there was some indication of additional impulsivity and mood lability.

Treatment Selection

Several aspects of the case supported initial pharmacologic treatment. First, the patient had a comorbid diagnosis of major depression. Second, the patient had relatively severe hair loss. Third, the patient described some, but not the majority, of her hair pulling as more driven and compulsive, with some hair pulling performed symmetrically. In light of the antidepressant, antiobsessional and presumably antitrichotillomanic properties of serotonin reuptake blockers, consideration of treatment with clomipramine or fluoxetine was made. Although clomipramine use was better supported by the literature, the patient had only partially responded to a previous trial of moderate dosage and adequate length. Side effects had prohibited an increase in dosage, and the patient was less willing to take this agent again. Fluoxetine was therefore selected. Lithium was also considered because of its potential benefit to TM and because the patient had some characteristics of mood lability and impulsiveness, although lithium was less expected to benefit her current depression.

The patient appeared sufficiently motivated to be an appropriate candidate for habit reversal. Her own attempts at behavioral intervention were deemed to have failed secondary to limited simultaneous techniques, inconsistent application, lack of support, and rapid frustration, all of which could be adequately addressed during behavior therapy. Habit reversal was deferred initially, however, so as to first adequately assess the efficacy of medication. Hypnosis was also considered but rejected by the patient as undesirable.

Treatment Course and Problems in Carrying Out Interventions

Fluoxetine was initiated at 20 mg orally each morning, following review of potential side effects with the patient. Three days after initiating treatment the patient called to report a sense of jitteriness since taking the medication. The patient was also frustrated with continued hair pulling. The patient was reassured that this side effect occasionally occurs and often resolves during the first week. Additionally, the patient was reminded that it might take weeks before a response was noted, which she acknowledged she had known but was having difficulty accepting. The patient called again at 1 week to report on her progress: she noted that the jitteriness had cleared and that she felt mildly more energetic, but that hair pulling continued at its previous level. Following some discussion, fluoxetine was increased to 40 mg on the same dosing schedule.

The patient was seen in the office in another week for follow-up. The medication increase had been tolerated without difficulty. Additionally, the patient was feeling less depressed and more energetic, and was sleeping better. Her appetite continued to be somewhat diminished, but this was not bothersome. It was discussed with the patient that her small appetite might now be related to the fluoxetine rather than her depression. The patient additionally estimated that the number of hair-pulling episodes had decreased by approximately 10% and that urges to pull were diminished. Her daily dose was increased to 60 mg each morning, with follow-up arranged for two weeks.

At the next follow-up (after 1 month of fluoxetine treatment), the patient reported complete clearing of her depression. Hair pulling had additionally improved such that she estimated a 50% reduction from baseline. Notably, the patient no longer experienced urges to pull out hair and denied any focused or compulsive hair pulling. Remaining hair pulling was of the automatic type in which the patient claimed she was unaware of her behavior. The patient's response suggested that the antiobsessional aspects of fluoxetine would be expected to benefit only the more compulsive aspects of her behavior and, since this hair pulling had resolved, further increases in fluoxetine dosage might be of less benefit. Remaining hair pulling seemed more "habitual," so the therapist decided to recommend additional treatment with the technique of habit reversal.

After some discussion about the expected benefit of habit reversal, the patient agreed to add this to her treatment program. She was given a treatment manual developed specifically for the treatment of TM with a modified version of habit reversal and cognitive-behavioral techniques and was instructed in exercises that would allow her to begin looking at the relationship of environmental and emotional cues to hair pulling. She received instruction on completing a hair-pulling dairy entry for each hair-pulling episode documenting the length of the episode, the number of hairs pulled, a rating of the strength of the hair-pulling urge, and associated activities, thoughts, and emotions.

The next session centered on reviewing the diary as well as looking at the negative consequences of the hair pulling. The patient noted that simple monitoring had reduced her hair pulling. Reflecting on her avoidance of certain recreational activities, notably swimming and sailing (for fear of the wind revealing her bald spot), as well as intimate relationships, had induced greater resolve to master control over her TM.

Over several additional sessions the patient was instructed in other aspects of habit reversal. The patient explored the separate components involved in her hair-pulling behavior; she learned that hair pulling often began while her elbow was resting on a surface (desk, arm of a chair) with her hand supporting her head, that she often rubbed her chin or tugged at her ear prior to her hand moving to the scalp or lashes, and that hair stroking and twirling generally preceded hair pulling. She was instructed to substitute a competing response of hand clenching instead of hair pulling and to practice this daily in front of a mirror as well as whenever she had an urge to pull or actually pulled hair. High-risk situations were identified, in which the patient paid extra attention to where her hands were and prophylactically executed the competing response. Progressive relaxation was taught; the patient gradually tensed and then relaxed various muscle groups until her body felt totally relaxed. The patient was instructed to practice these techniques twice daily and when encountering stressful situations.

Finally, her thoughts, particularly those pertaining to hair pulling, were explored, with cognitive restructuring applied when appropriate. The patient noted that realization of hair pulling was often followed by automatic thoughts that she would never get better, that she therefore might as well pull, and that she was a failure for not having complete control over her behavior. She acknowledged that these thoughts propagated continued hair pulling and found that rational restatements that reflected on the improvement she had already demonstrated and her success in controlling other aspects of her life (including new success in control over her TM) helped dismiss feelings of helplessness.

During her last session the difference between lapses and relapse was emphasized. The patient was told that occasional hair pulling might still be encountered (lapses) and that she should use the methods she had learned thus far when such situations arose. The patient was now occasionally twirling her hair but denied pulling. Hair regrowth was evident, which was commented on positively by the therapist. The regrowth was a new source of pride for the patient.

Outcome and Termination

The patient now had sustained several months devoid of depression and no longer pulled out her hair. She asked to try discontinuing the fluoxetine and, although some possibility of reemerging depressive symptoms remained, it was mutually decided to do so. She was encouraged to continue to practice relaxation techniques and to reinitiate other aspects of habit reversal if hair pulling returned. The patient agreed to call if there was any recurrence of depressive symptoms or TM.

Follow-Up and Maintenance

One month passed, at which time the patient called to report a 3-day period during which hair pulling resumed, triggered by a disagreement with an employee at work. She denied a return of depressive symptoms. An appointment was scheduled and the patient was seen several days later. When asked what interventions the patient had implemented in response to hair pulling, the patient confessed that she had made a meager effort to clench her hand (competing response) on the first day but had then abandoned any further efforts. The patient was encouraged to reexplore her thoughts at the time and easily discovered that she had equated her renewed hair pulling with an indication that she was bound to be chronically afflicted by the behavior and that any intervention was doomed to failure. The rest of the session challenged these notions, emphasizing the expected nature of the lapses (rather than relapse) she had experienced and her otherwise successful attempts at controlling hair pulling. The patient reflected favorably on this discussion and correctly volunteered that she also had attended only minimally to the techniques that had previously proved successful. She vowed to again begin behavioral monitoring, competing response substitution, relaxation techniques, and cognitive restructuring. The patient returned in 2 weeks to report complete elimination of hair pulling using these techniques. A phone contact 4 months later confirmed her continued success.

Summary

Trichotillomania consists of chronic hair pulling that results in visible hair loss and is not attributable to a psychotic process or an inflammatory scalp condition. Clinically relevant hair pulling may occur in approximately 2% of the population. Trichotillomania can involve any hair site and typically involves more than one; the most common sites are scalp, lashes, and brows. Hair pulling can be compulsive and focused, or automatic. Trichophagy (hair eating) is an associated behavior that in its most severe form can lead to the development of trichobezoars.

Psychiatric comorbidity, particularly mood, anxiety, eating, and substance abuse disorders, is common in cases of trichotillomania encountered clinically. A thorough psychiatric history is an essential component of the trichotillomania evaluation.

The literature on treatment remains scant. Serotonin reuptake inhibitors, particularly clomipramine and to a lesser extent fluoxetine, appear promising in the treatment of trichotillomania. Lithium, buspirone, tricyclic antidepressants, and monoamine oxidase inhibitors have also been reported as effective in some patients. Neuroleptics may have a role in select cases of trichotillomania. Appropriate pharmacotherapy should always take into account severity, phenomenology, and psychiatric comorbidity.

Habit reversal is a multicomponent method of behavior therapy which has been demonstrated empirically to be quite effective in the motivated patient. With special populations (e.g., young children and the mentally retarded), other behavioral techniques may be necessary. Hypnosis has additionally been reported as being effective. Irrespective of which intervention is selected, the therapist must provide understanding and support. An emphasis on expecting lapses (vs. relapses) is invaluable to helping the patient cope with the occasional episode of hair pulling that may follow successful intervention.

References

American Psychiatric Association (1987). *Diagnostic and statistical manual of mental disorders* (3rd ed., rev.). Washington, DC: Author.

Azrin, N. H., Nunn, R. G., & Frantz, S. E. (1980). Treatment of hair pulling (trichotillomania): A comparative study of habit reversal and negative practice training. *Journal of Behavior Therapy and Experimental Psychiatry, 11*, 13–20.

Barabasz, M. (1987). Trichotillomania: A new treatment. *International Journal of Clinical and Experimental Hypnosis, 35*, 146–154.

Benarroche, C. L. (1991). Discontinuation of fluoxetine in trichotillomania. In *New research program and abstracts: 144th annual meeting of the American Psychiatric Association* (p. 138). Washington, DC: American Psychiatric Association.

Bhatia, M. S., Singhal, P. K., Rastogi, V., Dhar, N. K., Nigam, V. R., & Taneja, S. B. (1991). Clinical profile of trichotillomania. *Journal of the Indian Medical Association, 89*, 137–139.

Black, D. W., & Blum, N. (1992). Trichotillomania treated with clomipramine and a topical steroid. *American Journal of Psychiatry, 149*, 842–843.

Chang, C. H., Lee, M. B., Chiang, Y. C., & Lü, Y. C. (1991). Trichotillomania: A clinical study of 36 patients. *Journal of the Formosan Medical Association, 90*, 176–180.

Childers, R. T. (1958). Report of two cases of trichotillomania of long standing duration and their response to chlorpromazine. *Journal of Clinical and Experimental Psychopathology and Quarterly Review of Psychiatry and Neurology, 19*, 141–144.

Christenson, G. A., Chernoff-Clementz, E., & Clementz, B. A. (1992). Personality and clinical characteristics in patients with trichotillomania. *Journal of Clinical Psychiatry, 53*, 407–413.

Christenson, G. A., Mackenzie, T. B., & Mitchell, J. E. (1991). Characteristics of 60 adult chronic hair pullers. *American Journal of Psychiatry, 148*, 365–370.

Christenson, G. A., Mackenzie, T. B., & Mitchell, J. E. (1992). Reply to Drs. Friman and Tattersall. *American Journal of Psychiatry, 149*, 284–285.

Christenson, G. A., Mackenzie, T. B., Mitchell, J. E., & Callies, A. L. (1991). A placebo-controlled double-blind crossover study of fluoxetine in trichotillomania. *American Journal of Psychiatry, 148*, 1566–1571.

Christenson, G. A., Pyle, R. L., & Mitchell, J. E. (1991). Estimated lifetime prevalence of trichotillomania in college students. *Journal of Clinical Psychology, 52*, 415–417.

Christenson, G. A., Popkin, M. K., Mackenzie, T. B., & Realmuto, G. M. (1991). Lithium treatment of chronic hair pulling. *Journal of Clinical Psychiatry, 52*, 116–120.

Cohen, N. S. (1990). The relapse prevention approach to the treatment of compulsive hair pulling. *OCD Newsletter, 4*, 7.

DeBakey, M., & Ochsner, A. (1938). Bezoars and concretions. *Surgery, 4*, 934–967.

De Luca, R. V., & Holborn, S. W. (1984). A comparison of relaxation training and competing response training to eliminate hair pulling and nail biting. *Journal of Behavior Therapy and Experimental Psychiatry, 15*, 67–70.

Friman, P. C., Finney, J. W., & Christophersen, E. R. (1984). Behavioral treatment of trichotillomania: An evaluative review. *Behavior Therapy, 15*, 249–265.

Friman, P. C., Rostain, A., Parrish, J. M., & Carey, W. B. (1990). Hair pulling. *Journal of the Academy of Child and Adolescent Psychiatry, 29*, 489–490.

Galski, T. J. (1981). The adjunctive use of hypnosis in the treatment of trichotillomania: A case report. *American Journal of Clinical Hypnosis, 23*, 198–201.

Gardner, G. G. (1978). Hypnotherapy in the management of childhood habit disorders. *Journal of Pediatrics, 92*, 838–840.

Ghaziuddin, M., Tsai, L. Y., & Ghaziuddin, N. (1991). Brief report: Haloperidol treatment of trichotillomania in a boy with autism and mental retardation. *Journal of Autism and Developmental Disorders, 21*, 365–371.

Greenberg, H. R., & Sarner, C. A. (1965). Trichotillomania: Symptom and syndrome. *Archives of General Psychiatry, 12,* 482–489.

Hall, J. R., & McGill, J. C. (1986). Hypnobehavioral treatment of self-destructive behavior: Trichotillomania and bulimia in the same patient. *American Journal of Clinical Hypnosis, 29,* 39–46.

Hallopeau, H. (1894). Sur un nouveau cas de trichotillomanie. *Annales de Dermatologie et de Syphiligraphie, 5,* 541–543.

Hynes, J. V. (1982). Hypnotic treatment of five adult cases of trichotillomania. *Australian Journal of Clinical and Experimental Hypnosis, 10,* 109–116.

Jonas, A. D. (1970). The importance of counterirritation in trichotillomania. *American Journal of Psychiatry, 126,* 1184–1185.

Krishnan, R. R., Davidson, J., & Miller, R. (1984). MAO inhibitor therapy in trichotillomania associated with depression: Case report. *Journal of Clinical Psychiatry, 45,* 267–268.

Monroe, J. T., & Abse, D. W. (1963). The psychopathology of trichotillomania and trichophagy. *Psychiatry, 26,* 95–103.

Muller, S. A. (1990). Trichotillomania: A histopathologic study in sixty-six patients. *Journal of the American Academy of Dermatology, 23,* 56–62.

Naylor, M. W., & Grossman, M. (1991). Trichotillomania and depression. *Journal of the American Academy of Child and Adolescent Psychiatry, 30,* 155–156.

Oguchi, T., & Miura, S. (1977). Trichotillomania: Its psychopathological aspect. *Comprehensive Psychiatry, 18,* 177–182.

Orange, A. P., Peereboom-Wynia, J. D. R., & De Raeymaecker, D. M. J. (1986). Trichotillomania in childhood. *Journal of the American Academy of Dermatology, 15,* 614–619.

Ottens, A. J. (1982). A cognitive-behavioral modification treatment of trichotillomania. *Journal of the American College of Health, 31,* 78–81.

Pollard, C. A., Ibe, I. O., Krojanker, D. N., Kitchen, A. D., Bronson, S. S., & Flynn, T. M. (1991). Clomipramine treatment of trichotillomania: A follow-up report on four cases. *Journal of Clinical Psychiatry, 52,* 128–130.

Rebora, A., Chiappara, G. M., Guarrera, M., & Parodi, A. (1990). Cheveux crépus acquis un cas féminin avec revue de la littérature. *Annales de Dermatologie et de Venereologie, 117,* 29–31.

Reeve, E. A., Bernstein, G. A., & Christenson G. A. (1992). Clinical characteristics and psychiatric comorbidity in children with trichotillomania. *Journal of the American Academy of Child and Adolescent Psychiatry, 31,* 132–138.

Reid, T. L. (1992). Treatment of generalized anxiety disorder and tirchotillomania with buspirone. *American Journal of Psychiatry, 149,* 573–574.

Rodalfa, E. R. (1986). The use of hypnosis in the multimodal treatment of trichotillomania: A case report. *Psychotherapy in Private Practice, 4,* 51–58.

Rosenbaum, M. S., & Ayllon, T. (1981). The habit reversal technique in treating trichotillomania. *Behavior Therapy, 12,* 473–481.

Rothbaum, B. O., & Ninan, P. (1992, November). *Treatment of trichotillomania: Behavior therapy versus clomipramine.* Paper presented at the convention of the Association for the Advancement of Behavior Therapy, Boston, MA.

Rowen, R. (1981). Hypnotic age regression in the treatment of a self-destructive habit: Trichotillomania. *American Journal of Clinical Hypnosis, 23,* 195–197.

Sachdeva, J. S., & Sidhu, B. S. (1987). Trichotillomania associated with depression. *Journal of the Indian Medical Association, 85,* 151–152.

Snyder, S. (1980). Trichotillomania treated with amitriptyline. *Journal of Nervous and Mental Disease, 168,* 505–507.

Spiegel, H., & Spiegel, D. (1978). *Trance and treatment.* New York: Basic Books.

Stein, D. J., & Hollander, E. (1992). Low-dose pimozide augmentation of serotonin reuptake blockers in the treatment of trichotillomania. *Journal of Clinical Psychiatry, 53,* 123–126.

Swedo, S. E., & Leonard, H. L. (1992). Trichotillomania: An obsessive compulsive spectrum disorder? *Psychiatric Clinics of North America, 15,* 777–790.

Swedo, S. E., Leonard, H. L., Rapoport, J. L., Lenane, M. C., Goldberger, E. L., & Cheslow, D. L. (1989). A double-blind comparison of clomipramine and desipramine in the treatment of trichotillomania (hair pulling). *New England Journal of Medicine, 321,* 497–501.

Swedo, S. E., & Rapoport, J. L. (1991). Annotation: Trichotillomania. *Journal of Child Psychology and Psychiatry, 32,* 401–409.

Swedo, S. E., Rapoport, J. L., Leonard, H. L., Schapiro, M. B., Rapoport, S. I., & Grady, C. L. (1991). Regional cerebral glucose metabolism of women with trichotillomania. *Archives of General Psychiatry, 48,* 828–833.

Tarnowski, K. J., Rosén, L. A., McGrath, M. L., & Drabman, R. S. (1987). A modified habit reversal procedure in a recalcitrant case of trichotillomania. *Journal of Behavior Therapy and Experimental Psychiatry, 18,* 157–163.

Task Force on DSM-IV: American Psychiatric Association (1991). *DSM-IV Options Book: Work in Progress.* Washington, DC: Author.

Weller, E. B., Weller, R. A., & Carr, S. (1989). Imipramine treatment of trichotillomania and coexisting depression in a seven-year-old. *Journal of the American Academy of Child and Adolescent Psychiatry, 28,* 952–953.

Wilens, T. E., Steingard, R., & Biederman, J. (1992). Clomipramine for comorbid conditions. *Journal of the American Academy of Child and Adolescent Psychiatry, 31,* 171.

Winchel, R. M., Jones, J. S., Stanley, B., Molcho, A., & Stanley, M. (1992). Clinical characteristics of trichotillomania and its response to fluoxetine. *Journal of Clinical Psychiatry, 53,* 304–308.

12

Posttraumatic Stress Disorder

Terence M. Keane, Lisa M. Fisher, Karen E. Krinsley, and Barbara L. Niles

Description of the Disorder

Clinical Features

Immediately following exposure to high-magnitude, life-threatening stressors (i.e., a traumatic event), most people develop an acute stress response that might include symptoms of arousal, anxiety, sadness, grief, agitation, irritability, sleep disturbance, and a host of psychophysiologic complaints (e.g., headaches, pains, stomach problems). For many individuals these symptoms remit over the days, weeks, and months that follow. In a sizeable minority of cases, individuals who are exposed to a traumatic event can develop a more persistent set of psychological symptoms now known as posttraumatic stress disorder (PTSD).

PTSD can be a severely debilitating psychological disorder and consists of several core symptom components. To meet diagnostic criteria for PTSD, an individual must be exposed to a traumatic event that would cause high levels of distress in most people. Typically, individuals experience overwhelming emotions at the time of the event, possibly even fearing for their own lives or those of others. Once the clinician determines that an event meets the criteria for being potentially traumatizing, then to meet criteria for PTSD a client must endorse symptoms of (a) reliving of the traumatic event, (b) emotional numbing and avoidance, and (c) physiological arousal. Clients who manifest each of these symptoms for a period of 1 month are eligible to receive the PTSD diagnosis.

To assess PTSD, clinicians conduct intensive diagnostic interviews, attempting to

Terence M. Keane, **Lisa M. Fisher**, **Karen E. Krinsley**, and **Barbara L. Niles** • National Center for PTSD–Behavioral Science Division, VA Medical Center, and Tufts University School of Medicine, Boston, Massachusetts 02130.

Handbook of Prescriptive Treatments for Adults, edited by Michel Hersen and Robert T. Ammerman. Plenum Press, New York, 1994.

make distinctions between symptoms of a disorder and psychological experiences that might be signs or indicators of a recovery process. Usually, these distinctions can be made by the extent to which these psychological experiences are persistent, aversive, and disabling. For example, individuals who survive a plane crash can be expected to have nightmares and intrusive thoughts of the disaster for a time after the experience. Yet if these psychological responses persist for a full year, causing an individual to function poorly at home and at work, emotionally and interpersonally, it is clear that these responses are symptoms of psychological disorder, passing the threshold for meeting this criterion.

Reliving experiences can include any or all of the following symptoms: nightmares that recapitulate the traumatic event or themes from the event; flashbacks or intense reliving of the event during the waking state; recurrent and intrusive thoughts about the event, particularly when the individual does not wish to think about the experience; and psychological distress when confronted with cues or reminders of the traumatic experience.

Emotional numbing is often manifested by diminished interest in previously enjoyed activities, and marked anhedonia. Social alienation and a sense of detachment from other people are also frequently observed symptoms. Numbing is also identifiable if there is a restricted range of emotional experiences. The absence of any positive emotions, such as love and feelings of contentment, is particularly noticeable. For some individuals, particularly children, there is a clear emphasis on the present, with little interest in preparation for the future and future roles.

Avoidance is also a key part of the PTSD symptom complex. People with PTSD attempt to avoid thoughts and feelings associated with the event as well as any activities or situations that would cue recollections of the experience. In some instances this avoidance is so extreme that memory for the event is either completely or partially impeded, resulting in a condition known as psychogenic amnesia.

Symptoms of arousal are also observed in cases of PTSD. The range of sleep disturbances, including trouble falling asleep, fitful sleep, and early morning awakening, can be part of the symptom picture. Accompanying these sleep problems can be irritability, anger, rage, concentration problems, hypervigilance for danger signs, startle reactions, and physiologic reactivity to cues of the traumatic event.

Associated Features

Generally, people with PTSD exhibit anxiety, depression, grief, and occasionally dissociative experiences. These symptoms, taken collectively with the criterion symptoms enumerated above, can render individuals who are affected significantly disabled. Other symptoms that are observed in PTSD are substance abuse, overwhelming feelings of guilt, and impulsive behavior. Individuals who were traumatized many years earlier can develop permanent alterations in personality that resemble any of a number of the recognized personality disorders (e.g., borderline, narcissistic, antisocial, or histrionic personality disorder). A meticulously collected history can detect those personality disorders that preceded and those that followed a traumatic life experience.

Epidemiology

In the past 10 years, studies of the prevalence of PTSD in the general population and in specific high-risk groups have contributed substantial new knowledge and an improved understanding of this disorder. Several key studies will be selectively reviewed in this section because of their importance, superior methodology, and sophisticated measurement. Others are included because they have established precedents for work in this area.

In 1987, Helzer, Robins, and McEvoy found that 1 to 2% of the general population reached criteria for PTSD, representing some 2.4 to 4.8 million cases of this disorder in the United States alone. These data were collected as a part of the Epidemiologic Catchment Area Study and are viewed by some as conservative estimates of PTSD, largely because of challenges to the measurement strategies employed (Keane & Penk, 1988). Notwithstanding the methodological concerns, this research study indicated that the prevalence of PTSD was at least as great as that of schizophrenia in the general population.

More recently, Breslau, Davis, Andreski, and Peterson (1991) found that approximately 39% of the members of a Health Maintenance Organization (HMO) were exposed to a traumatic event at some point in their lives. Of these, nearly 25% (9.2% of total) developed PTSD as a function of the high-magnitude stressor. These findings were striking because of the high rates of trauma exposure as well as the high lifetime prevalence rates of PTSD among both males and females.

In the National Women's Study, Kilpatrick, Edmunds, and Seymour (1992) found that 13% of a national sample of women reported at least one completed rape in their lifetime. Some 31% of these women ultimately developed PTSD, indicating that a significant proportion of women in our society are at risk for sexual assault and that a high percentage of them develop the disabling symptoms of PTSD.

Perhaps the most methodologically rigorous epidemiologic study of psychological problems ever conducted in the United States was the National Vietnam Veterans Readjustment Study (NVVRS; Kulka et al., 1988). These investigators employed a multimethod approach to case identification (Dohrenwend & Shrout, 1981) and also used multiple measures of PTSD to increase certainty. Using a nationally representative sampling procedure, the NVVRS found that the current rate of PTSD among Vietnam veterans was 15% and the lifetime rate was 30%. Having oversampled minorities in this study, the researchers estimated that among blacks the rate of current PTSD was 21%, whereas among Hispanics it was 28%. Nearly 18% of women who served in Vietnam had lifetime PTSD.

Following the volcanic explosion of Mount St. Helens, Shore, Tatum, and Vollmer (1986) examined the prevalence of psychological disorders in three groups stratified by stress exposure. Among those exposed to the highest levels of stress, 40% reported major psychological problems 3 to 4 years following the disaster. Moreover, McFarlane (1986) examined firefighters from the Australian Ash Wednesday bushfires and reported that 21% of these people had PTSD symptoms some 29 months after the event.

Similarly, the Beverly Hills Supper Club fire in Kentucky was studied by Green, Grace, Lindy, Titchener, and Lindy (1983). They learned that the survivors had high rates of psychological morbidity years after the fire, and they also established conceptual links among components of the stressor event, preexisting personality traits, and the posttrauma environment that were important in identifying people at greatest risk for continued psychosocial impairment.

It is clear that as the methodologies for measuring trauma exposure and PTSD become more sensitive, we are learning a great deal more about the prevalence of high-magnitude stressors in our society and also about the psychological effects of such exposure. High-risk populations continue to be studied in order to develop more information on which sound public policy can be based. At this time we can responsibly conclude that a significant proportion of the American population is likely to be exposed to at least one traumatic event and that, depending in part on the characteristics of the event, a significant proportion of survivors will develop PTSD.

Etiology

In PTSD, etiological factors are a component of the diagnostic criteria (i.e., the stressor criterion). Research to date across numerous types of traumatic events indicates that the severity of the disorder is in part a linear function of the event characteristics (i.e., frequency, intensity, or duration), with the most extreme events yielding the highest rates of psychological symptomatology.

Yet not all individuals exposed to high-magnitude stressors develop PTSD, and, accordingly, there must be other factors involved in determining who does and who does not develop PTSD on exposure to traumatic events. Moreover, some people can develop PTSD to events that are ostensibly of a lesser magnitude than would typically produce a psychological disorder.

To explain these observations, one must inevitably rely on a vulnerability-stress model of psychopathology (Zubin & Spring, 1977). Barlow (1988) categorized vulnerabilities as either genetic, physiologic, psychological, social, or possibly as involving an interaction of all these factors. A similar biopsychosocial model of vulnerability has been applied to the etiology of PTSD (Foy, Carroll, & Donahoe, 1987; Keane, 1985), taking into account numerous variables that might predispose someone, once exposed to a high-magnitude stressor, to develop PTSD.

Empirical support for these models comes from numerous studies. The NVVRS found that war zone stress exposure was the best predictor of psychological adjustment in their study, yet preexisting behavioral disturbances and antisocial patterns added to the prediction of PTSD. Clearly, preexisting psychopathology is an important risk factor for the development of PTSD, but other factors must play a part in determining who develops PTSD. Likely candidates to help us better understand the stressor–symptomatology relationship are biological variables, family and support variables, and preexisting cognitive schemas of the world (Janoff-Bulman, 1992). Future studies should examine pretrauma, trauma, and posttrauma factors in a systematic way so that the relative contributions of each can be more precisely determined.

Differential Diagnosis and Assessment

DSM-III-R and DSM-IV Categorization

Although there have been some changes in the diagnostic criteria for PTSD since the disorder was first recognized in the diagnostic nomenclature for psychiatry, the cardinal features—exposure to a traumatic event and reexperiencing of that event—have remained relatively unchanged. The most notable change in PTSD criteria from DSM-III-R to DSM-IV is the specificity of criterion A—the definition of the stressor or trauma. In order to meet criterion A in DSM-III-R, it was necessary for the person to experience a stressful event that the evaluator determined was "outside the range of usual human experience" (American Psychiatric Association, 1987, p. 250). In DSM-IV, in order for criterion A to be met, the individual must have experienced an event that involved "actual or threatened death or serious injury, or a threat to the physical integrity of oneself or others" and have had a response of "intense fear, helplessness, or horror" (American Psychiatric Association, 1991, p. H:17).

Criteria B (reexperiencing symptoms), C (avoidance and numbing), and D (increased arousal) remain relatively unchanged, with one important exception. As a result of data analyses conducted at several research laboratories, DSM-III-R criterion D-6 (physiologic reactivity upon exposure to reminders) is now considered a reexperiencing symptom rather than a symptom of hyperarousal. In order to meet criterion E, the disturbance must be of at least 1 month's duration. Criterion F, clinically significant distress or impairment in social or occupational functioning, is a new addition to the diagnostic criteria.

Under consideration for the DSM-IV was a new diagnostic category to include individuals suffering from the sequelae of prolonged and repeated trauma. Many clinicians and researchers believed that the diagnosis of PTSD failed to capture the full symptom picture of individuals who had been exposed to more extensive and ongoing trauma, such as childhood sexual abuse, domestic battering, or incarceration as a prisoner of war. "Complex PTSD" includes multiple symptoms: excessive somatization, dissociation, changes in affect and character traits, and a vulnerability to repeated harm. Although this constellation of symptoms was not included as a diagnostic category in DSM-IV, its description is included in the text preceding the PTSD diagnostic criteria. Its utility for clinicians will determine whether a new category or subcategory will be added to future editions of the DSM.

Differential Diagnosis

The hallmark feature of PTSD in both DSM-III-R and DSM-IV is reexperiencing of the traumatic event. These criterion B symptoms are specific to the diagnosis of PTSD, yet they can easily be mistaken to be symptoms of other disorders. For example, intrusive recollections can appear to be auditory hallucinations, and flashbacks can often be misconstrued to be psychotic episodes because of their dissociative qualities. For instance, the odor of burnt toast may trigger a flashback in a survivor of a fire so that the individual sees nonexistent flames and runs outside for safety. At times, both clinicians and clients may be unable to identify the subtle stimuli that induce the often dramatic responses. Without the identification of a stimulus, a reaction may appear random and is frequently considered a psychotic symptom. In these cases, sensitive questioning about the sights, sounds, odors, and thoughts occurring immediately prior to certain psychological symptoms may reveal a clear connection with a traumatic event.

In contrast to the reexperiencing criterion, criteria C and D contain many symptoms that are also found in affective disorders and in other anxiety disorders. For example, avoidance of activities, memory recall difficulties, feelings of detachment or estrangement, restricted range of affect, sleep disturbance, and difficulty concentrating are all consistent with a diagnosis of major depression. Irritability, hypervigilance, avoidance, and exaggerated startle response can suggest an anxiety disorder such as phobia or generalized anxiety. Some of the checking and rechecking for safety secondary to extreme hypervigilance can be mistaken for an obsessive-compulsive disorder. Many of these symptoms can occur alone or be part of other psychological disorders, and only when reexperiencing accompanies these symptoms is a diagnosis of PTSD indicated. These can be difficult differential diagnoses when clients report that their affective symptoms, anxiety, or obsessive-compulsive rituals began or were greatly exacerbated immediately following a traumatic event. However, reexperiencing the trauma through intrusive thoughts, psychological distress when exposed to reminders, flashbacks, or distressing dreams are what most clearly differentiate PTSD from other disorders.

There are other important differential diagnoses that must be made with PTSD. Avoidance of situations that arouse recollections of the trauma can be mistaken for simple phobia. Phobic avoidance can serve as a cue to the clinician to question the client further about his or her history; if a prior trauma is revealed, the clinician can then probe for other PTSD symptoms that may not have been previously reported. If the phobic behavior is coherently tied to the traumatic event, a diagnosis of simple phobia should not be conferred in addition to PTSD. For example, a combat veteran who was trapped inside a bunker for several hours after it collapsed on him now avoids going under low bridges or into basements. Although he may have enough symptoms to meet the diagnostic criteria for simple phobia, these symptoms should be considered part of his avoidance of reminders of the traumatic experience.

The frequent co-occurrence of other psychiatric disorders with PTSD has been widely documented in the scientific literature (Boudewyns, Albrecht, Talbert, & Hyer, 1991; Davidson & Fairbank, 1993; Keane & Wolfe, 1990; Kulka et al., 1990). The NVVRS (Kulka et al., 1990) found that 98.9% of the veterans diagnosed with PTSD in their sample met criteria for at least one other disorder at some point in their lives: 74% alcohol abuse or dependence, 43% generalized anxiety disorder, 26% major depression, 21% dysthymia, 11% drug abuse or dependence, 10% obsessive-compulsive disorder, and 8% panic disorder. Although the percentages vary somewhat from study to study, substance abuse, affective disorder, and other anxiety disorder diagnoses are consistently encountered in samples of subjects with PTSD from various types of traumas (Davidson & Fairbank, 1993). These comorbid disorders—especially psychoactive substance abuse disorders—greatly influence and complicate planning treatment interventions.

Assessment Strategies

The scientific literature on the assessment of PTSD has grown dramatically since the disorder was first identified, and numerous psychometrically sound instruments have been designed. These measures fall into three general categories: clinician-administered interviews, psychological tests, and psychophysiologic measurement. Over the last decade, it has been consistently acknowledged that none of these instruments is infallible. A multimethod approach (Malloy, Fairbank, & Keane, 1983), whereby all three types of assessment measures are used conjointly to define and describe the diagnostic picture, has been consistently regarded as the most effective approach to the diagnosis of PTSD, maximizing both sensitivity and specificity.

Clinician-Administered Structured Interviews. The Clinician-Administered PTSD Scale (CAPS; Blake et al., 1990) was developed to serve several functions in the assessment of PTSD. This instrument, which can be used to assess both current and lifetime diagnoses of PTSD, assesses the frequency of occurrence and the severity of each of the 17 DSM-III-R symptoms. The CAPS provides both continuous and dichotomous scores to suit the needs of the assessor. Although this measure provides much clinically useful information about the impact of each symptom on functioning, it requires substantial time to administer (45 to 90 minutes). Its main strength is in research, allowing the changing status of PTSD symptomatology to be determined over time.

If the clinician is simply interested in conferring diagnosis and a descriptive symptom picture is not needed, the Structured Clinical Interview for DSM-III-R (SCID; Spitzer, Williams, Gibbon, & First, 1989) may be more appropriate. The PTSD module of this instrument requires much less administration time (10 to 30 minutes) and provides information sufficient for diagnosis.

Psychological Tests. The Mississippi Scale for combat-related PTSD (Keane, Caddell, & Taylor, 1988) consists of 35 statements about PTSD symptoms and associated features. Individuals are asked to rate how accurate these statements are for them on a 5-point Likert-type scale. The summed score provides a continuous measure indicating severity of PTSD symptoms. This scale has been shown to have high test–retest reliability and good sensitivity and specificity in differentiating between subjects with and without PTSD (McFall, Smith, MacKay, & Tarver, 1990). A civilian version of this scale has been designed for use with clients who have experienced nonmilitary trauma; this civilian scale appears to have similar psychometric qualities.

Another useful aid in diagnosis is the PTSD scale of the Minnesota Multiphasic Personality Inventory (MMPI; Keane, Malloy, & Fairbank, 1984), which has diagnostic accuracy of 82% for combat-related PTSD. A similar scale from the MMPI-2 appears to perform equally well in distinguishing groups of patients with and without PTSD (Litz et al., 1991; Lyons & Keane, 1992).

The Impact of Event Scale (IES; Horowitz, Wilner, & Alvarez, 1979) is a widely used measure of intrusions (criterion B) and avoidance and numbing responses (criterion C). The IES has good internal consistency and test–retest reliability as well as high correlations with other indices of PTSD. One limitation of this instrument is that it measures only intrusions and avoidance and numbing and does not assess other aspects of the disorder.

An important advantage of the Penn Inventory (Hammerberg, 1992) is that it was developed and validated with both combat veterans and civilians who had been exposed to a traumatic event. This 26-item questionnaire has high sensitivity and specificity rates for both groups of traumatized individuals.

Psychophysiologic Measurement. An objective measurement of one of the symptoms of PTSD—physiologic reactivity to reminders of the trauma—can be obtained from psychophysiologic evaluations. In such an evaluation, the client's blood pressure, heart rate, electrodermal skin responsiveness, and muscle tension are measured during presentation of cues of the traumatic event and neutral cues. The results are then compared to determine physiologic reactivity to traumatic content. Several studies have demonstrated the utility of such an evaluation as an important aid in the diagnosis of PTSD (Blanchard, Kolb, Pallmeyer, & Gerardi, 1982; Malloy et al., 1983; Pitman, Orr, Forgue, deJong, & Claiborn, 1987).

Treatment

Evidence for Prescriptive Treatments

Treatment of PTSD typically involves the use of a multicomponent model. As we have seen, PTSD pervades many aspects of people's lives, adversely affecting their relationships and work, and sometimes influencing even the most basic daily needs (i.e., food, shelter, safety) (Kulka et al., 1988; Hearst, Newman, & Hulley, 1986; Herman, 1992).

Given the complexity of the clinical condition, there is a growing recognition that the treatment of PTSD involves multiple stages, often progressing systematically from one stage to the next (Herman, 1992; Scurfield, 1985). This should not suggest an inflexible, packaged treatment or a strict linear model, because survivors of trauma come into therapy with different needs, objectives, and resources. A stage model does, however, suggest that certain basic groundwork must be addressed in the areas of emotional and behavioral stabilization, trauma education, and positive coping skills before exposure to traumatic material should be tried. It also stresses the importance of appropriate aftercare and relapse prevention following exposure to, and processing of, traumatic material.

Behavior Therapy.   In light of the above caveats, this section will delineate a cognitive-behavioral treatment approach often used with PTSD. This model of care incorporates the following stages: (a) emotional and behavioral stabilization, (b) trauma education, (c) stress management, (d) trauma focus, (e) relapse prevention, and (f) aftercare. For each stage we will briefly review the rationale, relevant literature, and recommendations.

Emotional and Behavioral Stabilization.   For people with PTSD, traumatic events often leave in their wake dysfunctional coping strategies (Forsyth, Carey, Litz, & Fisher, 1991; Keane, Albano, & Blake, 1992), lack of trust (Munroe, 1991), and shattered beliefs in the safety of the world and the survivor's competence in it (Janoff-Bulman, 1992). Although many therapists are inclined to focus on the traumatic experiences early in treatment, Herman (1992) warns that reexposure to the traumatic events in therapy without creating a safe environment and a trusting relationship, and ensuring client control, may not only be doomed to failure but may, in fact, exacerbate rather than decrease symptoms in the survivor.

The therapist's first task, then, is to ensure that basic needs are met and safety issues are addressed, to create a therapeutic alliance, to address a basic acceptance of therapy, and to analyze current coping strategies.

Basic needs and safety issues.   In order to begin working on traumatic material, the survivor must be in a relatively safe environment. This includes adequate food, shelter, and protection from abuse. The abused spouse or homeless veteran cannot engage in work on traumatic experiences unless his or her basic needs are met. In fact, it can be dangerous to begin work on a traumatic life event prior to securing safety. The loss of hypervigilance while living on the streets or with an abusive spouse can lead to further trauma exposure. Herman (1992) recommends working with the survivor to create a support system that can help provide a safe environment. This support system can consist of friends, peers, relatives, or even professionals who appreciate the precarious nature of the client's environment.

Acceptance of therapy and creation of a therapeutic alliance. In work with PTSD clients, several factors can impede the progress of therapy. The violation of trust is basic to PTSD. Therefore, it is vital that a positive therapeutic alliance be established. Yet this is often difficult when working with traumatized clients; PTSD clients may have problems trusting or, alternately, they may be overly dependent. Moreover, therapists who listen to traumatic material may experience very strong emotions of their own, such as anger, frustration, or helplessness. At other times it appears that the client and therapist are drawn into replaying traumatic roles of victim and perpetrator, or ally and enemy. McCann and Pearlman (1991) describe these as the themes of trauma, and Herman (1992) also describes similar trauma roles. In addition to a positive alliance, it is necessary that the therapist and client establish some shared goals for therapy. At a minimum, they must agree to work together and plan how they will each respond to basic safety concerns.

Analysis of current coping strategies. The traumatized individual often learns to cope with life events and PTSD symptoms in maladaptive ways. Drug or alcohol dependence often co-occurs with PTSD; the substances may be used to cope with anxiety, intrusive thoughts, sleep disturbance, or social withdrawal (Keane & Wolfe, 1990; Sierles, Chen, McFarland, & Taylor, 1983; Sierles, Chen, Messing, Besyner, & Taylor, 1986). Violence or panic, depression, avoidance, and suicidal ideation are often present and may be the reactions to major life stressors (Green, Lindy, & Grace, 1988; Kulka et al., 1990). These deleterious coping strategies must be reduced prior to any work on trauma-related material.

Although combined treatment of substance dependence and PTSD is now becoming more accepted (Abueg & Fairbank, 1992), substance use—even in this comprehensive model—must first be stabilized through medical detoxification, behavioral treatment, the introduction of support systems, or medication, if necessary. Without first addressing problems in substance abuse, the trauma survivor cannot acquire alternate methods for addressing his or her symptomatology. As individuals progress through stages of therapy for trauma, it is crucial for them to rely on their own skills to manage the inevitable emotional reactions they will have to traumatic memories. Similarly, medication use in the stabilization phase may be necessary to deal with depression, rage, disorganized thinking, and panic. More details regarding medications used in the treatment of PTSD can be found in the pharmacotherapy section later in this chapter.

The emotional and behavioral stabilization phase may take one session or several months, depending on the survivor's history and emotional resources. An example of a short period of stabilization is seen in a woman who sought treatment after a car accident. She had many posttraumatic symptoms, including sleep difficulties, nightmares, intrusive thoughts, hyperarousal, and avoidance. However, she was an otherwise well-functioning person with a good support network. She was a married grandmother with a responsible job and supportive friends. In this case, stabilization was completed in less than one session. She readily made a therapeutic alliance and agreed to gradually begin driving again and to resist using alcohol to get to sleep at night. In contrast, another trauma survivor who was referred for treatment was a homeless veteran with severe early childhood and combat trauma. He was dependent on drugs and alcohol, had few social supports, and had significant legal problems. In his case, the first 2 years of therapy were primarily devoted to the first three stages of treatment: stabilization, education, and stress management.

Trauma Education. When the trauma client is safe and stabilized, education regarding the causes, course, and consequences of trauma exposure and PTSD can begin. In this stage the client learns about the symptoms of PTSD, both positive and negative (Keane, 1989), and about the common comorbid disorders. The client also learns about the effects of PTSD on the family, interpersonal relationships, and employment, as well as the possible physical and physiological effects. Trauma education can be accomplished by an individual therapist, through readings or videos, or, most powerfully, by other trauma survivors. A combination of these approaches is optimal. For the survivors of recent or uncomplicated trauma, this information may allow them to recognize symptoms and reactions as they happen and be less frightened by them. This tends to minimize the complexity of PTSD. In the treatment of more intense, persistent, and distant trauma, it may help the survivors to understand what has happened to them.

A client's reaction to the educational stage is generally one of surprise and relief. Often clients remark, "It's like you're reading my mind." Others say that they have been afraid to discuss these symptoms because they felt they would be considered crazy. Indeed, education for spouses and families of trauma survivors can be very useful by promoting enhanced understanding, prediction, and control for family members.

Stress Management. In order to cope with traumatic material, the survivor must not only avoid negative coping, but also employ positive coping strategies to deal with traumatic material and current life stressors. These strategies include relaxation techniques such as Jacobson's (1938) progressive relaxation, Wolpe's (1984) deep muscle relaxation, and Benson's (1975) relaxation response; biofeedback; cognitive techniques (Beck, 1972; Kilpatrick, Veronen, & Resick, 1979; Meichenbaum & Jaremko, 1983); skills training, including social skills, anger control, time management, and problem solving.

Relaxation techniques may be applied in several ways with PTSD. They may lower the overall level of anxiety or arousal and aid in sleep, and they may also be used as an alternate response when the individual is exposed to anxiety-provoking stimuli. The relaxation technique is introduced with an explanation of why it is useful and how it works. This is followed by training in the technique itself, which may center on muscle relaxation (as in Jacobson's technique), breathing (as in Benson's), or imagery. The type of relaxation chosen depends on the client's comfort and abilities as well as the symptoms being targeted. Muscle relaxation may be most effective with hyperarousal, whereas imagery may be more effective with intrusive thoughts. After learning the technique, the client practices in the therapy sessions and at home. After mastering the technique, the client may then start to use it in situations in which arousal would normally be high or which the client might normally avoid. Initial reports have been promising, but little controlled work evaluating the effects of relaxation therapy has been done specifically with a PTSD population. Hickling, Sison, and VanderPloeg (1986) found that 6 veterans with PTSD, for whom relaxation treatment was expected to be beneficial, improved on most measures after relaxation training. Peniston (1986) found reduced nightmares, flashbacks, and muscle tension as well as reduced hospital recidivism in 8 veterans treated with relaxation compared with a no-treatment control group. One of the reasons for the lack of controlled work on PTSD and relaxation is that in most PTSD treatment relaxation is used not alone but, rather, as a component of a more expansive treatment program.

Cognitive coping strategies are frequently used in the treatment of PTSD. Many theorists have proposed that cognitive changes take place after traumatic experiences. Lang (1977) and Foa and Kozak (1986) suggest that a fear memory network is central to symptoms of PTSD. They posit that fear can be reduced only when information is presented that is counter to the fear network that has been established. Chemtob, Roitblat, Hamada, Carlson, and Twentyman (1988) hypothesized that trauma survivors selectively scan their environment for information that confirms their world view. One task for therapy, then, is to challenge these fundamental views so that clients begin to perceive things differently. Although these theorists and others often see exposure as the key to cognitive reorientation, cognitive techniques are often used in conjunction with or as precursors to exposure, or as independent treatment techniques for PTSD.

Beck's (1972) cognitive restructuring has also been used with rape victims (Frank & Stewart, 1984). Central to Beck's approach is the hypothesis that the way individuals view the world (their cognitive assumptions) influences the way they feel. This therapy challenges maladaptive thinking and cognitive distortions, replacing them with more rational cognitions. Frank and Stewart used self-monitoring, identification of maladaptive cognitions, and assignments for practiced exposure for rape victims with PTSD symptoms. With this treatment, they reported a decrease in fear and depression and an increase in social adjustment among clients in the clinical trial.

Stress inoculation training (SIT; Meichenbaum & Jaremko, 1983) typically consists of three phases: an education phase, in which the client learns about the treatment rationale; a skill acquisition phase, during which a variety of skills are taught (e.g., assertiveness, relaxation, anger management, cognitive reappraisal, thought stopping); and a rehearsal and application phase, in which the client practices the new skills. In a randomized clinical study, Foa, Rothbaum, Riggs, and Murdock (1991) found that a modified version of SIT was superior to supportive counseling and to no treatment. In this study, exposure was found to be the most effective treatment at the follow-up assessment.

Resick and Schnicke (1992) developed a treatment package for rape victims based on information processing variables. The "cognitive processing therapy" begins by educating rape victims in the way rape affects beliefs and attitudes about oneself and the world. The posttrauma beliefs about the world are central to the PTSD symptoms manifested by the trauma survivor. The second phase of treatment is similar to stress inoculation, with an emphasis on changing maladaptive self-talk. The focus of the therapy is to develop more adaptive schemas about the world in a group therapy setting and through structured homework assignments. Resick and Schnicke (1992) found that compared to a wait-list control group, a cognitive processing therapy group improved on PTSD and depression measures and maintained improvement for 6 months.

As can be seen, most stress management treatments incorporate a number of factors: relaxation, cognitive restructuring, and skills training. And in most cases, some direct therapeutic exposures is also included as a key treatment component. Componential analyses to determine the effective ingredients for treatment would add to our understanding of the mechanisms of change.

Trauma Focus: Exposure-Based Therapy. Therapeutic exposure to traumatic experiences is often the core of PTSD therapy. However, it is only after the client is stabilized and has acquired sufficient coping skills that direct and continuous exposure to traumatic material is advisable. Traumatic material may come up many times in early phases of therapy, and it must be acknowledged and addressed, but prolonged trauma exposure should be delayed until safety and coping skills have been achieved. Instructions to the client that therapy will address the traumatic material once the client is prepared can be helpful and motivate compliance with earlier stages of the treatment process.

There are many rationales for exposure, coming from many different theoretical orientations. In the behavioral literature, there are several approaches to exposure. Systematic desensitization dates to Wolpe's (1956) seminal work on reciprocal inhibition. Here, certain behavioral responses are developed (e.g., relaxation) to inhibit the expression of emotional responses (e.g., fear). For PTSD, relaxation in the face of traumatic material can inhibit the arousal and anxiety normally experienced. Another behavioral origin is in flooding or implosive therapy. These techniques derive from the two-factor model of fear offered by Mowrer (1960). Treatment effectiveness is a function of extinction, in which continued exposure to a conditioned stimulus (trauma cues) in the absence of the unconditioned stimulus (e.g., an assault) eventually weakens the conditioned response (fear). For example, repeated exposure to the scene of a rape, without avoidance and without negative consequences, will eventually lead to decreased arousal. Generalization of the trauma response to many stimuli makes exposure a difficult task for the clinician. However, many of the stimuli are interdependent, and extinction to one memory of an assault can reduce arousal and negative emotions to other similar or related traumatic events. In cases in which an individual reports multiple traumatic events, realization of this principle of the extinction process can be encouraging to both the client and the therapist.

Cognitive theorists have proposed that exposure introduces new information to a closed link. For instance, Foa, Steketee, and Rothbaum (1989) have proposed that PTSD occurs because of an inability to process traumatic material. Foa and Kozak (1986) suggest that in order to reduce symptoms, the fear memory must be activated and new corrective information, incompatible with the traumatic memory, must be provided. Horowitz (1986) suggests that denial and the need to repeat certain aspects of trauma are central to PTSD. He also recommends some form of exposure to interrupt this process.

Exposure methods. Systematic desensitization has been used effectively in the treatment of PTSD. It generally consists of three components: (a) establishing an incompatible behavior (relaxation) to inhibit fear and avoidance responses, (b) establishing a graded hierarchy of feared images, and (c) facilitating graded exposure to the feared images while the client practices the relaxation techniques. At each step, the fear responses are replaced with more adaptive responses. Bower and Lambert (1985) found that veterans who used this technique showed decreased heart rate and muscle tension and less subjective anxiety when exposed to trauma stimuli.

Flooding and implosive therapy, based on the work of Stampfl and Levis (1967), involves directing the client to imagine repeatedly all aspects of the traumatic situation. The objective of the therapy is to have the client experience and keep experiencing the arousal until it extinguishes. Implosive therapy goes one step further by introducing beliefs or assumptions that may contribute to maintenance of anxiety symptoms. Fairbank, Gross, and Keane (1983), Keane and Kaloupek (1982), and Fairbank and Keane (1982) all found decreased arousal, depression, and intrusive thoughts after flooding treatment. Cooper and Clum (1989), in a group design, found decreased anxiety, sleep disturbance, and avoidance. Keane, Fairbank, Caddell, and

Zimering (1989), and Boudewyns and Hyer (1990), also found decreased physiologic responding, anxiety, fear, and depression after implosion treatments for PTSD. Each of these studies involved randomized, controlled designs.

Keane et al. (1992), in a review of the PTSD treatment literature, indicate that the exposure-based techniques appear to have the most positive effects on anxiety-based symptoms such as startle, arousal, and nightmares, whereas numbing, alienation, and restricted affect are less responsive to the exposure. This may suggest that a combination of exposure and skill-oriented group therapies would be useful.

Peer group exposure. There are many types of trauma peer groups: support, trauma focused, community focused. It is generally in later stages of therapy that trauma focus groups are most appropriate. Trauma focus groups have been employed with almost all trauma survivor populations: combat, abuse, disaster, rape, incest, political and ethnic persecution. These groups not only employ exposure to trauma material but also help survivors build trust and ties to one another. Herman (1992) defines these groups as being trauma-focused, homogeneous, and time-limited. She describes them as cohesive, closed, and goal directed. She recommends this model to allow the trauma survivor to have a safe place to explore the trauma for a prescribed amount of time and then to focus on future life directions.

Pharmacotherapy. A full review of the psychopharmacology of PTSD is beyond the scope of this chapter. Instead, we will outline the types of drugs that are commonly used or newly emerging and refer to the few placebo-controlled, double blind studies completed in this area (Solomon, Gerrity, & Muff, 1992).

There are several classes of medications used in the treatment of PTSD. Tricyclic and monoamine oxidase inhibitor (MAOI) antidepressants are widely used (Faustman & White, 1989; Wolf, Alavi, & Mosnaim, 1987). Tricyclics are often used for symptoms of PTSD and accompanying depression. There is much anecdotal evidence, and some data, to support their use. However, the efficacy of tricyclics for the treatment of PTSD has not yet been definitively demonstrated in double blind, placebo-controlled studies. Davidson, Kudler, and Smith (1990) found amitriptyline effective in depression but not on the general symptoms of PTSD. Reist, Kaufman, and Haier (1989) did not find significant effects of desipramine on PTSD symptoms. MAOIs have fared somewhat better in controlled trials. Frank, Kosten, Giller, and Dan (1988) and Kosten, Frank, and Dan (1991) found decreases in intrusive symptoms with phenelzine (and less so with the tricyclic imipramine). Other studies that found no improvement with MAOIs (Shestatzky, Greenberg, & Lerer, 1988), however, make it difficult to draw conclusions about the use of these medications in PTSD treatment.

Fluoxetine (a serotonin reuptake blocker) has recently been suggested to be effective in the treatment of PTSD, especially against the hyperarousal symptoms. Nagy, Morgan, Southwick, and Charney (in press) found fluoxetine to reduce the reexperiencing, avoidance, and hyperarousal symptoms of PTSD as well as panic attacks in an open clinical trial. These preliminary findings await a double blind placebo-controlled study for further clarification of fluoxetine's utility with PTSD. Such studies are in progress. Trazodone, an antidepressant with sedating qualities, is often prescribed to help alleviate the sleep difficulties associated with PTSD; no data on its usefulness have been published to date.

Antianxiety drugs are also used in the treatment of PTSD. One small controlled study found alprazolam helpful in reducing anxiety in people suffering from PTSD, but of no value over a placebo control for symptoms specific to PTSD (Braun,

Greenberg, Dasberg, & Lerer, 1990). Benzodiazepines have also been widely used, but there is concern about their addictive qualities. Buspirone is a medication with fewer side effects than the benzodiazepines, and consequently it is now being prescribed for anxiety, intrusive thoughts, and nightmares for PTSD clients. However, clinical trials documenting buspirone's efficacy have not yet appeared in the literature.

Beta-adrenergic blockers are another family of drugs that limit sympathetic reactions and are used to control some of the arousal reactions in PTSD. Preliminary evidence for propranolol suggests that it can be helpful for some of the PTSD symptoms (Kolb, Burris, & Griffiths, 1984).

Anticonvulsant mood-stabilizing medications have also been used to treat PTSD, especially to diminish impulsivity and aggression. Lithium and carbamazepine have long been used as adjunctive treatment with some patients. Valproic acid recently has also been suggested to be effective in the treatment of PTSD. Fesler (1991) reported that in open clinical trials, valproic acid reduced hyperarousal and avoidant symptoms as well as increasing sleep. Again, controlled clinical studies are not yet available.

In addition to the above-mentioned drugs, antipsychotic medications are still sometimes used for the most severe symptoms of flashbacks or voices, or as needed for sedation. Friedman (1988), in reviewing the literature on pharmacotherapy, noted that no single medication can address all symptoms of PTSD. Clinicians should attempt to identify key symptomatology and address those symptoms to ameliorate the severity of this disorder. His sensible recommendations hold true today.

Alternative Treatments.   Most alternative treatments involve some of the methods we have described. Exposure is central to many of them. Here, we will briefly discuss eye movement desensitization (EMDR), giving testimony, and other psychotherapies.

EMDR is a relatively new technique developed by Shapiro (1989a, b). The procedure is derived from Shapiro's clinical experience and is not theoretically based. In this procedure, the client is asked to maintain awareness of an image or memory, a negative self-statement, or a physical sensation. While he is doing this, the therapist stimulates the client's eye movements by having the client follow her fingers, which move rapidly across the visual field horizontally. More positive cognitions (e.g., coping statements) are inserted as the negative emotions lessen. Initial results with Vietnam veterans and rape and molestation victims found decreased subjective anxiety ratings and an increased belief in a more positive cognition as well as decreases in the presenting complaints when compared with findings with a placebo control treatment. More controlled studies of the procedure are currently under way. If it is found to be successful, it offers promise in that it is relatively short term and does not require a client to verbalize or stay with an image for an extended period, as do other forms of exposure therapy.

Giving testimony also uses exposure, recounting, or bearing witness to validate and empower the trauma survivor. It suggests that in mastering the material the victims gain control of their lives again. Giving testimony is a technique used most often with torture survivors and political prisoners. Agger and Jensen (1990) describe this approach, in which the victim tells, retells, and revises the account of the trauma until it is complete. This can be accomplished orally or in writing. After completion, there is a delivery ritual in which the account of the trauma is read aloud and signed by the victim and the therapist. Again, controlled research is lacking, but some of the principles we see in exposure also appear in this form of therapy. As one Vietnam veteran stated, "When I am able to face my whole year in 'Nam, when you believe me, and they believe me, and I believe in myself, then I can face anything."

Psychodynamic therapy and hypnotherapy also work at giving people access to their own traumatic material and integrating it into their lives. A description of these techniques is beyond the scope of this chapter. However, Brom, Kleber, and Defares (1989) compared psychodynamic therapy, hypnotherapy, desensitization, and a waiting list control and found all therapy method groups showed overall symptom improvement, compared to the control, with psychodynamic clients showing somewhat less avoidance and those in the other two therapy groups showing less intrusion.

Selecting Optimal Treatment Strategies

The stage model presented above suggests that at every juncture it is important to evaluate the current level of functioning of the client. Strengths, deficits, supports, and resources need to be assessed in order to decide the optimal direction in which to proceed. Once the client's needs and resources are understood, it is much easier to select the appropriate treatment for each stage. For example, Litz, Blake, Gerardi, and Keane (1990) outline decision-making rules for doing implosive therapy with PTSD clients. After polling experts in the field, they suggested that the client needs to be able to tolerate intense levels of arousal, be reactive to therapeutic memories, have imagery abilities, and have had effective treatment for comorbid diagnoses, as well as be motivated and compliant to the treatment.

Researchers and clinicians are now beginning to investigate whether trauma survivors with certain symptom clusters respond better to one kind of therapy than another. The inclusion of multiple components in the treatment of PTSD is clearly needed given the complexity of the disorder. Research will assist us in selecting interventions and determining the most effective sequence of the available interventions.

Problems in Carrying Out Interventions

Many difficulties in treatment have been indicated throughout this chapter. One difficulty inherent in a stage model is the need to recognize that treatment does not always proceed linearly. It may often be necessary to return to an earlier stage, one that the client previously mastered. For example, once trust has been established, the client may continue to test the trustworthiness of the therapist throughout therapy. Similarly, the PTSD client may also go back to less adaptive coping strategies in times of stress; alcohol use or suicidal ideation may emerge. Comorbid diagnoses such as substance abuse and depression can make interventions more complicated, and adequate treatment must be directed to these areas in order to address the multidimensional nature of PTSD.

Other factors that may raise challenges for therapy are anniversary dates and outside stressors. An anniversary date is the date or time of year that is associated with the traumatic event. If the therapist and client are unaware of these dates, it can often appear that progress is impeded for no reason. There can also be significant relapses and exacerbations of the client's condition at these times. Similarly, trauma survivors may be very sensitive to outside events that remind them of their trauma. A highly publicized assault may lead to increased symptoms in a rape victim, just as publicized military engagements may exacerbate symptoms in combat veterans. Addressing these issues directly in therapy is useful and provides increased control over symptoms as well as enhanced prediction of the event's effects.

Relapse Prevention

Much relapse prevention work is done throughout the therapy. Yet there are issues that the trauma survivor may not be ready to address until after the trauma focus work nears completion. These issues include establishing or reestablishing supportive and intimate relationships, pursuing vocational goals, and, if the client wishes, increasing his or her involvement in social or political activities. These are areas that are often hampered by the PTSD symptoms, and the trauma survivor may need help in developing them in order to maintain gains and make future progress.

Abueg and Fairbank (1992) describe a relapse prevention model for people with PTSD who are also substance abusers. It is a modification of Marlatt and Gordon's (1985) relapse prevention model. In a group therapy format, the clients identify their individual high-risk situations and learn how to cope with them as they arise. Practice and role playing are integral components of relapse prevention treatment modules.

When learning relapse prevention techniques, the survivor should appreciate the cyclical nature of PTSD. The condition is affected by external stressors, reminders or anniversary dates of the trauma, health, and other emotional factors. Accordingly, exacerbations can be expected. When clients finish the relapse prevention stage, they will have many tools to manage these periods of symptom exacerbation. However, aftercare is also important.

When formal treatment ends, the trauma survivor can benefit from continuing support systems. Systematic therapeutic follow-up is one method to ensure support. Here, contracts are arranged on a fixed time schedule or at anniversary dates. At these times, symptoms, activities, and supports are monitored. Any difficulty is detected, and interventions are made before a crisis ensues.

Perhaps more important at this stage is the integration of the client with the outside community. This can be achieved through community support groups and expanded social support systems. Many trauma survivors also find that community involvement in the form of volunteering or social activism is a final link that effectively connects them back to community and society.

Case Illustration

Case Description

Brian is a 43-year-old, divorced, African-American male Vietnam veteran who came to the hospital emergency room during the Persian Gulf War, presenting with vague homicidal ideation and fears of losing control. At the outset Brian was able to contract for safety and was then referred for an outpatient PTSD evaluation. In the initial interview he complained of increased feelings of rage, anxiety, and despair, and a fear that he would relapse to drug and alcohol use (the patient had been sober for 6 months). He described worsening nightmares of combat and decreased ability to sleep. Brian also reported that he had started carrying a gun again, after giving up this habit several years before. Brian stated that this visit was prompted by an unusually disturbing dissociative episode centered around seeing several Vietnamese youths.

He described a feeling of losing a sense of time and a feeling that he might have hurt the youths had he not been with a friend.

Brian's combat history included two 13-month tours in Vietnam with the Marine Corps, during which time he had been wounded twice. He described heavy combat exposure, including repeated search-and-destroy missions. More than half the Marines in his unit had been wounded or killed. Brian described as especially distressing the unavoidable killing of civilian women and children, and experienced both survivor guilt and guilt over his actions in combat. His combat report is corroborated by his discharge papers which list two Purple Hearts and a Bronze Star for bravery.

Admitting to an extensive history of violence since Vietnam, Brian had served two prison terms for assault and attempted murder. Moreover, he reported a lifetime history of polysubstance abuse, describing multiple admissions for detoxification in the last few years while denying any other type of treatment. Brian stated that this period of sobriety was the first time he was committed to remaining drug free. Unsure whether he could talk about his experiences in Vietnam, Brian agreed in desperation to participate in the psychological evaluation.

Brian's childhood had been marked by early experiences of racism and a familial history of alcoholism (his father, and possibly his mother). He denied any other childhood trauma; although Brian described his father as being a disciplinarian, he insisted that punishments were always appropriate and justified. Brian joined the Marines at 17, stating that he did so because he wanted to be a hero.

Differential Diagnosis and Assessment

Brian participated in a comprehensive assessment battery, which included: (a) an in-depth structured interview, including the Boston Clinical Interview, the CAPS, and the SCID; (b) multiple psychological tests (the MMPI-2, Mississippi Scale, BDI, STAI), and (c) a psychophysiologic assessment, which measured responsiveness to neutral and combat stimuli. The assessment lasted for 6 sessions; the goal was both diagnosis and an analysis of Brian's current coping resources and potential for violence. Sessions always started with a safety assessment. Once Brian was actively involved in the evaluation, his overt anxiety decreased and he was able to regularly contract for safety and sobriety. He agreed to stop carrying a weapon, although he continued to keep it at his apartment. He also agreed to resume attending AA/NA meetings daily.

Despite attempts to show minimal emotion, Brian became visibly anxious and tearful when revealing traumatic events, which he had agreed to do "as an experiment." However, he was guarded about relating his experiences in any depth and was concerned that he would be judged as crazy. Symptoms that particularly worried him included hearing voices. Inquiry revealed that these were voices of dead buddies from Vietnam, and that he heard the voices only during Vietnam-related dissociative experiences. Reassurance that these symptoms were part of PTSD and that he was not psychotic was helpful to him.

On the SCID, Brian met diagnostic criteria for (a) PTSD, combat-related; (b) major depression, recurrent, in partial remission; (c) polysubstance dependence, in remission; (d) alcohol dependence, in remission; and (e) borderline personality disorder. Because of his level of dissociation, the presence of borderline personality, and an early conduct disorder, childhood trauma was suspected. This issue was targeted for further exploration as treatment proceeded.

Treatment Selection

The final two formal assessment sessions included a discussion of treatment options; the patient preferred to continue in treatment, and a treatment contract was established initially for 6 months. Early goals focused on safety and stability, as well as relationship building.

During the discussion of treatment options, trauma education that was started in the formal assessment was continued in more detail. In this phase, different treatment options were discussed directly with the patient. Trauma exposure, "telling his story and his secrets," made intuitive sense to Brian, but it was agreed that his life was not yet stable enough for this phase and that he still had strong concerns about the therapist's ability to tolerate his stories. Instead, it was agreed that the initial focus of treatment would be on stress management and relationship building—especially trust issues. Exposure work would be added gradually. Despite Brian's 7 months of sobriety, his skills at coping with negative affect were poor, and it was noted that the PTSD reexperiencing led to increased urges to use drugs. Accordingly, relapse prevention with a specific link to trauma triggers was initiated. Anger management training was also started because of the patient's poor impulse control, history of violence, and fears of hurting others. A medication consultation was suggested, but Brian refused this option based on his drug-abuse history.

Treatment Course and Problems in Carrying Out Interventions

Treatment was conceptually based on the stage model just presented; however, as is often the case, treatment stages overlapped and were occasionally repeated. Therapy involved a continuous processing of the relationship between therapist and patient. This was an extended procedure, given the patient's history of poor or severed interpersonal relationships and his experience of relationships as aversive, always ending in punishment or death. Brian was quite fearful regarding his therapist's reactions to him and to the horrific material he revealed. He was concerned because the therapist was a young white woman, and he did not believe that she could ever understand his experiences. He was worried that she would be unable to tolerate the emotions expressed and that she would have nightmares of Brian's experiences. For a number of months, discussing the therapist's reaction to him and the converse was as important as the behavioral and emotional content areas discussed.

Exposure began early in therapy, but it was introduced as part of the trust-building process: Brian would reveal something traumatic about Vietnam and wait for the therapist's shock or rejection. For example, Brian revealed that he had regularly mutilated corpses and worn a necklace of ears. Brian was encouraged to discuss his beliefs about people's reactions to his story and his specific fears about the therapist's reactions. In addition, as Brian became more adept at identifying triggers for his anger and his urges for drugs, treatment naturally flowed into memories of things that happened in Vietnam.

Classic flooding or implosive therapy was not considered an option at this point, because of the patient's volatility and the extreme distress that he evidenced when discussing small incidents. The goal was gradual exposure of the traumatic memories in order to start to extinguish their affective power. Beginning in the second month of therapy, this goal was approached by encouraging Brian to share "secrets" he felt made him unacceptable and through weekly discussions of his most traumatic nightmares and dissociative images. Again, most important from his perspective was unconditional acceptance of him as a person regardless of the nature of his revelations. In addition, Brian was encouraged not to avoid material. For example, Brian would attempt to switch the focus to the therapist by making personal comments about her. As a rule, sessions did not terminate until he told a story with affect, rather than intellectualizing and removing himself from it or remaining so emotionally numb that nothing touched him. This segment of therapy, which lasted from approximately the second to the ninth month of treatment, was extremely anxiety arousing for the patient, and stress management techniques (e.g., relaxation, deep breathing) were used to help Brian continue to feel safe. Throughout the therapy, cognitive-behavioral techniques were employed to address the patient's dysfunctional schemas and distortions in appraisal. By the fifth month of treatment, Brian was beginning to notice spontaneously that it helped to address his traumas directly, and he described relief that someone else knew the worst. He started sharing more of himself with people outside of the therapy hour, and admitted to his therapy group and to his AA sponsor that he had been afraid in Vietnam. At first he felt overexposed and very threatened, but gradually he began to feel safer.

Trust in the therapeutic relationship was a continuing issue. About midway through treatment, Brian revealed that his father's mild beatings in fact had been severe physical abuse. After this disclosure, Brian did not keep his next appointment and then called to terminate therapy. After talking to the therapist, he continued in therapy. However, after one session dealing with childhood issues, Brian felt that he was able to contain these memories and chose to focus exclusively on combat trauma.

Given the long-standing and serious nature of Brian's problems, it was felt that a team approach would be helpful in his case. Accordingly, after 1 month of treatment Brian was referred to a Vietnam veterans group at a local veterans center. It was hoped that this referral would decrease Brian's isolation and feelings of separateness. Although Brian agreed to the referral, he had problems completing it and eventually admitted that the idea of a group terrified him. The referral was dropped at this time, but proposed again after 6 months of treatment. At this stage, Brian was less fearful of rejection when honest about his combat experience, and he also felt more ready to listen to the experiences of others. He joined a combat veterans group and in fact continued in this group even after individual therapy ended.

Brian had one relapse (to alcohol) in the fourth month of therapy, shortly after he revealed an atrocity committed in Vietnam. Brian called the therapist while drunk and despite significant threatening behavior, agreed to come in for detoxification. This incident was used to strengthen his commitment to sobriety and was reframed as a success (e.g., he drank for only 2 days and did not hurt anyone).

Outcome and Termination

After approximately 10 months, Brian began to comment regularly on improvements in his behavior and in the way he viewed himself. At this stage, discussion of termination began. Brian noted that he was no longer afraid of losing control, felt that he had the right to a decent life, had a new girlfriend, and was working steadily. He was more open about being a Vietnam combat veteran. In AA meetings he was talking about Vietnam as it related to his addiction.

One issue of concern was that the patient still had nightmares. He reported a significant decrease in frequency and distress level of intrusive thoughts while awake, and also noted that despite continued nightmares, he was not as actively violent at night and was able to sleep in the same bed with his girlfriend. Brian revealed that he was not ready to give up the nightmares, and felt that he wanted to stop changing before he lost himself completely.

Termination of therapy had been discussed from the beginning of treatment. Given the patient's multiple losses, termination was presented as a process, with no final end. Instead, after about one year, therapy gradually became less frequent. The patient was encouraged to see himself as changed and improved, but not necessarily cured, leaving the door open for returning with honor. Although Brian was offered treatment to focus on his childhood abuse, he refused this option, stating that he felt he had improved enough and that he did not want to undermine his recovery.

Follow-Up and Maintenance

Meetings decreased from once per week to once every 2 weeks for 2 months. At this point Brian wished to stop therapy, and he was encouraged to return in 6 months for follow-up, earlier if necessary. The model of PTSD as a cyclical disorder was presented to him, and he was encouraged to recontact the therapist if he had a temporary worsening or if he decided to work on another aspect of his life, such as his combat nightmares or his childhood abuse.

Brian regularly attended AA/NA meetings, had a sponsor, and was now sponsoring other members as well. At the 6-month follow-up he reported that his life was going well, but that he wanted to retain the option of seeing the therapist.

Ten months after termination, Brian did contact the therapist and reveal that he was struggling with trauma-related issues from his childhood. Brian recontracted for treatment with a focus on his early abuse, and with a goal of understanding how his childhood had influenced both his experience of Vietnam and his current functioning.

Summary

The treatment of PTSD is a complex, multidimensional process that involves numerous stages. Cognitive-behavioral treatments have yielded positive outcomes in clinical case studies, in single-subject designs, and in randomized clinical trials. Other conceptual models of treatment have yet to be empirically tested.

Given the pervasive nature of the PTSD symptom complex and its debilitating effects, comprehensive treatment of PTSD has included numerous behavioral and cognitive-behavioral techniques. The model proposed in this chapter is one that addresses the many needs of traumatized patients and clients. It includes (a) emotional and behavioral stabilization, (b) trauma education, (c) stress management, (d) trauma focus, (e) relapse prevention strategies, and (f) aftercare. This model is conceptually driven and has been, at least in part, empirically evaluated.

Future research on PTSD might include substantive outcome research in the form of clinical trials. Componential analyses would be particularly welcome. Longitudinal studies to determine the long-range impact of PTSD would add significant new knowledge to the field. Studies on the physiologic consequences of PTSD in terms of mortality, morbidity, and quality of life would provide a more complete understanding of the costs to society of PTSD.

Abueg, F. R., & Fairbank, J. A. (1992). Behavioral treatment of posttraumatic stress disorder and co-occurring substance abuse. In P. A. Saigh (Ed.), *Posttraumatic stress disorder: A behavioral approach to assessment and treatment* (pp. 111–145). New York: Macmillan.

Agger, I., & Jensen, S. J. (1990). Testimony as ritual and evidence in psychotherapy for political refugees. *Journal of Traumatic Stress, 3,* 115–130.

American Psychiatric Association (1987). *Diagnostic and statistical manual of mental disorders* (3rd ed., rev.). Washington, DC: Author.

American Psychiatric Association (1991). *DSM-IV options book: Work in progress.* Washington, DC: Author.

Barlow, D. H. (1988). *Anxiety and its disorders: The nature and treatment of anxiety and panic.* New York: Guilford.

Beck, A. T. (1972). *Depression: Causes and treatment.* Philadelphia: University of Pennsylvania Press.

Benson, H. (1975). *The relaxation response.* New York: William Morrow.

Blake, D. D., Weathers, F. W., Nagy, L. N., Kaloupek, D. G., Klauminzer, G., Charney, D. S., & Keane, T. M. (1990). A clinician rating scale for assessing current and lifetime PTSD: The CAPS-1. *The Behavior Therapist, 18,* 187–188.

Blanchard, E. B., Kolb, L. C., Pallmeyer, T. P., & Gerardi, R. J. (1982). A psychophysiological study of post-traumatic stress disorder in Vietnam veterans. *Psychiatric Quarterly, 54,* 220–229.

Boudewyns, P. A., Albrecht, J. W., Talbert, F. S., & Hyer, L. A. (1991). Comorbidity and treatment outcome of inpatients with chronic combat-related PTSD. *Hospital and Community Psychiatry, 42,* 847–849.

Boudewyns, P. A., & Hyer, L. (1990). Physiological response to combat memories and preliminary treatment outcome in Vietnam veteran PTSD patients treated with direct therapeutic exposure. *Behavior Therapy, 21,* 63–87.

Bower, G. R., & Lambert, J. A. (1985). Systematic desensitization therapy with post-traumatic stress disorder cases. In C. R. Figley (Ed.), *Trauma and its wake: Vol. 2. Traumatic stress theory, research, and intervention* (pp. 280–291). New York: Brunner/Mazel.

Braun, P., Greenberg, D., Dasberg H., & Lerer, B. (1990). Core symptoms of posttraumatic stress disorder unimproved by alprazolam treatment. *Journal of Clinical Psychiatry, 51,* 236–238.

Breslau, N., Davis, G. C., Andreski, P., & Peterson, E. (1991). Traumatic events and posttraumatic stress disorder in an urban population of young adults. *Archives of General Psychiatry, 48,* 216–222.

Brom, D., Kleber, R. J., & Defares, P. B. (1989). Brief psychotherapy for posttraumatic stress disorder. *Journal of Consulting and Clinical Psychology, 57,* 607–612.

Chemtob, C., Roitblat, H. L., Hamada, R. S., Carlson, S. G., & Twentyman, C. T. (1988). A cognitive action theory of post-traumatic stress disorder. *Journal of Anxiety Disorders, 2,* 253–275.

Cooper, N. A., & Clum, G. A. (1989). Imaginal flooding as a supplementary treatment for PTSD in combat veterans: A controlled study. *Behavior Therapy, 20,* 381–391.

Davidson, J., & Fairbank, J. A. (1993). The epidemiology of posttraumatic stress disorder. In J. R. T. Davidson and E. B. Foa (Eds.), *Posttraumatic stress disorder: DSM-IV and beyond* (pp. 147–172). Washington, DC: American Psychiatric Press.

Davidson, J. Kudler, H., & Smith, R. (1990). Treatment of posttraumatic stress disorder. *American Journal of Psychiatry, 47,* 259–266.

Dohrenwend, B. P., & Shrout, P. E. (1981). Toward the development of a two-stage procedure for case identification and classification in psychiatric epidemiology. *Research in Community and Mental Health, 2,* 295–323.

Fairbank, J. A., Gross, R. J., & Keane, T. M. (1983). Treatment of posttraumatic stress disorder: Evaluating outcome with a behavioral code. *Behavioral Modification, 7,* 557–568.

Fairbank, J. A., & Keane, T. M. (1982). Flooding for combat-related stress disorders: Assessment of anxiety reduction across traumatic memories. *Behavior Therapy, 13,* 499–510.

Faustman, W. O., & White, P. A. (1989). Diagnostic and psychopharmacology treatment characteristics of 536 inpatients with posttraumatic stress disorder. *Journal of Nervous and Mental Disease, 177,* 154–159.

Fesler, A. F. (1991). Valproate acid in combat-related posttraumatic stress disorder. *Journal of Clinical Psychiatry, 52,* 361–364.

Foa, E. B., & Kozak, M. J. (1986). Emotional processing of fear: Exposure to corrective information. *Psychological Bulletin, 99,* 20–35.

Foa, E. B., Rothbaum, B. O., Riggs, D. S., & Murdock, T. B. (1991). Treatment of PTSD in rape victims: A comparison between cognitive-behavioral procedures and counseling. *Journal of Consulting and Clinical Psychology, 59*, 715–723.

Foa, E. B., Steketee, G., & Rothbaum, B. (1989). Behavioral/cognitive conceptualizations of post-traumatic stress disorder. *Behavior Therapy, 20*, 155–176.

Forsyth, J. P., Carey, T., Litz, B. T., & Fisher, L. (1991, October). *Coping styles and comorbid symptomatology in combat-related PTSD.* Paper presented at the meeting of the International Society for Traumatic Stress Studies, Washington, DC.

Foy, D. W., Carroll, E. M., & Donahoe, C. P. (1987). Etiological factors in the development of PTSD in clinical samples of Vietnam combat veterans. *Journal of Clinical Psychology, 43*, 17–27.

Frank, E., & Stewart, B. D. (1984). Depressive symptoms in rape victims. *Journal of Affective Disorders, 1*, 269–277.

Frank, J. B., Kosten, T. R., Giller, E. L., & Dan, E. (1988). A randomized clinical trial of phenelzine and imipramine for post-traumatic stress disorder. *American Journal of Psychiatry, 145*, 1289–1291.

Friedman, M. J. (1988). Toward rational pharmacotherapy for posttraumatic stress disorder: An interim report. *American Journal of Psychiatry, 145*, 281–285.

Green, B., Grace, M., Lindy, J., Titchener, J., & Lindy, J. (1983). Levels of functional impairment following a civilian disaster: The Beverly Hills Supper Club fire. *Journal of Consulting and Clinical Psychology, 51*, 573–580.

Green, B., Lindy, J., & Grace, M. (1988). Long-term coping with combat stress. *Journal of Traumatic Stress, 1*, 399–418.

Hammerberg, M. (1992). Penn Inventory for posttraumatic stress disorder: Psychometric properties. *Psychological Assessment: A Journal of Consulting and Clinical Psychology, 4*, 67–76.

Hearst, N., Newman, T. B., & Hulley, S. B. (1986). Delayed effects of the military draft on mortality: A randomized natural experiment. *New England Journal of Medicine, 314*, 620–624.

Helzer, J. E., Robins, L. N., & McEvoy, L. (1987). Post-traumatic stress disorder in the general population: Findings of the Epidemiologic Catchment Area survey. *New England Journal of Medicine, 317*, 1630–1634.

Herman, J. L. (1992). *Trauma and recovery.* New York: Basic Books.

Hickling, E. J., Sison, G. F. P., & VanderPloeg, R. D. (1986). Treatment of posttraumatic stress disorder with relaxation and biofeedback training. *Behavior Therapy, 16*, 406–416.

Horowitz, M. J. (1986). *Stress response syndromes* (2nd ed.). New York: Jason Aronson.

Horowitz, M. J., Wilner, N. R., & Alvarez, W. (1979). Impact of Event Scale: A measure of subject stress. *Psychosomatic Medicine, 41*, 209–218.

Jacobson, E. (1938). *Progressive relaxation.* Chicago: Chicago Press.

Janoff-Bulman, R. (1992). *Shattered assumptions: Towards a new psychology of trauma.* New York: Free Press.

Keane, T. M. (1985). Defining traumatic stress: Some comments on the current terminological confusion. *Behavior Therapy, 16*, 419–423.

Keane, T. M. (1989). Post-traumatic stress disorder: Current status and future directions. *Behavior Therapy, 20*, 149–153.

Keane, T. M., Albano, A. M., & Blake, D. D. (1992). Current trends in the treatment of post-traumatic stress symptoms. In M. Basoglu (Ed.), *Torture and its consequences.* Cambridge, UK: Cambridge University Press.

Keane, T. M., Caddell, J. M., & Taylor, K. L. (1988). Mississippi Scale for Combat-Related Posttraumatic Stress Disorder: Three studies in reliability and validity. *Journal of Consulting and Clinical Psychology, 56*, 85–90.

Keane, T. M., Fairbank, J. A., Caddell, J. M., & Zimering, R. T. (1989). Implosive (flooding) therapy reduces symptom of PTSD in Vietnam veterans. *Behavior Therapy, 20*, 245–260.

Keane, T. M., & Kaloupek, D. G. (1982). Imaginal flooding in the treatment of a post-traumatic stress disorder. *Journal of Consulting and Clinical Psychology, 50*, 138–140.

Keane, T. M., Malloy, P. F., & Fairbank, J. A. (1984). Empirical development of an MMPI subscale for the assessment of combat-related post-traumatic stress disorder. *Journal of Consulting and Clinical Psychology, 5*, 888–891.

Keane, T. M., & Penk, W. E. (1988). Letter on prevalence of post-traumatic stress disorder (PTSD). *New England Journal of Medicine, 316*, 1152.

Keane, T. M., & Wolfe, J. (1990). Co-morbidity in post-traumatic stress disorder: An analysis of community and clinical studies. *Journal of Applied Social Psychology, 20*, 1776–1788.

Kilpatrick, D. G., Edmunds, C. N., & Seymour, A. K. (1992). *Rape in America: A report to the nation.* Arlington, VA: National Victims Center.

Kilpatrick, D. G., Veronen, L. J., & Resick, P. A. (1979). The aftermath of rape: Recent empirical findings. *American Journal of Orthopsychiatry, 49*, 658–669.

Kolb, L. C., Burris, B. C., & Griffiths, S. (1984). Propranolol and clonidine in treatment of the chronic post-traumatic stress disorders of war. In B. Van der Kolk (Ed.), *Post-traumatic stress disorder: Psychological and biological sequelae* (pp. 97–105). Washington DC: American Psychiatric Press.

Kosten, T., Frank, J. B., & Dan, E. (1991). Pharmacotherapy for post-traumatic stress disorder using phenelzine or imipramine. *Journal of Nervous and Mental Disease, 179*, 366–370.

Kulka, R. A., Schlenger, W. E., Fairbank, J. A., Hough, R. L., Jordan, B. K., Marmar, C. R., & Weiss, D. (1988). *National Vietnam Veterans Readjustment Study (NVVRS): Description, current status, and initial PTSD prevalence estimates.* Washington, DC: Veterans Administration.

Kulka, R. A., Schlenger, W. E., Fairbank, J. A., Hough, R. L., Jordan, B. K., Marmar, C. R., & Weiss, D. (1990). *Trauma and the Vietnam War generation.* New York: Brunner/Mazel.

Lang, P. J. (1977). Imagery in therapy: An information processing analysis of fear. *Behavior Therapy, 8*, 862–886.

Levis, D. J., & Hare, N. A. (1977). A review of the theoretical rationale and empirical support for the extinction approach of implosive (flooding) therapy. In M. Hersen, R. M. Eisler, & P. M. Miller (Eds.), *Progress in behavior modification* (Vol. 4, pp. 299–374). New York: Academic Press.

Litz, B. T., Blake, D. D., Gerardi, R. J., & Keane, T. M. (1990). Decision making guidelines for use of direct therapeutic exposure in the treatment of post-traumatic stress disorder. *The Behavior Therapist, 13*, 91–93.

Litz, B. T., Penk, W. E., Walsh, S., Hyer, L., Blake, D. D., Marx, B., Keane, T. M., & Bitman, D. (1991). Similarities and differences between MMPI and MMPI-2 applications to the assessment of post-traumatic stress disorder. *Journal of Personality Assessment, 57*, 238–253.

Lyons, J. A., & Keane, T. M. (1992). Keane PTSD scale: MMPI and MMPI-2 update. *Journal of Traumatic Stress, 5*, 111–117.

Malloy, P. F., Fairbank, J. A., & Keane, T. M. (1983). Validation of a multimethod assessment of post-traumatic stress disorders in Vietnam veterans. *Journal of Consulting and Clinical Psychology, 51*, 488–494.

Marlatt, G. A., & Gordon, J. R. (1985). *Relapse prevention.* New York: Guilford.

McCann, L., & Pearlman, L. A. (1991). *Psychological trauma and the adult survivor: Theory, therapy, and transformation.* New York: Brunner/Mazel.

McFall, M. E., Smith, D. E., MacKay, P. W., & Tarver, D. J. (1990). Reliability and validity of Mississippi Scale for combat-related posttraumatic stress disorder. *Psychological Assessment, 2*, 114–121.

McFarlane, A. C. (1986). Posttraumatic morbidity of a disaster: A study of cases presenting for psychiatric treatment. *Journal of Nervous and Mental Disease, 174*, 4–13.

Meichenbaum, D., & Jaremko, M. E. (1983). *Stress reduction and prevention.* New York: Plenum.

Mowrer, O. H. (1960). *Learning theory and behavior.* New York: Wiley.

Munroe, J. F. (1991). *Therapist traumatization from exposure to clients with combat-related post-traumatic stress disorder: Implications for administration and supervision.* Unpublished doctoral dissertation, Northeastern University, Boston, MA.

Nagy, L. M., Morgan, C. A., Southwick, S., & Charney, D. S. (in press). Open prospective trial of fluoxetine for post-traumatic stress disorder. *Journal of Clinical Psychopharmacology.*

Peniston, E. G. (1986). EMG biofeedback-assisted desensitization treatment for Vietnam combat veterans post-traumatic stress disorder. *Clinical Biofeedback and Health, 9*, 35–41.

Pitman, R. K., Orr, S. P., Forgue, D. F., deJong, J., & Claiborn, J. M. (1987). Psychophysiologic assessment of posttraumatic stress disorder imagery in Vietnam combat veterans. *Journal of General Psychiatry, 44*, 970–975.

Reist, C., Kaufman, C. D., & Haier, R. J. (1989). A controlled trial of desipramine in 18 men with post-traumatic stress disorder. *American Journal of Psychiatry, 146*, 513–516.

Resick, P. A., & Schnicke, M. K. (1992). Cognitive processing therapy for sexual assault victims. *Journal of Consulting and Clinical Psychology, 60*, 748–756.

Scurfield, R. S. (1985). Post-trauma stress assessment and treatment: Overview and formulations. In C. R. Figley (Ed.), *Trauma and its wake* (pp. 219–256). New York: Brunner/Mazel.

Shapiro, F. (1989a). Efficacy of eye movement desensitization procedure in the treatment of traumatic memories. *Journal of Behavior Therapy and Experimental Psychiatry, 20*(2), 199–223.

Shapiro, F. (1989b). Eye movement desensitization procedure: A new treatment for post traumatic stress disorder. *Journal of Behavior Therapy and Experimental Psychiatry, 20*(3), 211–217.

Shestatzky, M., Greenberg, D., & Lerer, B. (1988). A controlled trial of phenelzine in posttraumatic stress disorder. *Psychiatry Research, 24*, 149–155.

Shore, J. H., Tatum, E. L., & Vollmer, W. M. (1986). Psychiatric reactions to disaster: The Mount St. Helens experience. *American Journal of Psychiatry, 143,* 590–595.

Sierles, F. S., Chen, J., McFarland, R. E., & Taylor, M. A. (1983). Post-traumatic stress disorder and concurrent psychiatric illness. *American Journal of Psychiatry, 140,* 1177–1179.

Sierles, F. S., Chen, J., Messing, M. L., Besyner, T. K., & Taylor, M. A. (1986). Concurrent psychiatric illnesses in non-Hispanic outpatients diagnosed as having posttraumatic stress disorder. *Journal of Nervous and Mental Disease, 174,* 171–173.

Solomon, S. D., Gerrity, E. T., & Muff, A. M. (1992). Efficacy of treatments for posttraumatic stress disorder: An empirical review. *Journal of American Medical Association, 268,* 633–638.

Spitzer, R. L., Williams, J. B. W., Gibbon, M., & First, M. B. (1989). *Structured clinical interview for DSM-III-R—Non-patient edition (SCID-NP, Version 1.0).* Washington, DC: American Psychiatric Press.

Stampfl, T. G., & Levis, D. J. (1967). Essentials of implosive therapy: A learning-theory-based psychodynamic behavioral therapy. *Journal of Abnormal Psychology, 72,* 151–163.

Wolf, M. E., Alavi, A., & Mosnaim, A. D. (1987). Pharmacological interventions in Vietnam veterans with post-traumatic stress disorder. *Research Communications in Psychology, Psychiatry, and Behavior, 12,* 169–175.

Wolpe, J. (1956). *Psychotherapy by reciprocal inhibition.* Stanford, CA: Stanford University Press.

Wolpe, J. (1984). Deconditioning and ad hoc uses of relaxation: An overview. *Journal of Behavior Therapy and Experimental Psychiatry, 15,* 299–304.

Zubin, J., & Spring, B. (1977). Vulnerability: A new view of schizophrenia. *Journal of Abnormal Psychology, 86,* 103–126.

13

Generalized Anxiety Disorder

T. D. Borkovec and Lizabeth Roemer

Description of the Disorder

Generalized anxiety disorder (GAD) has undergone numerous transitions in definition. It was separated from panic disorder in DSM-III but remained a residual category
until DSM-III-R, wherein worry became its defining feature. Although research on the
disorder has been limited, considerable empirical investigation has occurred in the
last few years and a better understanding of its nature, functions, and effective
treatment is emerging.

Clinical Features

Generalized anxiety disorder is a chronic condition centrally defined in DSM-
III-R as excessive or unrealistic anxiety and worry about two or more life circumstances unrelated to other Axis I disorders and occurring more days than not over a
6-month period (American Psychiatric Association, 1987). The presence of 6 of 18
associated features involving vigilance and scanning, motor tension, and autonomic
hyperactivity is also required. Thus, the generally anxious individual experiences
more or less constant cognitive and somatic anxiety throughout the day. Unlike
phobic disorders, this anxiety is not triggered by easily identifiable or discrete
environmental stimuli, nor is it due to panic attacks. The principal changes proposed
for DSM-IV (American Psychiatric Association, 1993) include the deletion of "unrealistic" and the addition of "uncontrollable" in describing the worrying, and a simplification of the 18 associated symptoms to include only those six empirically found to be
highly characteristic of GAD: restlessness or feeling keyed up or on edge, being easily

---

T. D. Borkovec and **Lizabeth Roemer** • Department of Psychology, The Pennsylvania State University,
University Park, Pennsylvania 16802.

Handbook of Prescriptive Treatments for Adults, edited by Michel Hersen and Robert T. Ammerman.
Plenum Press, New York, 1994.

fatigued, having difficulty concentrating or mind going blank, irritability, muscle tension, and sleep disturbance.

Associated Features

Eighty-two percent of GAD cases meet criteria for other anxiety and depression disorders, the highest comorbidity rate among the anxiety disorders, and GAD is the most common additional diagnosis associated with other principal anxiety disorders (23%; Moras, DiNardo, Brown, & Barlow, submitted). The most common additional diagnoses among GAD clients (social and simple phobias) (Sanderson & Wetzler, 1991) share few of the GAD features, however, and co-occurrence of GAD and the anxiety disorder most similar to it in some ways (obsessive-compulsive disorder) is very rare (Brown, Moras, Zinbarg, & Barlow, 1993). Although additional diagnoses of depression occur among 29% of GAD patients, dysthymia and major depression are more common in both principal panic disorder with severe avoidance and obsessive-compulsive disorder (Brown & Barlow, 1992). Finally, some authors (e.g., Tollefson, Luxenberg, Valentine, Dunsmore, & Tollefson, 1991) have noted frequent comorbidity of irritable bowel syndrome and GAD.

Whereas earlier research suggested an absence of familial aggregation for GAD (e.g., Torgerson, 1983), more recent studies have found greater frequency of GAD and lower frequency of panic disorder among relatives of GAD probands than among relatives of panic disorder probands (e.g., Noyes et al., 1992).

Basic research has revealed distinctive features associated with GAD. Clients have a preattentive bias to diverse threat cues, especially those associated with their worries (Mathews, 1990), are more likely to interpret ambiguous material in a threatening way, and predict negative, low-probability events to be more likely (Butler & Mathews, 1983). Moreover, worrying about one topic increases the accessibility of worries related to other topics (Montalvo, Metzger, & Noll, 1989).

Worrying functions as a cognitive avoidance of perceived threat and is negatively reinforced in two ways. First, worry about low-probability events is usually followed by their nonoccurrence, leading to a superstitious engagement in worry. GAD subjects acknowledge such a possible function to a greater degree than control subjects (Roemer, Borkovec, Posa, & Lyonfields, 1991). Second, worry just prior to phobic images eliminates cardiovascular response to the images (Borkovec & Hu, 1990). Thus, GAD clients can escape or avoid somatic anxiety to fear material by worrying, giving meaning to their common report that worry helps them prepare for the worst. By doing so, however, they avoid complete functional exposure, prevent the processing of emotional material (Foa & Kozak, 1986), and thus perpetuate anxious meanings. The nature of worry provides clues to how it may function in this way. Worry is composed primarily of negative thoughts (as opposed to images), and GAD clients show greater negative thinking and less imagery than nonanxious individuals even during relaxation (Borkovec & Inz, 1990). Verbal articulation of emotional material does not produce the same degree of cardiovascular response that imagery of the same material does (Vrana, Cuthbert, & Lang, 1986). Indeed, it is the thought element of worry that suppresses physiologic response to phobic material (Borkovec, Lyonfields, Wiser, & Deihl, 1993). In fact, although muscle tension tends to be high, GAD clients display a *restriction* in variability of skin conductance and heart rate both during rest and in response to challenge (cf. Hoehn-Saric & McLeod, 1988), suggesting a deficiency in vagal tone and an autonomic inflexibility.

Because the perceived threats exist only in the future, thus precluding motoric avoidance, GAD clients have learned to use abstract worry for *cognitive* avoidance of their anxiety-provoking environments and anxious experience, a method that guarantees maintenance of their anxiety disorder. Worry breeds more worry; habit is continually strengthened so that clients become increasingly stuck in a worrisome pattern of responding. The resultant cognitive rigidity and associated autonomic rigidity are evident in the clients' constant predictions of negative events, reports that they always expect the worst, and such cognitive distortions as dichotomous thinking, personalization, mind reading, and overgeneralization.

Epidemiology

No adequate information on the prevalence of GAD as defined by DSM-III-R is available. Breslau and Davis (1985) and the NIMH Epidemiological Catchment Area investigation for its second wave (Blazer, Hughes, George, Swartz, & Boyer, 1991) both used the DSM-III definition and found lifetime prevalence of 9 and 5.8%, respectively. In the latter study, GAD tended to be more frequent among women, blacks, young adults, and persons with low income or occupational status. Such estimates led Rapee (1991) to argue that GAD may be one of the most common anxiety disorders, even though those affected make up only about 10% of people seeking treatment for anxiety of depression problems (Brown & Barlow, 1992).

In 10 therapy outcome studies of GAD, 65% of the clients were women, and the average age was 36 years (Borkovec & Whisman, in press). Age at onset ranges widely (Noyes, in press), tending on the average to be in the mid-teens to early 20s (Rapee, 1991). GAD occurs at an earlier age and with a more gradual onset than panic disorder (e.g., Noyes et al., 1992).

Etiology

Given the gradual onset of GAD, it is not surprising that 80% of patients are unable to recall specifically the onset of their problems (Rapee, 1985). The chronic nature of the disorder presents difficulties, then, to researchers interested in its precursors. Two studies have suggested historical contributors to the development of GAD. Torgerson (1986) found that GAD clients report experiencing the death of a parent before the age of 16 more often than panic disorder clients, and Blazer, Hughes, and George (1987) determined that a GAD diagnosis was more common among subjects who had experienced at least one unexpected negative life event. More recently, college students meeting DSM-III-R criteria for GAD reported a greater number of traumatic events than nonanxious subjects (Roemer et al., 1991). Traumatic events would reasonably lead to a view of the world as a dangerous, unpredictable, or uncontrollable place with which one may not be able to cope. However, retrospective data are suspect. Anxious individuals may be more likely to recall negative events or interpret an event as traumatic at the time of its occurrence. The latter possibility suggests that the origins of the disorder may arise even earlier in childhood. The child's attachment to a primary caregiver may play a crucial role. Bowlby (1973) proposed that an insecurely attached child will develop a working model of the world as a threatening place. Both GAD clients (Cassidy, 1992) and college students (Roemer et al., 1991) show signs of having been insecurely attached as children on self-report measure of attachment. Of course, difficulties remain with the possible unreliability of retrospective report, and it has yet to be determined whether such attachment patterns are distinctive of GAD or are common across anxiety disorders.

Differential Diagnosis and Assessment

DSM-III-R and DSM-IV Categorization

Debate surrounds the fate of GAD in DSM-IV, including its possible deletion or its movement to Axis II. The most likely recommendation (Barlow, personal communication, November 1992) will keep GAD as an Axis I disorder with the following features: (a) retention of worry as the cardinal aspect with a minimum 6-mouth duration; (b) elimination of the "unrealistic" criterion; (c) requirement that the worry be pervasive (i.e., about a number of events or activities unrelated to an Axis I disorder, and not part of posttraumatic stress disorder); (d) simplification of an 18-item list of associated symptoms; and (e) requirement that the worry be difficult to control and that the anxiety, worry, or physical symptoms significantly interfere with normal routine or cause marked distress. The diagnosis will be excluded if the generalized anxiety is due to substance-induced or secondary anxiety disorder or if the symptoms are present only during a mood disorder, psychotic disorder, or a pervasive developmental disorder. Finally, the overanxious child diagnosis will likely be subsumed under the GAD category in an effort to simplify the diagnostic system. Several changes are based on recent empirical information, some of which is summarized below.

GAD clients score higher on a trait measure of worry than do individuals with any other anxiety disorder (Brown, Antony, & Barlow, 1992), and trait-worry is statistically independent of other measures of anxiety and depression within GAD samples (Brown et al., 1992; Meyer, Miller, Metzger, & Borkovec, 1990). Assessors have found uncontrollability of worry and its interference with functioning to be present in 100% of GAD clients (Borkovec, 1992), and ratings of the severity of that interference distinguish GAD from other anxiety disorders (Borkovec, Shadick, & Hopkins, 1991). The pervasiveness of GAD worry is revealed by clients' report of a greater number of worry topics than nonanxious controls (5.2 vs. 1.2; Borkovec et al., 1991), by their greater likelihood of reporting excessive worry about minor things (92.5%, vs. 32–71% for those with other anxiety disorders and 0% for controls) (Barlow, 1988; Borkovec et al., 1991), and by the fact that, unlike nonanxious people, nearly one-third of their worry topics are not easily categorized into major themes (Shadick, Roemer, Hopkins, & Borkovec, 1991). Finally, GAD is characterized more by central nervous system (CNS) arousal (excessive muscle tension and vigilance and scanning) than by autonomic hyperactivity (Noyes et al., 1992). Thus, only three of the six most commonly found CNS-related symptoms (restlessness or feeling keyed up, easily fatigability, difficulty concentrating, irritability, muscle tension, and trouble sleeping) will be required for diagnosis.

Differential Diagnosis

Because of high comorbidity rates for GAD, several disorders (especially social and simple phobia) need to be considered carefully to accurately diagnose a principal GAD case. Because GAD is associated with low interrator reliability (kappa = 0.57) (Brown & Barlow, 1992), use of established structured interviews is highly recommended, and in research it is imperative that independent diagnostic interviews be conducted by two separate assessors to reduce the likelihood of false-positive cases.

One of the most important factors to consider in differential diagnosis is the focus of the client's worries (Rapee, 1991). If the worry clearly relates to another diagnosable Axis I disorder (e.g., panic attacks, weight gain), then that worry does not contribute to a GAD diagnostic decision. Given the diffuse nature of GAD worry, however, GAD clients frequently report worrying about phobic situations (particularly social ones) in addition to several other areas of life. The crucial distinction, then, is whether the worrying is truly pervasive and covers many life circumstances, in which case a GAD diagnosis would be appropriate.

GAD clients often report earlier periods of major depression or background dysthymia. It seems that their pattern of catastrophizing leads them at times to feel helpless and hopeless. To distinguish clients for whom GAD is principal, it is useful to obtain a history of the course of both the anxiety and the depression symptomatology. If GAD symptoms are present only during a depressive episode, diagnosis of GAD is inappropriate. In deciding whether GAD is the principal diagnosis, consider whether the anxiety preceded the onset of the depression, whether the depression occurs only when the anxiety is present, and whether the anxiety is currently more severe than the depression. GAD clients frequently indicate that their anxiety has always been present or that it precedes the emergence of depressive episodes. Some clients report that the depression has at times been worse than the anxiety but that it occurs less frequently and that it is the anxiety that they most want to change.

An additional diagnostic issue relates to posttraumatic stress disorder (PTSD). The possible role of past trauma in the etiology of some cases of GAD was mentioned earlier. Decisions rest on whether PTSD is diagnosable, and if so, what its severity level is relative to that of GAD. It is also useful to know whether the GAD symptoms were present prior to the occurrence of the traumatic event.

Clients often present with GAD symptoms when undergoing significantly stressful life experiences, and the anxiety and worry are reasonable reactions to these. Although the 6-month duration criterion reduces the likelihood of misdiagnosis, severe life conditions can persist even longer without adequate adjustment. Such cases, if diagnosed at all, are more properly placed under adjustment reactions, with reevaluation after the stressor has been removed. A few cases present greater difficulty; the assessor may remain uncertain whether the life events are severe enough to account for the disturbance or whether the worry and anxiety are truly excessive in their context. The presence of GAD symptoms prior to the event would lean toward principal GAD diagnosis.

Assessment Strategies

Our program uses the revised Anxiety Disorders Interview Schedule (ADIS-R; DiNardo & Barlow, 1988), a structured diagnostic interview covering the anxiety and mood disorders in detail and screening for such other disorders as psychosis and substance abuse. Other structured interviews that cover GAD include the Structured Clinical Interview for DSM-III-R (Spitzer, Williams, Gibbon, & First, 1990) and the Schedule for Affective Disorders and Schizophrenia (Endicott & Spitzer, 1978). The Hamilton Rating Scale for Anxiety (HARS) and the Hamilton Depression Rating Scale (HDRS) (Hamilton, 1959, 1960) can be included to provide assistance in distinguishing the severities of anxiety and depression symptoms and to generate assessor-determined measures for evaluating pretherapy to posttherapy change for clinical or research purposes.

Commonly used self-report instruments with GAD include the trait version of the State-Trait Anxiety Inventory (STAI; Spielberger, Gorsuch, Lushene, Vagg, & Jacobs, 1983) and the Beck Depression Inventory (BDI; Beck, Rush, Shaw, & Emery, 1978). The Penn State Worry Questionnaire (PSWQ; Meyer et al., 1990) is becoming increasingly popular because of its very good psychometric properties and its focus on the central defining feature of GAD. Finally, some measure of dysfunctional beliefs (e.g., the Dysfunctional Attitudes Scale; Weissman & Beck, 1978) is well recommended if cognitive therapy is likely to be one of the interventions used.

In order to assess fluctuations in daily anxiety level for functional analytic use in therapy, clients can complete a daily diary in which they rate four times a day their average level of anxious experience over the preceding few hours. They also monitor any acute episodes of anxiety and record details about the internal and external circumstances that surrounded the event to provide information on situations and responses contributing to their anxiety.

Treatment

Evidence for Prescriptive Treatments

Behavior Therapy. Early research in the treatment of GAD emphasized relaxation techniques, targeting the somatic aspects of anxious experience. The absence of clear and discrete fear-producing stimuli in the environment precluded the deployment of the exposure methods so effective in the treatment of phobias. Thus, the establishment of a generalized coping response that could be used any time anxiety was detected and the choice of relaxation as such a portable skill made sense. Subsequent basic research and clinical experience led to several developments. Recognition of the central role of cognitive and somatic anxiety cues resulted in increasing use of these internal stimuli in self-monitoring and imaginal exposure techniques. The latter tended toward a family of methods that included self-control desensitization (Goldfried, 1971), anxiety management training (Suinn & Richardson, 1971), and stress inoculation (Meichenbaum & Turk, 1973). All emphasized the rehearsal of coping strategies in response to in-session initiation of anxious experience and their application to naturally occurring anxiety, including in vivo exposures to problematic situations to facilitate extinction and to increase generalization of the strategies. Second, more thorough methods of applied relaxation were employed (e.g., Ost, 1987), including differential relaxation, cue-controlled relaxation and systematic training in application of relaxation to incipient anxiety cues. Third, given increasing evidence of the special role that conceptual activity plays in maintaining GAD, cognitive therapy (Beck & Emery, 1985) was incorporated to focus on self-statements and underlying dysfunctional beliefs that demonstrate a view of the world as a dangerous place and the client as an individual ineffective at coping with it.

This resulting package of behavioral and cognitive techniques is the most effective approach for GAD treatment based on existing empirical evidence (cf. Borkovec & Whisman, in press; Chambless & Gillis, 1993) The results of 11 outcome investigations on DSM-defined GAD indicate that the package consistently produces clinically significant improvements in both anxiety and depression, is associated with low dropout rates, and yields change clearly maintained at long-term follow-up.

Although differences in outcome have not always appeared between cognitive-behavioral therapy and elements of the total package or nonspecific factors alone, comparisons of effect size, degree of within-group change, and frequency of clients' meeting criteria for clinically significant change all favor the integrated package approach. In the most recent investigation (Borkovec & Costello, 1993), for example, the percentage of clients reaching high end-state functioning by 1-year follow-up was greatest for cognitive-behavioral therapy (58%), followed by applied relaxation (37.5%) and nondirective therapy (26.7%). Such figures also indicate that, despite progress in the development of treatment methods for GAD, not all clients are returned to normal levels, and further technique development is required.

Pharmacotherapy. Three types of medication have been evaluated in the pharmacologic treatment of GAD: benzodiazepines, azaspirones (mostly buspirone), and antidepressants (mostly imipramine), and existing empirical information documents some usefulness for each drug in acute (4- to 12-week) treatment. By far, the benzodiazepines have been the most thoroughly researched. Although these three classes differ in a number of ways (e.g., site of effect, mechanism of action, type and severity of side effects), research has yet to reveal differential efficacy or optimal matching of client characteristics to type of medication. A recent review by Schweizer and Rickels (in press) tentatively suggests that benzodiazepines may be favored for somatic symptoms, whereas buspirone or imipramine may be better for cognitive symptoms or when depression is part of the clinical picture.

One of the greatest general limitations of pharmacologic intervention for GAD is that anxiety symptoms very frequently return once medication is discontinued. For example, in two of the few drug studies that have evaluated long-term (1-year) follow-up after acute benzodiazepine treatment, relapse rates were found to be 63% (Rickels, Case, Downing, & Fridman, 1986) and 81% (Rickels, Case, & Diamond, 1980). These rates contrast vividly with the routine maintenance of improvement demonstrated for cognitive-behavioral therapies.

A second major limitation has to do with associated effects of medications. Side effects are common, resulting in frequent unacceptability by clients and high dropout rates in outcome trials. And although current evidence suggests that benzodiazepines and buspirone continue to have anxiolytic effects without dose escalation among those clients who continue to take them over considerable periods of time, physical dependence and withdrawal are nearly inevitable among clients chronically taking benzodiazepines. Consequently, there is need for careful, gradual tapering of medication to achieve discontinuation (Schweizer & Rickels, in press).

Because of these overall characteristics of pharmacologic interventions for GAD, Barlow (1988) has suggested that drug treatment be limited to very brief use during times of intense anxiety caused by environmental stressors, whereas Schweizer and Rickels (in press) have recommended that maintenance drug therapy for chronic GAD involve intermittent rather than continuous medication use, with buspirone preferred to benzodiazepines because of its greater safety, the lack of physical dependence, and the likely presence of antidepressant effects. So little adequate research exists, however, on the long-term efficacy of any medication for GAD that considerably more empirical information will be needed before confident assertions about drug intervention can be made.

Alternative Treatments. Two outcome investigations included nondirective (simple reflective listening) therapy alone as a comparison condition. In one

(Blowers, Cobb, & Mathews, 1987), this condition was superior to no treatment on a few measures, inferior to anxiety management training on some measures, and equivalent to the latter condition on several other assessments. In the Borkovec and Costello (1993) study, nondirective therapy was inferior to the other two conditions at posttherapy and 1-year follow-up, and many of its immediate treatment effects disappeared by follow-up. Even so, one-fourth of those in the nondirective group still met criteria for high end-state functioning a year after therapy, so the intervention may be specifically effective for a subset of clients. Whether a more thorough version of experiential therapy, with its focus on the allowance and acceptance of previously denied or suppressed emotional experience (Greenberg & Safran, 1987), might circumvent the apparent avoidance of affect demonstrated by GAD clients and thus facilitate emotional processing to yield significant change remains an as yet unresearched question.

The cognitive-behavioral package described above focuses primarily on learning to cope with the symptoms of anxiety via cognitive and relaxation strategies. The favorable outcomes of controlled protocol evaluations represent the degree of change possible with the use of a fairly rigid treatment; therapists in such trials are not allowed to use additional methods, even behavioral or cognitive ones, if those techniques are not specifically prescribed by the protocol manual. Demonstrated efficacy is thus likely to be a conservative estimate of what can be accomplished by the less restricted use of the various cognitive-behavioral methods available to the therapist and potentially very relevant to particular clients and their circumstances. For example, the use of assertion training, problem-solving training, marital therapy, parent management training, time management strategies, and study skill counseling might have made good clinical sense from a functional analytic point of view with some specific clients involved in our protocol studies. These methods could reasonably contribute to reducing the degree of worry and stress in daily living and should be incorporated into a general cognitive-behavioral treatment for GAD whenever appropriate.

Selecting Optimal Treatment Strategies

While keeping in mind the addition of tailored treatment elements for specific cases, we will describe the basic cognitive-behavioral package that we believe is currently the best available core therapy for GAD. Our description is a summary of the protocol treatment currently being evaluated in an experimental trial and is the second generation of the manual (Borkovec & Costello, 1993).

The degree of operational definition contained in protocol manuals notwithstanding, the therapeutic alliance is crucial for maximizing client motivation to change and willingness to expend the effort required. Our clients are told in Session 1 that the work will always be a collaborative effort, wherein we have expertise in the general principles of change and they are the experts about themselves and their own experience. Our role is to provide the techniques known nomothetically to be useful, and it is their role to discover through observation and experimentation how to translate those methods and their underlying metaphors into applications effective for their unique personalities and circumstances. Listening carefully to what the clients are communicating and adjusting interventions in response to their feedback represent therapist behaviors important to ensuring successful outcome.

Self-Monitoring and Early Cue Detection. Self-monitoring is basic to all else that follows in treatment. The rationale provided to the client emphasizes that anxiety is not just present or absent; it is a process over time that tends to spiral in response to detected threat and is self-reinforcing upon each occurrence. It is not our reactions that are problematic; our reactions to our reactions perpetuate the problem and are the targets for solution. The spiral occurs on the basis of both between-system and within-system interactions. A between-system interaction might involve, for example, an initial catastrophic image of a possible bad event, which leads to increased muscle tension, which produces restricted range of autonomic activity, which validates that something bad is actually going to happen, which activates worrisome thinking in an effort to escape somatic anxiety and avoid the occurrence of the future catastrophe. An example of within-system process is the chain of negative thinking that defines a worrisome episode. The longer one engages in worry, the more related and unrelated worry material is primed, the more this chain of association is strengthened in memory, and the more readily accessible it is upon next detection of threat. Over time, reinforced storage of these spirals yields stuck habits of responding any time an external or internal anxiety cue is detected, and they are increasingly organized to support dysfunctional beliefs about self, the world, and the future that predispose the individual to perceive threat in an increasing number of situations. Monitoring the spiral and its individual elements—images, worrisome thoughts, somatic reactions, affective experiences, possible behavioral reactions (such as subtle avoidance behavior, rushing, or procrastination), and the environments often associated with their initiation—and learning to catch them earlier and earlier in the sequence represent the very first goals of therapy. Coping responses will then be applied to cues detected early, with several advantages. At an early stage of the spiral, anxiety is less intense, and so coping responses are more effective. Short-circuiting of the spiral at an early stage also precludes further strengthening in memory of the entire habitual sequence. New associations, in contrast, are being strengthened. Early cues no longer mean only danger; they increasingly come to mean that it is time to deploy a coping response. Training in early cue detection uses imagery recall, role playing, periodic and frequent cueing of the client during the session whenever the therapist detects rising tension or anxiety, and encouragement to self-monitor during the week, looking for even earlier cues.

Emphasis on Flexibility in Coping.　Another general concept crucial in the treatment of GAD is the notion of flexibility. Because the client engages in stuck habits of thinking and rigid autonomic activity, the higher-order goal of therapy is to establish playful, experimental, and multiple coping responses. Thus, several types of methods will be incorporated into relaxation training, and during cognitive therapy multiple self-statements and alternative beliefs and perspectives will be encouraged for any given situation. In all instances the therapist asks the client to focus attention back on present-moment sensation or the task at hand after deploying coping responses, emphasizing that anxious experience is elicited largely by illusory images and thoughts about a future that does not now exist.

Applied Relaxation.　In the first session we provide an easily learned and rapidly effective relaxation method, so that the client has a coping response immediately available for rehearsal and application during the very first week. It involves diaphragmatic breathing, wherein the client learns to engage in slowed, paced breathing from the abdomen rather than the thorax. This technique not only provides a quick parasympathetic elicitor that targets somatic aspects of anxious responding, but also gives the client an attention-focusing device useful for terminating anxiety-provoking images and worrisome thoughts. Frequency of its application is emphasized, making use of temporal and behavioral reminders throughout the day and, of course, applying it in response to any detected early anxiety cues. Systematic training in progressive muscular relaxation as a means of increasing parasympathetic tone and strengthening the depth of the relaxation response begins in the second session and proceeds over sessions through combinations of major muscle groups and recall training (cf. Bernstein & Borkovec, 1973). It is accompanied by instructions to practice twice daily and eventually includes training in differential relaxation and cue-controlled relaxation. Later in therapy, clients are also introduced to guided imagery and mediational techniques and experiments to discover which methods work best under which circumstances and for which of the interacting systems involved in their particular spiral sequence. Distinctions are also made among the various moments when the usefulness of relaxation responses can be anticipated: just before, during, and in recovery just after a stressful event. Behavioral approach assignments are made whenever motoric avoidance is in evidence and as engineered opportunities to practice the developing coping responses. Throughout therapy, emphasis is placed on the concept of "moving toward" a deeply relaxed state (especially during daily applications) rather than achieving some ultimate, ideal state, and unique words that best represent a particular client's experience are used as metaphors to describe the adaptive state (e.g., "tranquility," "peace," "centered").

Eventually, the above methods are subsumed under the generic concept of "letting go" that will be applied metaphorically to other aspects of client experience later in therapy. Clients will be asked to begin letting go of anxious images, worrisome thoughts, and negative affect in a manner analogous to the releasing of muscle tension during the tensing phase of progressive relaxation training. They are told that this process involves first recognizing the internal event (to preclude automatic avoidance of it) and then detaching from it, allowing it to merely pass through their experience (in contrast to suppressing the experience, distracting oneself from it, or attaching to and dwelling on it). The latter is emphasized because of research indicating the difficulty of suppressing material (Wegner, Schneider, Carter, & White, 1987) and the increase in negative affect associated with suppressed material (Roemer & Borkovec, in press).

Self-Control Desensitization.   A further general concept is the importance of the systematic use of imagery methods. GAD clients use worry to suppress affect and physiological reactivity. Thus, imagery is an important vehicle for accessing affective meaning and for providing exposures to and processing of emotional material that is otherwise avoided. Second, establishing new, adaptive habits requires the frequent application of coping responses, particularly to earlier and earlier spiral cues.

Self-control desensitization (SCD) provides repeated opportunities to rehearse the deployment of the "letting go" reaction. It allows for the presentation of various internal cognitive (especially worry) and somatic anxiety cues to initiate anxious experience in the therapeutic setting, establishes their alternate meaning as cues for coping rather than for further spiraling, and increases the general habit strength of the various coping responses through practice. Numerous environmental situations commonly associated with stress or worry are used as the external context of the images, and various cognitive and somatic cues identified in assessment to be a frequent part of the client's anxious sequences are introduced into each image. As soon as the client begins to experience actual anxiety, the imagery proceeds to having the client imagine relaxing him- or herself while remaining in the situation, letting go of the anxiety, and engaging in alternate self-talk and shifts in perspective that have been developed during previous cognitive therapy portions of the session (see below). After eliminating the anxious experience, the client continues to imagine successfully coping with the situation for a while and then turns off the images altogether and focuses solely on deep relaxation in the office.

Repetitions of the same image continue until the client no longer feels anxiety in response to the anxiety-provoking image or is able to terminate anxiety rapidly with his or her coping responses, at which time new combinations of external and internal cues are presented. There is no attempt to exhaust possible situations or internal cues; rather, the goal is to provide a representative sampling of commonly encountered experiences. Images early in therapy are often taken from events that were problematic during the previous week, whereas anticipated events predominate in the content of images later in therapy. Clients also conduct their own SCD after each relaxation practice session at home, making use of images treated in prior sessions at first and later creating their own images that are more directly relevant to their current or upcoming circumstances. There are also times with particular clients when systematic desensitization may be useful. If a client is having difficulty eliminating anxiety to an imagined situation in SCD, or if the products of cognitive restructuring continue to not "feel true" for a particular situation, straightforward extinction through systematic desensitization can often break through the difficulty.

Cognitive Therapy. In cognitive therapy, we largely follow Beck and Emery's (1985) recommendations: (a) demonstrations of the causal role of perspectives, thoughts, and images in eliciting emotion; (b) identification of automatic thoughts, thought styles, and underlying beliefs; (c) viewing predictions and beliefs as hypotheses rather than as facts; (d) logical analysis of thoughts and beliefs and the use of probability, evidence, and behavioral experiments to test them; (e) use of decatastrophizing methods; (f) development of alternative (and especially multiple and flexible) thoughts and beliefs; and (g) therapist's dependence on Socratic method in each of the above steps to facilitate client confidence and competence. Particular emphasis is placed on worries; they reflect the major themes and negative predictions so characteristic of the disorder. Clients are often asked to stream their worries out loud so that we can examine their content and processes.

Characteristic worry streams are also used to initiate worry process in SCD. From the first or second session onward, clients are furthermore given a worry diary in which they identify each worry that occurs during the day and specify what outcomes they fear might happen. Once the actual outcome occurs, they provide scale ratings to reflect whether the outcome was worse or better than predicted and how well they coped. The purpose of this monitoring is multifold: (a) to facilitate the self-monitoring and detection of incipient worry processes; (b) to focus attention on actual outcomes and their discrepancy from predicted, feared outcomes; (c) to begin establishing a clear history of evidence about the world undistorted by dysfunctional styles such as negative filtering; and (d) to obtain evidence as to whether they can cope well with life, despite their overgeneralized belief that they are incapable of doing so.

Although any number of distorted beliefs may be revealed, our experience with GAD suggests that some styles are particularly salient: perfectionism, personalization, catastrophization, negative filtering, mind reading, and overgeneralization. And it is a rare GAD client for whom the word "should" does not make up a substantial percentage of his or her vocabulary. Very early in therapy, before conducting a full logical analysis of "shoulds" and other sources of potentially arbitrary rules, we highlight this tendency and suggest that the word can routinely be replaced with the word "could." Such substitution reminds clients about the all-important notions of choice and multiple possibilities (rather than singular necessity) and flexibility (rather than rigidity and stuck habit), and it removes much of the pressure that they often place on themselves.

Problems in Carrying Out Interventions

Because GAD is a chronic condition characterized by a general cognitive style of negative predictions, clients are often demoralized when they enter therapy and have difficulty believing that they can change. Many clients are also time-urgent, and adding tasks to an already busy schedule can result in compliance problems. The most useful approach to these potential problems is to provide as soon as possible strategies whose use yields some noticeable, even if small, effects both in the session and during daily life. Relaxation training usually produces a pleasant state; diaphragmatic breathing, quickly learned and applied, often results in reports by the second session that some success was achieved with its application. SCD is a good method for showing the client small but systematic changes: The time necessary to generate anxiety via imaginal threat cues routinely increases with repetition, and the time to eliminate the anxiety decreases. Early cognitive therapy would wisely aim at small cognitive distortions associated with mildly anxiety-provoking situations so that the client experiences a clear and convincing perspective shift and resulting anxiety reduction. If the therapist continues to emphasize that change will be gradual as habit strength grows and as applications are transferred to more situations, and if the daily diaries are systematically tracking small gains in process and outcome, then client motivation is likely to be increased and maintained. Most clients come to realize with therapist guidance and experiments outside of therapy that the time they invest now in learning to reduce their anxiety will pay off in greater productivity in their important life tasks in addition to greater tranquility.

Although the above problems can result in poor adherence to homework and practice, on the whole GAD clients are very compliant. In fact, successful therapy aims ultimately at reducing their frequent fear of negative evaluation by the therapist, and such issues are explicitly raised for intervention. Clients who, toward the end of therapy, are reporting failure to carry out assigned tasks without feeling guilty or are engineering their own tasks because they think them to be more useful than what the therapist recommended provide us with special joy.

Not all the interventions described earlier will have direct relevance for every client. It is important for the therapist to be sensitive to client feedback, to emphasize methods that are proving useful and not to insist on those that are not, and to work with the client to develop individualized meanings and applications from the available generic strategies. Insisting on the continued use of methods that the client finds of little value will only produce a poor therapeutic relationship. Given the variety of techniques available and our emphasis on flexibility, to do so is completely unnecessary.

Two subsets of GAD clients have a poor prognosis in this protocol therapy. The first group consists of those experiencing significant, realistic stress whose effects are superimposed on a GAD style of reacting. These stressors either enter the client's life after therapy has begun, or their significance becomes apparent only during the course of therapy. Our anecdotal observation in some cases is that clients do often seem to come up with methods such as greater assertion, more effective problem solving, or better parenting or spousal relationship behaviors on their own as they become more relaxed and realistic in their thinking. The restrictions of protocol therapy, however, do not allow us to implement such methods, nor can we directly help the client with significant life decisions aimed at producing more adaptive external circumstances to relieve the stress. Although our cognitive-behavioral interventions can provide some relief, there are limits to their effectiveness when severe, realistic stress exists.

The second subgroup is even more difficult. We have called this small minority of clients the "entitlement" group. Several sessions of therapy are required before we recognize their characteristics. Tension, anxiety, and worry are indeed the predominating emotional experiences, but their source is an underlying anger and frustration usually aimed at other people or the "system" in general. From their perspective, their stress is due to others who will not behave the way they wish them to behave or to a system (e.g., school or work institutions) that is not set up to meet their needs. No motivation to change themselves in any way derives from this perspective, and none of their thought styles are seen as distorted or maladaptive. Thus far, we have observed virtually no clinical improvement in this group of clients. Clearly, neither the underlying assumptions of our protocol therapy nor the rationale offered to these clients for it is conducive to creating a strong therapeutic alliance.

Relapse Prevention

Maintenance issues are addressed explicitly toward the end of therapy, but they also emerge throughout treatment. It is a rare client who does not experience a return of severe anxiety during the course of therapy, an event that is often viewed as a setback or is taken as evidence that he or she will never change. The therapist reminds the client that anxiety is a common and natural response, that novel events will always pull toward a reemergence of old habits, that the client already has evidence from prior weeks that what he or she is learning has been having an effect, and that he or she is always able to reengage his or her new coping strategies and develop his or her strength and effectiveness further. The hypothesis that he or she has lost all gains can be tested during the upcoming week.

Toward the end of therapy, images of future anxiety episodes and worries about relapse can be employed in SCD, and the therapist reminds the client that she now knows how to use SCD for any newly encountered situations. The therapist also uses reverse role plays and devil's advocate positions to reinforce independent use of generic cognitive strategies. Finally, one or two booster/fading sessions are held during the month after posttreatment assessment. Maintenance and relapse issues are once again covered, and clients are given an individually tailored handout that summarizes the specific steps of each intervention that was useful for them so that they can reinstitute at a future time any of the methods they have learned. The empirical literature regarding the durability of the effects of cognitive behavioral therapy with GAD is quite clear: immediate gains are routinely maintained and at times even further augmented by long-term follow-up (cf. Borkovec & Whisman, in press).

Case Illustration

Case Description

Susan, a 24-year-old unmarried woman, was in her last year of college, pursuing a degree in engineering. Excessive worry and anxiety had been a serious problem for the past $4\frac{1}{2}$ years and were accompanied by several distressing physical symptoms, particularly muscle tension and abdominal distress ("pit in my stomach"). She complained of constant difficulties coping with the stress of responsibilities at both school and work. Susan described experiencing intense worry regarding her perceived inability to cope in a variety of school-related situations that interfered with her performance (particularly by causing procrastination) such that she had had several failures, which in turn reinforced her lack of faith in her abilities. Her father had died 2 years previously, and this additional stressor had led to such difficulty completing her schoolwork that she withdrew from school after failing several classes. She was currently enrolled in school again but continued to experience constant worry and great difficulty in completing her work.

Differential Diagnosis and Assessment

Two independent assessors conducted the ADIS-R and agreed on a principal GAD diagnosis. Susan also received an additional diagnosis of social phobia, because many of her worries focused on social-evaluative concerns. GAD was considered principal because Susan worried about a broad range of topics, of which social situations were one subset. Excessive worry topics included getting her school work done, living up to her own sense of her potential, money, her job, procrastination, and many minor daily hassles. Assessment revealed a severity rating for GAD of 5.0 (between "definitely" and "markedly disturbing/disabling" on the 0- to 8-point assessor rating) and 4.0 for social phobia. Questionnaire scores included a HARS of 20.5, HDRS of 15, STAI of 57, BDI of 15, and PSWQ of 65.

Treatment Selection

Susan was a client in our current outcome study. Random assignment placed her in the group receiving cognitive-behavioral treatment, which included applied relaxation, SCD, and in-depth cognitive therapy. By protocol specification she received a total of 14 sessions prior to posttreatment assessment (four 2-hour and ten 90-minute sessions).

Treatment Course and Problems in Carrying Out Interventions

Session 1 was spent presenting our conceptualization of generalized anxiety and the rationale for the tripartite treatment package in the context of this conceptualization. The presentation was tied into what the therapist specifically knew about Susan's history and symptoms derived from the assessments. It was important for Susan to begin to see the way the spiral of anxiety worked in her daily functioning, with thoughts, images, affect, somatic sensations, and behaviors each contributing to her anxiety process over time. The therapist also emphasized specific, crucial habits that Susan had—for example, perceiving school assignments as representing a threat of failure, which led to images of professors confronting her about missed assignments, causing somatic sensations such as muscle tension and abdominal pain, which confirmed her initial perception of threat and interfered with her ability to concentrate on the task at hand.

The therapist described ways of changing these habits, emphasizing the importance of recognizing early cues in each system and targeting each system with a particular technique. The notions of flexibility and experimentation were stressed, with therapy providing many different alternative responses to change the overall habitual pattern of anxiety.

Within this framework of flexibly altering anxious patterns, the specific components of therapy were discussed. Susan and the therapist began identifying anxious automatic thoughts and styles and generating multiple alternative, less anxiety-provoking thoughts through logical analysis. Susan was also told that therapy would involve identifying somatic and imaginal cues and learning a variety of forms of relaxation to provide several coping responses to these cues. In addition, SCD was presented as a way to practice applying new cognitive and relaxation coping methods to identified cues in order to weaken previous anxious habits and strengthen newly developed habits of coping.

After being certain that Susan understood the rationale and answering her questions, the therapist introduced the first relaxation technique, diaphragmatic breathing. Susan noticed a difference in her anxiety level as soon as she tried the method.

At the end of session, Susan mentioned some of her anticipatory anxiety about therapy. She had been afraid she would have nothing to say or not be able to understand what the therapist was saying. She reported feeling better at this point, having made some conceptual connections and having recognized some anxiety cues already. This was explored as one example of how negative predictions are often unsubstantiated.

Session 2 included a review of the week, further training in thought identification, and presentation of progressive muscular relaxation. Susan indicated that she had noticed the whole cycle of anxiety for the first time during the previous week. In so doing, she recognized that her anticipatory fear was worse than the actual situation and began saying to herself, "This is not as bad as I think it's going to be," which she found calmed her down. In addition, she found that focusing on her breathing in stressful situations helped her think more clearly and stopped her habitual anxious spiral from increasing.

At the beginning of Session 3, a difficulty in complying with the homework was discussed. When Susan reported that she had not kept the daily diary, she stated that she knew that was "bad." Through imagery recall, Susan was able to identify that once she had missed one or two times of recording, every thought of the diary became associated with negative predictions that she would never be able to keep the diary well, and with negative thoughts about herself and her inability to get things done. This caused her to avoid any reminder of the diary and therefore to write entries less often, further strengthening negative associations to the diary. Describing this pattern in session led Susan to come up with some ways of changing it on her own. She decided (a) to make the diary more a part of her schedule so she would be less likely to forget about it initially, and (b) to remember that even if she did not complete her diary entries every day, she could still get many days completed instead of worsening the situation by giving up altogether. The therapist chose to address Susan's implicit fear of his disapproval in a later cognitive therapy session.

Later in the session, Susan and the therapist reviewed a printed list describing maladaptive thought styles and discussed the ones that seemed most relevant to her. She recognized her tendency toward catastrophizing, negative filtering, overgeneralization, dichotomous thinking, and thinking in terms of "shoulds." In response to the therapist's Socratic questioning regarding catastrophizing, Susan recognized a primary pattern to her anxiety: Her fear that things would go badly kept her from doing things, so that in the end things did go badly. This pattern occurred in several situations, such as completing the daily diary, getting schoolwork done, and meeting her professors when she was having problems in classes. She expressed excitement and relief at this realization:

Susan: I never really realized how it all tied in to that. I never really saw how I didn't get things started as a result of being so anxious of what the outcome would be.

Therapist: How does that make you feel?

Susan: I'm seeing where it's coming from. That if this is what's causing it, then now I can focus on how to change that, so that it won't be that way anymore. It makes me feel a lot better, more optimistic about getting through the semester. I'm feeling this way now, but if I start doing this other thing, I'm going to be able to deal with it better, start predicting the other way as opposed to the catastrophe thing.

Susan developed alternative thoughts to reflect this perspective shift and continued to explore this pattern during the next several sessions. Each session involved identifying maladaptive thoughts she had identified in situations during the week, treating these thoughts as hypotheses and developing alternative hypotheses to apply in similar situations during the next week. She responded to predictions that she would never get any work done by saying to herself, "I'll just do a little bit at a time." This change was made at several levels. She would use the alternative thoughts while planning work, making more realistic plans and realizing that if she did what she could she often did more than when she tried to do everything. Moreover, she would feel better while doing it. She also used this change in perspective moment-to-moment, taking many breaks while working on a particular project and thinking about how many pages she had read instead of how many remained.

These changes were enhanced by the continued relaxation training and its daily application, which were reducing Susan's general stress level. Susan experienced particular success with diaphragmatic breathing, which she began to find herself applying more automatically any time her anxiety level increased. Her ability to relax was leading her to think more clearly and therefore complete more work. This strengthened the validity of her alternative thought that she could get work done as opposed to the old predictions of never getting anything done. Self-control desensitization was used at the end of relaxation training on images of external and internal cues relevant to her anxious experience to further strengthen her relaxation applications.

During later sessions, Susan was periodically stopped and asked to rate her present anxiety level and then to let go of and relax away existing tension or anxiety in whatever way she chose. This encouraged early cue detection and provided multiple opportunities to rehearse applied relaxation. Susan used the metaphor of "letting go" of anxious thoughts and images in her applied relaxation, and in Session 5 described that this worked better for her than "pushing" thoughts away: ". . . Not so much worrying about putting this off and forgetting about it but just letting the anxiety go so that I can concentrate on something else. It's different. I'm not so worried then about how much more I'm going to have to do. I'm not worrying so much about that. It's actually easier to let it go than to push it aside."

As Susan found that her new strategies of letting go, practicing relaxation twice a day to strengthen the response, and generating alternative thoughts (particularly in response to her overgeneralized, catastrophic predictions of failure) were helping her to reduce her anxiety level and to get more work done, she began to choose more intensely anxiety-provoking images in SCD. In Session 7, for example, she used a scene of giving an upcoming class presentation, focusing on her fear that she would be unable to answer questions the teacher might ask. She coped with this anxiety in imagery by focusing on her breathing, letting go, and reminding herself that she knew a lot about the topic and could use her knowledge to come up with an answer as she had in previous presentations. She was also able, following decatastrophization of the fear, to generate alternative thoughts such as "Even if I fail this, I won't fail the class." At the beginning of Session 8, Susan was pleased to report that the presentation had gone very well and that she had not experienced the customary "pit" in her stomach.

By Session 9, Susan was coping well, generalizing her coping skills to a variety of situations. She found that in stressful situations she automatically looked for alternatives to her thoughts, focused on her breathing and letting go of anxiety, or both. She reported looking forward to the upcoming semester as an opportunity to try out her new way of being from the beginning of the term rather than from a position of being already behind, as she had been when she began therapy. Therapy at this point began to focus more on potential new situations. The anticipation of job interviews was approached at first using decatastrophization methods. As her fears at each level were identified, Susan quickly generated alternative perspectives (e.g., "I won't know an answer"—"I'll be able to come up with one or they'll learn what I don't know"; "I won't get the job"—"There are other jobs"; "I won't get any job"—"I'll go back to school"). Susan applied her new strategy of taking work a little at a time to the upcoming project of putting together her résumé.

During Session 10, attention was paid to issues of maintenance and relapse prevention, because Susan was continuing to feel relaxed, calm, and hopeful about the future. When asked what would happen if she felt anxious again in a situation, Susan said that she would still be able to use her new coping responses even if she exceeded her preferred level of anxiety. The therapist pointed out that given the strength and automatic nature of her new habits, it was unlikely old habits would reemerge even if the spirals started again. Susan enjoyed trying to imagine how she could work up her anxiety (e.g., in SCD) and realizing that coping statements and coping responses came to mind quickly and automatically.

Before Session 11 Susan missed several appointments. When she did arrive for the session, she was somewhat anxious and reported that she had found out that she might not be able to graduate, had to write a petition, and needed several professors to sign it. She felt anxious and jumpy when she first found out about this and felt the "pit" in her stomach again. However, that night she had actually sat down and started writing a draft of the petition, doing a little bit at a time. She was pleased to realize that although initially she had reacted in her old way, she had been able to cope later and reinstitute the new habits. The therapist reminded Susan that one can cope before, during, or after an anxious situation (or all three), another flexible aspect of this approach to anxiety.

As Susan continued to discuss the past several weeks, she recognized the cycle she had experienced before finding out about the graduation problem. She had been leaving some tasks until the last minute and was therefore choosing to miss her therapy sessions. She found herself thinking that she *should* have gone to therapy, that she wasn't working hard enough in therapy, and that now therapy wouldn't work. However, she also had responded to these thoughts by generating alternative perspectives, such as "I *could* have gone, but I made a choice to do my homework." She was pleased to notice later that not only did the products of therapy continue to work effectively even though she had missed sessions, but she actually demonstrated to herself her continued improvement in her coping quite well with the extremely unpredictable, anxiety-provoking situation of not graduating.

Susan was able in the session to identify the fears she had that her therapist would think less of her because of the missed sessions and to respond to this thought with the alternative perspective that what her therapist thought of her was less important than what she thought of herself and that she knew she was still working on coping with her anxiety even if her therapist might not think so. This internalized sense of herself was a very important shift in perspective for Susan, because much of her social-evaluative concern originated from her previous core belief that if people thought badly of her, they must be right.

The next three sessions were spent continuing maintenance and generalization training. Susan's feelings about leaving therapy were also discussed. She would miss the support of the therapeutic relationship, but she was feeling confident now in her ability to continue the progress she had made and knew it was time to fly on her own.

Outcome and Termination

At posttreatment assessment Susan no longer met diagnostic criteria for GAD and received a GAD symptom severity rating of 2.5 ("mild anxiety"). The severity rating of social phobia was 1.5 (less than "mild"). Her other scores included 5.5 on the HARS, 3.5 on the HDRS, 36 on the STAI, 3 on the BDI, and 46 on the PSWQ. All of these scores were within nonanxious norms and indicated high end-state functioning.

Following the assessment Susan had one more session to finalize termination and maintenance issues. Susan was feeling very pleased with the changes she had made and optimistic about her future. Although she still did not know whether she would graduate, she felt comfortable with that uncertainty and confident that she would be all right either way.

Follow-Up and Maintenance

Susan let our staff know several months later that she had in fact graduated and was doing well. At her 6-month follow-up, her GAD severity rating had further decreased, to 2.0. The severity rating of social phobia was 1.5. She had a HARS rating of 2.0, a HDRS rating of 3.0, a STAI score of 34, a BDI score of 3, and a PSWQ score of 45.

Summary

Our understanding of the nature of generalized anxiety has increased greatly over the past few years. GAD clients are characterized by a rigid perception of the world as a threatening place, leading to habitual responses of verbal-linguistic worry which avoids imaginal activity, suppresses somatic experience, and results in autonomic rigidity. In this context, cognitive-behavioral treatment characterized by flexibility and the targeting of cognitive, imaginal, somatic, and behavioral systems with multiple relaxation and cognitive coping strategies is quite effective in providing anxiety and worry relief that is maintained at long-term follow-up. However, because many clients continue to experience residual anxiety after treatment, it is clear that further progress remains to be made.

ACKNOWLEDGMENT. Preparation of this chapter was supported in part by Grant MH-39172 from the National Institute of Mental Health to the senior author.

References

American Psychiatric Association (1987). *Diagnostic and statistical manual of mental disorders.* Washington, DC: Author.

American Psychiatric Association (1993). *DSM-IV draft criteria.* Washington, DC: Author.

Barlow, D. H. (1988). *Anxiety and its disorders.* New York: Guilford.

Beck, A. T., & Emery, G. (1985). *Anxiety disorders and phobias: A cognitive perspective.* New York: Basic Books.

Beck, A. T., Rush, A. J., Shaw, B. F., & Emery, G. (1978). *Cognitive therapy of depression.* New York: Guilford.

Bernstein, D. A., & Borkovec, T. D. (1973). *Progressive relaxation training.* Champaign, Il: Research Press.

Blazer, D., Hughes, D., & George, L. K. (1987). Stressful life events and the onset of a generalized anxiety syndrome. *American Journal of Psychiatry, 144,* 1178–1183.

Blazer, D. G., Hughes, D., George, L. K., Swartz, M., & Boyer, R. (1991). Generalized anxiety disorder. In L. N. Robins & D. A. Regier (Eds.), *Psychiatric disorders in America: The Epidemiological Catchment Area Study* (pp. 180–203). New York: Free Press.

Blowers, C., Cobb, J., & Mathews, A. (1987). Generalized anxiety: A controlled treatment study. *Behaviour Research and Therapy, 25,* 493–502.

Borkovec, T. D. (1992, December). *Psychological processes in generalized anxiety disorder.* Paper presented at the annual meeting of the American College of Neuropsychopharmacology, San Juan, Puerto Rico.

Borkovec, T. D., & Costello, E. (1993). Efficacy of applied relaxation and cognitive behavioral therapy in the treatment of generalized anxiety disorder. *Journal of Consulting and Clinical Psychology, 61,* 611–619.

Borkovec, T. D., & Hu, S. (1990). The effect of worry on cardiovascular response to phobic imagery. *Behaviour Research and Therapy, 28,* 69–73.

Borkovec, T. D., & Inz, J. (1990). The nature of worry in generalized anxiety disorder: A predominance of thought activity. *Behaviour Research and Therapy, 28,* 153–158.

Borkovec, T. D., Lyonfields, J. D., Wiser, S., & Deihl, L. (1993). The role of worrisome thinking in the suppression of cardiovascular response to phobic imagery. *Behaviour Research and Therapy, 31,* 321–324.

Borkovec, T. D., Shadick, R. N., & Hopkins, M. (1991). The nature of normal versus pathological worry. In R. Rapee & D. H. Barlow (Eds.), *Chronic anxiety and generalized anxiety disorder,* (pp. 29–51). New York: Guilford.

Borkovec, T. D., & Whisman, M. A. (in press). Psychosocial treatment for generalized anxiety disorder. In M. Mavissakalian & R. F. Prien (Eds.), *Anxiety disorders: Psychosocial and pharmacological treatments.* Washington, DC: American Psychiatric Association.

Bowlby, J. (1973). *Separation: Anxiety and anger.* New York: Basic Books.

Breslau, N., & Davis, G. C. (1985). DSM-III generalised anxiety disorder: An empirical investigation of more stringent criteria. *Psychiatry Research, 14,* 231–238.

Brown, T. A., Antony, M. M., & Barlow, D. H. (1992). Psychometric properties of the Penn State Worry Questionnaire in a clinical anxiety disorders sample. *Behaviour Research and Therapy, 30,* 33–37.

Brown, T. A., & Barlow, D. H. (1992). Comorbidity among anxiety disorders: Implications for treatment and DSM-IV. *Journal of Consulting and Clinical Psychology, 60,* 835–844.

Brown, T. A., Moras, K., Zinbarg, R. E., & Barlow, D. H. (1993). Diagnostic and symptom distinguishability of generalized anxiety disorder and obsessive-compulsive disorder. *Behavior Therapy, 24,* 227–241.

Butler, G., & Mathews, A. (1983). Anticipatory anxiety and risk perception. *Cognitive Therapy and Research, 11,* 551–565.

Cassidy, J. (1992). *Generalized anxiety disorder and attachment: Emotion and cognition.* Paper presented at the Rochester Symposium on Developmental Psychopathology, Rochester, NY.

Chambless, D. L., & Gillis, M. M. (1993). Cognitive therapy of anxiety disorders. *Journal of Consulting and Clinical Psychology, 61,* 248–260.

DiNardo, P. A., & Barlow, D. H. (1988). *Anxiety Disorders Interview Schedule—Revised (ADIS-R).* Albany, NY: Phobia and Anxiety Disorders Clinic, State University of New York.

Endicott, J., & Spitzer, R. L. (1978). A diagnostic interview: The schedule for affective disorders and schizophrenia. *Archives of General Psychiatry, 35,* 837–844.

Foa, E. B., & Kozak, M. J. (1986). Emotional processing of fear: Exposure to corrective information. *Psychological Bulletin, 99,* 20–35.

Goldfried, M. R. (1971). Systematic desensitization as training in self-control. *Journal of Consulting and Clinical Psychology, 37,* 228–234.

Greenberg, L. S., & Safran, J. D. (1987). *Emotion in psychotherapy.* New York: Guilford.

Hamilton, M. (1959). The assessment of anxiety states by rating. *British Journal of Medical Psychology, 32,* 50–55.

Hamilton, M. (1960). A rating scale for depression. *Journal of Neurology, Neurosurgery and Psychiatry, 23,* 56–62.

Hoehn-Saric, R., & McLeod, O. R. (1988). The peripheral sympathetic nervous system: Its role in normal and pathologic anxiety. *Psychiatric Clinics of North America, 11,* 375–386.

Mathews, A. (1990). Why worry? The cognitive function of anxiety. *Behaviour Research and Therapy, 28,* 455–468.

Meichenbaum, D. H., & Turk, D. (1973). *Stress inoculation: A skills training approach to anxiety management.* Unpublished manuscript, University of Waterloo, Ontario, Canada.

Meyer, T. J., Miller, M. L., Metzger, R. L., & Borkovec, T. D. (1990). Development and validation of the Penn State Worry Questionnaire. *Behaviour Research and Therapy, 28,* 487–496.

Montalvo, A., Metzger, R. L., & Noll, J. A. (1989, November). *The network structure of worry in memory.* Paper presented at the North Carolina Cognition Group, Davidson, NC.

Noyes, R. (in press). Natural course of anxiety disorders. In M. R. Mavissakalian & R. F. Prien (Eds.), *Anxiety disorders: Psychological and pharmacological treatments.* Washington, DC: American Psychiatric Association.

Noyes, R., Woodman, C., Garvey, M. J., Cook, B. L., Suelzer, M., Clancy, J., & Anderson, D. J. (1992). Generalized anxiety disorder vs. panic disorder: Distinguishing characteristics and patterns of comorbidity. *Journal of Nervous and Mental Disease, 180,* 369–379.

Ost, L. (1987). Applied relaxation: Description of a coping technique and review of controlled studies. *Behaviour Research and Therapy, 25,* 397–409.

Rapee, R. (1985). Distinctions between panic disorder and generalized anxiety disorder: Clinical presentation. *Australian and New Zealand Journal of Psychiatry, 19,* 227–232.

Rapee, R. M. (1991). Generalized anxiety disorder: A review of clinical features and theoretical concepts. *Clinical Psychology Review, 11,* 419–440.

Rickels, K., Case, W. G., & Diamond, L. (1980). Relapse after short-term drug therapy in neurotic outpatients. *International Pharmacopsychiatry, 15,* 186–192.

Rickels, K., Case, W. G., Downing, R. W., & Fridman, R. (1986). One-year follow-up of anxious patients treated with diazepam. *Journal of Clinical Psychopharmacology, 6,* 32–36.

Roemer, L., & Borkovec, T. D. (in press). The effects of suppressing thoughts about emotional material. *Journal of Abnormal Psychology.*

Roemer, L., Borkovec, M., Posa, S., & Lyonfields, J. D. (1991, November). *Generalized anxiety disorder in an analogue population: The role of past trauma.* Paper presented at the annual convention of the Association for Advancement of Behavior Therapy, New York.

Sanderson, W. C., & Wetzler, S. (1991). Chronic anxiety and generalized anxiety disorder: Issues in comorbidity. In R. Rapee & D. H. Barlow (Eds.), *Chronic anxiety and generalized anxiety disorder.* New York: Guilford.

Schweizer, E., & Rickels, K. (in press). Generalized anxiety disorder: Pharmacological treatment. In M. Mavissakalian & R. F. Prien (Eds.), *Anxiety disorders: Psychological and pharmacological treatments.* Washington, DC: American Psychiatric Association.

Shadick, R. N., Roemer, L., Hopkins, M., & Borkovec, T. D. (1991, November). *The nature of worrisome thoughts*. Paper presented at the annual convention of the Association for Advancement of Behavior Therapy, New York.

Spielberger, C. D., Gorsuch, R. L., Lushene, R., Vagg, P. R., & Jacobs, G. A. (1983). *Manual for the State-Trait Anxiety Inventory (Form Y)*. Palo Alto, CA: Consulting Psychologists Press.

Spitzer, R. L., Williams, J. B. W., Gibbon, M., & First, M. B. (1990). *Structured Clinical Interview for DSM-III-R–Patient Edition (SCID-P, Version 1.0)*. Washington DC: American Psychiatric Press.

Suinn, R. M., & Richardson, R. (1971). Anxiety management training: A nonspecific behavior therapy program for anxiety control. *Behavior Therapy, 2*, 498–510.

Tollefson, G. D., Luxenberg, M., Valentine, R., Dunsmore, G., & Tollefson, S. L. (1991). An open label trial of alprazolam in comorbid irritable bowel syndrome and generalized anxiety disorder. *Journal of Clinical Psychiatry, 52*, 502–508.

Torgerson, S. (1983). Genetic factors in anxiety disorders. *Archives of General Psychiatry, 40*, 1085–1089.

Torgerson, S. (1986). Childhood and family characteristics in panic and generalized anxiety disorders. *American Journal of Psychiatry, 143*, 630–632.

Vrana, S. R., Cuthbert, B. N., & Lang, P. J. (1986). Fear imagery and text processing. *Psychophysiology, 23*, 247–253.

Wegner, D. M., Schneider, D. J., Carter, S. R., & White, T. L. (1987). Paradoxical effects of thought suppression. *Journal of Personality and Social Psychology, 53*, 5–13.

Weissman, A. N., & Beck, A. T. (1978, November). *Development and validation of the dysfunctional attitudes scale: A preliminary investigation*. Paper presented at the annual meeting of the American Education Association, Toronto.

14

Somatization Disorder

Pamela E. Parker and Charles V. Ford

Description of the Disorder

Clinical Features

The concept of somatization disorder (SD) has evolved from hysteria and Briquet's syndrome and is the current term applied to a specific type of illness behavior (Ford, 1983). By definition, patients with this disorder have multiple bodily complaints that cannot be explained physiologically. These complaints have origins from a variety of body systems, such as cardiac, renal, pulmonary, and genitourinary. The disorder must have been present for years and is diagnosed retrospectively with symptoms beginning before the age of 30.

Patients with SD seek care from a large number of physicians ("doctor shopping"), often concurrently, and are frequently referred to medical specialists. They characteristically provide ambiguous, vague, or nonphysiologic medical histories. They receive multiple medications and are subject to surgical and invasive diagnostic procedures, even when indications are marginal or nonexistent. It is not unusual for the patient to report a history of numerous surgical operations, often of the pelvic organs (DeVaul & Faillace, 1980). Multiple hospitalizations are the rule, and the patient frequently "carries" one diagnosis or more of chronic systemic disease (e.g., systemic lupus erythematosus) despite few or no confirmatory laboratory findings. Because of doctors' energetic propensity to seek relief of discomfort, patients with SD are commonly prescribed addicting medications, including benzodiazepines, narcotics, and barbiturates (now less stylish).

Pamela E. Parker • Department of Psychiatry, College of Community Health Sciences, University of Alabama, Tuscaloosa, Alabama 35487-0326.   **Charles V. Ford** • Department of Psychiatry and Behavioral Neurobiology, School of Medicine, University of Alabama at Birmingham, Birmingham, Alabama 35294-0018.

Handbook of Prescriptive Treatments for Adults, edited by Michel Hersen and Robert T. Ammerman. Plenum Press, New York, 1994.

Somatization disorder usually has a predictable course. In the patient's early adulthood, when symptoms are beginning, the patient's physicians make a concerted effort to identify physiologic pathology, leading to multiple medical tests, many of which may be invasive. The patient becomes increasingly involved in medical care, with intermittent surgical interventions or procedures expected to relieve symptoms. Symptoms recur, leading to a resumption of investigative attempts. To a varying degree, the patient's physicians develop suspicions of SD, which may be already obscured by iatrogenic pathology. A psychiatrist is usually consulted when the patient's physician feels he or she has exhausted the physiologic possibilities. This may occur in early adulthood if the patient has had a large number of procedures, but is more likely in middle age. If the patient's course has been more insidious, a psychiatric evaluation may never be sought.

Associated Features

In addition to multiple unexplained physical symptoms, the SD patient usually has a history of psychiatric symptoms. Anxiety, depression, drug abuse, suicidal gestures, and brief psychiatric hospitalizations are commonly reported (or discovered in the patient's thick medical record). Furthermore, there is almost always evidence of social dysfunction. Employment and educational histories are poor, there may be suggestions of a criminal record, marital discord is common (an alcoholic spouse is frequently found), and there may be difficulties with children, landlords, and creditors.

Somatization disorder is usually comorbid with one or more other DSM-III-R Axis I disorders. Liskow, Pennick, DeSouza, and Gabrielli (1986) studied 78 patients with SD and found that only 1 patient did not meet diagnostic criteria for one or more additional psychiatric disorders. Among the most frequently found were panic disorder, 45%; obsessive-compulsive disorder, 27%; drug dependence, 27%; and alcohol abuse, 17%. Smith (1991) reported that 92% of the patients in his study had a lifetime history of major depression and an additional 9% had dysthymia. Further, 66% had a diagnosable anxiety disorder and 23% showed alcohol abuse, dependence, or both.

Personality disorders are frequently comorbid with SD. Rost, Akins, Brown, and Smith (1992), using a structured clinical interview to diagnose personality disorders, found that 23.4% of a group of patients with SD had one personality diagnosis and 37.2% had two or more personality diagnoses. The most common personality disorders, in decreasing frequency, were avoidant, paranoid, self-defeating, obsessive-compulsive, schizotypal, histrionic, and borderline.

Some medical disorders are associated with a higher-than-average incidence of somatization. These include irritable bowel syndrome (Liss, Alpers, & Woodruff, 1973; Young, Alpers, Norland, & Woodruff, 1976), polycystic ovary disease (Orenstein, Raskind, Wyllie, Raskind, & Soules, 1986), and patients undergoing non-cancer-related hysterectomy (Martin, Roberts, & Clayton, 1980).

In severe cases of SD, patients may receive so many invasive procedures that they develop iatrogenic physiologic pathology far greater than the original illness.

Epidemiology

Prevalence of SD has been studied in a variety of settings. For example, prevalence in the general population as determined by the Epidemiologic Catchment Areas (ECA) studies ranged from 0 to 0.7% at six different sites and averaged about 0.1% (Escobar, Swartz, Rubio-Stipec, & Mann, 1991). These figures were considerably lower than those originally reported by Farley, Woodruff, and Guze (1968). However, Escobar and colleagues (1991) defined a subsyndromal form of the disorder (four unexplained symptoms for males and six for females) that was 50 to 100 times more prevalent than the full-blown syndrome. These persons had characteristics similar to those in patients with the full disorder but less extreme, suggesting that somatization is a dimensional disorder with SD being the most extreme form. Increased prevalence rates for subsyndromal SD were associated with increasing age, female gender, and less education.

DeGruy, Columbia, and Dickinson (1987) found that up to 5% of patients seen in an academic family practice setting had SD and another 4% were borderline for the disorder. A significant proportion of these patients included lower-socioeconomic-status unmarried women with children.

Etiology

The causes of SD have long been debated. Until recently, psychosocial factors have been implicated—patients often had been raised in families where marital disruption, somatization, and substance, physical, and sexual abuse were common. The same families that produced females with SD produced males with antisocial personality disorder, thereby suggesting a link between the two diagnoses (Guze, Woodruff, & Clayton, 1971).

However, recent studies have challenged the psychological theories. Auditory evoked potentials in SD patients (Gordon, Kraiuhin, Meares, & Howson, 1986) indicate an abnormality in cortical functioning. James and colleagues (James, Gordon, Kraiuhin, & Meares, 1989; James et al., 1987) demonstrated an abnormality of attention in SD patients. Electroencephalographic abnormalities in the right frontal region have been discovered by Drake, Padamadan, and Pakainis (1988). Similarly, Gorman, Liebowitz, Fyer, and Stein (1989) have proposed a "neuroanatomical hypothesis" for somatized anxiety that bears a close resemblance to the strict criteria for SD.

Genetic studies by Torgersen (1986) reflect a surprisingly low concordance rate of 29% in monozygotic twins and 10% in dizygotic twins. However, there seems to be a pairing of somatization disorder with anxiety disorders, depression, or both: one monozygotic twin may have SD and the other anxiety or depression.

All etiological explanations of SD must take into account that symptoms are precipitated by psychosocial stressors, and these may be not only a reaction to stress but also a coping mechanism. Katon et al. (in press) point out that many of the factors associated with somatization—including anhedonia, social withdrawal, and despair—may be mutually reinforcing, making it difficult to distinguish the cause from the effect. It is probable that SD represents a final common symptom pathway for a number of different etiologic factors (Ford, 1992).

Differential Diagnosis and Assessment

DSM-III-R and DSM-IV Categorization

Somatization disorder is classified in DSM-III-R as one of the somatoform disorders (American Psychiatric Association, 1987). Diagnostic criteria for SD require 13 unexplained physical symptoms (from a list of 37), the first of which must have begun before the age of 30.

According to Yutzy, Pribor, Cloninger, and Guze (1992), DSM-IV will address a number of cumbersome aspects of the DSM-III-R criteria for SD. Reanalysis of data from Cloninger and colleagues' (1986) studies suggests that the criteria can be significantly reduced while continuing to identify patients who meet the original Feighner criteria for Briquet's syndrome.

Katon et al. (1991) have also called for changes in DSM-IV, noting that somatization as a symptom complex secondary to other psychiatric disorders has been overlooked in the diagnostic approaches.

Differential Diagnosis

The most obvious differential diagnosis in the evaluation of SD is physical treatable disease. Unfortunately, many so-called organic illnesses lack clear biological markers, a dilemma often ascribed only to psychiatric disease. Examples include systemic lupus erythematosus, rheumatoid arthritis, fibromyalgia, and migraine headaches.

Although we attempt diagnostically to distinguish the somatizing disorders from one another, in actuality it is not so simple to do so (Nadelson, 1985; Ford, 1992). Malingering and factitious disorders must be ruled out. Somatoform pain disorder can usually be identified by its nonmigratory presentation. Classically, chronic pain recurs in the same location over many years, with back pain, headache, pelvic pain, and abdominal pain being among the more common sites. The discomforts of SD more characteristically occur in changing locations in the body, sometimes changing even within a single episode. Conversion disorder, by definition, involves a loss of function often unassociated with pain.

For nonpsychiatrists, the distinction between somatization disorder and hypochondriasis has been the most vague, resulting from the common presentation of physical complaints. A closer look, however, shows the two to be quite different, and the distinction affects management. For the hypochondriacal patient, fear of an illness, usually a specific illness, is more prominent than physical discomforts. Associated obsessive features of hypochondriasis are also quite different and do not reflect the more dramatic aspects (e.g., acting out) often found in SD.

The differential diagnosis of SD must include possibilities of depression, panic disorder, and psychosis, which are thought to be etiological in many cases. Some believe that somatization is a symptom complex caused by underlying panic disorder (Sheehan & Sheehan, 1982) or depression (Orenstein, 1989). Psychotic disorders such as schizophrenia and organic psychosis must also be recognized and treated.

Assessment Strategies

The systems review required to investigate all possible complaints may necessitate a lengthy interview (45 to 60 minutes), and therefore several screening tests have been developed. If the DSM-III-R screening index (at least two symptoms from a list of seven) is used, then a patient with a positive screen has a 69% chance of having the disorder. Similarly, a patient with a negative screen has an 81% chance of *not* having SD (Smith & Brown, 1990).

Assessment of SD occurs simultaneously along two tracks, looking carefully at past history while addressing the current complaints. The disorder must be diagnosed in retrospect; therefore, a detailed medical history from the patient (and relatives or friends) is imperative. The patient's description of another physician's evaluation may be skewed, and it is most helpful to review previous records whenever possible. The threads of the biopsychosocial tangle must be teased out. In these cases, an accurate assessment often depends on history available from a family member or friend who knew the patient in early adulthood and can clarify the course of illness and illness behavior before it became complicated, often with iatrogenic disease. Assessment of the patient's psychological sophistication will have an impact on management.

The psychiatrist may be asked to evaluate the patient at the point at which the primary physician starts to question the need for invasive procedures. The psychiatrist must be prepared to discuss with the primary physician not only the psychiatric findings, but also their role in medical illness.

Because the diagnostic/therapeutic relationship begins as soon as the doctor and patient have contact with each other, the physician must be ever alert to the style of the interaction, even in history gathering. The SD patient often provides a history of dramatic illness with the use of colorful terms (e.g., "The pain is like liquid fire poured into my belly").

The treatment of any existing depression, panic, alcoholism or other substance abuse, or psychosis may clarify the diagnosis, either by resolving the symptomatic presentation or by allowing the remaining symptoms to emerge.

Treatment

Evidence for Prescriptive Treatments

Treatment approaches for this widely heterogeneous disorder must necessarily be fitted to the needs of the specific patient. The SD patient is seen most frequently in a primary care setting and resists referral to mental health settings. Thus, the best care of the patient occurs in the hands of the primary physician. The therapeutic strategy includes: (a) respect for general management guidelines by the patient's medical/surgical physicians; (b) specific interventions, often pharmacologic, for comorbid psychiatric disorders; (c) behavior therapy techniques, employed primarily by the patient's primary care physicians, aimed at helping the patient recognize the origins of the somatic distress (reattribution) and at reducing the factors that reinforce somatization; and (d) when available, the provision of group experiences that reduce the patient's need for somatization. An individual patient may require one or more of these interventions. Each will be discussed separately.

Smith, Monson, and Ray (1986) demonstrated that a single letter detailing a few basic management principles reduces by half the medical care utilization of SD patients. Presumably, such decreased medical utilization leads to decreased morbidity, although this remains to be systematically demonstrated. The principles are: (a) establishment of a relationship with one primary physician; (b) avoidance of comments or implication to the patient that "It's all in your head"; (c) avoidance of invasive diagnostic/therapeutic procedures except in the face of objective findings; (d) frequently scheduled office visits that are not contingent on the development of new symptoms; and (e) at least a partial physical examination, investigating each new complaint, at every office visit. These principles serve to provide a nonadversarial, cooperative doctor–patient relationship that helps reduce need for somatic symptoms as a means of communication, as well as reducing the likelihood of iatrogenic morbidity. Hospitalization should be diligently avoided, with the possible exception of some medical–psychiatric units prepared to handle somatization problems (Abbey & Lipowski, 1987; Stoudemire, Brown, McCleod, Stewart, & Houpt, 1983).

As with many physical complaints that have a significant psychological component, SD treatment actually begins in the assessment phase. A brusque, uninterested interview style that does not allow patients to verbalize complaints may annoy them, exacerbating the drive to find physicians who will diagnose a disorder requiring further procedures and medications. It puts the patient in the defensive stance and encourages more "doctor shopping." Allowing the patient to ventilate physical complaints is essential to establishing rapport. Great care must be taken to avoid any insinuation that the complaint is "all in your head" or that "nothing is wrong." The primary physician must be alert to the emergence and proper evaluation of new symptoms, because the diagnosis of SD does not rule out the presence of physiologic illness.

Behavior Therapy. Data from controlled studies that demonstrate the therapeutic effectiveness of behavior therapy techniques for SD are not available. However, proposals for use of these therapeutic interventions seem so eminently reasonable that they are recommended as a component of the overall treatment plan.

Morrison (1978, 1990) suggests several techniques, incorporating behavior therapy principles, that propose to reduce somatizing behavior. These include:

1. Reduction of reinforcement for symptoms. This includes involving the family in the treatment plan so that they will not repetitively respond to the patient's symptoms by actions such as rushing her to the emergency room. The family should be advised that the patient is particularly sensitive to discomforts, and although the patient may be uncomfortable, she must have support in coping. As in dealing with the patient, the family should never be told that the complaints are "all in her head."
2. Teaching the patient to deal with symptoms by nonmedical therapies that puts him in control of the symptoms and their treatment—for example, use of heating pads or cold compresses for headaches or muscle pain.
3. Changing the focus from somatic concerns to real-life psychosocial problems—for example, encouraging participation in an Al-Anon group to learn how to deal with an alcoholic spouse.
4. Emphasis on behaviors that allow for a more open expression or more appropriate sublimation of emotional distress—for example, the patient may be encouraged to recognize anger and then to go running rather than engage in a self-destructive somatic behavior.
5. Physician's use of praise to reinforce more healthy nonsomatizing behaviors.

Goldberg, Gask, and O'Dowd (1989) have suggested a three-stage approach for interviews with patients who somatize. From a practical standpoint, however, these three stages will need to be implemented progressively over numerous visits by the SD patient to the primary care physician. The first stage is to establish rapport and to make sure that the patient feels understood. This is accomplished by taking a full history of the symptoms and those factors that may exacerbate them, exploring health beliefs, obtaining a psychosocial history, and performing a focused physical examination. Stage two is devoted to "changing the agenda," and is accomplished by providing feedback of results of the physical examination, acknowledging the reality of the patient's pain, and reframing the patient's complaint in terms of her other symptoms and the link to life events. The third and final stage is to make the link between the patient's emotions and symptoms. This is accomplished by explanations of the physiologic aspects of anxiety and depression (e.g., muscle tension and fatigue), practical demonstrations (e.g., production of muscle pain by the fatigue of holding a book with an outstretched arm), and relating the patient's symptoms to life events and the here-and-now situations. A further technique is that of projection, which involves getting the patient to describe the relationship of a family member's symptoms (e.g., "sick headaches") to life situations. Patients can often recognize in others that which they cannot see in themselves. Through these various techniques, employed in a stepwise manner, the somatizing patient is taught how to reattribute bodily symptoms as manifestations of psychosocial stress rather than as physical disease. This opens the door for more effective psychotherapeutic interventions.

Specific Interventions for Comorbid Psychiatric Disorders. As noted earlier, SD is almost always associated with one or more psychiatric comorbid diagnoses. Whether these are Axis I or Axis II (personality) disorders, they must be identified, and treatment (management) of them coordinated into the treatment plan. An exhaustive review of these possibilities is beyond the scope of this chapter. However, several comorbid conditions are very common and deserve comment.

Major depression (either current or in the history) is a factor in at least 50% of SD cases (Smith, 1992). The primary treatment is pharmacologic, although cognitive-behavioral therapy and interpersonal therapy may also play a therapeutic role. Because many SD patients have a propensity for acting out (e.g., suicidal gestures), caution should be used in the prescription of these medications. Tricyclic antidepressants have a relatively low therapeutic/lethal dose ratio, and, when indicated, should be prescribed in small quantities. They are particularly useful for concurrent irritable bowel syndrome (Steinhart, Wong, & Zarr, 1981). The more recently released specific serotonin reuptake inhibitors (SSRIs) are usually well tolerated and provide less risk of a fatal overdose. With successful treatment of an underlying depression, the patient's physical complaints and medical utilization may be significantly reduced.

Panic disorder is also a frequent comorbid diagnosis in the SD patient, and successful control of panic attacks may, as with treatment of depression, significantly reduce physical complaints and comorbid phobias (Noyes, Reich, Clancy, & O'Gorman, 1986). Panic disorder can be effectively treated with tricyclic antidepressants, SSRIs, and several of the benzodiazepines. Caution must be employed in the prescription of the last because many SD patients have a personal or family history of substance abuse and thus are at increased risk for benzodiazepine habituation (Morrison, 1990). When they are indicated, prescriptions for the benzodiazepines must be closely monitored.

Alcoholism or other forms of substance abuse or dependence are frequently comorbid with SD. Further, the spouse or other family members may be alcoholic. Treatment of any other psychiatric disorder is difficult, if not impossible, in the face of ongoing chemical dependency. Hospitalization for detoxification, referral to a drug rehabilitation program, active involvement with Alcoholics Anonymous and associated groups for family members (e.g., Al-Anon), or some combination of these may be an essential component of an overall treatment plan.

Personality disorders, particularly borderline personality disorder, are frequently comorbid with SD. Management principles must include consideration of behaviors associated with severe personality disturbance, such as suicidal gestures, drug dependency, poor or abusive child care, manipulations, self-mutilative behaviors including factitious disease, lying, and alternating idealization and devaluation of the treatment team. Open and frequent communication among the various members of the patient's health care treatment team, including *all* physicians, is necessary to avoid splitting behaviors and fragmentation of treatment goals. The patient, for example, may be seeking habituating medications from several physicians simultaneously or withholding or distorting information in an effort to seek further diagnostic tests or surgical operations (Ford, 1983).

In brief, the treatment of somatization disorder generally involves treatment of one or more concurrent psychiatric disorders. This may create some therapeutic dilemmas, in that all medications, including psychotropic agents, should be used sparingly with these patients. The prescription of *any* medication reinforces the patient's somatic interpretations of his psychosocial stressors.

Group Therapy. Use of groups for somatizing patients has been described by a number of clinicians (Ford, 1984). Outcomes of such a relatively simple and inexpensive intervention have been favorable and markedly cost effective because of savings created by the patients' decreased medical utilization. Two types of groups have been described, a specific focused group and general supportive self-help groups.

Valko (1976) described a focused weekly group for patients with hysteria (somatization disorder) that emphasized education about the disorder and mutual support, similar to that provided in small meetings of Alcoholics Anonymous. Patients learned to relate their symptoms to stress and over a relatively short period markedly reduced their utilization of psychiatric and medical facilities. Symptoms did tend to recur with cessation of the group, but improvement could be sustained if return group visits were scheduled monthly.

Most of the group therapies described for somatizing patients have been less focused and have had the relatively simple goal of providing social support. Although fundamental changes in patients' coping styles are minimal, the support provided, which often extends outside the therapy hours, decreases the patients' need to turn to medical care as an alternate social support system. Consequently, these patients, when attending group sessions, tend to significantly reduce their use of medical facilities (Ford, 1984).

Alternative Treatments. As the history is reviewed, any unusual features should be noted. Occasionally a patient will present with adequate psychological insight to be a candidate for psychotherapy. However, unless the patient volunteers the possibility that psychological factors are playing a role, the suggestion of psychotherapy is likely to be counterproductive.

For severe somatizers, hospitalization on a medical–psychiatric unit that emphasizes a variety of intensive group therapy may prove efficacious in breaking through the patient's resistances and use of somatization (Abbey & Lipowski, 1987).

Problems in Carrying Out Interventions

Perhaps the greatest challenge in the management of SD is the eternal scrutiny involved in avoiding medical tests while remaining alert to medical disease. Attentive care often saps the energy of the physician, and even physicians with remarkable patience find themselves losing their temper or giving in to the patient's demands for more diagnostic procedures. Close follow-up of the patient should lessen the physician's need for scrutiny and ease the challenge.

The American medical system (or lack thereof) may be the single most confounding factor. In a system in which people highly value their privacy and freedom, it is very difficult to limit the doctor shopping and the resultant "polypharmacy" of the somatizer. Some family practice physicians have been able to limit doctor shopping by establishing good rapport with the patient and then explaining that it is countertherapeutic for the patient to receive medications from other physicians while under his or her care. Some physicians explain to the patient that they can no longer care for the patient if all referrals are not made through him or her.

Even if the physician is able to carry through with a program of conducting frequent outpatient visits, establishing good rapport, and limiting use of multiple physicians, he or she may find some difficulty in billing and reimbursement; procedure codes and reimbursement schedules are not designed for the somatizer. Therefore, the physician may have difficulty qualifying his or her treatment plan with insurance companies, even though these measures will drastically reduce costs.

Case Illustration

Case Description

A 54-year-old man was referred by his primary care physician to a psychiatrist for evaluation of depression. The patient, a blue-collar worker at a local factory, had completed high school in a rural community and with his wife reared two children. Two older brothers were known to be alcoholic. The patient's wife noted that even his mother had commented on his being a "chronic complainer," and that he had multiple unexplained physical symptoms that began in adolescence.

The patient had suffered a stroke one year previously, which initially left him with mild motor impairment in his left arm. His workplace had then granted him early retirement. His impairment had slowly resolved, but he continued to have multiple somatic complaints, fatigue, negativism, anhedonia, and occasional emotional outbursts. Physical complaints included left arm pain, intermittent nausea, shortness of breath, headache, painful joints, difficulty urinating (nonspecific), fullness in his throat, back pain, occasional right-sided weakness, and coughing spells.

He was prescribed a low dosage of amitriptyline, but 3 days later he called to say that dry mouth, sedation, and constipation were overwhelming. He refused to continue the medication at any dosage and was lost to follow-up.

Several months later, the patient's wife again sought psychiatric care for him because of his psychomotor retardation and expressions of death wishes. The patient was evaluated and placed on a regimen of nortriptyline, 10 mg at bedtime. One week later the dosage was increased to 25 mg at bedtime, with clear resolution of psychomotor retardation and improvement of mood. His wife noted that his multiple bodily complaints had markedly decreased. After one month of treatment with nortriptyline, 50 mg at bedtime, the patient's left-sided weakness had lessened, sleep patterns had returned to normal, multiple joint pain had resolved, anhedonia and chronic fatigue were resolving, and he was generally in better spirits. He continued to complain of shortness of breath, headache, and left arm tingling, paresthesia, and mild weakness.

The patient's wife noted that although he had been prone to physical complaints, she had usually been able to encourage him to work. Discussion with the patient's family physician revealed that he was indeed a frequent utilizer of the medical system, and his wife had indeed played a major role in decreasing and deflecting illness behavior.

The patient was seen monthly for 30-minute visits. Somatic complaints continued, but he functioned at a higher level. He was reassured about his shortness of breath and chest pain. After one year the patient's wife requested extended time between visits, because she had to drive the patient 90 minutes to the appointments. The appointments were then spaced 2 months apart. But before the initial 2 months had elapsed, the patient's wife called, saying that her husband had complained for 48 hours of intense back pain, which had been evaluated by the internist with multiple scans and chemistry workups—all without any determination of cause. He had been sent home with acetaminophen as the only pharmacologic intervention and was seen again by the psychiatrist, who increased the nortriptyline dosage to 75 mg daily. Visits were rescheduled at 1 month intervals.

The patient did well for about 6 months, when the patient's wife reported intensification of complaints of shortness of breath and several emotional outbursts. During one of these episodes the patient had thrown a coffee pot at his grown daughter, who was visiting in their home. There was no apparent precipitant for his behavior. The patient had no clear explanation for this behavior but insisted that it had been warranted.

The patient was referred to the pulmonary division for complete evaluation of shortness of breath, which revealed no abnormalities. With concern that his shortness of breath might be a somatic delusion and that his behavioral outburst might also have roots in an organic psychotic process, the psychiatrist added fluphenazine, 1 mg daily, to the patient's regimen. The patient's wife reported improvement within several days. Monthly appointments continued, and the patient continued to complain of shortness of breath, headaches, left-sided pain, pain in his neck, and fatigue. His complaints lacked the previous intensity, and he was stable for many months. His psychiatrist listened to the complaints and offered reassurance. His primary physician also continued to see him regularly and performed a brief physical exam each visit. The pharmacologic regimen was not changed.

One year later, at a routine appointment, the patient complained to the psychiatrist of pain in the joint of his great toe. Although his complaint was in keeping with the style of previous complaints of joint pain, he was uncharacteristically insistent that this particular toe was so painful that he could not walk. His wife acknowledged that he had in fact been limping for several days, a behavior that she had tried to ignore. The patient's complaints had only intensified, however, and he was quite specific as to the site of pain and the positions in which it occurred.

Referral to the emergency room that same day for evaluation revealed nearly total disintegration of the joint, probably a result of previous injury. An orthopedic surgeon was consulted, and surgical correction was completed during the following week. The patient tolerated the procedure well, resumed psychiatric appointments once a month, and continued to take nortriptyline and fluphenazine with success.

Differential Diagnosis and Assessment

The differential diagnosis of this patient's symptoms included somatoform pain disorder, depression, somatization disorder, organic psychosis, and numerous nonpsychiatric diagnoses—including poststroke neuralgia—for his bodily complaints. Somatization disorder could be diagnosed on the basis of history alone. Although the "organic workup" was appropriately performed prior to referral to the psychiatrist, continued assessment and consideration of the possibility of physiologic disease was imperative to good management. The psychiatrist was cognizant of the subtle but real change in the character of the patient's joint symptoms. This change initiated a new diagnostic workup that disclosed genuine underlying physical disease.

Treatment Selection

The scheduling of regular appointments with both the primary physician and the psychiatrist allowed stabilization of the patient's condition and gratification of his psychological needs. Use of antidepressant and antipsychotic agents allowed those somatic symptoms that resulted from depression and psychosis to resolve, leaving a manageable profile of complaints.

The patient initially warranted a diagnosis of both depression and SD. Treatment of depression led to resolution of many of the somatic complaints as well.

Treatment Course and Problems in Carrying Out Interventions

Treatment was initially impaired by the patient's sensitivity to side effects of amitriptyline, which might have been avoided by initiation with a lower dosage of medication. Many somatizing patients are exquisitely sensitive to medication side effects, and the physician is cautioned to initially use low dosages (Barsky, 1979).

Another challenge for the patient's physicians was the presence of existing disease. Particularly, because the consequences of stroke can be only partially predicted from radiologic evidence, it was impossible to know exactly which symptoms resulted from brain injury. However, existence of previous somatizing behavior was confirmatory of SD. The patient's wife had previously been able to provide behavioral interventions that prevented his SD from coming to the attention of a psychiatrist. Repeated and unnecessary medical testing may have been a temptation for the internist and the psychiatrist, but frequently scheduled visits allowed physicians involved to have a better concept of the patient's baseline functioning and therefore to keep invasive procedures and studies to a minimum.

Outcome and Termination

This man with SD has continued to have periodic unexplained physical symptoms mixed in among his genuine medical problems. As with all SD patients, his physicians never harbored any delusions of "cure." Thus, he has never been discharged from the original medical–psychiatric management plan.

Follow-Up and Maintenance

Patients with SD have a pervasive lifelong disorder. It can be managed, and symptomatic expression reduced, by continuing to follow the patient at regular intervals. It was clear that this patient required at least monthly medical visits in order to maintain reasonable control of his tendency to somatize. With each individual patient frequency of scheduled office visits must be titrated. Some patients may require weekly visits, whereas others may do well when seen as infrequently as every 2 months.

Summary

Somatization disorder is a symptom complex resulting from highly heterogeneous etiologies. It has no doubt remained illusive in both diagnosis and management because of its protean nature. A number of different treatment modalities have been described. This varied menu reflects the heterogeneous nature of the disorder. Each patient requires an individual assessment of treatment needs, and most will require more than one of the proposed therapeutic modalities. Therefore, treatment relies first on the management of underlying disorders that can be identified. When somatizing behavior is the remaining symptom, treatment relies basically on a psychosocial approach combined with the wary eye of the primary physician, who must be ever alert to the possibility of new physiologic disease. The demands on the physician reach beyond the usual training of any specialty (although family medicine programs probably come closest to meeting the need), thereby leaving many to feel that they are unable to manage the patient. Furthermore, the traditions of medicine in the United States do little to assist the physician, because the patient is free to see multiple doctors without knowledge of the primary physician, opening the door for polysubstance abuse. Recent research suggests that biological diatheses to somatization will emerge that may point more clearly to pharmacologic intervention(s).

Successful management of somatization disorder is important in an economic community that can no longer stand the strain of unnecessary medical costs. Although the individual physician may see the somatizer as potential income from procedures, the public has a vested interest in encouraging proper use of medical care.

References

Abbey, S. E., & Lipowski, Z. J. (1987). Comprehensive management of persistent somatization: An innovative treatment program. *Psychotherapy and Psychosomatics, 48*, 110–115.

American Psychiatric Association (1987). *Diagnostic and statistical manual of mental disorders*, (3rd ed., rev.). Washington, DC: Author.

Barsky, A. J., III. (1979). Patients who amplify bodily sensations. *Annals of Internal Medicine, 91*(1), 63–70.

Cloninger, C. R., Martin, R. L., Guze, S. B., & Clayton, P. J. (1986). A prospective follow-up and family study of somatization in men and women. *American Journal of Psychiatry, 143*, 873–878.

deGruy, F., Columbia, L., & Dickinson, P. (1987). Somatization disorder in a family practice. *Journal of Family Practice, 25*, 45–51.

Devaul, R. A., & Faillace, L. A. (1980). Surgery proneness: A review and clinical assessment. *Psychosomatics, 32*, 295–299.

Drake, M. E., Padamadan, H., & Pakainis, A. (1988). EEG frequency analysis in conversion and somatoform disorder. *Clinical Electroencephalography, 19*, 123–128.

Escobar, J. I., Swartz, M., Rubio-Stipec, M., & Mann, P. (1991). Medically unexplained symptoms: Distribution, risk factors and co-morbidity. In L.J. Kirmayer & J. M. Robbins (Eds.), *Current concepts of somatization, research and clinical perspectives* (pp. 63–78). Washington, DC: American Psychiatric Press.

Farley, J., Woodruff, R. A., & Guze, S. B. (1968). The prevalence of hysteria and conversion symptoms. *British Journal of Psychiatry, 114*, 1121–1125.

Ford, C. V. (1983). *The somatizing disorders: Illness as a way of life*. New York: Elsevier Biomedical.

Ford, C. V. (1984). Somatizing disorders. In H. B. Roback (Ed.), *Helping patients and their families cope with medical problems* (pp. 39–59). San Francisco: Jossey-Bass.

Ford, C. V. (1992). Illness as a life style: The role of somatization in medical practice. *Spine, 17*, S338–S343.

Goldberg, D., Gask, L., & O'Dowd, T. (1989). The treatment of somatization: Teaching techniques of reattribution. *Journal of Psychosomatic Research, 33*, 689–695.

Gordon, E., Kraiuhin, C., Meares, R., & Howson, A. (1986). Auditory evoked response potentials in somatization disorder. *Journal of Psychiatric Research, 20*, 237–248.

Gorman, J. M., Liebowitz, M. R., Fyer, A. J., & Stein, J. (1989). A neuroanatomical hypothesis for panic disorder. *American Journal of Psychiatry, 146*, 148–161.

Guze, S. B., Woodruff, R. A, & Clayton, P. J. (1971). Hysteria and antisocial behavior: Further evidence of an association. *American Journal of Psychiatry, 127*, 957–960.

James, L., Gordon, E., Kraiuhin, C., & Meares, R. (1989). Selective attention and auditory event-related potentials in somatization disorder. *Comprehensive Psychiatry, 30*, 84–89.

James, L., Singer, A., Zurnyski, Y., Gordon, E., Kraiuhin, C. J., Harris, A., Howson, A. J., & Meares, R. (1987). Evoked response potentials and regional cerebral blood flow in somatization disorder. *Psychotherapy and Psychosomatics, 47*, 190–196.

Katon, W., Lin, E., von Korff, M., Russo, J., Lipscomb, P., & Bush, T. (1991). Somatization: A spectrum of severity. *American Journal of Psychiatry, 148*, 34–40.

Liskow, B. I., Pennick, E. C., DeSouza, C., & Gabrielli, W. (1986). Is Briquet's syndrome a heterogeneous disorder? *American Journal of Psychiatry, 143*(5), 334–338.

Liss, J. L., Alpers, E., & Woodruff, R. A., Jr. (1973). The irritable colon syndrome and psychiatric illness. *Diseases of the Nervous System, 34*, 151–157.

Martin, R. L., Roberts, W. V., and Clayton, P. J. (1980). Psychiatric status after hysterectomy. *Journal of the American Medical Association, 244*, 350–353.

Mechanic, D., & Volkart, E. F. H. (1961). Illness behavior and the sick role. *American Sociological Review, 26*(1), 51–58.

Morrison, J. (1990). Managing somatization disorder. *Disease-a-Month, 36*(10), 537–591.

Morrison, J. R. (1978). Management of Briquet's syndrome (hysteria). *Western Journal of Medicine, 128*, 482–487.

Nadelson, T. (1985). False patients/real patients: A spectrum of disease presentation. *Psychotherapy and Psychosomatics, 44*, 175–184.

Noyes, R., Reich, S., Clancy, J., & O'Gorman, T. W. (1986). Reduction in hypochondriasis with treatment of panic disorder. *British Journal of Psychiatry, 149*, 631–635.

Orenstein, H. (1989). Briquet's syndrome in association with depression and panic: A reconceptualization of Briquet's syndrome. *American Journal of Psychiatry, 146*, 334–338.

Orenstein, H., Raskind, M. A., Wyllie, E., Raskind, W. H., & Soules, M. R. (1986). Polysymptomatic complaints and Briquet's syndrome in polycystic ovary disease. *American Journal of Psychiatry, 143*, 768–771.

Rost, K. M., Akins, R. N., Brown, F. W., & Smith, G. R. (1992). The co-morbidity of DSM-III-R personality disorders in somatization disorder. *General Hospital Psychiatry, 14*, 322–326.

Sheehan, D. V., & Sheehan, K. H. (1982). The classification of anxiety and hysterical states. II: Toward a more heuristic classification. *Journal of Clinical Psychopharmacology, 6*(2), 386–393.

Smith, G. R., Jr. (1991). *Somatization disorder in the medical setting.* Washington, DC: American Psychiatric Association Press.

Smith, G. R., Jr. (1992). The epidemiology and treatment of depression when it coexists with somatoform disorders, somatization, or pain. *General Hospital Psychiatry, 14*, 265–272.

Smith, G. R., Jr., Monson, R. A., & Ray, D. C. (1986). Psychiatric consultation in somatization disorder. *New England Journal of Medicine, 314*, 1407–1413.

Smith, G. R., Jr., & Brown, F. W. (1990). Screening indexes in DSM-III-R somatization disorder. *General Hospital Psychiatry, 12*, 148–152.

Steinhart, M. J., Wong, P. Y., & Zarr, M. L. (1981). Therapeutic usefulness of amitriptyline in spastic colon syndrome. *International Journal of Psychiatry in Medicine, 11*, 45–57.

Stoudemire, A., Brown, T. J., McCleod, M., Stewart, B., & Houpt, J. L. (1983). The combined medical specialties unit: An innovative approach to patient care. *North Carolina Medical Journal, 44*, 365–367.

Torgersen, S. (1986). Genetics of somatoform disorders. *Archives of General Psychiatry, 43*, 502–505.

Valko, R. J. (1976). Group therapy for patients with hysteria (Briquet's disorder). *Diseases of the Nervous System, 37*, 484–487.

Young, S. J., Alpers, D. H., Norland, D. D., & Woodruff, R. A., Jr. (1976). Psychiatric illness and the irritable bowel syndrome. *Gastroenterology, 70*, 162–166.

Yutzy, S. H., Pribor, E. F., Cloninger, R. C., & Guze, S. B. (1992). Reconsidering the criteria for somatization disorder. *Hospital and Community Psychiatry, 43*(11), 1075–1076.

15

Multiple Personality Disorder

Philip M. Coons

Description of the Disorder

Clinical Features

Multiple personality disorder (MPD), which has been described elsewhere (Coons, Bowman, & Milstein, 1988; Kluft, 1991b; Putnam, 1989; Putnam, Guroff, Silberman, Barban, & Post, 1986; Ross, 1989), is a polysymptomatic disorder which most often presents in women who report histories of long-standing and severe physical and sexual abuse beginning in early childhood. Depression most commonly overlies the more subtle dissociative symptomatology. Loewenstein (1991a) best articulated the polysymptomatic nature of MPD by dividing the syndrome into symptom clusters, including process, amnesic, autohypnotic, posttraumatic, somatoform, and affective symptoms. The dissociative symptoms will be described first, even though they are more subtle and have prompted one expert to call for a radical change in the way MPD is diagnosed (Nakdimen, 1992).

Alter Personality States.   In MPD the personality is split into two or more personality states or personalities, at least two of which recurrently take full control of the person's behavior. These personalities have their own relatively enduring pattern of perception about the self and the environment. They may differ in age, gender, sexual orientation, affect, mannerisms, attitude, dress, voice quality, and handwriting style. The number of personalities may range from 2 to 100 or more, but the mean is 7 to 13, with a mode of 3. Most commonly the other personalities have different first names, but sometimes the personalities have different last names, are unnamed, or are named by their particular function, such as "observer" or "protector." The transition between personality states is usually sudden and is often triggered

Philip M. Coons • Larue D. Carter Memorial Hospital, Indiana University, Indianapolis, Indiana 46202.

Handbook of Prescriptive Treatments for Adults, edited by Michel Hersen and Robert T. Ammerman. Plenum Press, New York, 1994.

by either psychic distress or other personally meaningful cues. These switches are often subtle and include fluctuations in affect, feelings, and behaviors (Franklin, 1990). For example, a brief stare or eye roll is often followed by a posture and affect change during the switch from one personality to another. This switch may be heralded by either a headache or feelings of derealization or depersonalization, or it may occur without warning.

Amnesia. Amnesia is invariably present in MPD, although it may be hidden. Most commonly, the host personality is initially unaware that alter personalities exist. These alters may have varying degrees of awareness of one another. In about half of MPD patients, there exists an alter, variously labeled a memory trace or inner self-helper, that appears to have a completely intact memory. Some personalities are capable of a process called coconsciousness, or being aware of what is transpiring while another personality is in control. However, the host personality and many alters are usually unaware of events when other alters are "out," and they perceive these intervals as lost periods of times, or at least as time distortion. Sometimes these lost periods appear to be short fugue states. Being told by others of disremembered and disavowed behaviors, such as drinking, drug abuse, self-mutilation, provocative dressing, and becoming enraged, is nearly a universal experience. Some persons with MPD are such poor time keepers that they are unaware of lost time. Others may be aware of time lost but reluctant to disclose it because of fear of being labeled "crazy." If the clinician takes a careful chronological history, there are usually varying degrees of amnesia present for childhood events, such as child abuse.

Associated Features

MPD presents with depression, suicidality, or both in 80 to 90% of patients (Coons et al., 1988; Putnam et al., 1986). Somatoform symptoms may include headaches, conversion phenomena, pseudoseizures, and a variety of other physical complaints that may represent either somatic memories or underlying anxiety, which may reach panic proportions. Symptoms of posttraumatic stress disorder (PTSD) are nearly universal; the most troubling of these are intrusive recollections, nightmares, and flashbacks of previous trauma.

Because depressive and posttraumatic symptoms are so common in MPD, many individuals qualify for comorbid affective disorder and PTSD diagnoses. In addition, because acting out is so common in MPD, many individuals also quality for a personality disorder diagnosis, most frequently borderline personality disorder.

Auditory hallucinations, sometimes of either a derogatory or a command nature, are experienced by 30 to 70% of persons with MPD. These voices are usually experienced as inner voices or internal conversations, occasionally arguments. These types of experiences must be carefully differentiated from psychotic hallucinations.

The personalities may exhibit profound psychophysiologic differences. Differences in heart rate, blood pressure, respiration, visual acuity, and galvanic skin response have been reported, as well as differential response to medication. Persons with MPD have also been reported to have neurophysiologic differences among their various personalities. These include differences in electroencephalographic and electromyographic findings, visual evoked potentials, regional cerebral blood flow, and brain electrical mapping (Miller & Triggiano, 1992). The current research on such differences suffers, however, from its largely uncontrolled and sometimes anecdotal nature.

Ross (1991) recently reviewed the epidemiology of MPD. Once thought to be a rare syndrome, MPD has been increasingly diagnosed since it was accepted as an official diagnosis in DSM-III (American Psychiatric Association, 1980). The current prevalence of MPD is 2 to 4% in psychiatric patients, whether inpatient or outpatient. MPD patients are more commonly women (85 to 95%), perhaps because of the greater incidence of sexual abuse in women. It is speculated that MPD may be underdiagnosed in men because males with MPD are more prone to criminal activities and subsequent incarceration, thus never entering the mental health system (Loewenstein & Putnam, 1990). Age at first diagnosis is usually in the third or fourth decade, but MPD has been reported in both adolescents and children (Hornstein & Putnam, 1992). Childhood dissociative symptoms are usually quite subtle and confused with creation of imaginary playmates and other forms of fantasy. MPD can occur regardless of race and occupational and social level (Putnam et al., 1986) and even occurs cross-culturally (Coons, Bowman, Kluft, & Milstein, 1991).

Etiology

The etiology of MPD is almost invariably linked to repetitive childhood trauma, predominantly sexual or physical abuse, or both. The Putnam et al. (1986) and the Coons et al. (1988) studies reported a 85 to 95% incidence of child abuse. Only 2% of patients report no previous trauma of any kind. Although several studies have demonstrated that MPD is more common in first-degree biological relatives of affected individuals than in the general population, reasons for this are unclear and require further study. Either there is a genetic predisposition to dissociation, or dissociation occurs regularly in response to severe repetitive child abuse that is transmitted from generation to generation. Bliss (1986) has proposed that MPD is an autohypnotic method of coping with the emotional distress accompanying the experience of severe trauma. Ludwig (1984) has proposed that MPD is an example of state-dependent learning. Certainly the use of fantasy (Young, 1988) and suggestibility (Kluft, 1989a) have a role in the production of MPD symptoms, but it is unknown to what extent these factors are important. The evidence that MPD results from iatrogenesis (Aldridge-Morris, 1989), social role playing (Spanos, Weekes, & Bertrand, 1985), or temporal lobe epilepsy (Schenk & Bear, 1981) is limited and unconvincing, except in forensic cases, where a combination of iatrogenesis and role playing may occur (Coons, 1989, 1991).

Differential Diagnosis and Assessment

DSM-III-R and DSM-IV Categorization

The current DSM-III-R criteria for MPD include the following:

A. The existence within the person of two or more distinct personalities or personality states (each with its own relatively enduring pattern of perceiving, relating to, and thinking about the environment and the self).

B. At least two of these personalities or personality states recurrently take full control of the person's behavior (American Psychiatric Association, 1987).

These criteria have been justly criticized for being too broad and have actually resulted in the misdiagnosis of MPD by inexperienced clinicians who have mistaken hypnotic states and role playing for alter personality states. Consequently, amnesia will be added as a diagnostic criterion in DSM-IV (American Psychiatric Association, 1991).

Differential Diagnosis

Because of the hidden nature of dissociation and polysymptomatology of MPD, differential diagnosis can be a formidable task. Since there are several excellent reviews of the differential diagnosis of MPD (Coons, 1984, in press; Kluft, 1991b; Loewenstein, 1991a; Putnam, 1989; Ross, 1989), only the salient points will be summarized here.

Dissociative Disorders.   MPD must be differentiated from the other dissociative disorders. If symptoms of identity alteration are present, the diagnosis of psychogenic amnesia, psychogenic fugue, or depersonalization disorder cannot be made. If identity alteration occurs, either MPD or dissociative disorder not otherwise specified (DDNOS) is present. In psychogenic fugue new identity formation is possible in a prolonged fugue, but there is no switching back and forth between identities. In depersonalization disorder there may be limited identity disturbance, but there is no amnesia. There are no definitive criteria to distinguish MPD from DDNOS. In clinical practice, however, one finds little or no amnesia in DDNOS and there is much fluidity among ego states. Often these ego states never assume complete executive control of the individual. Currently most children with severe dissociative disorders would probably be diagnosed with DDNOS, because the symptoms of childhood dissociative disorder are extremely subtle and fall short of criteria needed to diagnose MPD in adults (Hornstein & Putnam, 1992).

Nondissociative Disorders.   In distinguishing MPD from the nondissociative disorders, the clinician must remember that MPD is comorbid with many psychiatric disorders, including major depression, dysthymia, PTSD, various somatoform disorders, eating disorders, sexual dysfunctions, drug and alcohol abuse, and borderline personality disorder (Coons et al., 1988).

MPD is probably most often misdiagnosed as schizophrenia because of auditory hallucinations. In the schizophrenic, however, these hallucinations are usually experienced as external. The person with MPD does not experience primary symptoms of schizophrenia, such as marked ambivalence, bizarre autistic thinking, flat or inappropriate affect, and loose, illogical associations. Kluft (1987) showed that persons with MPD frequently exhibit the Schneiderian first-rank symptoms of made thoughts, feelings, and behaviors (i.e., symptoms experienced as being imposed from outside the person), but these do not have the bizarre nature found in the schizophrenic.

The frequent mood shifts seen in MPD, which are usually associated with switches between personality states, are frequently mistaken for the mood shifts and switches in borderline personality disorder and bipolar disorder, respectively. However, the relatively brief duration of the mood shifts and presence of other dissociative symptoms should alert the clinician to the possibility of MPD.

At least two organic conditions may be confused with MPD. The blackouts characteristic of drug and alcohol abuse may be mistaken for amnesic episodes in MPD. Likewise, the memory loss and depersonalization present in partial complex seizures may also be mistaken for a dissociative disorder. To complicate matters further, these conditions can be comorbid with MPD. Careful history taking should tease out pertinent details in the former case, but a videoelectroencephalogram is the only certain way of distinguishing partial complex seizures from pseudoseizures sometimes present in MPD.

Perhaps the greatest challenge is to distinguish factitious or malingered MPD from genuine MPD. The clinician should be very suspicious of malingering in forensic contexts, especially in murder defendants, among whom there has been a recent epidemic of feigning MPD to try to diminish criminal responsibility (Coons, 1991). Contrary to popular opinion, MPD is easy to feign, and novice clinicians are especially prone to accept this clever ruse because of their unfamiliarity with dissociative symptoms. Although factitious MPD is less common in clinical situations, it still occurs in about 1 out of 11 individuals in whom MPD is suspected (Coons, 1992). The key to distinguishing genuine from simulated MPD is taking a very thorough history and obtaining collateral interviews and old records. Persons with genuine MPD will usually have evidence of prior dissociative symptoms; those who simulate MPD will not. In addition, in simulated MPD, there is an overdramatization of symptoms, inconsistency in personality presentations from one examination to the next, and evidence of other symptoms common to factitious disorders or malingering, such as refusal to allow the collection of collateral data, lying, inconsistent stories, and lack of symptomatology when the person is unaware of being observed.

Assessment Strategies

Screening Instruments.   The Dissociative Experiences Scale (DES; Bernstein & Putnam, 1986) is one of a number of dissociation screening instruments developed during the last decade (Coons, in press). It consists of a series of 28 questions about various aspects of dissociative symptomatology, including amnesia, fugue, depersonalization, derealization, and identity alteration. It is self-administered in about 10 minutes. Scores range from 0 to 100, and a normal score ranges from 1 to 10 (slightly higher in adolescents). Scores above 20 indicate a high probability of dissociation. Novice clinicians may use this instrument as preliminary to further inquiry about dissociative symptoms.

The Clinical Interview.   The clinical interview and mental status examination are by far the most important tools in the diagnosis of MPD. It is imperative that the clinician take an extremely thorough history, including present and past psychiatric problems, medical history, family history, and social history. As this is done, the polysymptomatic nature of MPD quickly becomes apparent. Like other psychiatric symptoms, each type of dissociative symptom, including amnesia, fugue, depersonalization, derealization, and identity alteration, should be thoroughly explored as to onset, quality, duration, frequency, severity, and possible precipitants. If a detailed chronological life history is taken, periods of amnesia will often become apparent.

The clinician should develop a repertoire of questions regarding dissociation, especially identity alteration. I ask about internal splits or struggles, use of different names by self or others, different handwriting styles, inner conversations or voices, and disremembered behaviors such as angry outbursts and sexual indiscretions. There are several good sources of such questions (Bernstein & Putnam, 1986; Loewenstein, 1991a; Steinberg, Rounsaville, & Cicchetti, 1990).

Keen observational skills are required for the mental status examination. The clinician should observe for evidence of dissociation, such as subtle changes in mood, attitude, dress, and tone of voice; sudden shifts in posture, identity, and transference; spontaneous age regression or childlike behavior; references to self in other than first person; talking to self; intrainterview amnesia; and eye rolling, staring, or other trancelike behaviors.

Once the history taking is complete, the clinician should ask to speak to different personality states, if evidence of spontaneous dissociation has not already been observed. If present, the different personalities can describe themselves and amnesic patterns may be explored. If personality states do not manifest themselves spontaneously after being asked to do so, often asking the patient to close her eyes and relax will allow her to dissociate into another alter as its name is called. If these maneuvers fail, and MPD is still suspected, the judicious use of hypnosis may be successful (Kluft, 1982). Failing hypnosis, use of sodium amytal should be considered (Coons, 1984, in press).

Structured Interview.   The recently developed Structured Interview for Dissociative Disorders (SCID-D; Steinberg, Rounsaville, & Cicchetti, 1990) is an excellent instrument for novice clinicians to use while developing a repertoire of questions about dissociation. In patients with dissociative disorders, the SCID-D takes 60 to 90 minutes to administer. A shorter version, the mini-SCID-D, is also available.

Collateral Information and Interviews.   Two useful techniques for either confirming or negating an MPD diagnosis are the acquisition of previous psychiatric and/or legal records, and a collateral interview with someone well-acquainted with the patient. These maneuvers may reveal good descriptions of dissociative behavior if it exists, or, alternately, reveal evidence of factitious disorder or malingering.

Psychological Testing.   Psychological testing alone has not proven useful in diagnosing MPD, but it may provide diagnostic clues and is certainly useful in differential diagnosis. Most research on psychological testing with MPD has been conducted with the Minnesota Multiphasic Personality Inventory (MMPI) and the Rorschach. Characteristic MMPI profiles include critical items denoting amnesia and a "floating profile" with high F and Sc scales (Coons & Sterne, 1986). Rorschach response patterns are psychologically complex, with evidence of a highly developed self-observing capacity and unusual or highly intellectualized and obsessive thinking (Armstrong & Loewenstein, 1990).

Physical Examination and Laboratory Testing.   Occasionally the physical and neurological examination will reveal evidence of either conversion or self-mutilation. Alternately, absence of evidence of prior abuse described by the patient, such as old fractures, skin mutilation, or pregnancies, may indicated simulation. There are no current laboratory examinations or biological markers for MPD. Current research on various brain imaging techniques may eventually prove useful, however, in differentiating real from simulated MPD.

Evidence for Prescriptive Treatments

Behavior Therapy.   There are only three case reports concerning the use of behavioral techniques in MPD. In the first reported use of behavior therapy in MPD, Kohlenberg (1973) described a 51-year-old man with diagnoses of both schizophrenia and MPD. He exhibited three personality states, consisting primarily of different rates of speech that were labeled "high, medium, and low" by the treating clinician. Using a token system of reinforcement, it was shown that frequency of appearance of these states could be increased. Likewise, frequency could be decreased by offering no reinforcement. This study is flawed by the lack of diagnostic criteria for either MPD or schizophrenia and the lack of follow-up. Even in bonafide MPD cases, Kluft (1984, 1991b) cautions, ignoring personality states exhibited by persons with MPD results in no therapeutic gain. Ignoring a suicidal personality may result in recurrent hospitalizations, or even death, as I have observed in one recent case.

Price and Hess (1979) reported on a 31-year-old woman who developed a "transient dual personality" during desensitization therapy for phobia and panic. Because this alter was quite angry, the primary personality was taught how to express anger using role-playing techniques. Although the alter apparently integrated, this report suffers from lack of adequate follow-up.

In the next case, a combination of pharmacotherapy, psychodynamic psychotherapy, and cognitive therapy was used over a $3\frac{1}{2}$-year period, culminating in a successful integration (Caddy, 1985). The cognitive techniques used by Caddy included progressive muscle relaxation training and biofeedback to reduce tension and anxiety, education and in vivo systematic desensitization to decrease phobic symptoms, the encouragement of a repertoire of assertive behaviors in the primary personality, and a cognitive analysis of the patient's low self-esteem.

Cognitive Analysis.   Both Ross and Gahan (1988) and Fine (1988) have elaborated on the use of cognitive-behavioral techniques in the treatment of MPD. These techniques attempt to decrease the many cognitive distortions present in affected patients. Such cognitive distortions appear to be the result of dichotomous thinking, selective abstraction, arbitrary inference, overgeneralization and undergeneralization, catastrophizing and minimization, time distortion, excessive responsibility and excessive irresponsibility, circular thinking, and misassuming causality (Fine, 1988). These cognitive distortions may result in such symptoms as feelings of worthlessness, minimization of behavior, feelings of separateness, distrust, time distortion, denial of abuse, and inability to express anger (Ross & Gahan, 1988). Treatment of these cognitive errors involves working with the primary and alter personalities by helping them to empathize with and accept the experiences of the others, and teaching them various interpersonal behaviors such as how to be assertive, handle anger, and deal with sexuality.

Hospital Milieu Management.   Andreason and Seidel (1992) described three hospitalized patients with MPD in whom increased structure and limit setting resulted in improvement. All received psychodynamic psychotherapy, pharmacotherapy, and hypnosis in addition to milieu management. In the first case, a 30-year-old woman stopped her self-mutilation and anorexic weight loss in order to avoid transfer to a state hospital. In the second, a 25-year-old woman was transferred from an unstructured open unit, where the focus had been on catharsis and abreaction, to a regimented, locked residential unit where the focus was on her suicidal and self-mutilatory behavior. After 18 months of this regimen she was discharged, and at 1-year follow-up she had no further self-destructive behavior. The last individual, a 34-year-old woman, was arrested repeatedly for theft. Following each crime she would request admission to a mental health facility. Finally, a judge threatened her with jail if her thefts persisted. At 1-year follow-up she had not been rearrested.

The previous cases build upon articles written by several clinicians experienced in the inpatient treatment of MPD (Ganaway, 1989; Kluft, 1991a; Lewin, 1991; Sakheim, Hess, & Chivas, 1988; Steinmeyer, 1991). These authors emphasize the following points about milieu management: (a) the treatment focus must be on target symptoms in order to avoid staff splitting over belief/disbelief in MPD; (b) abreactive work should be deemphasized if the patient is seriously self-destructive; (c) limits must be firm and nonpunitive; (d) the MPD patient should not be treated as a special patient; (e) consistently providing the same primary care staff may help avoid dependency on others; (f) MPD patients should not be allowed to avoid ward and other activities; (g) the entire person should be held responsible for self-destructive and other disruptive behaviors; and (h) restraint should be used carefully and judiciously to treat self-destructive behavior.

Pharmacotherapy.   Although the literature is replete with single case reports and other anecdotal reports of the use of medication in MPD, only one well-designed open trial has been conducted (Loewenstein, Hornstein, & Farber, 1988). Moreover, there are numerous anecdotal reports of different personality states within a single MPD patient who experience different side effects and therapeutic responses to the same medication (Miller & Triggiano, 1992). Therefore, caution is advised in the prescription of pharmacologic agents in MPD. It is best to treat specific target symptoms, titrate medication dosages slowly and carefully, and reevaluate for therapeutic response frequently. Medication should be used for target symptoms present across the entire personality system rather than those confined to single alters (Loewenstein, 1991b). There are no data to suggest that maintenance medication is indicated at this time. Despite the present paucity of literature, the pharmacologic treatment of MPD should be considered a sometimes valuable adjunctive treatment.

Symptoms of Depression.   Because of the frequent co-occurrence of depressive disorders with MPD, antidepressants have been prescribed frequently and, when used, judged effective in 50% of individual cases (Coons, 1986). Caution is urged, however, with use of monoamine oxidase inhibitors (MAOIs) and lithium carbonate, both of which require strict patient compliance.

Symptoms of Posttraumatic Stress Disorder.   In the Loewenstein et al. (1988) study, clonazepam decreased the intrusive posttraumatic symptoms in a group of 5 patients with MPD and PTSD. Presumably, many of the different antidepressant and antianxiety agents used to treat intrusive PTSD symptoms may also be useful in the treatment of PTSD symptoms associated with MPD. A recent review of pharmacotherapy for PTSD described the use of tricyclics, MAOIs, carbamazepine, beta-blockers, alpha-2 agonists, benzodiazepines, and lithium carbonate (Davidson, 1992). Caution is strongly urged, however, because of the paucity of studies on their use in MPD.

Symptoms of Anxiety and Sleeplessness. Benzodiazepines and sedative-hypnotic agents are increasingly being prescribed to patients with MPD (Loewenstein, 1991b). However, because of the frequent co-occurrence of substance abuse problems in MPD patients and the lack of any well-controlled, blind trials of such agents, their use should probably be restricted to patients not demonstrating substance abuse and showing acute symptomatology. These agents should be withdrawn when symptoms have subsided or acute crises have run their course.

Psychotic-like Symptoms. Although antipsychotic drugs are frequently tried in patients with MPD, presumably for hallucinatory experiences, they are rarely judged to be effective (Coons, 1986). Antipsychotic medications are indicated for the rare brief psychosis associated with MPD (Coons, 1986), or occasionally at low dosages to control severe PTSD symptoms that have not responded to more commonly used medications.

Alternative Treatments. The alternative treatments, primarily long-term psychodynamic psychotherapy and hypnosis, are used most frequently in the treatment of MPD because of the disappointing response to behavior therapy and the mixed response to pharmacotherapy.

Psychodynamic Psychotherapy. The treatment of MPD can best be divided into three stages, including beginning, middle, and termination phases. A number of different tasks must be accomplished during each. Both Putnam (1989) and Kluft (1991b) provide excellent descriptions of the psychotherapy of MPD.

During the initial interviews the history gathering process should be used to make a diagnosis. Care should be exercised, however, in sharing this diagnosis with the patient, since a premature disclosure may cause the patient to fearfully flee therapy. It is best to explain in the patient's own words what is happening and offer a brief description of how trauma causes dissociation.

Also during these initial interviews, the clinician attempts to establish a therapeutic rapport with the patient. This process can be very difficult, because the MPD patient often comes into treatment with a great deal of distrust secondary to having been abused by major caregivers, usually parents or other parental figures. The trust issue may extend into later phases of therapy, particularly if borderline dynamics are present and the patient vacillates between love and hate for the therapist. Initially these affective alterations may be a test of the therapist to determine if he or she really cares.

The final task of the initial phase of treatment is the gathering of sufficient history and description of the primary and alter personality states. This should include learning the name, age, gender, origin, and function of each personality state. Not all personality states are fully developed, so this information may be incomplete in certain instances. Care must be taken not to prolong this phase; therapist fascination is thought to reinforce the dissociative process.

Most of the real work in the treatment of MPD occurs during the middle phase of therapy, which lasts a minimum of 1 to 2 years. Patients are usually seen once or twice a week for 45- to 60-minute sessions. An extended session or emergency sessions for crises are occasionally necessary. In a hospital setting, treatment may proceed on a more frequent basis. However, in my experience, when treatment extends to more than 5 hours per week, serious transferential and countertransferential problems usually exist.

A major task in the middle phase of treatment involves helping the primary personality deal with dissociated affects, thoughts, and impulses. Here, one might work on issues such as the expression of anger and coping with depression or sexuality. The therapist should be careful not to "play favorites" among personality states or try to banish alters who behave in ways unacceptable to the therapist. A neutral stance with firm limit setting is advocated.

Another major task of the middle phase of therapy is to uncover, abreact, and work through various traumatic incidents. Care should be exercised, however, to avoid this plan until sufficient rapport has been achieved or the patient has established an adequate support system. Abreaction should not be considered the major focus of treatment, because it is painful, arduous, and often quite destabilizing for the patient. Abreaction should be carefully paced in order to maintain both functioning in interpersonal relationships and employment.

A third major task is to continue rapport building with other alters and establish a cooperative relationship among them. For some persons with MPD, this often brings order to their lives for the first time.

A final task of this phase of treatment is working toward dissolving amnesic barriers among different alters. Lessening of amnesic barriers generally proceeds with abreaction; when traumas are abreacted, the need for amnesia lessens. Decreasing amnesia can be enhanced by several methods. Describing to the primary personality what occurs when other alters are in control is one method. Encouraging the keeping of a daily journal can also provide useful information for alters about other, unknown personalities. The use of audio and video recordings is another useful way to provide knowledge, but these methods should be used cautiously; premature use may unduly frighten the primary personality and cause her to flee therapy.

Although integration of dissociated feelings, impulses, and experiences begins with initiation of therapy and continues throughout, the actual fusion of personality states does not usually take place until well into the middle phase of treatment. As trauma is abreacted and worked through, amnesic barriers fall, and the primary self learns how to deal with dissociated aspects of the self, the need to dissociate lessens. Usually, alter personalities begin to fuse spontaneously.

The final phase of treatment includes the fusion of the remaining personality states. Final integration generally involves significant grief because of the loss of a familiar method of adaptation, without which the person might have either become psychotic or committed suicide. During this phase nondissociative defenses must be added to the patient's armamentarium of coping defenses. Follow-up is recommended to ensure that dissociation does not recur.

Hypnosis. Hypnosis can be a valuable adjunct to the therapeutic process. Although hypnosis may be used in any phase of treatment, it should be used infrequently in diagnosis and not used at all in forensic investigations of criminal defendants, so as to avoid suggesting the production of dissociative symptoms, which are then used to evade criminal responsibility (Coons, 1991). Kluft (1982) has described the use of hypnosis in MPD for the following purposes: encouragement of communication and cooperation among alters, abreaction and working through of trauma, decreasing amnesic barriers, and fusion of alters. Hypnotic techniques used are varied and include use of the affect bridge, posthypnotic suggestion, age regression and progression, and use of various distancing techniques to lessen the painfulness of abreaction.

A great variety of other therapeutic techniques have been used in individuals with MPD. These include group therapy (Caul, 1984; Coons & Bradley, 1985), art therapy (Frye, 1990), family and marital therapy (Sachs, Frischoltz, & Wood, 1988), occupational therapy (Skinner, 1990), field trips (Tudor, 1989), restraint therapy (Lamberti & Cummings, 1992), and electroconvulsive therapy for severe depression unresponsive to medication (Bowman & Coons, 1992). The interested reader should consult the appropriate sources for more information about these techniques.

Selecting Optimal Treatment Strategies

Currently the optimal treatment strategy for MPD includes primarily the use of long-term psychodynamic psychotherapy combined with the setting of firm limits and maintenance of therapeutic boundaries. Useful adjunctive treatments include hypnosis and pharmacotherapy. Although there are a variety of other treatment techniques available, these should be carefully chosen.

Problems in Carrying Out Interventions

There are numerous pitfalls to the treatment of MPD. These include undue skepticism about the diagnosis of MPD (Dell, 1988), numerous types of patient resistances (Chu 1988a, 1988b), therapist boundary violations (Greaves, 1988; Watkins & Watkins, 1984), and iatrogenesis (Coons, 1989; Fine, 1988). In addition, special problems may be encountered in dealing with malevolent ego states (Watkins & Watkins, 1988), in treating the older patient (Kluft, 1988a) or extremely complex patient (Kluft, 1988b), or in pacing the therapy to avoid undue morbidity (Kluft, 1989b). Space prevents discussing all these techniques in detail, so only two major problem areas will be discussed: the maintenance of proper therapeutic boundaries and use of proper abreactive technique.

Therapeutic Boundaries. The violation of therapeutic boundaries is a common problem among clinicians who treat MPD and appears to be most common in those who are not solidly grounded in the principles of psychodynamic psychotherapy. These boundary violations take many forms, including treating the patient free of charge or at a greatly reduced fee, allowing the patient to fall far behind in payments, frequently extending the therapy hour, seeing the patient after regular office hours, spending more than 5 hours per week in therapy with the patient, holding hands with or hugging the patient (in extreme cases this has extended to actual sexual contact), inviting the patient to the therapist's home or vice versa, sharing intimate details of one's life with the patient, making frequent nontherapeutic excursions with the patient, writing books with patients before successful completion of therapy, using unusual forms of therapy such as reparenting, pursuing excessive advocacy on the patient's behalf (such as encouraging lawsuits), and inviting the patient into one's home to babysit or do yard work or other jobs.

These therapeutic boundary violations ultimately reinforce the MPD patient's dependency and desire to be loved and accepted, and can bolster her dissociative defenses. Ultimately the therapist becomes worn out by increasing patient demands and may withdraw from the therapeutic relationship.

Avoidance of boundary problems may be averted by a thorough understanding of psychodynamics and training in psychodynamic psychotherapy along with the imposition of firm therapeutic limits. Feeling sorry for, trying to love back into health, or being fascinated by the MPD patient should be warning signals for the cautious therapist. Consultation with a clinician experienced in the treatment of MPD may be quite useful in helping the clinician who is embroiled in boundary difficulties.

Abreaction. Another major mistake of a clinician's inexperience in the treatment of MPD is to engage in premature therapeutic abreaction of painful material. If material is abreacted before the patient is ready, or if the therapeutic focus is on abreaction exclusively, the patient will usually regress into a nonfunctional state and hospitalization may be necessary. If abreaction continues to be a major focus, further regression will occur, with subsequent prolonged or repeated hospitalizations. An additional danger is for the unprepared clinician to fall victim to the painful abreacted material and then withdraw from the therapeutic relationship. As I have said, in order to avoid these catastrophic outcomes, the clinician and patient must initially ensure that a stable support system is present and that depressive and PTSD symptoms are fairly well stabilized before beginning abreactive work. Abreactive work should then be carefully paced to prevent compromised functioning.

Relapse Prevention

The prognosis for recovery from MPD is presumed to be good to excellent. Unfortunately, there are no long-term follow-up studies to support this assumption. Two investigators have reported therapeutic gains at $3\frac{1}{2}$ and 3 years, respectively (Coons, 1986; Ross, 1989). These therapeutic gains included improved functioning and lessening of amnesia as well as integration, partial or complete in many patients. Dropout rates are in the range of 15 to 25%. Kluft (1984) described 33 patients who had been solidly integrated for 27 months. These patients became integrated in a mean of 22 months. Unfortunately, Kluft did not comment on the other patients in his treatment cohort who were either still in treatment or were therapy dropouts.

The current state of knowledge about MPD treatment does not allow prediction of which patients will ultimately integrate and which will relapse after integration. Kluft's (1984) integration criteria consist of continuity of memory, absence of signs of dissociation, subjective sense of unity, absence of alters upon hypnotic reexploration, and an acknowledgment of attitudes and memories that were previously dissociated. He advised a 6- to 24-month period of follow-up to detect those susceptible to relapse. In those who are truly integrated, relapse usually occurs because of further trauma and, unfortunately, there is little we can do to prevent this.

Case Illustration

Case Description

Roberta Louise Kelso (fictitious name) was a 26-year-old married woman when she presented for treatment 6 years ago. She was referred by a social worker from a local community mental health center. This clinician had suspected that her patient had a dissociative disorder because she exhibited brief trancelike staring episodes during therapy sessions, especially when discussing memories of previous child abuse. On several occasions Mrs. Kelso had called her therapist but had not subsequently remembered their telephone conversations. During one therapy session she appeared very regressed and childlike and crawled under a table.

Roberta had had her first contact with mental health professionals at age 19, when she presented with symptoms of depression to her university student health service following a broken romance. She was diagnosed with adjustment disorder with depression; her depression responded to imipramine 150 mg per day and supportive psychotherapy. Although she continued to have bouts of depression, she did not seek treatment again until age 24, when she was seen at a community mental health center for depression and marital problems, which followed a particularly violent rape. The examining psychiatrist diagnosed her as having a borderline personality disorder because of her temper outbursts, substance abuse, binge eating, affective instability, and self-mutilation. After 6 months of supportive psychotherapy and marital counseling, she became markedly depressed and suicidal. She was admitted for a 5-week hospitalization and treatment of major depression with psychosis. In addition to standard antidepressant therapy, she was treated with haloperidol for derogatory auditory hallucinations.

When I saw Mrs. Kelso, she gave a history of depression extending into childhood as far back as she could remember. Symptoms of depression included sleeplessness, low energy, variable appetite, low self-esteem, and intermittent suicidal ideation. Although she was taking lithium carbonate, this had not seemed to alter her depressive symptoms.

In discussing her memory difficulties she reluctantly admitted that she had lost periods of time, which varied from a few minutes to as long as several hours. She was vague about onset of these episodes but admitted that she often lost track of time and could remember nothing before age 9. On two occasions she had found herself in places where she had not intended to go. Once she found herself unexpectedly in a shopping mall, and on another occasion found herself in a city 3 hours distant from her home. In the latter case she had always assumed that alcohol intoxication at a fraternity party was to blame for this one-day fugue. She almost always felt depersonalized prior to her amnesic episodes. After these episodes she almost always had a headache.

Mrs. Kelso felt as though she were split into at least two different parts, in that she often felt small and childlike. She could not remember crawling under the table in her therapist's office, nor could she remember the numerous angry outbursts that she had with her husband. When asked about the use of different names, she remembered that her father used to call her Bobbie and that a stranger had recently stopped her at a shopping mall and called her Rita. She reluctantly admitted that she had heard voices inside her head since childhood. During the past several years these voices had become mostly derogatory and sometimes instructed her to take an overdose or cut her arms. She could not remember the antidepressant overdose that had precipitated her psychiatric hospitalization and had only a hazy remembrance of feeling compelled on numerous occasions to self-mutilate after discussing her sexual abuse in psychotherapy.

Mrs. Kelso had many symptoms indicative of PTSD, including intrusive memories, flashbacks, and nightmares. She avoided sexual relations with her husband and television talk shows or movies about violence or child abuse. When she and her husband had sex, she experienced flashbacks involving incest with her father. These flashbacks had begun after she was raped by a stranger just prior to seeking therapy with her social worker. Her amnesic episodes intensified and became more frequent at this time.

Mrs. Kelso was employed as a legal secretary but was finding it more difficult to work because of her amnesic episodes and increasing depressive and posttraumatic stress symptoms. Prior to her marriage at age 23, she had graduated from high school and had attended a local community college for 2 years. She had been raised as a mainline Protestant but stopped attending church as her sexual abuse memories emerged and she became angry at God for allowing her abuse.

Her medical history revealed a succession of visits to a gynecologist for pelvic pain and painful, irregular menses, but no organic cause was found. She was fearful of starting a family because she felt she might hurt her baby in one of her angry outbursts.

She had begun abusing alcohol at age 14 and by the time she was 16 had experimented with marijuana and her mother's sleeping pills. Her substance abuse enabled her to escape the painful reality of her father's frequent physical and verbal abuse.

Mrs. Kelso was the eldest of three daughters. Her father worked as a laborer for the railroad and had been physically abused by his father. He was alcoholic, as were his father and two of his brothers. Her mother was a homemaker and a nurse's aide on the evening shift at a nursing home. She was rather passive and was frequently the target of her husband's drunken rages. She was unaware that her husband was sexually abusing his two eldest daughters. Roberta's sexual abuse started with fondling at about age 5, graduated to sexual intercourse at age 13, and continued until she left home.

She was thrown out of the house when she became pregnant at age 18. Subsequently she married the father but lost the baby at 3 months' gestation after her husband beat her severely. She separated from him and went to live with her maternal grandparents, where she stayed until her second marriage. She put herself through school by working part-time as a secretary and through various educational grants.

Differential Diagnosis and Assessment

On her first visit Roberta was given the DES and scored 40. She was asked to clarify her answers on all items on which she scored 15 or above. When asked about the use of different names, she mentioned Bobbie and Rita and also remembered that she had had three imaginary playmates as a child—Robert, Bobbi, and Tina. On her second visit she dissociated spontaneously into a childish part who said her name was Robbi but refused to speak further. Following Roberta's return to executive control, she was asked to relax and close her eyes while I called forth other personality states. She was reluctant to do this at first, but finally agreed at the urging of her therapist. Rita emerged first and revealed that she often drank heavily and that she knew something of at least five other personality states besides Roberta.

Her MMPI revealed an F scale of 85 and an Sc scale of 90, the two highest respective validity and clinical scales. A sleep-deprived EEG with nasopharyngeal leads was normal and showed no evidence of seizure activity. A consultant neurologist found a normal neurological presentation except for a hysterical hemianesthesia. Evidence of previous self-mutilation could be seen in the many superficial scares on her forearms. Previous psychiatric records were requested and revealed that although she had never been diagnosed with MPD, there were complaints of both memory loss and depersonalization during her psychiatric hospitalization.

Initial psychiatric diagnoses included MPD, dysthymic disorder with history of a single major depression, PTSD, and previous drug and alcohol abuse. Although she had many symptoms consistent with borderline personality disorder, Axis II diagnoses were deferred because of the overlap with symptoms of MPD. A seizure disorder was ruled out by the neurological consultation and EEG.

Treatment Selection

Her therapist felt ill equipped to continue therapy with Mrs. Kelso, being unfamiliar with the treatment of MPD. Mrs. Kelso agreed to begin therapy with me, and we initially contracted to see each other twice weekly for 50-minute sessions. I explained to her the need for psychodynamic psychotherapy, use of adjunctive therapies such as medication and hypnosis, and probable course of treatment. Her lithium carbonate was stopped, and, because she was so disturbed by sleeplessness and the intrusive imagery of her PTSD, she was started on a course of trazodone, which was gradually titrated to a dose of 250 mg at bedtime.

Treatment Course and Problems in Carrying Out Interventions

The initial several months of therapy were spent developing a therapeutic rapport and becoming familiar with her personality system. A total of nine personality states were discovered. There were seven female and two male personality states, ranging in age from 5 to 26. These personality states included Roberta, the original or host personality; Louise, a rescuer personality; Bobby, a 13-year-old boy; Bobbi, a 26-year-old female personality who enjoyed sex with her husband; Rita, an 18-year-old rebellious personality who drank heavily; Blue, a 19-year-old depressed personality; Robbi, a 5-year-old girl who was extremely fearful; Robert, a very angry male twin of Rita; and Spirit, her memory trace personality. Robbi had emerged when the sexual abuse first began, and Bobby emerged when it graduated to sexual intercourse. Both Roberta and Robbi were amnesic for their other personality states. The twins were co-conscious with each other but had no awareness of the other alters. Spirit, Louise, and Bobbi were co-conscious with all of the others.

During the first 6 months of treatment, the major therapeutic focus was on strengthening her supportive relationships. Her husband was invited to a session, where the diagnosis and treatment were explained. He attended several more conjoint sessions, where he learned not to reinforce his wife's dissociation by playing with her 5-year-old alter and giving birthday gifts to all of her alters. Their sexual relationship was explored, and the couple was cautioned that abreactive work might decrease the frequency and enjoyment of sex.

Three months into therapy, Roberta joined a local MPD self-help group. She derived a great deal of information about her illness from this experience and was glad to know that there were others like her. She stopped going, however, because the group was dominated by persons reluctant to relinquish their multiplicity.

During the second and third years of treatment, therapy forged ahead on several fronts. Work with the primary personality focused on helping her deal with dissociated affects and impulses, including depression, anger, and sexuality. As she became better at dealing with these issues, she dissociated less. Abreactive work involved working with Roberta regarding the rape, and all of the alters regarding the child abuse. Amnesic barriers were lowered by her keeping a daily journal initially and later by the use of audio- and videotaping.

A major focus early in therapy was in ensuring that Roberta be allowed to do secretarial work without interruption by the alters. This cooperative agreement resulted in a new sense of mastery and increased self-esteem for Roberta. Cooperation also involved the alters deciding together what issues would be addressed in therapy and how time would be shared outside of work.

Hypnotherapy was of major benefit. Initially hypnosis was used to talk to difficult-to-access alters, but this became unnecessary later in therapy as Roberta gained more control over dissociation. Hypnosis was used to abreact painful memories through use of the affect bridge and various distancing techniques. Hypnosis also facilitated communication among the various alters.

Two major problem areas were encountered during treatment. The first involved excessive dependency on the therapist, manifested in frequent phone calls for reassurance, requests for hugs, and extra time, and so forth. This was dealt with both by expressing empathy and by educating Roberta about proper therapeutic boundaries. The other major problem was a resistance that developed to the idea of integration and the belief that some alters would "die" in the process of integration. Over time the alters gradually accepted the idea that nothing is lost through integration, whereas troubling dissociative symptoms disappear.

Outcome and Termination

During the fourth year of therapy, Roberta's alter personality states finally began to fuse with one another. This happened spontaneously for most, but was facilitated by hypnosis with the remaining two. During this process, Roberta mourned the loss of her "friends" who had helped her cope with repeated trauma. I continued to see her for 6 months after she became totally fused, first on a bimonthly basis and then on a monthly basis for the final 3 months. During this time we discussed termination issues and Roberta worked on reinforcing her nondissociative defenses.

Follow-Up and Maintenance

We remained in touch occasionally by phone and letter for the next year. Unfortunately, Roberta was the victim of a purse snatching and was battered badly when she tried to resist. Although she began dissociating again, the fragment that split off remained unnamed. I began seeing her weekly and continued for the next 3 months. She reintegrated easily as we discussed her recent assault. During the last 2 years we have continued to correspond by letter since she moved. She reports no further dissociation.

Summary

Multiple personality disorder is a polysymptomatic syndrome characterized by affective, posttraumatic, and somatic symptoms, as well as dissociative amnesia and identity alteration. It is found in 2 to 4% of psychiatric patients and is linked etiologically to repetitive childhood trauma, particularly abuse. The disorder must be differentiated from schizophrenia, bipolar disorder, malingering, and the other dissociative disorders.

The diagnosis of MPD is made on the basis of history and clinical findings. Use of collateral data cannot be overemphasized. The Dissociative Experiences Scale is a useful screening instrument for dissociative symptoms, and the Structured Clinical Interview for Dissociative Disorders can further elucidate dissociative symptoms. The Rorschach and Minnesota Multiphasic Personality Inventory can add immense detail to the evaluation, but neither has been useful in making an initial diagnosis.

The treatment of MPD consists of traditional psychodynamic psychotherapy coupled with the maintenance of therapeutic boundaries and firm limit setting. Certain behavioral techniques, pharmacotherapy, and hypnosis are valuable therapeutic adjuncts. A variety of other treatment techniques have been woven into this therapeutic fabric. Follow-up studies are urgently needed to test the efficacy of various treatment modalities.

References

Aldridge-Morris, R. (1989). *Multiple personality: An exercise in deception.* Hillsdale, NJ: Erlbaum.

American Psychiatric Association (1980). *Diagnostic and statistical manual of mental disorders* (3rd ed., pp. 257–259). Washington, DC: Author.

American Psychiatric Association (1987). *Diagnostic and statistical manual of mental disorders* (3rd ed., rev., pp. 269–272). Washington, DC: Author.

American Psychiatric Association (1991). *DSM-IV options book: Work in progress, 9/1/91* (p. K2). Washington, DC: Author.

Andreason, P. J., & Seidel, J. A. (1992). Behavioral techniques in the treatment of patients with multiple personality disorder. *Annals of Clinical Psychiatry, 4,* 29–32.

Armstrong, J. G., & Loewenstein, R. J. (1990). Characteristics of patients with multiple personality and dissociative disorders on psychological testing. *Journal of Nervous and Mental Disease, 178,* 448–454.

Bernstein, E. M., & Putnam, F. W. (1986). Development, reliability, and validity of a dissociation scale. *Journal of Nervous and Mental Disease, 174,* 727–735.

Bliss, E. L. (1986). *Multiple personality, allied disorders, and hypnosis.* New York: Oxford University Press.

Bowman, E. S., & Coons, P. M. (1992). The use of electroconvulsive therapy in patients with dissociative disorders. *Journal of Nervous and Mental Disease, 180,* 524–528.

Caddy, G. R. (1985). Cognitive behavior therapy in the treatment of multiple personality. *Behavior Modification, 9,* 267–292.

Caul, D. (1984). Group and videotape techniques for multiple personality disorder. *Psychiatric Annals, 14,* 43–50.

Chu, J. A. (1988a). Some aspects of resistance in the treatment of multiple personality disorder. *Dissociation, 1(2),* 34–38.

Chu, J. A. (1988b). Ten traps for therapists in the treatment of trauma survivors. *Dissociation, 1(4),* 24–32.

Coons, P. M. (1984). The differential diagnosis of multiple personality: A comprehensive review. *Psychiatric Clinics of North America, 7,* 51–67.

Coons, P. M. (1986). Treatment progress in 20 patients with multiple personality disorder. *Journal of Nervous and Mental Disease, 174,* 715–721.

Coons, P. M. (1989). Iatrogenic factors in the misdiagnosis of multiple personality disorder. *Dissociation, 2,* 70–76.

Coons, P. M. (1991). Iatrogenesis and malingering of multiple personality disorder in the forensic evaluation of homicide defendants. *Psychiatric Clinics of North America, 14,* 757–768.

Coons, P. M. (1992). Factitious or malingered MPD: Eleven cases. *Proceedings of the Ninth International Conference on Multiple Personality/Dissociative States* (p. 153). Chicago: Rush-Presbyterian-St. Luke's Medical Center.

Coons, P. M. (in press). The clinical interview and differential diagnosis of multiple personality disorder. In J. A. Turkus & B. M. Cohen (Eds.), *Multiple personality disorder: Continuum of care.* New York: Jason Aronson.

Coons, P. M., Bowman, E. S., Kluft, R. P., & Milstein, V. (1991). The cross-cultural occurrence of MPD: Additional cases from a recent survey. *Dissociation, 4,* 124–128.

Coons, P. M., Bowman, E. S., & Milstein, V. (1988). Multiple personality disorder: A clinical investigation of 50 cases. *Journal of Nervous and Mental Disease, 176,* 519–527.

Coons, P. M., & Bradley, K. (1985). Group psychotherapy with multiple personality patients. *Journal of Nervous and Mental Disease, 173,* 515–521.

Coons, P. M., & Sterne, A. (1986). Initial and followup psychological testing on a group of patients with multiple personality disorder. *Psychological Reports, 58,* 43–49.

Davidson, J. (1992). Drug therapy in post-traumatic stress disorder. *British Journal of Psychiatry, 160,* 309–314.

Dell, P. F. (1988). Professional skepticism about multiple personality. *Journal of Nervous and Mental Disease, 176,* 528–531.

Fine, C. G. (1988). Thoughts on the cognitive perceptual substrates of multiple personality disorder. *Dissociation, 1*(4), 5–10.

Franklin, J. (1990). The diagnosis of multiple personality disorder based on subtle dissociative signs. *Journal of Nervous and Mental Disease, 178,* 4–14.

Frye, B. (1990). Art and multiple personality disorder: An expressive framework for occupational therapy. *American Journal of Occupational Therapy, 44,* 1013–1022.

Ganaway, G. (1989). Establishing safety and stability within the inpatient milieu. *Trauma and Recovery Newsletter* (Vol. 2, No. 2, pp. 2–5). Akron, OH: Akron General Medical Center.

Greaves, G. B. (1988). Common errors in the treatment of multiple personality disorder. *Dissociation, 1*(1), 61–66.

Hornstein, N., & Putnam, F. W. (1992). Clinical phenomenology of child and adolescent dissociative disorders. *Journal of the American Academy of Child and Adolescent Psychiatry, 31,* 1077–1085.

Kluft, R. P. (1982). Varieties of hypnotic interventions in the treatment of multiple personality. *American Journal of Clinical Hypnosis, 24,* 232–240.

Kluft, R. P. (1984). Treatment of multiple personality disorder: A study of 33 cases. *Psychiatric Clinics of North America, 7,* 9–29.

Kluft, R. P. (1987). First-rank symptoms as a diagnostic clue to multiple personality disorder. *American Journal of Psychiatry, 144,* 293–298.

Kluft, R. P. (1988a). On treating the older patient with multiple personality disorder: "Race against time" or "make haste slowly." *American Journal of Clinical Hypnosis, 30,* 257–266.

Kluft, R. P. (1988b). The phenomenology and treatment of the extremely complex multiple personality disorder. *Dissociation, 1*(4), 47–58.

Kluft, R. P. (1989a). Iatrogenic creation of new alter personalities. *Dissociation, 2,* 83–91.

Kluft, R. P. (1989b). Playing for time: Temporizing techniques in the treatment of multiple personality disorder. *American Journal of Clinical Hypnosis, 32,* 90–98.

Kluft, R. P. (1991a). Hospital treatment of multiple personality disorder: An overview. *Psychiatric Clinics of North America, 14,* 695–719.

Kluft, R. P. (1991b). Multiple personality disorder. In A. Tasman & S. M. Goldfinger (Eds.), *American Psychiatric Press review of psychiatry* (Vol. 10, pp. 161–168). Washington, DC: American Psychiatric Press.

Kohlenberg, R. T. (1973). Behavioristic approach to multiple personality: A case study. *Behavior Therapy, 4,* 137–140.

Lamberti, J. S., & Cummings, S. (1992). Hands-on restraint in the treatment of multiple personality disorder. *Hospital and Community Psychiatry, 43,* 283–284.

Lewin, R. A. (1991). Preliminary thoughts on milieu treatment of patients with multiple personality disorder. *Psychiatric Hospital, 22,* 161–163.

Loewenstein, R. J. (1991a). An office mental status examination for complex chronic dissociative symptoms and multiple personality disorder. *Psychiatric Clinics of North America, 14,* 567–604.

Loewenstein, R. J. (1991b). Rational psychopharmacotherapy in the treatment of multiple personality disorder. *Psychiatric Clinics of North America, 14,* 721–740.

Loewenstein, R. J., Hornstein, N., & Farber, B. (1988). Open trial of clonazepam in the treatment of post-traumatic symptoms in multiple personality disorder. *Dissociation, 1*(3), 3–12.

Loewenstein, R. J., & Putnam, F. W. (1990). The clinical phenomenology of males with multiple personality disorder: A report of 21 cases. *Dissociation, 3,* 135–143.

Ludwig, A. M. (1984). Intoxication and sobriety: Implications for understanding multiple personality. *Psychiatric Clinics of North America, 7,* 161–169.

Miller, S. D., & Triggiano, P. G. (1992). The psychophysiological investigation of multiple personality disorder: A review and update. *American Journal of Clinical Hypnosis, 35,* 47–61.

Nakdimen, K. A. (1992). Diagnostic criteria for multiple personality disorder [Letter to the editor]. *American Journal of Psychiatry, 149,* 576–577.

Price, J., & Hess, N. C. (1979). Behavior therapy as precipitant and treatment of a case of dual personality. *Australian and New Zealand Journal of Psychiatry, 13,* 63–66.

Putnam, F. W. (1989). *The diagnosis and treatment of multiple personality disorder.* New York: Guilford.

Putnam, F. W., Guroff, J. J., Silberman, E. K., Barban, L., & Post, R. M. (1986). The clinical phenomenology of multiple personality disorder: A review of 100 recent cases. *Journal of Clinical Psychiatry, 47,* 285–293.

Ross, C. A. (1989). *Multiple personality disorder: Diagnosis, clinical features, and treatment.* New York: Wiley.

Ross, C. A. (1991). Epidemiology of multiple personality disorder and dissociation. *Psychiatric Clinics of North America, 14,* 503–517.

Ross, C. A., & Gahan, P. (1988). Cognitive analysis of multiple personality disorder. *American Journal of Psychotherapy, 42,* 40–52.

Sachs, R., Frischoltz, E. J., & Wood, J. I. (1988). Marital and family therapy in the treatment of multiple personality disorder. *Journal of Marital and Family Therapy, 14,* 249–259.

Sakheim, D. K., Hess, E. P., & Chivas, A. (1988). General principles for short-term inpatient work with multiple personality disorder patients. *Psychotherapy, 25,* 117–124.

Schenk, L., & Bear, D. (1981). Multiple personality and related dissociative phenomena in patients with temporal lobe epilepsy. *American Journal of Psychiatry, 138,* 1311–1315.

Skinner, S. T. (1990). Occupational therapy in patients with multiple personality disorder: Personal reflections. *American Journal of Occupational Therapy, 44,* 1024–1027.

Spanos, N. P., Weekes, J. R., & Bertrand, L. D. (1985). Multiple personality disorder: A social psychological perspective. *Journal of Abnormal Psychology, 94,* 326–376.

Steinberg, M., Rounsaville, B., & Cicchetti, D. (1990). The structured clinical interview for DSM-III-R dissociative disorders: Preliminary report on a new diagnostic instrument. *American Journal of Psychiatry, 149,* 76–82.

Steinmeyer, S. M. (1991). Some hard-learned lessons in milieu management of multiple personality disorder. *Psychiatric Hospital, 22,* 1–4.

Tudor, T. G. (1989). Field trips in the treatment of multiple personality disorder. *The Psychotherapy Patient, 6,* 197–213.

Watkins, J. G., & Watkins, H. H. (1984). Hazards to the therapist in the treatment of multiple personalities. *Psychiatric Clinics of North America, 7,* 111–119.

Watkins, J. G., & Watkins, H. H. (1988). The management of malevolent ego states in multiple personality disorder. *Dissociation, 1*(1), 67–72.

Young, W. C. (1988). Observations on fantasy in the formation of multiple personality disorder. *Dissociation, 1*(3), 13–20.

16

Paraphilias and Gender Identity Disorders

Nathaniel McConaghy

Description of the Disorders

The terms *paraphilias* and *gender identity disorders* are currently employed for conditions previously referred to as sexual deviations, behaviors seen as deviating from those currently socially acceptable. With recent changes in social values, some, such as masturbation or homosexuality, have ceased to be classified as deviations.

Clinical Features

Exhibitionism is the most common paraphilia for which subjects are charged or seek treatment. It typically takes the form of unsolicited exposure of their genitals by postpubertal males to one or a few females, usually strangers around the age of puberty. The behavior commonly commences in adolescence, when it is experienced as sexually exciting. When in adulthood subjects seek treatment, as they find they are unable to cease the behavior in the situations where they have previously carried it out, they usually report that the excitement is largely nonsexual but, rather, a state of heightened arousal approaching panic. It is extremely rarely carried out by women (Grob, 1985).

Voyeurism appears to be a related paraphilia, in that it is also extremely rare in women and commences in adolescence, when it is experienced as sexually exciting, whereas in adulthood, when it has become compulsive, the excitement is largely nonsexual. Its best-known form has been termed *peeping*: the looking by males into a

Nathaniel McConaghy • Psychiatric Unit, Prince of Wales Hospital, Randwick, New South Wales. 2031 Australia.

Handbook of Prescriptive Treatments for Adults, edited by Michel Hersen and Robert T. Ammerman. Plenum Press, New York, 1994.

private area to observe without her consent a partially or completely nude woman. Forms of voyeurism less likely to come to attention are the observing by heterosexual men of heterosexual couples having intercourse in parked automobiles and by homosexual men of homosexual activity in public lavatories or steam baths. In its most common form, *coprophilia* is the observing of subjects urinating or defecating; in some cases it is the planned overhearing of these behaviors.

Pedophilia, sexual activity by postpubertal with prepubertal subjects, is the most commonly treated paraphilia after exhibitionism. It is carried out by a significant number of women; unlike men, however, they are usually not regarded as offenders, possibly in part because male child partners of women do not usually regard the experience negatively. Russell's decision (1986) that pedophilic activity was abusive whether or not the children considered their reactions neutral or positive appears to be generally applied only to adult sexual activity with girls.

Most males offend against only male or female children, not both. Homosexual offenders commonly commence pedophilic activity in adolescence. In adulthood, when they seek treatment or are charged, most report having had a large number of victims who were strangers or casual acquaintances. A similar history is given by hebephiles, men sexually attracted to pubertal or immediately postpubertal boys. The offenses of heterosexual pedophiles commonly commence in adulthood, with one or a few victims who are related or well known to them.

The obtaining of sexual excitement from the infliction of pain or humiliation is termed *sadism*, and from the experience of pain or humiliation, *masochism*. These behaviors rarely lead to seeking of treatment or criminal charges, and information concerning the behaviors is largely obtained from investigation of members of "S & M" clubs, 20 to 30% of whom were female (McConaghy, 1993). Over 50% of the men and 21% of the women were aware of sadomasochistic interest by age 14. Beating, bondage, and fetishistic practices were common, and more extreme and dangerous practices rare.

It was suggested in DSM-III-R (American Psychiatric Association, 1987) that fewer than 10% of rapists had sexual sadism. They inflicted suffering on the victim far in excess of that necessary for compliance and found the visible pain of the victim sexually arousing. Knight and Prentky (1990) were unable to substantiate this distinction between sadistic and nonsadistic rapists, consistent with the finding that a significant percentage of men considered normal are aroused by descriptions of rape in which the woman experiences pain or is humiliated (Malamuth & Check, 1983; Pfaus, Myronuk, & Jacobs, 1986).

Fetishists are almost invariably male and in childhood commonly experience a strong interest in particular objects, most commonly clothing or footwear (the interest becoming associated with sexual arousal disproportionate to that produced by secondary sexual characteristics at puberty). The subject's wearing the clothing of the opposite sex is termed *transvestic fetishism*. At least in some pubertal and adolescent boys, transvestic fetishism will be followed by the adult form of transvestism. When the object was a body part, such as hair, feet, or hands, or a deformity or mutilation, the condition was termed *partialism* in DSM-IV draft criteria (American Psychiatric Association, 1993).

Frotteurism is defined by some researchers as the pressing of the subject's penis against the body of an unknown woman, and toucheurism as the intimate touching of an unknown woman (Freund, 1990). Both are carried out in public, usually in crowded situations.

Although some degree of feeling like a member of and wishing to belong to the opposite sex is associated with homosexual feelings in adults (McConaghy, 1987a), the term *gender identity disorder* is restricted to those adults with an urge to cross-dress (transvestism). The development of an operation to convert male to female genitalia led to recognition that some men with this urge wished to live permanently as women. They, and the smaller number of women who sought some degree of sex conversion to live permanently as men, were termed *transsexuals*. Transvestism was restricted to the condition of those men who were satisfied to cross-dress periodically. Members of both groups report cross-dressing in childhood, but during puberty typically transvestites, unlike transsexuals, experience sexual arousal with cross-dressing. The intensity of sexual arousal decreases in adulthood, when most transvestites say cross-dressing is associated with feeling relaxed, relieved of responsibility, and sensual, elegant, and beautiful (Buhrich, 1977). However, if they resist desires to cross-dress when stimulated to do so, they experience increased tension, which appears responsible for the compulsive quality of the behavior. Transvestites are predominantly heterosexual and usually marry. Some seek sex conversion in middle age. Periodic cross-dressing to feel masculine appears not to have been reported in women.

Transsexuals are typically attracted to members of their own biological sex. Presence of marked wishes to be of the opposite sex accompanied by extreme opposite-sex behavior in childhood—in boys, dressing in female clothes, using cosmetics and jewelry, and walking and posturing like girls, and in girls, marked tomboyism—is termed *gender identity disorder of childhood*. It is probably incorrectly considered categorically different from the milder forms of opposite sex–linked behaviors, called sissiness and tomboyism by the lay public (McConaghy, 1993).

Associated Features

When exhibitionists and voyeurs present for treatment in adulthood, most are in satisfactory sexual relationships and report a stable work history, appearing to show no obvious personality problems (Langevin & Lang, 1987; Smukler & Schiebel, 1975). Male homosexual pedophiles and hebephiles, although commonly of average intelligence or above, report an inability to find any social or sexual interest in adults of either sex. Male heterosexual pedophiles are more likely to be heavy drinkers and of lower socioeconomic class, to have had little schooling, and to have committed other criminal offenses (McConaghy, 1993). Members of sadomasochistic clubs have been found to be of above average intelligence and social status. The women are more likely to be bisexual, most of the men being predominantly heterosexual (Breslow, Evans, & Langley, 1985; Moser & Livitt, 1987). Transvestites tend to be of higher socioeconomic class than transsexuals and more stable in their relationships and occupation than male (but not female) transsexuals. The degree of opposite sex–linked behavior in male but not female children correlates with their degree of homosexual (compared to heterosexual) feeling in adulthood (McConaghy, 1987a). At this time the majority of boys exhibiting the high degree of opposite sex–linked behaviors present in gender identity disorder identify as homosexual (Zuger, 1966, 1984). Less information is available about the outcome of girls with the disorder.

Epidemiology

Information concerning the prevalence of sexually deviant behaviors is limited. It was not investigated in surveys of mental disorder in representative community samples (McConaghy, 1993). Person, Terestman, Myers, Goldberg, and Salvadori (1989) reported an investigation of the sexual activities of male university students over the previous 3 months. Four percent reported exhibiting in public; 4% watching others make love; 3% being tied and bound during sexual activities; 1% dressing in the clothes of the opposite sex; 1% degrading a sexual partner; and 1% being whipped or beaten by a partner. Twenty-one percent reported a lifetime prevalence of having exhibited in public; the lifetime prevalence of the other practices was not stated. Templeman and Stinnett (1991) found that 65% of 57 male undergraduates had engaged in some form of sexual misconduct, although only 2 had been arrested for sexual offenses. Two others had been in trouble with parents, school, or employers for their sexual behavior. Voyeurism was the most common offense, reported by 42%; frottage was reported by 35% and making obscene phone calls by 8%. Only one subject reported exhibitionism, which appears inconsistent with the generally stated finding that this is the most common offense for which men are charged or seek treatment (McConaghy, 1993). The students were raised and educated in primarily rural environments, where this offense may be more rarely carried out, because the possibility of being recognized would be greater than in urban environments. Three (5%) revealed coercive sexual behaviors, consistent with the percentage of male students reporting the use of some physical force to obtain sexual acts in the United States and Australia (McConaghy, 1993). Two reported sexual contacts with girls younger than 12, and a further 3 sexual contact with girls aged 13 to 15 when they were more than 20 years of age.

Prevalence of sexually arousing paraphilic fantasies and possibly of urges to act on them is much higher. Studies of normal men revealed that more than 30% reported sexual fantasies of tying up and of raping a woman, and 10 to 20% of torturing or beating up a woman (Crepault & Couture, 1980; Person et al., 1989). Of Australian and United States university students asked about the likelihood of their carrying out sexual acts if there was no possibility of the acts being discovered, the percentage of men reporting some likelihood of using force on or raping a postpubertal person or of having sexual activity with a child was 32 to 41%, 14 to 18%, and 14 to 16%, respectively (Malamuth,1989; McConaghy, Zamir, & Manicavasagar, 1993). Women students in the United States studies were not asked these questions; 2%, 0, and 4% of the Australian women reported some likelihood of carrying out these behaviors.

Women were reported to be perpetrators of pedophilia in from 4% (Russell, 1983) to 19% of offenses against girls and from 17% (Finkelhor, 1985) to 75% (Fromuth & Burkhart, 1989) of offenses against boys. Women were assailants in 25% of sexual assaults of adults analyzed in a supplementary study of the Los Angeles NIMH Epidemiologic Catchment Area survey (Sorenson, Stein, Siegel, Golding, & Burnam, 1987). However, women rarely seek treatment or are charged with sexual assault or pedophilia. They were convicted of 1% of sexual offenses and 1.5% of acts of indecency against children in Britain (O'Connor, 1987).

In a national survey of 2,000 subjects (Hunt, 1974), sexual pleasure was obtained by 4.8% of men and 2.1% of women by inflicting pain and by 2.5% of men and 4.6% of women by receiving pain. In Person et al.'s (1989) investigation of university students' sexual experience in the prior 3 months, 4 to 6% of women reported sexual acts in which they were forced to submit, bound, and degraded, and 1% reported being tortured, beaten, or whipped, or torturing a partner. A smaller percentage of men reported similar experiences. Although it was not stated that the subjects were consenting, this was implied by their being described as sadomasochistic and presented in relation to reports of a much higher percentage of the students having sexual fantasies of these acts. Penile circumference assessment of paraphilias in 66 normal controls demonstrated clinically significant tendencies to sadism (defined as nonsexual violence against fully clothed females) in 5%, pedophilia in 18%, and at least one paraphilia in 28% (Fedora et al., 1992).

No attempt appears to have been made to determine the prevalence of gender identity disorders in children, or the percentage of men who identify as transvestites. In the study of Person et al. (1989), 4% of female and 1% of male university students reported dressing in the clothes of the opposite sex in the previous 3 months. The motivation for the behavior was not reported, but 3% of the men and 2% of the women reported recent sexual fantasies of dressing in clothes of the opposite sex. Fifteen of 138 male medical students but none of 58 female medical students reported that they had obtained sexual arousal from dressing in the external or underclothes of the opposite sex (McConaghy, 1982).

The reported prevalence of transsexualism has steadily increased since the condition was recognized. Estimated rates for male-to-female and female-to-male transsexualism, respectively, were 1 in 100,000 and 1 in 400,000 in the United States in 1968; 1 in 37,000 and 1 in 100,000 in Sweden in 1968 and in the United Kingdom in 1974; 1 in 45,000 and 1 in 200,000 in the Netherlands in 1980; 1 in 26,000 and 1 in 100,000 in the Netherlands in 1983; and 1 in 18,000 and 1 in 54,000 in the Netherlands in 1986 (Eklund, Gooren, & Bezemer, 1988). The highest figure as yet reported was a prevalence of 1 in 2,900 for male and 1 in 8,300 for female Singapore-born transsexuals (Tsoi, 1988). Eklund et al. (1988) pointed out the ratio of male-to-female and female-to-male transsexuals tended to remain constant at about 3:1. There was no trend for the age of subjects seeking treatment to be younger in the more recent studies, which they argued would be the case if the true prevalence of transsexualism had risen. They believed more transsexuals to be seeking sex conversion because of the increasingly benevolent social climate concerning the procedure.

Etiology

The etiology of sexual deviations is best understood by combining three current models commonly seen as independent: the stimulus control, cognitive, and psychiatric-psychopathological models (McConaghy, 1993). The stimulus control model proposed that deviant behaviors are motivated by sexual arousal to the relevant deviant stimuli. One of its inadequacies was pointed out when it was found that men who had received aversive therapy were able to control homosexual behaviors they had experienced as compulsive, while continuing to be aware of their homosexual feelings (McConaghy, 1976). The theory was modified by the suggestion that behavior completion mechanisms (BCMs) are established in the brain for behaviors that are carried out repeatedly. When a person is exposed to a stimulus for the behavior (i.e., a situation in which he or she previously carried out the behavior), the BCM for that behavior is activated. The BCM then monitors incoming stimuli to determine that the behavior is being completed. If it is not, the BCM stimulates the brain arousal system, with a resultant increase in heart rate, sweating, and feelings of generalized excitement, tension, or anxiety, which can be experienced as sufficiently unpleasant for the person to feel driven to complete the behavior. Aversive therapy was considered to act by inhibiting the BCM for the related stimuli (McConaghy, 1980). The BCM modification also accounted for the observation that with the repetition of such deviations as exhibitionism, voyeurism, and transvestism, subjects report the carrying out of the behaviors to be accompanied by increased generalized excitement rather than sexual arousal. Sexual arousal would appear to still play some part in their motivation, as its reduction by testosterone-reducing agents appear effective in their treatment.

The BCM modification of the stimulus control hypothesis predicts that sexual behaviors carried out repeatedly may become compulsive. A significant percentage of normal subjects experience some sexual arousal to deviant stimuli in imagination, and evidence cited earlier indicates that a high percentage of male adolescents express this arousal in behaviors at least occasionally (either seeking out situations where such expression is possible or encountering them fortuitously). In some this behavior could therefore be expected to become compulsively driven by these situations, so that if the subjects subsequently attempted to cease the behaviors, they would find this difficult or impossible.

The stimulus control model in relation to sexual offenses against women (and to a lesser extent children) was criticized on the basis that such offenses were not sexually motivated but were an expression of men's cognitions that they must maintain power over and dominate women to preserve the social system of male patriarchy. Palmer (1988) critically reviewed and rejected the arguments that sexual assault was not sexually motivated. Proponents of the cognitive model of sexual deviations (Herman, 1990) ignored the evidence cited earlier that men are victims of one-third of sexually coercive acts and that women carry out a significant percentage of them. The radical feminist version proposed that all men were likely to sexually assault women (Palmer, 1988). To account for the fact that only a small percentage do, other theorists considered that men's likelihood of assaulting women was determined by the degree to which they held rape-supportive cognitions, including those labeled "rape myths" (e.g., that many women have an unconscious wish to be sexually coerced and unconsciously set up situations that provoke such coercion). However, neither incarcerated rapists (Stermac, Segal, & Gilles, 1990) nor sexually assaultive male adolescents (Ageton, 1983) differed from controls in the degree to which they held rape-supportive cognitions. Such cognitions may not differentiate rapists from nonrapists, but may determine social values that increase the prevalence of rape. Cultures that idealize male toughness, encourage interpersonal violence, and give women little political or economic power are associated with high levels of rape (Herman, 1990; Stermac et al., 1990). It was considered that these features characterized United States society and the official figures of incidence of rape as reported to authorities is higher in this than in other Western societies. However, as community studies such as those of Ageton (1983) and Koss and Oros (1982) reveal, incidence of rape reported to authorities provides a poor index of its actual incidence (McConaghy, 1993).

The psychiatric-psychopathological model postulates that offenders may be driven by compulsive impulses, are psychiatrically disordered, or act under the influence of alcohol, and that some victims may have a vulnerability that increases their likelihood of being sexually coerced. Herman (1990) considered that following the initiation of sexual assault by rape-supportive cognitions, addiction to the behavior could develop and require treatment. The psychodynamic model advanced by Groth, Burgess, and Holmstrom (1977) appears to be widely accepted, possibly because of its compatibility with the cognitive theory that rape was not primarily sexually motivated. Groth et al. (1977) distinguished anger and power rapists. Power rapists did not desire to harm their victims but to control them to alleviate doubts of their own sexual adequacy and masculinity, or their sense of identity and effectiveness. Anger rapists expressed anger, rage, contempt, and hatred for their victims by abusing them with profane language, beating them, sexually assaulting them, and forcing them to perform or submit to additional degrading acts, either as an expression of their hostility and rage toward women or because they found pleasure, thrills, and excitation in the suffering of the victim. Data that sexual offenders, particularly child molesters, frequently report having been themselves sexually abused in childhood were criticized as lacking appropriate comparison groups and employing vague definition of childhood sexual abuse (Herman, 1990). Also, Freund, Watson, and Dickey (1990) argued that such offenders may give this history in the hope of obtaining more lenient legal treatment, or unconsciously exaggerate remembered events to reduce feelings of guilt.

The most consistent finding concerning the personality of rapists and child molesters is that a high percentage show evidence of psychopathy, consistent with the finding that a significant number of convicted sex offenders have been convicted also for nonsexual offenses (Ageton, 1983; Knight, Rosenberg, & Schneider, 1985). Ageton, in her study of a representative sample of adolescents, found that sexually assaultive males were basically delinquent youths. About half had been drinking or taking drugs prior to the assault, and female victims considered the offender's drunkenness to have been a major factor in precipitating their assault. Marshall and Barbaree (1990a) found that police and victims confirmed alcohol intoxication in 70% of rapists. Supportive of the victim vulnerability hypothesis, prior to their assault, victims compared to controls showed statistically significant increased evidence of delinquency (Ageton, 1983) and statistically significant higher prevalences of major depression, alcohol and drug abuse, antisocial personality, and phobia (Burnam, et al., 1988). Of 412 university students, lesbian and gay students were three times as likely to report sexual victimization as their heterosexual colleagues (Duncan, 1990).

The current empirical evidence would appear most compatible with a theory that sexual deviations are motivated by sexual arousal to cues for the deviant behaviors, but that an interaction of social attitudes, fortuitous circumstances, personality factors, drug use, and physiologic mechanisms maintaining habitual behaviors determines whether this motivation is expressed in behaviors, and, if so, whether the behaviors are carried out rarely or repeatedly and compulsively.

Differential Diagnosis and Assessment

DSM-III-R and DSM-IV Categorization

The DSM-III-R categorization of sexual disorders stated that the term *paraphilia* was preferable to sexual deviation, as it correctly emphasizes that the deviation (para) lies in that to which the person is attracted (philia). This appears to be contradicted by the later statement in DSM-III-R that the imagery in a paraphilic fantasy is frequently the stimulus for sexual excitement in people without a paraphilia. It is further stated in DSM-III-R, as well as in the DSM-IV draft criteria (American Psychiatric Association, 1993), that the diagnosis is made only if the person has acted on the paraphilic urges or is markedly distressed by them, a statement included in each of the diagnostic criteria provided for the paraphilias described earlier, along with a description and a requirement that the urges have been experienced for a period of at least 6 months. DSM-IV draft criteria describe the urges in exhibitionism and voyeurism as sexual.

Transvestism and transsexualism were categorized in DSM-III-R together with gender identity disorder of childhood as gender identity disorders, and included in the disorders usually first evident in infancy, childhood, or adolescence. Transvestism received the cumbersome title of gender identity disorder of adolescence or adulthood, nontranssexual type (GIDAANT). The diagnostic criteria for GIDAANT included persistent or recurrent cross-dressing in the role of the other sex, either in fantasy or actuality, but not for the purposes of sexual excitement (as in transvestic fetishism). This exclusion was criticized in view of the evidence that some degree of sexual arousal to cross-dressing is shown by most transvestites, although many do not wish to acknowledge it (Blanchard, Clemmensen, & Steiner, 1987, McConaghy, 1993). Also, controversy exists as to whether all or only a subgroup of transvestites become increasingly dissatisfied with their biological sex. A number of significant differences in the clinical features of the transvestites who in middle age desired physical sex conversion as compared with those who did not led Buhrich and McConaghy (1977b) to suggest that those desiring sex conversion be classified as marginal transvestites, and those not desiring it, nuclear transvestites. The fact that the two groups did not differ in mean age was considered to indicate that nuclear transvestites do not develop into marginal transvestites. Other workers have also reported differences in the clinical features of the two groups (McConaghy, 1993).

These controversies do not seem to challenge the existence of major differences between the clinical conditions of most transvestites and transsexuals (Buhrich & McConaghy, 1977c) and between both and gender disorder of childhood. However, it was decided in the options for DSM-IV (American Psychiatric Association, 1991) that the distinctions were artificial and cumbersome and all three are incorporated in the DSM-IV draft criteria in a single broad category of gender identity disorder. This disorder is characterized by such features as desire to be of the opposite sex, frequent passing as the opposite sex, or desire to live as or be treated as the opposite sex, along with persistent discomfort with one's assigned sex or sense of inappropriateness in that gender role. It would appear that the latter feelings are not shown by a number of transvestites. Sixty-nine percent of 504 subscribers to *Transvestia*, a magazine for heterosexual cross-dressers, felt that they were men who had a feminine side seeking expression, and 72% hoped to expand their activities and develop their feminine self more fully (Prince & Bentler, 1972). Forty-four percent preferred their masculine self to their feminine self (Prince & Bentler, 1972).

It would seem unfortunate that the DSM-IV draft criteria ignore the frequently expressed and strongly held conviction of transvestites that their condition differs markedly from that of transsexuals, and of both groups that they differ from homosexuals (Buhrich & McConaghy, 1977a; Prince & Bentler, 1972). In the DSM-IV draft criteria, the history of sexual attraction to males, females, or both is to be specified, but no diagnostic significance is attached to the difference. Typically transsexuals are predominantly attracted to members of their own biological sex, are single, and seek sex conversion in late adolescence or early adulthood. Marginal transvestites are attracted to members of the opposite biological sex, are married, and seek sex conversion in middle age. Most male subjects with gender identity disorder in childhood identify themselves in adulthood as homosexual rather than as transvestite or transsexual. These differences would appear of importance in the etiology of the conditions, as well as their management. The failure to distinguish them in the DSM-IV draft criteria makes it likely that clinicians will retain the terms *transsexual* and *transvestite*.

325

**Paraphilias and
Gender Identity
Disorders**

Differential Diagnosis

In clinical practice differential diagnosis of the paraphilias rarely presents difficulties. Although it has been reported that many paraphiliacs reveal with appropriate questioning that they carried out deviations additional to that with which they presented (Freund & Blanchard, 1986), frequency of the behaviors was not given, so that in many subjects they may have been isolated acts. As discussed earlier, it is possible that the majority of adolescents have carried out sexually deviant acts on one or more occasions. In my experience, offenders seeking treatment report having carried out mainly the same deviant behavior, although some have occasionally carried out additional ones (McConaghy, Blaszczynski, Armstrong, & Kidson, 1989). If they have been charged repeatedly, it was usually for the same form of deviation. Although the DSM classifications include the necessity for deviant urges to have been experienced for at least 6 months, with most paraphilias the subjects have been aware of them since adolescence. Some men who have sexually offended against female children report no awareness of an urge to do so, except on the occasion or occasions of actual occurrence. In practice their behavior is nevertheless classified as pedophilia.

Controversy persists concerning the criteria that justify diagnosing as transsexual subjects seeking sex conversion. As stated above, this controversy is unlikely to be resolved by acceptance of the alternate DSM-IV options term of gender identity disorder. Fortunately, the controversy is of little practical significance. There is virtual unanimity that sex conversion be recommended for all subjects who have maintained an emotionally and occupationally stable life as a member of the opposite sex for at least 1, and preferably 2, years (McConaghy, 1993).

Assessment Strategies

The unstructured interview appears to remain the major assessment method for diagnosis and evaluation of paraphilias and gender identity disorders, despite criticism of the reliability of diagnoses reached in this way (Matarazzo, 1983). In none of the studies published from 1989 to 1991 in the *Archives of Sexual Behavior*, a major sexuality research journal, were structured interviews used to reach diagnoses of sexual disorders. In only two was reference made to the employment of DSM-III or DSM-III-R criteria. Failure to use DSM-III criteria could be due, in the case of the paraphilias, to the criteria's adding little of relevance to the descriptions currently accepted by clinicians, and, in the case of the gender disorders, to the controversies concerning them. The reluctance of clinicians to replace unstructured with structured diagnostic interviews possibly reflects failure of the proponents of the latter to demonstrate that their use increases diagnostic validity (McConaghy, 1993). Increased validity would seem necessary to offset loss of the flexibility of the unstructured interview, wherein clinicians can vary the nature and order of their questions as seems appropriate in light of patients' responses and behavior—for example, if they show signs of guilt, embarrassment, or reluctance to talk when particular topics are introduced.

In addition to increasing the likelihood of obtaining useful historical information, the flexibility of the unstructured interview allows the clinician to obtain impressions useful in determining the nature of the patients' personalities. If interviews are commenced nondirectively by the clinician's adopting a listening approach and asking a minimum of questions, patients have the opportunity to take charge. The extent to which they do so allows their confidence, assertiveness, and dominance to be assessed. Determining the presence of significant personality disorders, in particular psychopathy, borderline personality, or inadequate dependency, is as important as determining the nature of patients' sexual difficulties, because these disorders markedly influence not only patients' ability to provide accurate information, but also their motivation to change their behaviors, and the nature of the relationship they attempt to establish with the clinician. If this relationship is handled inappropriately, lack of compliance with or major disruption of the treatment plan can result. During the unstructured interview the treatment process can also be initiated, because such an interview permits the establishment of a relationship in which the patient's confidence and trust in the clinician's abilities are maximized.

Use of structured procedures additional to the diagnostic interview, such as rating scales or diary cards with which the patient records the intensity of sexual urges or frequency of sexual behaviors, are at times reported in research studies. Evidence has been advanced indicating that such procedures can reduce patient compliance (Reading, 1983) and may be of limited validity (McConaghy, in press; Taylor, Agras, Schneider, & Allen, 1983). Apart from its intuitive use as part of the unstructured interview, structured use of observational assessment has been reported of exhibitionist behavior, and of the effeminate behavior of adult males by clinicians, and of boys by clinicians, teachers, or parents (McConaghy, 1988).

Physiologic measures of sexual arousal in paraphiliacs and the gender disordered have largely been restricted to measures of subjects' penile volume or circumference responses to sexual stimuli. In its original form, using penile volume responses to pictures of male and female nudes, the assessment was repeatedly shown to correctly identify a high percentage of individuals as predominantly either heterosexual or homosexual (McConaghy, 1992). Although penile volume responses were recorded within 10 to 15 seconds of exposure to the erotic stimulus and penile circumference responses required at least 2 minutes of exposure, the responses were regarded as equivalent, and it was accepted without supporting research that the findings validating penile volume assessment of sexual orientation validated the use of penile circumference responses. Several years later it was reported that for penile circumference responses to correctly identify most predominantly heterosexual or homosexual men, it is necessary to use the more powerful erotic stimuli of moving films of men and women involved in homosexual activity rather than pictures of single male and female nudes. In the meantime, penile circumference responses to the latter stimuli had become generally accepted in single case studies as the major outcome measure of change in subjects' heterosexual and homosexual feelings.

On the basis of a small number of studies reporting that their penile circumference responses to audiotaped descriptions of sexual activities or pictures of male and female nudes of various ages could identify paraphiliacs, these responses became widely employed in the diagnosis and assessment of change with treatment of individual pedophiles and rapists. This use has continued to be recommended (McAnulty & Adams, 1992), despite subsequent studies with larger subject numbers that failed to discriminate these paraphiliacs from controls (McConaghy, 1989). However, other workers, apparently independently of the author's repeated criticisms, appear to have recently come to the same conclusion as to the limited validity of penile circumference assessment of deviant sexual urges: "If behaviorists are to maintain [their] exaggerated faith in erectile measurements, they must solve the experimental riddle of demonstrating the relevance of changing such indices to the maintenance of offensive behavior and, particularly, to the issue of treatment benefits" (Marshall & Barbaree, 1990b, p. 382).

Monitoring the degree of reduction of paraphiliac subjects' serum testosterone levels provides an accurate measure of the reduction in the intensity of their deviant sexual urges (McConaghy, Blaszczynski, & Kidson, 1988).

Treatment

Evidence for Prescriptive Treatments

Behavior Therapy. Behavior therapy as it was introduced for treatment of paraphilias in the 1960s was based on the concepts that these sexual behaviors were under stimulus control and that such control could be modified by conditioning procedures. Evaluation of the procedures mainly investigated male subjects seeking to reduce homosexual and increase heterosexual feelings. Freund (1960) investigated the use of aversive therapy, in which subjects viewed pictures of dressed and nude men while experiencing nausea and vomiting produced by emetic chemicals. Although the therapy was designed as a classical conditioning procedure, presumably with the aim of replacing sexual arousal with aversion to homosexual stimuli, Freund reported that the majority of subjects continued to report greater homosexual than heterosexual feelings, and loss of homosexual feelings was extremely rare. However, it appears that a number of his subjects reduced the frequency of homosexual activity. Other workers, who mainly employed electric shock as the aversive stimulus, also reported reduction in the subjects' homosexual feelings and behaviors (McConaghy, 1977). The belief that the procedure acted by conditioning to produce an aversive response to homosexual stimuli continued to be accepted throughout the 1960s, although the presence of this aversive response was rarely noted. Finally, at the end of the decade, its absence was emphasized and the suggestion was made that the procedure might not act by conditioning. This suggestion was tested in one of a series of studies evaluating aversive therapy by McConaghy and his colleagues (McConaghy, 1976), in which the validated assessment of the subjects' penile volume responses to moving pictures of nude men and women was used as an outcome measure in addition to the subjects' reported changes in feelings and behavior. It was shown that the same reduction in reported homosexual feelings and behavior followed a backward as a forward aversive procedure (that is, one in which the aversive stimulus preceded rather than followed the stimulus eliciting homosexual feelings). Because backward conditioning is less effective, it was concluded that reduction in homosexual feelings and behavior was not produced by conditioning. It was also found that there was no meaningful alteration in treated subjects' penile volume responses to pictures of nude men and women, indicating that the behavioral changes were not due to alterations in the subjects' homosexual or heterosexual arousability. This was consistent with the subjects' reports that though they still were aware of attraction to men they encountered, if they wished they could cease to fantasize about them, and could cease homosexual behaviors that prior to treatment they had experienced as compulsive.

As discussed earlier, the paradoxical finding that subjects could control homosexual behaviors without reduction in homosexual arousability led to the advancement of the hypothesis that a neurophysiologic behavior completion mechanism independent of sexual arousal contributed to the compulsiveness of habitual sexual behaviors by activating the arousal system, producing a feeling of tension or anxiety until the behavior was carried out. This hypothesis concerning the motivation of compulsive behaviors provided an explanation for reports in the 1960s and 1970s of the efficacy of the anxiety-reducing therapy of systematic desensitization, both in single case studies of exhibitionists and in comparison studies with aversive therapy in groups of homosexuals (McConaghy, 1990b). Possibly because of the absence of a rationale for systematic desensitization therapy alone, an aversive procedure that incorporates it, termed *covert sensitization* (Cautela, 1967), has become the preferred treatment in North America for compulsive sexual behaviors. With it, the patient is trained to relax and then to visualize carrying out the behavior he wishes to control. He then visualizes an aversive stimulus, such as being overcome with nausea. Maletzky (1973) attempted to enhance the efficacy of the procedure by "assisting" the aversive image with a noxious smell. In a review of the use of covert sensitization, Lichstein and Hung (1980) pointed out the lack of investigations of its efficacy that controlled adequately for expectancy effects. Also, most of those using single case design tended to discount the subjects' self-reports and rely on the invalid assessment of penile circumference responses to pictures of nude men and women as measures of changes in homosexual and heterosexual arousability (McConaghy, 1990b).

On the basis of the behavior completion hypothesis, a modification of systematic desensitization termed *imaginal desensitization* was developed (McConaghy, Armstrong, Blaszczynski, & Allcock, 1983). The procedure was similar to covert sensitization except that while relaxed the subject did not visualize terminating the unwanted behavior followed by an aversive stimulus, but instead visualized leaving the situation without carrying out the unwanted behavior but remaining relaxed and feeling in control; that is, no aversive images were incorporated. The aim was that with repetition of the treatment, the subject would learn to relax rather than become aroused in response to the cues for completion of the behavior, and hence be able to control the compulsive urge. Imaginal desensitization proved superior to covert sensitization in treatment of 20 subjects with compulsive homosexuality or paraphilias, who were randomly allocated to one or the other of the two therapies (McConaghy, Armstrong, & Blaszczynski, 1985). No attempts have been made to replicate or reject this finding, and aversive procedures appear to remain the initial behavioral treatment of choice in North America.

In general, behavior therapists in North America followed the operant conditioning model they developed, which tended to use single case designs in evaluative studies and to prefer physiologic measures to subjects' self-report of behavioral change in assessing treatment outcome (McConaghy, 1987b, 1990b). Response of paraphilias to behavioral therapies was therefore largely determined by change in the subjects' penile circumference responses to paraphiliac stimuli. Unlike penile volume responses, which are recorded within 10 to 15 seconds of erotic stimulus onset and which, as Freund (1963) reported, only a few men could modify to the extent that they would be misclassified in terms of their sexual orientation, penile circumference responses require a minimum of a few minutes of exposure to erotic stimuli. This allows subjects time to fantasize alternative stimuli, which could account for such findings as the ability of some subjects to reduce their penile circumference responses to arousing stimuli (Laws & Rubin, 1969) and for normal subjects to influence their responses to pictures of children so as to appear pedophilic (Quinsey & Bergersen, 1976). When subjects are being treated with aversive therapy for paraphilias, it is likely that a number, consciously or unconsciously, will modify their responses so as not to respond to the deviant stimuli. This could account for the failure of such changes to correlate with the treated subjects' behavioral outcome (Marshall & Barbaree, 1988; Rice, Quinsey, & Harris, 1991).

When for whatever reason subjects' paraphilic penile circumference responses do not change following covert sensitization and electric shock aversive therapy, satiation therapy has been recommended (Marshall, Earls, Segal, & Darke, 1983). The subject is instructed to masturbate continuously for 1 hour, whether or not he ejaculates during that time, while verbalizing every variation he can imagine concerning his deviant fantasies. The procedure can be carried out under supervision or at home, where the subject records his verbalization so that the therapist can check that he was following the instructions given. Change in subjects' penile circumference responses to paraphiliac stimuli appear to be considered acceptable evidence of the treatment's efficacy (Laws & Marshall, 1991).

The most commonly employed behavioral techniques to increase paraphiliacs' heterosexual arousability is termed *orgasmic* or *masturbatory reconditioning* or *retraining*. In its original form the subject was asked to masturbate and to report when orgasm was imminent, whereupon he was shown the picture of an attractive, scantily dressed woman until he reported ejaculation. Ten years after its introduction, Conrad and Winzce (1976) pointed out that the evidence of its efficacy had not gone beyond the case study level. In their own evaluation they relied upon the invalid penile circumference responses to pictures of nudes to assess subjects' heterosexual arousal. Laws and Marshall (1991) distinguished between the commonly used variation, in which the subjects used deviant fantasies initially, and directed masturbation, in which they were instructed to use exclusively heterosexual fantasies from the commencement of masturbation. Laws and Marshall believed that there were inadequate data to support the efficacy of the thematic shift procedure, but there was some evidence that directed masturbation might be effective. They ignored the fact that such evidence was largely based on changes in the invalid assessment of sexual arousal by penile circumference responses to pictures of nude women. Evidence indicating that organic reconditioning was likely to be ineffective was reported in an investigation of men who sought treatment for compulsive homosexual feelings (McConaghy, 1978). The valid penile volume assessment of their balance of heterosexual to homosexual feelings was employed. Men who had repeatedly experienced orgasm in the presence of female cues, namely female sexual partners, showed no evidence of increased heterosexual arousability compared to men without this experience.

In the last decade social skills and assertive training have also been employed with the aim of improving paraphilic subjects' heterosocial skills. These therapies usually were incorporated in multimodal approaches, which included one or more of the behavior therapies reviewed, which aimed to reduce deviant preferences, as well as cognitive therapies discussed subsequently. James (1978) found that addition of social skills training, sex education, and training in dating behavior and interpretation of women's nonverbal communication produced little improvement in homosexual subjects' ability to develop heterosexual relationships.

Studies in the 1960s reported that emetic and electric shock aversive therapy enabled about 50% of transvestites to cease cross-dressing behaviors (McConaghy, 1993). There appears to be little recent information concerning behavior therapy for the condition. Similarly, there appears to be no follow-up of earlier isolated reports of the efficacy of behavioral procedures for transsexuals. Aversive therapy was combined with modification of female-specific patterns of sitting, walking, and standing by modeling and videotape feedback, with reinforcement by verbal praise when the patterns changed in the masculine direction (McConaghy, 1993). The few subjects seeking sex conversion who accepted such behavioral approaches were considered atypical (Green, 1978). Reinforcement of masculine behavior and withdrawal of reinforcement for feminine behaviors were reported to be successful in single case studies of gender-disordered children. Other workers reported similar success by admitting such children to a child psychiatric unit, without attempting to encourage same-sex behaviors (McConaghy, 1990b).

Pharmacotherapy. Use of pharmacotherapy in the treatment of paraphilias has mainly aimed at reduction of the intensity of the subjects' sexual urges. In the past the phenothiazine thioridazine was employed after reduction in sexual urges was noted as a side effect of its use with psychiatric patients. However, in view of the lack of certainty of the effect and the likelihood of other severe side effects, the drug appears to have been replaced by chemicals that have the specific action of lowering the subjects' testosterone levels. High correlations were reported (McConaghy et al., 1988) between the degree of reduction of subjects' testosterone levels and of deviant sexual urges following administration of medroxyprogesterone acetate (MPA), the chemical generally used for this purpose in North America. No long-term placebo-controlled trials of MPA therapy have been conducted. Gagne (1981) found no relapse over 2 years in 40 of 48 sex offenders who initially received MPA 200 mg intramuscularly 2 to 3 times weekly, reduced to 100 mg weekly to monthly as a maintenance dose. Gagne reported that the patients generally became impotent for some period, and all reported side effects that included fatigue, weight gain, hot and cold flashes, headache, and insomnia. In contrast Langevin et al. (1979) reported disappointing results in a comparison of MPA and assertive training. Of the 37 exhibitionists treated, 20 dropped out of treatment. Of the remainder, 6 of 12 treated with assertive training and 1 of 5 treated with MPA and assertive training recidivated. Of the 10 who had not recidivated, 7 had urges to expose.

In light of the behavior completion model of compulsive sexuality, it was suggested (McConaghy et al., 1988) that MPA, by reducing the strength of the patients' deviant sexual urges, allowed them to control these urges in the presence of cues that provoked them. Over time the behavior completion mechanisms for the deviant behaviors would therefore be extinguished, so that when treatment ceased, most patients would not experience returning deviant urges as compulsive. Other workers had reported persistence of the therapeutic effect of androgen-suppressing chemicals following their withdrawal (Bradford, 1990). The hypothesis stimulated investigation of the use of a short period of MPA therapy at a dose sufficient to reduce the intensity of the subjects' deviant urges to render them controllable, while not producing impotence. Thirty sex offenders were randomly allocated, 10 to receive MPA alone, 10 imaginal desensitization alone, and 10 the combined therapies (McConaghy et al., 1988). The dosage of MPA was 150 mg every 2 weeks for 2 months and then monthly for 4 months, which on average reduced subjects' testosterone levels to about 30% of pretreatment levels. Only 2 of the 20 subjects treated with MPA reported some degree of impotence, which caused them to reduce their frequency of intercourse and which disappeared with cessation of the medication. There was no significant difference in response to the three treatments at 1-year follow-up, no deviant behavior being reported by 7 subjects following imaginal desensitization alone, by 8 following MPA alone, and by 9 following the combined treatment. Four of the 6 patients who did not respond to the initial therapy responded to the alternative therapy, 2 requiring addition of electric shock aversion therapy. The results were comparable to those of the high-dose prolonged therapy used by Gagne (1981).

Alternative Treatments.   The major alternative treatments to behavior therapy and pharmacotherapy currently employed are cognitive therapies. Use of castration, considered to act by reduction of subjects' blood testosterone levels, was critically reviewed by Heim and Hursch (1979). Although it was never evaluated in appropriate comparison studies, and some offenders continued to achieve erections for many years following castration, it would seem that the majority of those treated did not reoffend. Ethical objections to the procedure appear to have resulted in the employment of pharmacotherapy when reduction in subjects' testosterone is considered appropriate.

Watson's rejection of the role of mental processes in behavior, an approach maintained by Skinner (McConaghy, 1987b), influenced psychologists who adopted an operant conditioning approach to ignore their treated subjects' cognitions. Behavior therapists, mainly those working outside North America, who based their approach on Pavlovian theory considered it essential to investigate and modify their subjects' cognitions, consistent with the importance given cognitive processes in Pavlovian theory. Wolpe (1958), in his seminal monograph, "Psychotherapy by Reciprocal Inhibition," emphasized that correction of subjects' faulty beliefs was a necessary component of the behavior therapy he practiced. Subsequently, most behaviorally oriented psychologists in North America have come to accept the need for this component. The return to the approach traditionally adopted by both lay people and scientists in explaining human behavior had inconsistently been termed the cognitive revolution in psychotherapy (Mahoney, 1977), rather than the cognitive reaction. Some therapists adopt one of the available systematic cognitive approaches, such as rational-emotive therapy, developed by Ellis (1973). However, there is no convincing evidence that any of these systematic approaches is more effective than another, or than the less systematic cognitive corrections incorporated into the initial and subsequent interviews accompanying the administration of behavioral techniques in the model described by Wolpe.

The content of the cognitive changes most commonly advocated for treatment of sex offenders against women and children is based on the theory that the offenses are expressions of men's need to dominate women and children. The aim of treatment is to make the offender aware of and then eliminate cognitions supportive of rape and child sexual abuse and to accept total responsibility for his behavior rather than attribute it to the victim. He is also encouraged to develop understanding of the harmful effects of his behavior on his victims and empathy with their experiences, by such techniques as being confronted by them, or writing accounts of the victim's emotional experience of the offense. Some behaviorally oriented workers (Quinsey & Earls, 1990) have suggested that such cognitive therapies for sex offenders may not require the addition of behavioral approaches, arguing that in view of the variety of behavioral treatments used to modify sexual arousal patterns, all of which appeared at least somewhat effective, all may act nonspecifically. Other workers who accept the cognitive perspective on the initiation of sexual assault just described (Herman, 1990) have considered that addiction to it could develop secondarily and require specific treatment, such as painstaking documentation of the offender's sexual fantasy and arousal, his modus operandi for securing access to his victims and evading detection, his preferred sexual activities, and his system of excuses and rationalizations, and changes in these must be closely monitored.

Herman (1990) was critical of treatments based on psychodynamic formulations, such as those of Groth discussed earlier, which describe rapists as committing their crimes in efforts to combat deep-seated feelings of insecurity and vulnerability or to express wishes for virility, masculinity, and dominance. She considered such formulations to result in the victimizer being seen as a victim, no longer an object of fear but of pity, and in the risk that the would-be therapist would accept the offender's rationalizations for his crimes as well as supplying him with new ones. This risk could be reduced by the requirement that a victim impact statement describing the offender's crime be available in the case record before any form of treatment is attempted, and it should be frequently reviewed to counteract tendencies toward denial and minimization of the offense, which patient and therapist may share.

The availability of the wide variety of behavioral and cognitive techniques described, the failure to investigate the limited empirical evidence that imaginal desensitization is superior to aversive procedures in giving subjects control over paraphilic urges, and the absence of evidence of differential suitability of the techniques for different patient groups have resulted in widespread acceptance that a selection be used in multimodal form, the particular selection being determined by the clinical experience and theoretical beliefs of the therapist.

Quinsey (1986) reported on the response of self-referred sex offenders treated with covert sensitization and masturbatory satiation, cognitive restructuring, social and assertiveness skills, and sex education: 89% of 44 contacted at 6 months and 79% of 19 contacted at 12 months under confidential conditions reported no recidivism. Travin, Bluestone, Coleman, Cullen, and Melella (1986) reported a lower rate of recidivism over a shorter follow-up period with similar therapy in more highly selected sex offenders. These results were not superior to those reported with therapy focused mainly on the use of imaginal desensitization with brief nonstructured cognitive restructuring carried out during follow-up interviews (McConaghy et al., 1985, 1988). However, such comparisons cannot be accepted as meaningful in view of the lack of control of subject differences. McConaghy et al. (1985, 1988) treated all subjects who sought help for deviant urges they could not control in a cost-free program tailored to allow those employed to continue to work. The selection procedures and cost of the other programs were not specified, as is usual.

Rice et al. (1991), in a 6-year follow-up study, reported failure of a multimodal program incorporating electric shock aversive therapy to reduce recidivism in 50 extrafamilial child molesters who received the therapy in addition to the institutional regimen of a maximum security psychiatric institution. Their outcome was compared with that of 86 child molesters who received the regimen only. However, the 50 were not randomly selected from the total group of offenders, and the authors had doubts about the comparability of the two groups.

Failure to use random allocation also rendered uninterpretable potentially valuable treatment comparison studies by Marshall and Barbaree (1988) and Marshall, Eccles, and Barbaree (1991). In these studies the comparison subjects were denied treatment because they lived too far away from the clinic to permit regular attendance. Marshall et al. (1991) argued that because the groups did not differ on a few demographic variables, they could be treated as if the subjects were randomly allocated. However, the groups could have differed on numerous other variables that might have affected the outcome. Also, differences in location may have offered different opportunities for reoffending or being detected if reoffenses occurred. A further problem with the design of the studies is that untreated controls are an unsatisfactory comparison group. Probably the most consistent finding of meta-analyses of psychotherapies has been the marked superiority of the outcome of subjects who received placebo therapy compared to that of untreated controls. The latter group often deteriorated over the period of investigation, possibly due to their negative reaction to not being offered treatment (McConaghy, 1990a, 1993). Many of the sex offenders I have interviewed initially expressed their resentment that they had never been offered adequate treatment previously.

Using a multimodal cognitive behavioral program similar to that reported by Quinsey (1986), Marshall and Barbaree (1988) compared the outcome for 58 untreated child molesters with 68 treated over the period 1976 to 1984. Five percent of the treated group reoffended in 1 to 2 years, and 25% by 4 years. Reoffense rate was significantly lower than that of the untreated subjects only after 4 years, by which time 60% of the untreated group had reoffended. Similar multimodal therapy was administered to 23 of 44 exhibitionists (Marshall et al., 1991). In a follow-up of more than 8 years, 39% of the treated and 57% of the untreated subjects reoffended, either being charged or being reported in police files for exhibiting without being charged. Marshall et al. (1991) also treated a subsequent group of 17 exhibitionists from 1984 to 1987 with a multimodal procedure that the authors stated shifted the major focus from sexual deviance to changing cognitions. It dispensed with aversive therapy by electric shock but retained covert sensitization. Covert sensitization produced control of compulsive sexual behavior equal to that achieved with electric shock aversive therapy (McConaghy, Armstrong, & Blaszczynski, 1981). In a 4-year follow-up of the exhibitionists, Marshall et al. (1991) reported that 23% reoffended. The authors justified comparison with the earlier treated group on the basis that of those who reoffended in the 8-year follow-up, 91% did so in the first 4 years. They compared the combined responses of the earlier treated and untreated groups with the later treated group, to report that the later treated group showed a statistically significantly superior response. If their response was compared only with that of the earlier treated group, however, the difference was not statistically significant (Exact Test). However, the difference in relapse rates following the two different multimodal procedures (23% and 39%) would be clinically meaningful if replicated, and it is unfortunate that the possibility cannot be excluded that the difference was due to variation in the two groups of subjects who sought and were selected for treatment during the earlier and later periods. Certainly, the results of comparison studies of this sort are urgently needed provided subjects are randomly allocated to the different procedures currently in use. There would appear to be no ethical objection to random allocation to different treatments when there is no acceptable evidence that one is superior to another.

Regarding alternative treatment for gender disorders, Prince and Bentler (1972) reported that psychotherapy brought about a temporary cure in only 5% of transvestites who sought treatment, and 53% considered it a waste of time and money. Croughan, Saghir, Cohen, & Robins (1981) reported that treatment, mainly psychotherapy alone, played virtually no role in bringing about periods of abstinence from cross-dressing in the transvestites they investigated. There also appears to be widespread agreement that psychotherapy is rarely accepted as an alternative to sex conversion by transsexuals (McConaghy, 1993).

Selecting Optimal Treatment Strategies

As the previous discussion indicated, there is insufficient empirical evidence to select optimal strategies for treatment of subjects with sexually deviant behaviors, so they are determined by the individual clinician on the basis of his or her experience. My practice is that while interviewing the patient to determine the nature of his problem and the possible presence of significant personality disorder, I also establish what the patient wants from treatment and decide to what extent this is appropriate and achievable and whether it is in the interest of the patient or the community that he be encouraged to adopt additional aims. In view of my belief in the efficacy of imaginal desensitization in giving patients control over sexual urges they experience as compulsive, I attempt to determine if they wish to cease their paraphilic behaviors but find this difficult or impossible. If this is the major problem (as is usually the case with exhibitionists, voyeurs, and transvestites, and is true of some pedophiles), and if apart from the paraphilia they report a satisfactory occupational, sexual, and social life, I proceed to offer them the choice of either imaginal desensitization or medroxy-progestrone (MPA) therapy. My expectation is that with either treatment the majority of these subjects will report a marked reduction in the intensity of deviant urges, and the ability to control them. In view of the evidence that there are no effective procedures that alter subjects' sexual preferences, I do not employ strategies aimed at such alteration (McConaghy, 1976, 1980). More recently other workers, apparently independently of the author's findings and conclusions, have adopted a similar aim. Marshall et al. (1991) recommend that cognitive-behavioral programs treating rapists and exhibitionists shift their emphasis from a sexual deviant orientation toward social, cognitive, and attitudinal problems. However, in their program they retain aversive procedures, suggesting they were at some level aware of the possible existence of compulsive sexual behaviors that were driven by mechanisms other than the deviant sexual urges.

If the subject chooses imaginal desensitization, he is asked to describe four situations in which he commonly carried out the compulsive activities or thought of doing so. Influenced by previous experience in treating phobic patients with systematic desensitization, I consider that the necessary information concerning these situations can be obtained from the patients within a few minutes and detailed analysis of the compulsive behaviors is not required. The subject's descriptions of typical situations is altered in that he does not feel impelled to carry out the compulsive behaviors, but leaves the situation in a relaxed state without having done so. For this reason it was recently suggested that the treatment would be better called alternative behavior completion (ABC). A typical scenario for an exhibitionist would be: "You are walking along a quiet street and see a teenaged girl walking toward you. As she approaches, the thought of exposing yourself comes into your mind. You realize the urge is not strong and you can control it. You walk past her without exposing."

As ABC was administered in the evaluative studies reviewed, in the first session of about 20 minutes' duration, the subject was given brief training in relaxation. With systematic desensitization, patients were initially trained over several hours in a progressive muscular relaxation procedure (Wolpe, 1958). I found from clinical experience that this training could be markedly curtailed without apparent loss of therapeutic efficacy. With the modified procedure, the patient lies comfortably on a couch in a darkened room, with his arms by his sides and his eyes closed. He is then asked to clench his fists and concentrate on the tension in them. After about 20 seconds he is asked to relax them and concentrate on the sensation of his hands feeling limp and heavy. He is then asked similarly to tense and then relax progressively his arms, legs, stomach, neck, and facial muscles, while concentrating on the accompanying feeling of tension or relaxation. He is finally asked to tense further any muscle groups that feel tense and then to relax them and to signal by raising the index finger visible to the therapist when he feels relaxed. This procedure is carried out within 5 minutes with the therapist conveying complete conviction that the patient will be relaxed at its termination. It is extremely rare for patients not to signal that they are relaxed.

When the patient signals he is relaxed, the therapist instructs the patient to visualize performing the first behavior of one of the scenarios and to signal when he is doing so and is relaxed. Once he does so, after a few seconds the therapist instructs him to visualize performing the next behavior in the scenario and to signal when he is doing so and is relaxed, and so on until the patient signals he is visualizing leaving the situation without having carried out the compulsive behavior and is feeling relaxed. In the form evaluated in the studies reviewed, ABC was administered in this manner in a total of 14 sessions over 1 week. Currently, to render the procedure more cost-effective, I audiotape the initial and two or three subsequent personally administered sessions and encourage the patient to listen to the tape a few times a week between the sessions. In this form the treatment is carried out over several weeks, with the patient gradually reducing the frequency with which he listens to the tape. Although my clinical impression is that this form is equally effective, it has not been evaluated in comparison studies.

If the patient chooses MPA as the initial therapy, prior to its commencement at a dosage of 150 mg intramuscularly every 2 weeks, his serum testosterone level is estimated between 11:00 A.M. and noon to control for fluctuations that occur throughout the day. If prior to the third injection he reports that deviant urges are still strong, blood is taken for a further testosterone estimation and the dose is doubled. Usually when the result becomes available it is found that the level has not been reduced to about 30% of the pretreatment level, and the higher dose is maintained. If prior to the third injection he reports good control but some degree of impotence, testosterone estimation is again made and the medication resumed at a lower dose after a few weeks when his potency has returned. In these subjects it is usually found that the initial dose level reduced their serum testosterone level to about 10% of the pretreatment level. If the subject who receives initial MPA therapy reports continuance of strong urges for more than 2 weeks after his serum testosterone level is reduced to below 30%, or the subject who receives initial ABC reports similarly after 8 sessions of individually administered or taped sessions, I suggest the addition of the other therapy. If his urges persist I recommend the still further addition of electric shock aversive therapy.

This treatment program has proved effective in giving good control to virtually all subjects with compulsions to carry out sexually deviant urges that they could not cease. The few who did not respond showed ambivalent motivation about ceasing the behaviors, usually in association with marked personality disorder of a borderline or psychopathic nature, or mental impairment.

For subjects, often those with dependent or avoidant personalities, who in addition to their compulsive paraphilic behaviors report inadequacies in their relationships due to social or sexual phobias or lack of assertiveness, I recommend ABC. In addition to scenarios dealing with their deviant sexual urges, others are added in which they act out the behaviors about which they are anxious. Subjects are then encouraged to perform these behaviors in homework sessions. However, my experience with these and related behavioral procedures, such as social skills training is that although patients report feeling more relaxed in social situations, they do not show significant improvement in their social and sexual relationships. This has led me to recommend addition of surrogate therapy for those with marked fears about engaging in sexual relationships.

A few of the patients are confident that their deviant behavior has not been compulsive and that they could easily cease it in the future. The major aim of treatment is then to encourage them to explore their motivation for carrying out the behavior in the past and to develop cognitions that will motivate them to cease the behavior in the future. These patients are most commonly offenders against children or adolescents. A number of homosexual pedophiles or hebephiles who appear ethical and responsible in other areas of their lives believe that their deviant sexual behavior should be socially accepted. Heterosexual pedophiles tend to fall into two groups. Members of one also appear ethical and responsible; their offense occurred in a situation where they fortuitously were alone with the victim and suddenly became aware of and impulsively acted on a feeling of sexual arousal toward her. They are extremely guilty about and highly motivated not to repeat the behavior. Members of the second group give a history indicative of low ethical standards, often associated with a socially and educationally deprived development, and evidence of psychopathic personality or intellectual impairment. They are commonly unemployed, drink heavily, and are at home alone during the day, when their offenses took place repeatedly with a relative or child of neighbors. While one attempts to develop appropriate cognitions in the latter group of subjects and in homosexual pedophiles and hebephiles, reduction of their sexual interest with MPA is advisable.

Problems in Carrying Out Interventions

Personality disorders, intellectual impairment, psychosis that has not fully responded to treatment, or some combination of these presents major problems in both assessment and treatment. Patients with personality disorders are likely to distort their history, those with psychopathy to make a favorable impression, and those with borderline disorder to emotionally involve the therapist to elicit sympathy, sexual interest, or alarm at the severity of their problem (in the last case at times by reporting sexually aggressive behaviors that it proves impossible to obtain evidence of their ever having performed). Patients with psychosis or intellectual impairment are commonly unable to give adequate details of their past behaviors. Also, the therapist may feel uncertain of their ability to give informed consent to treatment procedures, and will need to decide whether to obtain opinions concerning this from independent professionals, in addition to the judgment of the patients' legal guardians.

In treating patients with personality disorders, in addition to instituting the program described, my practice has been to inform them that I believe they have a personality problem that will require more intensive help. I will guarantee to see them regularly for as long as necessary at a frequency we both agree is acceptable. My aim is to gain their respect over time, with the hope that this will motivate them to wish to maintain my approval and, where appropriate, increase their self-esteem (as they come to believe that someone they respect shows concern for them sufficient to go on seeing them indefinitely). At the same time I encourage them to correct faulty cognitions concerning their evaluation of themselves and the behavior of others and guide and reinforce their attempts to develop stable and satisfying occupational, leisure, social, and sexual activities. In treating patients with intellectual impairment or psychosis, their difficulty in establishing and maintaining cognitions motivating cessation of deviant behaviors needs to be taken into account. For this reason it is commonly advisable to employ prolonged administration of MPA. Some patients who receive MPA for longer than 6 months begin to show a reduced response. It is therefore necessary to monitor the testosterone levels of these patients every few months to detect any increase. If any is found, the dose of MPA can be increased or other chemicals that reduce testosterone levels added.

Programs that treat offenders are not available in many areas, possibly in part reflecting the view I have frequently heard from some therapists that such offenders should be treated only as criminals. Some patients seeking treatment therefore come considerable distances. This can present a problem in maintaining adequate evaluation of their behaviors over the prolonged period required for follow-up.

The mandatory reporting of child sexual abuse requires the therapist to depart from his usual practice of preserving the confidentiality of information given him by patients, a practice relied on to increase the likelihood of the patient's providing valid information. The dissatisfaction of some therapists with this requirement is evidenced by the fact that it was not met in 36% of their last cases by 327 workers in Boston child abuse agencies (Finkelhor, 1984).

Relapse Prevention

George and Marlatt (1989) recommended that a cognitive procedure termed relapse prevention, developed to treat addictive disorders, be extended to treat sex offenders. They consider that the aim of multimodal treatment packages in common use is to produce an effect so powerful it will not wear off, that there is little recognition that maintenance may require qualitatively different analyses and interventions, and that multimodal procedures are administered by the therapist, whereas maintenance procedures need to be administered by the patient. A feature of relapse prevention is the use of acronyms. The sex offender is considered to control his behavior until he encounters a high-risk situation (HRS), identified as an emotional state rather than a situation in which he has previously offended. The latter HRS is the one considered important in stimulus control models. If offenders in HRSs "lapse" (i.e., willfully fantasize sexual offending), the effect of the lapse, the abstinence violation effect (AVE), will depend on the offenders' cognitive attributions of the cause of the lapse and their affective reactions to this attribution. Decreased self-efficacy and pleasurable sensations associated with the lapse will increase the likelihood of "relapse," or offending. To help offenders handle HRSs, they prepare life autobiographies and self-monitor deviant urges. The therapist may need to confront offenders concerning their apparently irrelevant decisions (AIDs) or seemingly unimportant behaviors that lead to errors (SUBTLE). These are behaviors that enable the offender unconsciously to seek out HRSs. Examples are pedophiles who seek jobs that involve contact with children, reporting such benevolent reasons for their choice as their commitment to helping children, or rapists who leave home in the early morning to jog. Other avoidance strategies include recognizing and handling the PIG—the problem of immediate gratification—that inches the offender closer to relapse.

Skills training to recognize HRSs, PIGs, and AIDs, and, where appropriate, to develop assertiveness, stress management, relaxation training, anger management, enhancement of empathy for victims, and communication skills and general social or dating skills are incorporated in relapse prevention along with homework assignments to enhance self-efficacy (George & Marlatt, 1989). The final thrust is to teach the offender to achieve and maintain a balanced lifestyle. Positive addictions to regular exercise and substitute indulgences are encouraged. In practice relapse prevention is added to multimodal procedures currently in use (Laws, 1989), but no empirical evidence has been produced that they add to their efficacy. Such evidence could be difficult to obtain; clearly it would not be easy to separate out what was specific to relapse prevention from the components of current multimodal approaches.

Case Illustration

Case Description

Mr. N.S. was a 33-year-old apparently intellectually impaired man with a history of sexually assaultive behavior. When asked why he had come to see me, he commenced a rambling account of a walk he took with another man. Although after a time I pointed out repeatedly that I could not see the relevance of his story, he continued it; finally I interviewed him with the social worker who had accompanied him and learned that he had taken the walk on a picnic with other patients from a church residential service for subjects with developmental disabilities. The walk terminated in his coercing a 19-year-old intellectually impaired man into fellating him.

When I asked him whether he had used force on the other man, he replied that he had not used enough force to strangle him. He was unable to give any meaningful account of his past life, but the records available reported he had shown evidence of behavioral disturbance before age 2, following an apparently normal pregnancy, labor, and development until that age. He had said simple words soon after his first birthday, and sang some songs. At about 18 months he had appeared to withdraw, and stopped speaking completely and communicated by gestures. No problems with toileting, eating, or sleeping were noted. At 4 years of age he had been considered to be deaf and attended a class for the partially deaf, until it was decided that his hearing was intact. At the age of 6 he had attended a preschool, where he showed little attempt to mix with his peers. He had been seen by a child psychiatrist, who considered him to have autistic tendencies and recommended therapy. His parents had separated by this stage, and N.S. was living with his mother, who did not accept the recommendation. His father had taken him to see the psychiatrist again when he was 10. It was then noted that he had very poor speech, which was delivered in a high, monotonous tone. He was manneristic, his drawings were infantile, he was obsessively preoccupied with his reflection in the mirror, and he objected to change. He shrank from personal contact with adults and was reported to disrupt his school class by tearing up books and throwing milk, chairs, and other objects at the teacher and other children. Psychological assessment found his IQ to be 51 and concluded that he had great difficulty with auditory reception, association, and expression, but that he was stronger in visual performance. It was decided that he had experienced an infantile psychosis, which had gradually remitted but left him with intellectual and probable perceptual difficulties. He then lived with his father until he was aged 14, when at his father's request he was admitted to a psychiatric institution.

When he was 17 his behavior in the institution was reported to be at times provocative, but generally cheerful and outgoing. He carried out domestic chores if supervised to prevent his being distracted, and his major problem was stated to be sex role conflict. No details were given concerning this, however. He was discharged to the care of his mother when he was 18, but she sought residential placement for him when he was 23. Since then he had been under the supervision of the residential service and had lived in a number of their residential facilities, being shifted each time his behavior toward other residents became unacceptable. Following training in living skills, he was able to obtain part-time employment as a cleaner. He visited his mother every second weekend and his father infrequently.

From the time of his original residential placement it was noted that he showed no heterosexual interest, but sought homosexual contacts whenever possible, behaving coercively if the partner was not cooperative, destroying food or possessions the other valued, and using force with weaker males. On one occasion he was given a trial of living with women and a male educator, but he commenced stealing their underwear and was aggressive and destructive when the educator explained that he could not accept N.S.'s sexual advances. He had been dismissed from one job 18 months prior for persistent unwanted sexual advances to other employees. When some months earlier the residential service could no longer find any of their facilities that were suitable, they arranged for placement in a boarding house that mainly accommodated adult males with psychiatric conditions. The service continued to supervise his activities and arrange his attendance at social gatherings. Consultations had been arranged with both psychiatrists and psychologists but had not produced any immediate change in his behavior, and he had not persisted in attending. His social worker felt that the staff and occupants of the boarding house where he was staying had reached the limits of their tolerance of his behavior, but it did not appear possible to find other accommodations for him. In view of his mental state he had not been legally charged until the present, but his most recent victim indicated that he wished that this action be taken.

Differential Diagnosis and Assessment

The major diagnostic problem N.S. presented was whether his behavior was due in part to an active psychosis that might respond to antipsychotic medication. However, although in the interview he volunteered little of relevance, his answers to questions indicated that he understood them. Despite his tendency to minimize the extent of his coercive and destructive behaviors or to justify them, he showed no evidence of delusional thinking or of hallucinations. A second problem was to assess his motivation. Despite his tendency to minimize his inappropriate behaviors, when challenged he agreed that he had pressured or forced men to let him have sex with them and that this behavior was causing him problems. He was able to understand that he might be charged with sexual assault and this could lead to his being jailed. He also understood that this outcome was less likely if by the time he appeared in court, information was available that he was receiving treatment that appeared effective in enabling him to control his inappropriate behaviors. Although he showed no evidence of guilt, this consideration appeared to persuade him he would benefit by accepting treatment and attempting to cease the behaviors.

In view of the persistence of his unacceptable behaviors despite counseling, it seemed unlikely that he would respond completely to a cognitive-behavioral program without the addition of an agent such as MPA, which would reduce the intensity of his sexual urges. The possibility of its use raised the further diagnostic problem of whether he was capable of informed consent. I believed that he was able to understand my explanation that this treatment would make his interest in sex much less, but he would still be able to have sex with willing partners. In addition, I asked his social worker to discuss the treatment with him in a later session so as to form an opinion concerning informed consent, and also requested the psychiatrist who referred him to see him again and give me his opinion.

Treatment Selection

In view of the lack of evidence of active psychosis, use of antipsychotics was not considered appropriate. With agreement of N.S.'s social worker and the referring psychiatrist that he was capable of giving informed consent, it was decided to use MPA. However, in view of the severity of his problem and his lack of strong motivation to control it, addition of ABC was considered advisable. Although he lived some distance from the therapist's office, his social worker agreed that she could accompany him if his assessment and treatment consultations were not too frequent. It was agreed that provided he responded satisfactorily, consultations could be scheduled every 2 weeks for 4 sessions and then at 4-week intervals until his response was sufficiently maintained. She also agreed to liaise with the manager of N.S.'s boarding-house to obtain his assessment of the client's behavior and to request him to supervise the client's listening to the audiotape of ABC sessions.

After N.S.'s serum testosterone level was estimated between 11:00 A.M. and noon, MPA was commenced at a level of 150 mg intramuscularly every 2 weeks. At the same consultation a session of ABC was also administered and audiotaped so that N.S. could listen to it at his boarding house between consultations. In the ABC session after being trained to relax, N.S. was instructed to visualize scenarios in which when he wanted to have sex with a male who was not interested, he would leave him alone and not go on making physical advances or using force. In addition, he visualized scenarios involving control of his anger if rejected and not stealing or destroying property of the rejecting male.

Treatment Course and Problems in Carrying Out Interventions

When he was seen 2 weeks later, as in previous interviews he did not volunteer anything meaningful, but he agreed on direct questioning that his sexual feelings weren't strong. His social worker said that he had continued to ask men at the boarding house for sex on a number of occasions but had accepted their refusal. The manager of the boarding house had supervised his listening to the tape three times a week. In the session of ABC, which was then administered, additional scenarios were incorporated in which he was asked to visualize not asking the same man for sex if he had been refused in the last few weeks. When he was seen on the occasion of his third injection, it was reported that he had been less persistent in approaching men at the boarding house and that his behavior was considered acceptable if it remained at that level. He was instructed to continue listening to one or the other of the two tapes twice weekly. His serum testosterone estimate of 6.4 ng/ml had been received by this time, but as he appeared to be responding satisfactorily it was not considered necessary to put the patient to the expense of determining the degree to which the level had been reduced.

N.S. continued to attend scheduled consultations with his social worker, and when after his fourth biweekly injection of MPA the reports of his behavior continued to be satisfactory, it was decided to follow the usual practice of reducing frequency of injections to once every 4 weeks. The theory justifying this procedure was that the learned excitement resulting from his not completing the unacceptable behaviors in response to the situations which stimulated them should have begun to lessen as he continued not to carry out the behaviors while remaining relaxed. With such reduction in excitement he should be able to control the behaviors in the period toward the end of the 4 weeks, when his testosterone level would be increasing toward a normal range and the biological urge would be greater. This experience of control of the stronger urge would enable further learning to take place.

Outcome and Termination

Reports of his behavior remained satisfactory, and 2 months after the frequency of the injections was reduced he appeared in court on the charge of sexual assault for the offense that had led to his being referred for treatment. He was placed on a bond of good behavior for 3 years and was directed to continue treatment. In the following 2 months, during which he continued to receive MPA, 150 mg, at 4-week intervals, reports of his behavior continued to be satisfactory.

With well-motivated patients who can be relied on to report the presence and strength of urges to carry out unacceptable sexual behaviors, it is my practice—if they report easily controllable or absent urges after 6 months of MPA therapy—to give them a trial without it. However, because N.S. could not reliably report the presence of such urges, I decided to reduce the frequency of injections to every 5th week for the next 4 months. When his behavior continued to be reported as satisfactory over this period, frequency of injections was further reduced to every 6 weeks. His behavior remained satisfactory for a further 6 months. Because over this period his serum testosterone would have returned to its normal level for the latter part of the 6 weeks between injections, it was concluded that he had learned to control his sexual urges adequately and the injections were ceased. He was instructed to continue to listen to one or the other of the two tapes at weekly intervals, and I reduced the frequency of the consultations to three monthly.

Follow-Up and Maintenance

At the second of the three monthly consultations, it was reported that a physically attractive young male had recently come to live in the boarding house and N.S. had commenced to distress him with repeated requests for sexual activity despite being instructed by the manager and his social worker that this was unacceptable. I discussed N.S.'s behavior with him, pointing out that he could be charged with this behavior and that it would be a breach of his bond, possibly leading to a jail sentence. He accepted my recommendation to resume MPA therapy, and a further session of ABC dealing with the current behavior was taped, which he was to listen to three times a week. The injections were recommenced at 2-week intervals. Again, cessation of his unacceptable behavior was reported. After four injections their frequency was again reduced to once every 4 weeks, but it was decided to maintain him on this dosage for at least a year. Currently, he has been taking this does for 8 months and listens to the tape weekly while his behavior continues to be reported as satisfactory.

Summary

Clinical features of exhibitionists, voyeurs, pedophiles, sadomasochists, rapists, fetishists, transvestites, transsexuals, and gender-disordered children are briefly described, and the prevalence of their conditions and that of related fantasies discussed. It is suggested that their etiology is best understood as an interaction of stimulus control, cognitive processes, and psychiatric-psychopathological factors. The categorization of these conditions in DSM-III-R and DSM-IV and their differential diagnosis are reviewed. In regard to assessment, the value of the unstructured interview is emphasized and that of penile response measurement questioned.

Evidence is reviewed that aversive therapy does not alter deviant sexual motivation but increases the treated subject's ability to control unacceptable deviant behavior, and that imaginal desensitization is more effective in this respect than aversive procedures currently in use, such as covert sensitization. The value of techniques such as masturbatory reconditioning in increasing heterosexual arousability is questioned. Reduction of subjects' deviant urges correlates strongly with reduction of their serum testosterone levels by pharmacotherapy with medroxyprogesterone. Reduction to 30% of the pretreatment levels allows most subjects to cease unacceptable deviant behaviors while maintaining acceptable sexual activity. After 6 months of such therapy the majority can continue to control the deviant urges following its cessation.

Use of cognitive approaches, commonly based on the model that male sexual aggression is motivated by urges to dominate women or children rather than by sexual urges, is discussed. Cognitive approaches are usually employed in multimodal form combined with aversive procedures, social and assertiveness skills, and sex education. Studies evaluating such multimodal treatment with child molesters and exhibitionists were flawed by use of untreated rather than placebo-treated controls and failure to employ random allocation. Selection of optimal treatment strategies and problems in their administration are discussed, followed by a description of relapse prevention. The therapy of an apparently intellectually impaired sexually assaultive male with a combination of imaginal desensitization and medroxyprogesterone is reported.

References

Ageton, S. S. (1983). *Sexual assault among adolescents.* Lexington, MA: Lexington Books.
American Psychiatric Association (1987). *Diagnostic and statistical manual of mental disorders* (3rd ed., rev.). Washington, DC: Author.

American Psychiatric Association (1991). *DSM-IV options book: Work in progress 9/1/91*. Washington, DC: Author.

American Psychiatric Association (1993). *DSM-IV draft criteria 3/1/93*. Washington, DC: Author.

Blanchard, R., Clemmensen, L. H., & Steiner, B. W. (1987). Heterosexual and homosexual gender dysphoria. *Archives of Sexual Behavior, 16*, 139–152.

Bradford, J. M. W. (1990). The antiandrogen and hormonal treatment of sex offenders. In W. L. Marshall, D. R. Laws, & H. E. Barbaree (Eds.), *Handbook of sexual assault* (pp. 297–310). New York: Plenum.

Breslow, N., Evans, L., & Langley, J. (1985). On the prevalence and roles of females in the sadomasochistic subculture: Report of an empirical study. *Archives of Sexual Behavior, 14*, 303–319.

Buhrich, N. (1977). *Clinical study of heterosexual male transvestism*. Unpublished doctoral thesis, University of New South Wales, Sydney, Australia.

Buhrich, N., & McConaghy, N. (1977a). Clinical comparison of transvestism and transsexualism. *Australian and New Zealand Journal of Psychiatry, 6*, 83–86.

Buhrich, N., & McConaghy, N. (1977b). The clinical syndromes of femmiphilic transvestism. *Archives of Sexual Behavior, 6*, 397–412.

Buhrich, N., & McConaghy, N. (1977c). The discrete syndromes of transvestism and transsexualism. *Archives of Sexual Behavior, 6*, 483–495.

Burnam, M. A., Stein, J. A., Golding, J. M., Siegel, J. M., Sorenson, S. B., Forsythe, A. B., & Telles, C. A. (1988). Sexual assault and mental disorders in a community population. *Journal of Consulting and Clinical Psychology, 56*, 843–850.

Cautela, J. R. (1967). Covert sensitization. *Psychological Reports, 20*, 459–468.

Conrad, S. R., & Winzce, J. P. (1976). Orgasmic reconditioning: A controlled study of its effects upon the sexual arousal and behavior of adult male homosexuals. *Behavior Therapy, 7*, 155–166.

Crepault, C., & Couture, M. (1980). Men's erotic fantasies. *Archives of Sexual Behavior, 9*, 565–581.

Croughan, J. L., Saghir, M., Cohen, R., & Robins, E. (1981). A comparison of treated and untreated male cross-dressers. *Archives of Sexual Behavior, 10*, 515–528.

Duncan, D. F. (1990). Prevalence of sexual assault victimization among heterosexual and gay/lesbian university students. *Psychological Reports, 66*, 65–66.

Eklund, P. L. E., Gooren, L. J. G., & Bezemer, P. D. (1988). Prevalence of transsexualism in the Netherlands. *British Journal of Psychiatry, 152*, 638–640.

Ellis, A. (1973). *Humanistic psychotherapy: The rational-emotive approach*. New York: Crown and McGraw-Hill.

Fedora, O., Reddon, J. R., Morrison, J. W., Fedora, S. K., Pascoe, H., & Yeudall, L. T. (1992). Sadism and other paraphilias in normal controls and aggressive and nonaggressive sex offenders. *Archives of Sexual Behavior, 21*, 1–15.

Finkelhor, D. (1984). *Child sexual abuse: New theory and research*. New York: Free Press.

Finkelhor, D. (1985). Sexual abuse of boys. In A. W . Burgess (Ed.), *Rape and sexual assault* (pp. 97–103). New York: Garland.

Freund, K. (1960). Some problems in the treatment of homosexuality. In H. J. Eysenck (Ed.), *Behaviour therapy and the neuroses* (pp. 312–326). Oxford: Pergamon.

Freund, K. (1963). A laboratory method of diagnosing predominance of homo- or hetero-erotic interest in the male. *Behaviour Research and Therapy, 12*, 355–359.

Freund, K. (1990). Courtship disorder. In W. L. Marshall, D. R. Laws, & H. E. Barbaree (Eds.), *Handbook of sexual assault* (pp. 195–207). New York: Plenum.

Freund, K., & Blanchard, R. (1986). The concept of courtship disorder. *Journal of Sex and Marital Therapy, 12*, 79–92.

Freund, K., Watson, R., & Dickey, R. (1990). Does sexual abuse in childhood cause pedophilia: An exploratory study. *Archives of Sexual Behavior, 19*, 557–568.

Fromuth, M. E., & Burkhart, B. R. (1989). Long-term physiological correlates of childhood sexual abuse in two samples of college men. *Child Abuse and Neglect, 13*, 533–542.

Gagne, P. (1981). Treatment of sex offenders with MPA acetate. *American Journal of Psychiatry, 138*, 644–646.

George, W. H., & Marlatt, G. A. (1989). Introduction. In D. R. Laws (Ed.), *Relapse prevention with sex offenders* (pp. 1–33). New York: Guilford.

Green, R. (1978). Open forum. *Archives of Sexual Behavior, 7*, 387–415.

Grob, C. S. (1985). Female exhibitionism. *Journal of Nervous and Mental Disease, 173*, 253–256.

Groth, A. N., Burgess, A. W., & Holmstrom, L. L. (1977). Rape: Power, anger and sexuality. *American Journal of Psychiatry, 134*, 1239–1243.

Heim, N., & Hursch, C. J. (1979). Castration of sex offenders: Treatment or punishment? A review and critique of recent European literature. *Archives of Sexual Behavior, 8,* 281–304.

Herman, J. L. (1990). Sex offenders: A feminist perspective. In W. L. Marshall, D. R. Laws, & H. E. Barbaree (Eds.), *Handbook of sexual assault* (pp. 177–193). New York: Plenum.

Hunt, M. (1974). *Sexual behavior in the 1970's.* New York: Dell.

James, S. (1978). Treatment of homosexuality. II: Superiority or desensitization arousal as compared with anticipatory avoidance conditioning: Results of a controlled trial. *Behavior Therapy, 9,* 28–36.

Knight, R. A., & Prentky, R. A. (1990). Classifying sexual offenders. In W. L. Marshall, D. R. Laws, & H. E. Barbaree (Eds.), *Handbook of sexual assault* (pp. 23–52). New York: Plenum.

Knight, R. A., Rosenberg, R., & Schneider, B. A. (1985). Classification of sexual offenders: Perspectives, methods, and validation. In A. W. Burgess (Ed.), *Rape and sexual assault* (pp. 222–293). New York: Garland.

Koss, M. P., & Oros, C. J. (1982). Sexual experiences survey: A research instrument investigating sexual aggression and victimization. *Journal of Consulting and Clinical Psychology, 50,* 455–457.

Langevin, R., & Lang, R. A. (1987). The courtship disorders. In G. D. Wilson (Ed.), *Variant sexuality: Research and theory* (pp. 202–228). London: Croom Helm.

Langevin, R., Paitich, D., Hucker, S., Newman, S., Ramsay, G., Pope, S., Gelles, G., & Anderson, C. (1979). The effect of assertiveness training, provera and sex of therapist in the treatment of genital exhibitionism. *Journal of Behavior Therapy and Experimental Psychiatry, 10,* 275–282.

Laws, D. R. (Ed.). (1989). *Relapse prevention with sex offenders.* New York: Guilford.

Laws, D. R., & Marshall, W. L. (1991). Masturbatory reconditioning with sexual deviates: An evaluative review. *Advances in Behaviour Research and Therapy, 13,* 13–25.

Laws, D. R., & Rubin, H. H. (1969). Instructional control of an autonomic sexual response. *Journal of Applied Behavior Analysis, 2,* 93–99.

Lichstein, K. L., & Hung, J. H. F. (1980). Covert sensitization: An examination of covert and overt parameters. *Behavioral Engineering, 6,* 1–18.

Mahoney, M. J. (1977). Reflections on the cognitive-learning trend in psychotherapy. *American Psychologist, 32,* 5–13.

Malamuth, N. M. (1989). The attraction to sexual aggression scale: II. *Journal of Sex Research, 26,* 324–354.

Malamuth, N. M., & Check, J. V. P. (1983). Sexual arousal to rape depictions: Individual differences. *Journal of Abnormal Psychology, 92,* 55–67.

Maletzky, B. M. (1973). "Assisted" covert sensitization: A preliminary report. *Behavior Therapy, 4,* 117–119.

Marshall, W. L., & Barbaree, H. E. (1988). The long-term evaluation of a behavioral treatment program for child molesters. *Behaviour Research and Therapy, 26,* 499–511.

Marshall, W. L., & Barbaree, H. E. (1990a). An integrated theory of the etiology of sexual offending. In W. L. Marshall, D. R. Laws, & H. E. Barbaree (Eds.), *Handbook of sexual assault* (pp. 257–275). New York: Plenum.

Marshall, W. L. & Barbaree, H. E. (1990b). Outcome of comprehensive cognitive-behavioral treatment programs. In W. L. Marshall, D. R. Laws, & H. E. Barbaree (Eds.), *Handbook of sexual assault* (pp. 363–385). New York: Plenum.

Marshall, W. L., Eccles, A., & Barbaree, H. E. (1991). The treatment of exhibitionists: a focus on sexual deviance versus cognitive and relationship features. *Behaviour Research and Therapy, 29,* 129–135.

Marshall, W. L., Earls, C. M., Segal, Z., & Darke, J. (1983). A behavioral program for the assessment and treatment of sexual aggressors. In K. D. Craig & R. J. McMahon (Eds.), *Advances in clinical behavior therapy* (pp. 148–174). New York: Brunner/Mazel.

Matarazzo, J. D. (1983). The reliability of psychiatric and psychological diagnosis. *Clinical Psychology Review, 3,* 103–145.

McAnulty, R. D., & Adams, H. E. (1992). Validity and ethics of penile circumference measures of sexual arousal: A reply to McConaghy. *Archives of Sexual Behavior, 21,* 101–119.

McConaghy, N. (1976). Is a homosexual orientation irreversible? *British Journal of Psychiatry, 129,* 556–563.

McConaghy, N. (1977). Behavioral treatment in homosexuality. In M. Hersen, R. M. Eisler, & P. M. Miller (Eds.), *Progress in behavior modification* (Vol. 5, pp. 309–380). New York: Academic.

McConaghy, N. (1978). Heterosexual experience, marital status and orientation of homosexual males. *Archives of Sexual Behavior, 7,* 575–581.

McConaghy, N. (1980). Behavior completion mechanisms rather than primary drives maintain behavioral patterns. *Activitas Nervòsa Superior* (Prague), *22,* 138–151.

McConaghy, N. (1982). Sexual deviation. In A. S. Bellack, M. Hersen, & A. E. Kazdin (Eds.), *International handbook of behavior therapy and modification* (pp. 683–716). New York: Plenum.

McConaghy, N. (1987a). Heterosexuality/homosexuality: Dichotomy or continuum. *Archives of Sexual Behavior, 16*, 411–424.

McConaghy, N. (1987b). A learning approach. In J. H. Geer & W. T. O'Donohue (Eds.), *Theories of human sexuality* (pp. 287–333). New York: Plenum.

McConaghy, N. (1988). Sexual dysfunction and deviation. In A. S. Bellack & M. Hersen (Eds.), *Behavioral assessment* (3rd ed., pp. 490–541). New York: Pergamon.

McConaghy, N. (1989). Validity and ethics of penile circumference measures of sexual arousal: A critical review. *Archives of Sexual Behavior, 18*, 357–369.

McConaghy, N. (1990a). Can reliance be placed on a single meta-analysis? *Australian and New Zealand Journal of Psychiatry, 24*, 405–415.

McConaghy, N. (1990b). Sexual deviation. In A. S. Bellack, M. Hersen, & A. E. Kazdin (Eds.), *International handbook of behavior therapy and modification* (2nd ed., pp. 565–580). New York: Plenum.

McConaghy, N. (1992). Validity and ethics of penile circumference measures of sexual arousal: A response to McAnulty and Adams. *Archives of Sexual Behavior, 21*, 187–195.

McConaghy, N. (1993). *Sexual behavior: Problems and management.* New York: Plenum.

McConaghy, N. (in press). Sexual dysfunctions and deviations. In M. Hersen & S. M. Turner (Eds.), *Diagnostic interviewing* (2nd ed.). New York: Plenum.

McConaghy, N., Armstrong, M. S., & Blaszczynski, A. (1981). Controlled comparison of aversive therapy and covert sensitization in compulsive homosexuality. *Behaviour Research and Therapy, 19*, 425–434.

McConaghy, N., Armstrong, M. S., & Blaszczynski, A. (1985). Expectancy, covert sensitization and imaginal desensitization in compulsive sexuality. *Acta Psychiatrica Scandinavica, 72*, 176–187.

McConaghy, N., Armstrong, M. S., Blaszczynski, A., & Allcock, C. (1983). Controlled comparison of aversive therapy and imaginal desensitization in compulsive gambling. *British Journal of Psychiatry, 142*, 366–372.

McConaghy, N., Blaszczynski, A., Armstrong, M. S., & Kidson, W. (1989). Resistance to treatment of adolescent sexual offenders. *Archives of Sexual Behavior, 18*, 97–107.

McConaghy, N. Blaszczynski, A., & Kidson, W. (1988). Treatment of sex offenders with imaginal desensitization and/or MPA. *Acta Psychiatrica Scandinavica, 77*, 199–206.

McConaghy, N., Zamir, R., & Manicavasagar, V. (1993). Non-sexist sexual experiences survey and scale of attraction to sexual aggression. *Australian and New Zealand Journal of Psychiatry, 27*, 686–693.

Moser, C., & Levitt, E. E. (1987). An exploratory-descriptive study of a sadomasochistically oriented sample. *Journal of Sex Research, 23*, 322–337.

O'Connor, A. A. (1987). Female sex offenders. *British Journal of Psychiatry, 150*, 615–620.

Palmer, C. T. (1988). Twelve reasons why rape is not sexually motivated: A skeptical examination. *Journal of Sex Research, 25*, 512–530.

Person, E. S., Terestman, N., Myers, W. A., Goldberg, E. L., & Salvadori, C. (1989). Gender differences in sexual behaviors and fantasies in a college population. *Journal of Sex and Marital Therapy, 15*, 187–198.

Pfaus, J. G., Myronuk, L. D. S., & Jacobs, W. J. (1986). Soundtrack contents and depicted sexual violence. *Archives of Sexual Behavior, 15*, 231–237.

Prince, V., & Bentler, P. M. (1972). Survey of 504 cases of transvestism. *Psychological Reports, 32*, 903–917.

Quinsey, V. L. (1986). Men who have sex with children. In D. N. Weisstub (Ed.), *Law and mental health: International perspectives* (Vol. 2, pp. 140–172). New York: Pergamon.

Quinsey, V. L., & Bergersen, S. G. (1976). Instructional control of penile circumference in assessment of sexual preference. *Behavior Therapy, 7*, 489–493.

Quinsey, V. L., & Earls, C. M. (1990). The modification of sexual preferences. In W. L. Marshall, D. R. Laws, & H. E. Barbaree (Eds.), *Handbook of sexual assault* (pp. 279–295). New York: Plenum.

Reading, A. E. (1983). A comparison of the accuracy and reactivity of methods of monitoring male sexual behavior. *Journal of Behavioral Assessment, 5*, 11–23.

Rice, M. E., Quinsey, V. L., & Harris, G. T. (1991). Sexual recidivism among child molesters released from a maximum security psychiatric institution. *Journal of Consulting and Clinical Psychology, 59*, 381–386.

Russell, D. E. H. (1983). The incidence and prevalence of intrafamilial and extrafamilial sexual abuse of female children. *Child Abuse and Neglect, 7*, 133–146.

Russell, D. E. H. (1986). *The secret trauma: Incest in the lives of girls and women.* New York: Basic Books.

Smukler, A. J., & Schiebel, D. (1975). Personality characteristics of exhibitionists. *Diseases of the Nervous System, 36*, 600–603.

Sorenson, S. B., Stein, J. A., Siegel, J. M., Golding, J. M., and Burnam, M. A. (1987). The prevalence of adult sexual assault. *American Journal of Epidemiology, 126*, 1154–1164.

Stermac, L.E., Segal, Z. V., & Gillis, R. (1990). Social and cultural factors in sexual assault. In W. L. Marshall, D. R. Laws, & H. E. Barbaree (Eds.), *Handbook of sexual assault* (pp. 143–159). New York: Plenum.

Taylor, C. B., Agras, W. S., Schneider, J. A., & Allen, R. A. (1983). Adherence to instructions in practice relaxation exercises. *Journal of Consulting and Clinical Psychology, 51,* 952–953.

Templeman, T. L., & Stinnett, R. D. (1991). Patterns of sexual arousal and history in a "normal" sample of young men. *Archives of Sexual Behavior, 20,* 137–150.

Travin, S., Bluestone, H., Coleman, E., Cullen, K., & Melella, J. (1986). Pedophile types and treatment perspectives. *Journal of Forensic Sciences, 31,* 614–620.

Tsoi, W. F. (1988). The prevalence of transsexualism in Singapore. *Acta Psychiatrica Scandinavica, 78,* 501–504.

Wolpe, J. (1958). *Psychotherapy by reciprocal inhibition.* Stanford, CA: Stanford University Press.

Zuger, B. (1966). Effeminate behavior present in boys from early childhood. I: The clinical syndrome and follow-up studies. *Journal of Pediatrics, 69,* 1098–1107.

Zuger, B. (1984). Early effeminate behavior in boys: Outcome and significance for homosexuality. *Journal of Nervous and Mental Disease, 172,* 90–97.

17

Male Erectile Disorder

Michael P. Carey, Larry J. Lantinga, and Dennis J. Krauss

Description of the Disorder

Male erectile disorder involves a persistent and recurrent difficulty in which a man cannot attain or maintain an erection that is sufficient for intromission and subsequent sexual activity. Expressions such as "I can't get it up anymore," "I've lost my manhood," and "It's dead down there" all capture the typical client's view of this disorder.

Male erectile disorder is often referred to as "impotence" by many professionals, the lay media, and the general public. Although briefer, the term *impotence* is less descriptive (e.g., it has often been used to describe premature ejaculation and other complaints) than male erectile disorder and is, in our view, unnecessarily pejorative. After all, the first two meanings of the word *impotent*, according to *Webster's New World Dictionary* (1982), are: "1. lacking physical strength; weak; 2. ineffective, powerless, or helpless" (p. 706). Therefore, along with others (e.g., participants at the 1992 Consensus Development Conference on Impotence sponsored by the National Institutes of Health), we prefer the use of the term *male erectile disorder*.

Clinical Features

Typically, male erectile disorder is diagnosed when one of the following scenarios develops: (a) a man cannot obtain an erection of adequate rigidity to allow intromis-

Michael P. Carey • Department of Psychology and Center for Health and Behavior, Syracuse University, Syracuse, New York 13244-2340.   **Larry J. Lantinga** • Psychology Service, Syracuse Department of Veterans Affairs Medical Center, and Department of Psychiatry, SUNY Health Science Center at Syracuse, Syracuse, New York 13210.   **Dennis J. Krauss** • Urology Section, Surgical Service, Syracuse Department of Veterans Affairs Medical Center, and Department of Urology, SUNY Health Science Center at Syracuse, Syracuse, New York 13210.

Handbook of Prescriptive Treatments for Adults, edited by Michel Hersen and Robert T. Ammerman. Plenum Press, New York, 1994.

sion, (b) a man can achieve an erection that is adequate (or "usable") but loses this erection prior to or soon after intromission (and before orgasm), or (c) a man can obtain and maintain erections on some but not all occasions. Male erectile disorder can be classified as *lifelong* (when it has occurred during the man's entire sexual life; also referred to by some authors as "primary") or *acquired* (when it develops after a period of satisfactory sexual functioning; also known as "secondary"), and as *generalized* (occurs across all partners, sexual activities, and situations) versus *situational* (limited to certain partners, sexual activities, or situations).

It is important to distinguish male erectile disorder from other sexual health problems that men can experience. *Hypoactive sexual desire disorder* refers to a persistent lack of sexual fantasies and interest in being sexually active. Typically, this difficulty arises in the context of a dyadic relationship wherein a partner prefers sexual activity much more often than does the man who receives the diagnosis. Men with this disorder can obtain erections when they want to—but the "problem" is that they often have little interest in sex. *Premature ejaculation* refers to a difficulty, common among younger men, in which a man is able to achieve adequate erections but ejaculates earlier than he would like. *Retrograde ejaculation* occurs when a man achieves an erection and ejaculates within a comfortable time frame, but the ejaculatory fluid travels backward (into the bladder) rather than forward and out the urethra. This difficulty is more common among older men who have a neurologic deficit involving the bladder neck (e.g., diabetes) or who have taken medication (e.g., anti-alpha-adrenergic drugs) or had surgery (e.g., prostatectomy). *Inhibited male orgasm* is a rare condition in which a man does not reach organism despite adequate desire, arousal, and stimulation. Typically the man has no difficulty obtaining an erection and participating in sexual intercourse. *Priapism* is also a rare condition and refers to a persistent and often painful erection (*not* associated with erotic stimulation), which may occur for a variety of reasons. Most cases involve vascular or neurologic conditions, or reflect side effects of medication (e.g., trazodone, heparin). *Infertility* is a much more common condition in which a heterosexual couple cannot conceive a child after one year of regular intercourse without using contraceptives. Typically the man has no problem obtaining and maintaining an erection. For more information on these difficulties, interested readers can consult Spark (1991), Wincze and Carey (1991), and Zilbergeld (1992).

Associated Features

Men experiencing erection problems are often anxious, embarrassed, discouraged, and depressed; in extreme cases, these men will confide that they have even had suicidal thoughts as a result of their erectile difficulties. Zilbergeld (1992) provided the following illustration from one of his clients, a 38-year-old man: "I have trouble sleeping and I can't concentrate at work. All I think about day and night is my problem, about how I can't do the job anymore. I feel limp and weak, just like my dick" (p. 439).

Because of the discouragement they feel, many men will try self-help "remedies" such as using drugs (e.g., alcohol, cocaine, and the so-called aphrodisiacs), viewing erotica, or initiating an affair. Some will visit a prostitute "to see if it works" under "optimal conditions." These attempts usually fail and result in additional despair as well as other secondary problems. For example, men in relationships will often report relationship discord, whereas unattached men describe increased social isolation because they see no point in dating if they are unable to obtain an erection. Because of their desperation, many men with male erectile disorder are vulnerable to scams or rip-offs that promise fantastic erections.

Epidemiology

Prevalence. The plethora of advertisements, self-aids, professional products and services, magazine articles, and talk shows devoted to male erectile disorder suggests that this is a very common problem. In one year (1985), according to the National Center for Health Statistics (cited in Krane, Goldstein, & Saenz de Tejada, 1989), male erectile disorder accounted for more than 400,000 outpatient visits to physicians (alone) and more than 30,000 hospital admissions, costing approximately $150 million. Despite these calculations, scientific estimates of the prevalence of male erectile disorder have been scant. Evidence that is available arises from two sources: community-based (i.e., general population) studies and clinical samples.

Community-Based Estimates. The most recent large-scale field study of mental disorders [the Epidemiologic Catchment Area studies conducted by the National Institute of Mental Health (Regier et al., 1984)] did not include male erectile disorder as one of the conditions assessed. Therefore, we have to rely on other sources to estimate the prevalence of male erectile disorder in the general population. Based on her clinical practice, Kaplan (1974) estimated that as many as 50% of all men will experience erectile difficulties as adults. After reviewing the scientific literature, Spector and Carey (1990) provided a more conservative estimate, namely that between 4 and 9% of the adult male population were experiencing the disorder. Consistent with the higher end of this range, Krane et al. (1989) estimated that 10 million American males have erectile disorder.

Clinic-Based Estimates. It is also possible to estimate the prevalence of the disorder based on the clinical treatment literature. Spector and Carey (1990) also reviewed this literature and found that erectile disorder was the most common presenting complaint at sex therapy clinics. For example, Masters and Johnson (1970) reported that 50% of men requesting treatment at their institute in St. Louis complained of secondary (i.e., acquired) erectile disorder, and 8% complained of primary (i.e., lifelong) erectile disorder. Frank, Anderson, and Kupfer (1976) and Bancroft and Coles (1976) found, respectively, that 36 and 40% of males presenting for sex therapy had erectile disorder as their primary complaint. Hawton (1982) replicated the Bancroft and Coles (1976) study (in the same clinic, several years later) and observed that male erectile disorder accounted for 53% of the presenting problems at this clinic. More recently, Renshaw (1988), at her clinic in Chicago, reported that 3.5% of her clients complained of lifelong erectile disorder and 48% complained of acquired erectile disorder. It should be noted that the figures just cited are from specialty sex therapy clinics. It is likely that an even larger number of men present initially to private practitioners, or to nonspecialized clinics located in departments of psychology, psychiatry, urology, or medicine. Unfortunately, systematic data are not yet available from these settings.

Risk Factors. It is probably safe to say that not all men are at equal risk for male erectile disorder. Chronic illnesses such as diabetes, cancer, cardiovascular diseases, end-stage renal disease, chronic obstructive pulmonary disease, and multiple sclerosis have all been associated with higher rates of male erectile disorder (Schover & Jensen, 1988). Mental disorders including Alzheimer's disease, major depression, and schizophrenia often impair sexual functioning, as do numerous prescription medications, alcohol, and illegal drugs (Segraves & Segraves, 1992). Recent evidence suggests that even long-term cigarette smoking can place men at greater risk of erection problems (Shabsigh, Fishman, Schum, & Dunn, 1991).

It has long been suspected that advancing age increases a man's risk of erectile disorder. Kinsey, Pomeroy, and Martin (1948) found that erectile disorder occurs in less than 1% of the male population before age 19, increasing to 25% by age 75. More recent data have confirmed this relationship. Weizman and Hart (1987) reported that 36% of their sample of older men (range, 60 to 71 years of age) experienced erection difficulties despite being otherwise physically and psychologically healthy, as well as happily married. They also noted that, fortunately, sexual interest and activity continued in these men despite their erectile disorder. In the recently completed Massachusetts Male Aging Study (McKinlay, 1992), conducted with 1,709 men between the ages of 40 and 70 years, the prevalence of male erectile disorder increased from 5% to 15% as men aged. However, it should be noted that aging per se did not explain most cases of male erectile disorder; rather, other modifiable para-aging phenomena (e.g., vascular disease, cigarette smoking) were implicated.

Etiology

Male erectile disorder can be caused by many factors. Most common are neurologic, vascular, psychological, and relationship causes. Buvat and his colleagues have noted that at least two "causes" have been found in two-thirds of all cases of male erectile disorder (Buvat, Buvat-Herbaut, Lemaire, Marcolin, & Quittelier, 1990). Therefore, it is essential to adopt a biopsychosocial model when evaluating and treating male erectile disorder; that is, one should assume that biological, psychological, and social forces can contribute—separately and in combination—to cause male erectile disorder (Wincze & Carey, 1991). In some instances a single causal agent may be strong enough to prevent erections. Such cases are relatively easy to recognize, assess, and (sometimes) treat. More often, however, there exists a combination of subtle forces that work together to impair erectile capacity. In explaining this kind of model to clients, we have sometimes used Domeena Renshaw's metaphor of weights anchoring down an erect penis (Krauss, Lantinga, & Kelly, 1990). A single weight (representing, for example, alcohol use prior to sexual intercourse) may not be sufficient to pull down an erect penis in a young, healthy man in a healthy relationship. However, the combined effects of several factors (e.g., alcohol use, atherosclerosis, depressed affect, and poor communication between partners) might be sufficient to impair erections in a middle-aged man.

We have previously hypothesized that the "final" effect of several risk factors may be "negatively" synergistic (rather than just additive); in other words, when multiple risk factors are present, the net effect may be more than just the sum of the individual factors (Carey, Wincze, & Meisler, 1993). For example, Leiblum and Rosen (1991) reviewed literature that suggests that lowered social status (resulting from failure experiences) may actually reduce circulating levels of testosterone. The corollary of this hypothesis is that treatment may have a greater effect than originally anticipated (i.e., based on an analysis of the likely *direct* effects of the intervention) because of a kind of "positive" synergism. Thus, the problem and the intervention might be thought of as biopsychosocial *patterns* going in different directions (one toward sexual dysfunction and the other toward sexual satisfaction).

Finally, a biopsychosocial model such as this allows for multiple pathways to the clinical endpoint of male erectile disorder. Erection problems can result from a plethora of combinations of risk factors. The model also helps explain how narrowly trained clinicians looking for a causal agent from within their particular perspective, discipline, or paradigm might actually find it—but treatment fails because it has addressed only one of several causal factors. A model such as this requires a multimodal assessment and treatment strategy.

Differential Diagnosis and Assessment

DSM-III-R and DSM-IV Categorization

The DSM-III-R (American Psychiatric Association, 1987) defines male erectile disorder as either (a) "persistent or recurrent partial or complete failure in a male to attain or maintain erection until completion of the sexual activity," or (b) "persistent or recurrent lack of a subjective sense of sexual excitement and pleasure in a male during sexual activity" (p. 294). This diagnosis was not used if the erection problem occurred exclusively during the course of another Axis I disorder (other than a sexual dysfunction), such as major depression. This definition will be changed in DSM-IV (American Psychiatric Association, 1993). Now male erectile disorder refers to the "persistent or recurrent inability to attain or maintain an adequate erection until completion of the sexual activity." Use of this diagnosis requires that the erection problem causes "marked distress or interpersonal difficulty." As with DSM-III-R, male erectile disorder would not be diagnosed with DSM-IV if the erection problems were the result of another psychological disorder (e.g., major depression) or substance abuse.

Differential Diagnosis

For many of the clients we see, the diagnosis of male erectile disorder creates three interesting challenges. The first and easiest involves distinguishing among the various sexual problems that men may experience. Previously, we described six conditions (hypoactive sexual desire disorder, premature ejaculation, retrograde ejaculation, inhibited male orgasm, priapism, and infertility) that clients can confuse with male erectile disorder. It is important to determine which problem(s) the client is experiencing and, equally important, to explain the correct diagnosis to the client.

The second challenge occurs in the context of comorbidity and involves determining which of several psychological conditions is primary. For example, in a man who has both hypoactive sexual desire disorder and male erectile disorder, either disorder may be primary—that is, a man's interest in sex may be diminished because he has difficulty obtaining usable erections, or a man may have difficulty getting an erection because he has no interest in his partner or in sex in general. Other common examples include the comorbidity of depression and personality disorders with male erectile disorder. In these cases we have found that a careful history taking can often help us establish clinical hypotheses that can be tested during subsequent assessment and therapy (cf. Carey, Flasher, Maisto, & Turkat, 1984). However, it may be necessary to make a provisional diagnosis until more data are available.

A third challenge occurs once the disorder is confidently diagnosed as male erectile disorder. This challenge is to formulate the case: that is, to determine which causal factors are most important (this will determine the most appropriate treatment). This formulation needs to be done in such a way that the problem is *not* framed as either solely an organic (i.e., biologically caused) or functional (i.e., psychologically caused) one.

Assessment Strategies

Evaluation of male erectile disorder begins with an understanding of the physiology of erections. The four stages of penile erection include (a) initiation (neurogenic: cognitive, reflexive, or emotional), (b) vascular filling (arteriogenic), (c) storage (veno-occlusive), and (d) release (neurogenic or malfunction of earlier mechanisms). Each stage requires careful evaluation.

Interview. We have found that two sessions devoted to obtaining the history is usually adequate. If the client is in a relationship and the partner is willing to come in, separate interviews should be conducted with each partner. All couples are told that it is more helpful and efficient to undergo initial interviews separately, even though the overall emphasis will be on the couple. Furthermore, couples are told that at times it may be helpful to deal with either person alone in order to work through specific issues. By making these statements at the outset, one establishes conditions that will allow for working through problems that present later during therapy.

Assessment should always begin with an appropriate introduction for the client. During this time the assessment structure and content should be outlined. We prefer to do this while both partners are present. After the introductory remarks, the couple should be invited to ask questions. The remainder of the first session is spent interviewing the man with erectile disorder alone. The goals of this first session include establishing rapport and obtaining a general description of erection problem, a thorough psychosocial history, and a description of other life concerns.

Throughout the interview it is useful to notice how comfortably the client discusses his erection problem. Use probes and directive comments to keep the client on target. Generally, we find information from the adult years to be most important. We ask about significant relationships and events; areas to be addressed include self-esteem, marriage/relationship history, and sexual experiences. Inquire about any unusual sexual experiences, psychiatric history, or treatment. Finally, acquire details regarding the current sexual situation, including sexual and nonsexual experiences in the current relationship, recent changes in sexual functioning and satisfaction, flexibility in sexual attitudes and behaviors, extramarital affairs, strengths and weaknesses of partner, and likes and dislikes of partner's sexual behavior. We also find it helpful to obtain a brief medical history, including significant diseases, surgery, medical care, and congenital disorders. We pay particular attention to the medical history after age 20 and are sure to ask if the client is taking prescribed medication. We also determine the client's habits regarding the use of nicotine, alcohol, and other nonprescription drugs.

Throughout the history you should be sensitive to potential covert issues. Ask if there are any issues that the client does not want discussed in front of his partner. We believe strongly in creating an interview environment in which each partner can be assured of confidentiality. Without separate and confidential interviews, crucial information may remain hidden. Provide the client with a second opportunity to reveal anything he or she thinks may be relevant. You might ask: "Is there anything else that you would like to tell me about yourself that I have not asked but that you think I should know?" These suggestions provide useful information, but for more detailed guidelines to interviewing, consult Wincze and Carey (1991).

Physical Examination. A physical examination should be completed by a physician who has remained current with developments in the evaluation of male erectile disorder (see Buvat et al., 1990). An examination should be a routine part of all evaluations. It should include evaluation of the vibratory sense on the penis (i.e., biothesiometry) and neurologic testing to evaluate cerebral and spinal cord function as well as peripheral nerve function. Because it is not yet practical to repair damaged nerves, direct measurement of the autonomic nerves is not common in clinical practice, although it is an important area of research. Laboratory studies should be ordered selectively, because routine endocrine evaluation is expensive and fewer than 5% of men presenting with male erectile disorder actually have hypogonadism; thus, the consensus among physicians is to order the blood work only if the patient has low sexual desire and abnormally small testes (Johnson & Jarow, 1992).

More detailed medical evaluation is done if the client wants to try injection therapy via the corpora cavernosa, or if the client desires a precise diagnosis. In the former case, the man must have a test injection to see if he will respond and to determine the appropriate therapeutic dose. Some clients need visual sexual stimulation, self-stimulation, or both in order to get the full benefit of the injection (Donatucci & Lue, 1992). The comfort and ambience of the surroundings in which he is given the test injection can play an important role in his ability to respond. If his sympathetic nerves are in a "fight-or-flight" mode, he will not be able to get sufficient smooth muscle relaxation to achieve the pharmacologically stimulated erection.

To establish a precise diagnosis, more invasive testing is necessary. Ultrasonic measurement of arterial blood flow in the corpora cavernosa (before and after pharmacologic injection), arteriography, and dynamic infusion cavernosometry and cavernosography (these procedures measure pressures and document by x-ray the problems with the veno-occlusive mechanism) are complex diagnostic procedures that can evaluate the vascular system more precisely. These procedures tend to be complex and expensive but are necessary if surgery on the vascular system is being considered.

Self-Report Measures. Standardized paper-and-pencil questionnaires that can be completed quickly by clients and easily scored can provide helpful information during the initial assessment and as therapy progresses. We often send out a brief battery of measures in advance of the first session (along with directions to our office, parking suggestions, and information on fees). We encourage clients to complete this information before the first session in order to prepare them for the session as well as provide some initial clinical material to guide the clinical interview. We also use questionnaires to monitor progress in therapy. A third way in which we sometimes use questionnaires is the method of paired reports for couples where we suspect such problems as communication difficulties or mismatched sexual scripts. With this method, the same questionnaire is completed twice by each partner: first for himself, and a second time as he believes his partner would complete it. This allows one to examine the agreement between partners as well as the amount of understanding that they have for each other's preferences or views. Use of this paired reports method can be very diagnostic of and therapeutic for dyadic problems (Carey et al., 1993).

Psychophysiologic Assessment. Psychophysiologic assessment can be a powerful tool. This approach tends to be less susceptible to the distortions and biases that can occur with interviews and questionnaires. In addition, psychophysiologic measures allow one to better understand the physiologic underpinnings, and sometimes the actual mechanisms, of the disorder. Two approaches are worthy of attention. The first approach is the physiologic recording of nocturnal penile tumescence (NPT) during sleep (Meisler & Carey, 1990). This can be done in a full sleep laboratory or even in an outpatient setting. Briefly, the rationale for this procedure is as follows: If a man can obtain an erection during sleep (which most men do two to four times per night) but cannot obtain an erection during partner stimulation, it is assumed that the source of the erectile disorder is primarily psychosocial. In contrast, if a man cannot obtain an erection at night, it is assumed that his disorder is primarily a product of biological factors. However, NPT can be suppressed by psychological causes (e.g., depression; see Thase et al., 1988) and should never be used as the only source of diagnostic information.

A second approach is the physiologic recording of penile tumescence in response to erotic stimulation. Indeed, it is the lack of such a response that is often reported as the problem in erectile disorder. Such daytime arousal studies or visual sexual stimulation studies, as they have been called, have proven valuable in the assessment process. We have found that some dysfunctional men who view erotic stimulation experienced full erection responses even though those men reported an inability to obtain an erection. Such data can be vital in formulating a case.

Case Formulation. One of the more challenging aspects of the assessment of male erectile disorder is integrating data obtained from the multidisciplinary approach (see Carey et al., 1984). Although it may be tempting to identify a single cause that demands a specific treatment, this is usually not possible given the many pathways by which male erectile disorder can emerge. Therefore, we strive to present a case formulation that includes all relevant biological, psychological, and social risk factors. By doing this we have laid the groundwork should additional information become available or further developments occur. Moreover, this comprehensive approach to case formulation will give the client confidence that you have considered all possibilities. This is an opportunity to communicate to the client that he, too, should also think about his problem in a multifaceted, biopsychosocial framework.

Treatment

Evidence for Prescriptive Treatments

Behavior Therapy. Although Wolpe (1958) and others had used behavioral techniques to treat sexual problems, it was Masters and Johnson (1970) who established behavioral sex therapy as a legitimate clinical specialty. Although they did not describe themselves as "behavior therapists," the structured homework exercises they prescribed, the short duration of their interventions, and their willingness to collect data to evaluate their work clearly reflected a behavioral influence.

Masters and Johnson (1970) reported good success with sex therapy for acquired male erectile disorder. Their approach emphasized sensate focus exercises as prescribed and monitored by a male and female co-therapist team; therapy occurred during an intensive 2-week period. Their findings indicate that only 26.3% of their subjects were identified as treatment failures at the end of therapy. Of the "non-failures" the relapse rate was 11.1%. However, the scientific aspects of this work have been criticized. In a scathing critique of this research, Zilbergeld and Evans (1980) summarized it as follows: "Our conclusion in brief: Masters and Johnson's sex-therapy research is so flawed by methodological errors and slipshod reporting that it fails to meet customary standards—and their own—for evaluation. This raises serious questions about the effectiveness of the 10-year-old discipline they created" (p. 29).

Since Masters and Johnson's pioneering work in the 1960s and 1970s, many behavioral and cognitive-behavioral clinicians have contributed to the development and evaluation of sex therapy in the treatment of male erectile disorder. Current cognitive-behavioral approaches (e.g., Wincze & Carey, 1991) tend to be multimodal, involving therapeutic use of sensate focus exercises and other sexual skills training approaches, education (including bibliotherapy), stimulus control procedures, relationship enhancement techniques (including communication skills training), cognitive restructuring and, most recently, health promotion strategies.

The effectiveness of these treatment programs has been evaluated and, as with psychotherapy research in general, the scientific evidence for the efficacy of the treatment programs tends to be less substantial than we would like. When one searches the treatment outcome literature, one finds mostly small-scale studies that tend not to be methodologically rigorous. The vast majority of these are studies of male and female clients with a variety of "sexual disorders" rather than focused studies of men with male erectile disorder. Outcome tends to be assessed in vague, global ways, often relying on therapist judgment or the use of nonstandardized self-report instruments. There are exceptions, of course, and it is the stronger studies that we have chosen to summarize.

Kilmann and his colleagues (1987) provide data from a study of 20 middle-aged men (mean, 51 years of age) with erectile disorder and their partners. The mean duration of the dysfunction was 5 years. Couples were assigned to 1 of 5 conditions: Communication Technique Training (including effective listening skills, self-assertion, sexual initiations and refusals), Sexual Technique Training (including sensate focus exercises), Combination Training, Attention-Placebo control, or No-Treatment control. Couples in the 3 treatment groups and the attention-placebo condition met in twice-weekly sessions for a total of 20 hours. Outcome was determined by asking the clients to complete four self-report measures. Collapsing across these four measures revealed an 80% success rate, with no significant differences among the 3 treatment conditions (not surprising given the small number of subjects in each condition).

Hawton, Catalan, and Fagg (1992) reported data from 36 couples presenting to a Sexual Dysfunction Clinic in the National Health Service setting of the United Kingdom. Couples (mean age, 43.2 years) participated in a multimodal treatment program, including Masters and Johnson–styled sensate focus exercises. They received an average of 12 sessions (range, 4 to 30) with a single therapist. Twenty-five (69.4%) couples completed treatment, nine (25%) dropped out, and two couples (5.6%) were terminated by the therapist because of poor progress. According to therapist ratings, 69.4% of the couples were able to engage in intercourse with only minor difficulties following therapy.

Based on these and other studies (see review by Mohr & Beutler 1990), what can we conclude about the effectiveness of cognitive-behavioral treatments for male erectile disorder? In general, sex therapy appears to be a worthwhile intervention for younger men without significant pathophysiology or comorbid psychopathology, who are in a stable relationship with a healthy, sexually functional partner. Presence of alcohol or drug use, other psychopathology, rigid beliefs about masculinity, and dyadic distress all reduce the likely effectiveness of sex therapy. Reluctance to participate in psychologically based therapy and premature termination remain common in this area (Hawton et al., 1992; Tiefer & Melman, 1987).

Pharmacotherapy

Self-injection Therapy. Self-injection of therapeutic drugs (e.g., papaverine, phentolamine, prostaglandin E_1) has become one of the most common ways that urologists treat male erectile disorder. This treatment is based on the notion that these substances can cause the cavernosal and arterial smooth muscle to relax, thereby facilitating an erection.

Complications of self-injection therapy include pain and bleeding at the injection site, pharmacologically induced prolonged erection, infection, and scarring of the corpora cavernosa. Prolonged erections can last for more than 4 hours and must be reversed by needle aspiration of some blood from the corpora and then injection of another medication that will cause smooth muscle contraction (e.g., phenylephrine, epinephrine, dopamine).

Recently, much research has been completed to evaluate the efficacy, safety, and patient acceptance of self-injection therapy. For example, in a short-term follow-up study, Althof et al. (1987) found that, within 6 months of home-based (i.e., self-injection) therapy, 35% of the men in the program had dropped out. Unfortunately, the authors did not complete a detailed study of attrition. It is suspected that many dropped out early because of objections to the injection procedure itself. Of those who remained in the program, 26% reported periodic bruising at the injection site, and plaque-like nodules were detected in 21% of the patients.

In a later study, Althof and his colleagues (1991) assessed the long-term effects of self-injected papaverine and phentolamine in 42 men and their partners. Over the course of the study, men were injecting themselves an average of five times a month, with 84% of these injections producing satisfactory erections. Improvements were noted in the quality of the erections, sexual satisfaction, and frequency of intercourse; decreases in psychiatric symptoms were also reported. The dropout rate was high (57%), however, due to side effects such as fibrotic nodules, abnormal liver function values, and bruising.

A significant psychological concern regarding papaverine injections (and other medically based interventions) involves the impact that such injections can have on the partner. For most individuals, it is very arousing and affirming to watch their partners' arousal grow as a result of their sexual attractiveness or skills. Relatedly, a partner's lack of erection can initiate a fear that one is no longer attractive or sexually desirable to the partner and cannot "turn him on." If erections are caused by injection rather than foreplay, a primary source of psychological feedback may be lost, and one's concerns about desirability can be exacerbated. The consequences may be a decline in arousal; thus, partners should be encouraged to communicate that they are attracted to and desirous of each other.

Overall, however, self-injection therapy appears to be an effective treatment for erectile disorder in men who have significant physiologic risk factors and are willing to learn how to give self-injections. Not all men (or their partners) accept this treatment (Althof et al., 1991; Sidi, Pratap, & Chen, 1988), however, because of frustration with trial dosing, unwillingness to inject, and concerns about cost or side effects.

Yohimbine. Yohimbine hydrochloride is an alpha-2-adrenoreceptor blocker believed to increase erections by increasing blood flow into the penis and decreasing outflow (Meyer, 1988). Unlike vasoactive substances (which are self-injected and act locally in the penile tissue), yohimbine is taken orally and is believed to exercise its effects centrally. It has a half-life of 35 minutes and produces many peripheral autonomic changes (e.g., increased heart rate) in addition to the desired effect of increased erections. Yohimbine gained notoriety through Davidson's work with rats (Clark, Smith, & Davidson, 1984), in which he demonstrated an increase in sexual activity of laboratory rats who ingested yohimbine.

At least five controlled studies have attempted to clarify the exact effect of yohimbine on humans. For example, Susset et al. (1989) reported a modest improvement in the erectile functioning among sexually dysfunctional men. Those who responded best were younger, with less organicity and with relatively recent onset of erectile problems. In contrast, Morales et al. (1987) reported no difference between yohimbine and placebo in the treatment of "organic impotence." Overall, however, the available data suggest that yohimbine may be effective in milder instances of male erectile disorder in which subtle organic and psychosocial risk factors are operative (Segraves & Segraves, 1992). Fortunately, yohimbine has few (if any) side effects when taken at clinical levels.

Testosterone. Testosterone is used when clients have hypogonadism. However, it should be noted that these endocrine problems are rarely the cause of male erectile disorder. When indicated, depot injections should be given approximately every 3 weeks. Oral forms have a risk of hepatotoxicity. However, because testosterone enanthate is an anabolic steroid, it has many potential side effects and should not be used cavalierly. Testosterone can stimulate the growth of a preexisting prostate cancer and elevate the red blood count (Krauss, Taub, Lantinga, Dunsky, & Kelly, 1991). Generally speaking, this should not be a common treatment for male erectile disorder.

Alternative Treatments

External Suction/Constriction Devices. A number of external suction devices have been designed and evaluated during the past decade. These devices induce an erection by creating a vacuum around the penis. This vacuum is created within a plastic cylinder by creating a suction force of 175 to 300 mmHg via hand or battery pump for 3 to 7 minutes. This vacuum will cause enough inflow of blood and swelling to make the penis firm enough (i.e., 454 gm of buckling force) for intromission. A rubber ring is then placed around the base of the penis prior to removal of the cylinder so that the erection is maintained. The ring must be removed (with attached handles or strings) within 30 minutes to avoid side effects. These devices are very appealing because they are relatively noninvasive and can be used by most men with erection problems.

In a recent review of studies evaluating the effectiveness of these devices, Althof and Turner (1992) concluded that 90% of all men treated, regardless of the purported etiology, were able to achieve erections sufficient for intercourse by employing these devices. In one study (Turner et al., 1990), men used the device in order to have intercourse an average of four times a month, with satisfactory erections occurring 78% of the time. The men also reported increased psychological adjustment as a consequence of this treatment at 6- and 12-month follow-up sessions. According to some authors (e.g., Althof & Turner, 1992), client acceptance for vacuum therapy is higher than for self-injection therapy. In addition, the side effects (with correct use) are few.

Penile Prostheses. Surgical implantation of prosthetic devices is still widely used. For example, during 1989, United States surgeons implanted an estimated 27,500 prostheses (Spark, 1991). These ingenious technological inventions can be semirigid, malleable, articulating, inflatable, and hydraulically malleable (Krauss, 1987). Prostheses are thought to be effective and dependable; they are well tolerated by clients and partners. The disadvantages of these prostheses include the necessity of surgery with its cost and risks, including complications such as infection, urethral injury, postsurgical pain, erosion, and mechanical breakdown. The last-mentioned problem has been much less common with recent models (Krauss, 1987).

Research evaluating the efficacy of prostheses has tended to be positive. However, much of the available data have come from studies that are methodologically flawed. Common problems include reliance on unvalidated and global measures of postsurgical adjustment and satisfaction, failure to assess partner acceptance of the prosthesis, retrospective designs with low patient response rates, and inadequate follow-up intervals. Recent studies have lessened some of these flaws. For example, Krauss, Lantinga, Carey, Meisler, and Kelly (1989) completed a prospective, longitudinal study of 19 implant recipients and their partners. The findings suggested that most patients and partners were satisfied with their prosthesis one year after surgery, although use of the prosthesis was sometimes accompanied by short-term complications (e.g., general discomfort or disappointment with size). Satisfaction tended to be lower among spouses than patients. Frequency of sexual intercourse increased during the follow-up period, but there were no changes in sexual desire. Neither dyadic nor psychological adjustment changed significantly during this period.

In an earlier but more fine-grained study, Meisler, Carey, Krauss, and Lantinga (1988) reported on two heterosexual couples in which the man received an implant. Both couples underwent a presurgical evaluation in which the patient and sexual partner were assessed on a number of psychological, dyadic, and sexual functioning variables. The surgery was performed and the couples' subsequent satisfaction with the prosthesis as well as their psychological, dyadic, and sexual adjustment were measured 6 and 12 months after surgery. Despite many similarities in medical aspects of the surgery, for one couple a successful outcome was evidenced, whereas the other couple demonstrated a therapeutic failure despite the technical success of the surgery. Several psychosocial differences between the couples were identified: The couple with the negative outcome had a history of previous psychiatric treatment, history of poor sexual adjustment for the partner, poor dyadic adjustment, and poor communication. Findings such as these highlight the need for presurgical assessment, even when a clear physiologic cause for the male erectile disorder is present.

The consensus in the field is that selection and preparation of clients for a prosthesis are extremely important (Melman & Tiefer, 1992). Increasingly it is recognized that follow-up care must include attention to psychosocial as well as medical complications.

Selecting Optimal Treatment Strategies

Given the wide array of legitimate therapeutic options, it can be difficult for clients and clinicians alike to make choices among them. In our practice, we attempt to balance the following principles with our clients as we make choices about treatment: First, to the extent possible, we try to match the intervention with the hypothesized etiology. Thus, if the evaluation data indicate that dyadic distress is the primary cause for the disorder, we try to target the dyadic problem in therapy. If the data reveal a venous leakage problem, we would advise a medical solution (e.g., prosthesis). Often, however, multiple risk factors are present and no clear-cut etiology can be established. Thus, a second principle is educate the client about the options and allow him (and his partner) to choose the approach most consistent with their values. Of course, this choice should be appropriate and defensible to our professional colleagues. Third, we prefer to begin with the least invasive intervention. Thus, we would prefer to start with a vacuum device before initiating surgery for an implant.

It is often appropriate to combine medical and psychological approaches. Earlier we mentioned the need for careful follow-up care with penile prosthesis recipients. Some men who receive implants may now be able to achieve firm erections, but this may not result in a healthy sexual relationship if the client and his partner are still having difficulty communicating and are using sex in a struggle for control in the relationship. Similarly, it may be appropriate to use a vacuum device or self-injection therapy to enhance sex therapy in carefully selected couples (see Kaplan, 1990). In all cases we remind clients that sex is not just intercourse, and encourage them to enhance other aspects of their relationship (see Wincze & Carey, 1991; Zilbergeld, 1992).

Problems in Carrying Out Interventions

Every specialty area has its unique problems or challenges; the sexuality area is no different. It may even be that the treatment of male erectile disorder is more challenging than most, because it involves a socially sensitive area and it usually involves two people! Nevertheless, here are a few of the common problems we encounter.

Preference for a Quick Fix. Most men experiencing male erectile disorder have a prior history of "trouble-free erections on demand" with little or no effort involved. This history predisposes them to expect a quick and easy fix for their problems. In addition, much of the advertising directed at men with male erectile disorder offers "quick and easy cures." When the so-called "fix" requires some pain and discomfort (e.g., self-injections or penile prosthetic surgery) or sustained effort (e.g., a course of sex or couples therapy), some clients become impatient or noncompliant. Open and honest communication with the client and, if appropriate, the partner about the nature of the assessment process and the prescribed treatments can go a long way toward establishing and maintaining reasonable treatment expectations. We find that the time used to explain the rationale for a selected treatment is well spent and often increases compliance.

Competing Beliefs. Occasionally, the client and partner will have competing beliefs regarding sexuality. Such disparate belief systems have usually been present from the beginning of the relationship, but the stress associated with the current disorder will often highlight such conflict and bring it out into the open. Such differences can be minor (e.g., occasional disagreement about the timing of sexual encounters), or they can be significant in their disruptive capabilities (e.g., frequent arguments about the partner's unwillingness to employ erotic aids, or bitter confrontations regarding the role of oral sex in the relationship). We make every effort to assume a value-neutral stance in our assessment and treatment efforts, seldom taking sides when the client and partner have competing beliefs that are affecting their sexuality. When we believe that such differences will interfere significantly with outcome, we make them a focus of prescribed treatment and provide a therapeutic forum within which the couple can learn to compromise and adjust. This is best accomplished within the context of the more psychosocially oriented treatments of couples, sex therapy, or both.

Alcohol and Drug Use. Acute intoxication from many substances (e.g., alcohol, barbiturates) can produce situational, transient male erectile disorder (Segraves & Segraves, 1992). Also, prolonged abuse of many substances (e.g., alcohol) can result in chronic sexual problems, including male erectile disorder, often because of hepatic dysfunction (Salaspuro, 1989). These risk factors associated with male erectile disorder, however, are not the only way in which substance abuse and dependence can adversely affect sexual functioning. The profound disruption of the dyadic relationship that typically occurs when one or both partners are experiencing substance abuse/dependence problems (Bean-Bayog, 1986) can adversely affect most efforts to assess and treat male erectile disorder. Thus, a thorough biopsychosocial assessment must include an examination for possible substance abuse/dependence disorders. When significant problems in this domain are diagnosed, we recommend referring the client or couple for appropriate substance abuse therapy as part of the comprehensive treatment plan developed.

Single Men. Clients without current sexual partners pose difficulties when the prescribed treatment modality involves a couples approach (e.g., sex therapy). We believe that the use of so-called sexual surrogates raises ethical concerns and we do not subscribe to this strategy. When sex therapy is part of our treatment recommendation for clients without partners, we make extensive use of office- and homework-based guided imagery in place of the more traditional couples-based pleasuring exercises and relationship enhancement techniques.

Unwilling Partners. The most comprehensive and sophisticated assessment and treatment strategies are doomed to failure if one of the partners is an unwilling participant in the process. For example, we have documented cases of surgically successful penile prosthesis surgery but ultimate treatment failure due to unwilling partner participation (Krauss, Bogin, & Culebras, 1983; Meisler et al. 1988). We cannot foresee all possible sources of partner or client noncompliance, but involving both partners in the assessment and treatment process from the very beginning can minimize problems of a partner's feeling left out of the decision-making process. When the client refuses initially to involve his partner in the assessment and treatment process, we stress the importance of doing so and make every effort to persuade him to change his mind. We do not refuse to assess and treat if the client chooses to exclude his partner, but we proceed with caution in such instances.

Relapse Prevention

Researchers have not paid much attention to relapse following treatment for male erectile disorder. Despite Masters and Johnson's (1970) optimistic report that only

11.1% of the "nonfailures" in their study relapsed, most practitioners believe that relapse is very high among men treated for male erectile disorder (Mohr & Beutler, 1990). Therefore, after concluding a course of treatment, it is wise to schedule booster sessions (every 3 or 6 months) to check in with clients and assess maintenance of gains as well as the emergence of new problems or concerns. We try to help clients to understand the value of such booster sessions without undermining their positive expectancies or confidence.

Case Illustration

Case Description

Presenting Problem.   Mr. George Hansen (a pseudonym) is a 54-year-old married white man who was referred to our Sexual Health Clinic (an interdisciplinary medical center–based clinic staffed by a urologist, psychologists, and a nurse practitioner) by his family practice physician for evaluation and treatment of "impotence." During a recent routine physical examination, Mr. Hansen, with considerable reluctance, had informed his physician that he was having difficulty satisfying his wife and that his interest in sex was diminishing.

Sexual Health Clinic Intake.   Hr. Hansen completed our paper-and-pencil questionnaire before an office visit with our physician and nurse practitioner. During the office visit, he provided his medical history and underwent a comprehensive physical exam. Laboratory tests were ordered at this time. Mr. Hansen and his wife then met with the clinic psychologist to complete a psychosocial history and brief psychological testing.

Upon detailed inquiry, Mr. Hansen reported that about 5 to 6 years prior he had begun to experience occasional difficulties achieving a "normal erection." Often, it took longer for the erections to occur and he seemed to lose the erections more quickly, especially if distracted by his concerns that he might not be able to perform adequately. Since then, his erectile capabilities had seemed to worsen gradually. At the time of the interview, his best obtainable erections during sexual activity with his partner were 40 to 50% of "normal" and were rarely firm enough for intromission. He was experiencing some morning erections that were larger (60 to 75% of normal), but they quickly dissipated. Masturbation produced erections of about 75% of normal that, he said, were probably firm enough for intromission. He was still able to ejaculate and reported only some mild decrease in force. He was not concerned about the size or shape of his penis. Mr. Hansen reported that he had had less desire for sex for the past several months and was concerned that something might be wrong; despite this he said he experienced frequent sexual fantasies. He had never experienced any sexual problems prior to 6 years prior.

History: Medical and Surgical.   Mr. Hansen reported that he was currently being treated for systolic hypertension, angina pectoris, intermittent claudication of the legs, and gout. The hypertension onset had been approximately 10 years prior, the angina approximately 7 years prior, the intermittent claudication about 2 years prior, and the gout about 3 years prior. Previous surgeries included an appendectomy at age 24 and a cholesystectomy at age 49. Current regular medications include hydrochlorothiazide (a diuretic and antihypertensive), alpha-methyldopa (an antihyperten-sive), allopurinal (used in the treatment of gout), diltiazem hydrochloride (a calcium-channel blocker used in the treatment of angina pectoris), and nitroglycerin as needed. Mr. Hansen had stopped smoking 10 years earlier. He and his wife drank an occasional glass of wine when dining out. Neither had ever abused alcohol or other drugs.

History: Psychosocial. Mr. Hansen reported a normal childhood with no history of abuse or deprivation. He was one of three children born to his parents, who were deceased; his father died of coronary disease and his mother as a result of a stroke. Mr. and Mrs. Hansen had been married for 30 years and had two grown daughters, both of whom lived outside the home. Mr. Hansen had a bachelor's degree and was an accountant. He was on recent partial disability secondary to his coronary condition and was working as a part-time inventory clerk, a job he thought beneath him. Mrs. Hansen was a high school graduate. She returned to the work force after her daughters entered high school. She had worked as an executive secretary and had been promoted recently to a managerial position with a significant increase in salary and responsibility.

Mr. and Mrs. Hansen had been in brief marital therapy about 12 years prior to address problems caused by Mr. Hansen's "workaholic tendencies." They reported that the therapy seemed to help "in improving the communication difficulties, while reducing the arguments." Mr. Hansen reported that he had not been very happy since he was forced to retire. He felt dissatisfied and less useful and had not been pleased with himself. No other histories of psychiatric problems or treatments were reported.

History: Sexual. Mr. Hansen reported that his first sexual experience was with a prostitute during his military service (he requested that we not reveal that information to his wife, who was unaware of this history). He had dated occasionally before his first and only marriage, which had occurred when he and his wife were each 24 years of age. He reported no history of sexual trauma or injury. Mr. Hansen's interest in sex had been less than normal for him for several months; before that, his interest level was normal. He said that he had experienced rapid ejaculation on occasion in the past but that it always occurred after periods of prolonged sexual abstinence and he never considered it problematic. Mr. Hansen reported that he always believed they had a very good marriage, although lately he had been feeling somewhat distant from Mrs. Hansen and had a vague feeling that he was losing her. He had not discussed his feelings with her. Mrs. Hansen reported one previous sexual partner before their marriage. She reported no history of sexual trauma or injury, nor did she report any history of or any current difficulties with painful intercourse, problems with sexual desire, or difficulty with orgasm. Mrs. Hansen said that she was supportive of her husband's efforts to deal with his sexual difficulties. She said that he seemed to overreact to the situation and worried about it more than necessary. She felt they had a good marriage with no major problems.

Physical Examination and Laboratory Findings. Physical examination re-vealed a slightly overweight, well-developed, and well-nourished man in no acute distress. Pertinent physical findings included: a normal male hair pattern, normal thyroid function, no gynecomastia, normal scrotum and penis, slightly atrophic testes, good rectal sphincter tone, and a small, benign feeling prostate. Findings of neurologic examination, especially concentrating on the lumbosacral area, were within normal limits. His pedal pulses were weak. Testosterone, luteinizing hormone, and follicle-stimulating hormone values were all well within normal limits (the blood work was ordered because of Mr. Hansen's report of low sexual desire and his small testes). We did not conduct intracavernosal pharmacologic testing because the Hansens chose, after discussing the treatment options, to try first the external suction device.

Differential Diagnosis and Assessment

Based on all available data, we found Mr. Hansen to be experiencing male erectile disorder. Despite his self-report of deficient desire and low rate of sexual activity, we ruled out hypoactive sexual desire disorder because Mr. Hansen was experiencing sexual fantasies regularly. Despite occasional instances of premature ejaculation, Mr. Hansen's symptoms did not meet the criteria for that diagnosis. A differential diagnosis we considered was that of major depressive disorder with accompanying erectile dysfunction. We ultimately ruled that out based on a more detailed interview by our psychologist team member, who decided that Mr. Hansen's symptoms did not meet the criteria for that disorder.

Risk Factors. We identified the following risk factors associated with Mr. Hansen's erectile disorder:

Medical Problems. Mr. Hansen has vascular disease, as evidenced by his coronary artery disease (the source of his angina) and by his peripheral vascular disease (the source of his intermittent claudication and poor pedal pulses). Consultation with his cardiologist revealed a significant level of pathology associated with his coronary artery disease and a prognosis that included probable future coronary artery bypass surgery. As well as affecting the coronary arteries, Mr. Hansen's vascular disease was no doubt causing reduced blood flow to the penis and was thus adversely affecting his erectile capabilities.

Medication Side Effects. Mr. Hansen's medication regimen was also contributing to the etiology of his erectile disorder. Allopurinol for gout has less than a 1% incidence of erectile disorder as a side effect; the diltiazem also has a very low reported incidence of erectile disorder as a side effect. However, Mr. Hansen's antihypertensive medication was probably adversely affecting his erections. Methyldopa, especially in combination with hydrochlorothiazide, has been linked directly to erectile dysfunction (Croog, Levine, Sudilovsky, Baume, & Cline, 1988).

Psychosocial Risk Factors. Symptoms of depression and low self-esteem were troubling Mr. Hansen. His score on the Center for Epidemiological Studies Depression Scale (CES-D) was above the mean, indicating a moderate degree of depression. Although he did not link these concerns with his male erectile disorder, we believed that they were strongly associated. His forced disability retirement and the associated loss of self-esteem, accompanied by his partner's recent career successes, had led to feelings of inadequacy and failure, and a resultant estrangement from his partner. His recently acquired part-time job was not meeting Mr. Hansen's needs for a sense of success and contribution. His feelings of inadequacy as a professional and "bread-winner" were exacerbated by his feelings of inadequacy as husband and lover.

Another risk factor was the Hansens' troubled dyadic relationship. As part of our usual assessment process, the Hansens each completed the Dyadic Adjustment Scale

(Spanier, 1989). Their total scale scores suggested strongly that their relationship was troubled. The Dyadic Consensus subscale showed the presence of disagreements between the partners on matters important to the relationship, namely, work roles and expectations. For the early years of their marriage, they had what would be considered a traditional sex-role relationship, with Mr. Hansen working outside the home and Mrs. Hansen staying home and caring for the children. Mr. Hansen's medical problems and work limitations, and Mrs. Hansen's successful reentry into a meaningful career, shook to the very foundation their traditional roles. The couple was unable to address these issues themselves and withdrew from each other further. This estrangement was also played out in their sexual behavior, creating feelings of dislike and avoidance, as evidenced, for example, by Mr. Hansen's declining sexual desire for his partner. The Dyadic Satisfaction subscale was also abnormal, indicating elevated amounts of tension in the relationship and dissatisfaction with its present state. Significant abnormalities were also evidenced in the Affectional Expression subscale, showing their mutual dissatisfaction with the current expression of affection and sex in the relationship. Their scores on the Dyadic Cohesion subscale, however, were very positive, indicating interests and activities shared by the couple.

Case Formulation.   Upon completion of our biopsychosocial assessment, we met as a team and agreed on the following case formulation: Mr. Hansen's male erectile disorder had multiple causes. His serious vascular disease had apparently compromised penile blood flow, thus reducing erectile capabilities. His medication regimen, as well, had further reduced his erectile capacity. His vascular disease was not reversible and his medications, after previous unsuccessful trials of other antihypertensives, were deemed absolutely necessary. Thus, we decided that some biologically based intervention was necessary to overcome these risk factors. We met with the Hansens and offered them the choice between self-injection therapy and an external suction device. The Hansens chose the external suction device, after expressing reservations about using needles for self-injection.

Serious issues were also troubling this relationship, and we believed that these difficulties, if unresolved, would continue to adversely affect Mr. Hansen's erectile capabilities. We believed that Mr. Hansen's depressive symptoms were also interacting with his erectile disorder, and we wanted to ensure that subsequent treatment could address that issue as well.

Treatment Selection

Consistent with our strategy of prescribing treatments based on the identified risk factors, we recommended the following treatments for the Hansens. Our physician prescribed an external suction device. We referred the Hansens to a psychologist for short-term marital therapy to address their communication, sex-role, and affectional difficulties. The psychologist was an experienced sex therapist, so the issue of reduced sexual attraction could be addressed; he was also able to further assess and treat Mr. Hansen's depressive symptoms.

Treatment Course and Problems in Carrying Out Interventions

The Hansens agreed to our treatment recommendations and eagerly purchased the device. They tried to use it, and called us soon after with some problems. It quickly became apparent that they had not followed all the enclosed instructions for its use and were experiencing difficulties that were easily resolved with appropriate information and reassurance. The couple agreed to accept our referral for marital/sex therapy. However, they delayed following through with our recommendations for several weeks, in an apparent attempt to determine if the "quick fix" of the device would be sufficient. The couple realized that despite the restoration of erectile capabilities, they were still experiencing problems with their relationship and they eventually entered therapy.

Outcome and Termination

Six months later, we contacted the Hansens to see how they were doing. Mr. Hansen reported that he could achieve and maintain consistently usable erections with the assistance of the external suction device. He reported satisfaction with the device, as did Mrs. Hansen. Both reported that they were communicating better, arguing less, and feeling more connected than they had in many months. We agreed that no additional follow-up was necessary unless significant new problems arose.

Summary

Male erectile disorder is a condition in which a man is unable to achieve or maintain an erection during sexual activity. This disorder often has a profound and negative effect on the client's self-esteem and is likely to impair an existing dyadic relationship or decrease the client's willingness to develop new relationships. Evidence suggests that male erectile disorder is the most common male sexual dysfunction for which treatment is sought. Many medical disorders place a man at increased risk for the disorder, including those that compromise the hormonal, vascular, and neurologic systems involved in sexual responding. Psychological and relationship risk factors are also common and they often co-occur with physiologic risk factors, making diagnosis and assessment quite challenging. Therefore, we advocate a multidisciplinary evaluation in almost all cases. This evaluation should include a comprehensive medical, sexual, psychological, and relationship history as well as a physical examination by a qualified urologist. Selective use of self-report questionnaires and psychophysiologic testing is also advised. Treatment options include cognitive-behavioral sex therapy, self-injection therapy, yohimbine, testosterone, external suction and constriction devices, and penile prostheses. Because many treatment options are available, we encourage an approach that is matched to the hypothesized etiology of the disorder, consistent with the client's values and goals, and least invasive. We also encourage a combined use of medical and psychosocial interventions, and the inclusion of the client's partner in both assessment and treatment.

References

Althof, S. E., & Turner, L. A. (1992). Self-injection therapy and external vacuum devices in the treatment of erectile dysfunction: Methods and outcome. In R. C. Rosen & S. R. Leiblum (Eds.), *Erectile disorders: Assessment and treatment* (pp. 283–309). New York: Guilford.

Althof, S. E., Turner, L. A., Levine, S. B., Risen, C., Bodner, D., Kursh, E., & Resnick, M. I. (1991). Sexual, psychological, and marital impact of self-injection and papaverine and phentolamine: A long-term prospective study. *Journal of Sex and Marital Therapy, 17,* 101–112.

Althof, S. E., Turner, L. A., Levine, S. B., Risen, C., Kursh, E., Bodner, D., & Resnick, M. (1987). Intracavernosal injection in the treatment of impotence: A prospective study of sexual, psychological, and marital functioning. *Journal of Sex and Marital Therapy, 13,* 155–167.

American Psychiatric Association (1987). *Diagnostic and statistical manual of mental disorders* (3rd ed., rev.). Washington, DC: Author.

American Psychiatric Association (1993). *DSM-IV draft criteria.* Washington, DC: Author.

Bancroft, J., & Coles, L. (1976). Three years' experience in a sexual problems clinic. *British Medical Journal, 1,* 1575–1577.

Bean-Bayog, M. (1986). Psychopathology produced by alcoholism. In R. E. Meyer (Ed.), *Psychopathology and addictive disorders* (pp. 334–345). New York: Guilford.

Buvat, J., Buvat-Herbaut, M., Lemaire, A., Marcolin, G., & Quittelier, E. (1990). Recent developments in the clinical assessment and diagnosis of erectile dysfunction. *Annual Review of Sex Research,* 265–308.

Carey, M. P., Flasher, L. V., Maisto, S. A., & Turkat, I. D. (1984). The a priori approach to psychological assessment. *Professional Psychology: Research and Practice, 15,* 515–527.

Carey, M. P., Wincze, J. P., & Meisler, A. W. (1993). Sexual dysfunction: Male erectile disorder. In D. H. Barlow (Ed.), *Clinical handbook of psychological disorders* (2nd ed., pp. 442–480). New York: Guilford.

Clark, J., Smith, E., & Davidson, J. (1984). Enhancement of sexual motivation in male rats by yohimbine. *Science, 225,* 847–848.

Croog, S. H., Levine, S., Sudilovsky, A., Baume, R. M., & Cline, J. (1988). Sexual symptoms in hypertensive patients: A clinical trial of antihypertensive medications. *Archives of Internal Medicine, 148,* 788–794.

Donatucci, C. F., & Lue, T. F. (1992). The combined intracavernous injection and stimulation test: Diagnostic accuracy. *Journal of Urology, 148,* 61–62.

Frank, E., Anderson, C., & Kupfer, D. J. (1976). Profiles of couples seeking sex therapy and marital therapy. *American Journal of Psychiatry, 113,* 559–562.

Hawton, K. (1982). The behavioural treatment of sexual dysfunction. *British Journal of Psychiatry, 140,* 94–101.

Hawton, K., Catalan, J., & Fagg, J. (1992). Sex therapy for erectile dysfunction: Characteristics of couples, treatment outcome, and prognostic factors. *Archives of Sexual Behavior, 21,* 161–175.

Johnson, A. R., & Jarow, J. P. (1992). Is routine endocrine testing of impotent men necessary? *Journal of Urology, 147,* 1542–1544.

Kaplan, H. S. (1974). *The new sex therapy.* New York: Brunner/Mazel.

Kaplan, H. S. (1990). The combined use of sex therapy and intrapenile injections in the treatment of impotence. *Journal of Sex and Marital Therapy, 16,* 195–207.

Kilmann, P. R., Milan, R. J., Boland, J. P., Nankin, H. R., Davidson, E., West, M. O., Sabalis, R. F., Caid, C., & Devine, J. M. (1987). Group treatment of secondary erectile dysfunction. *Journal of Sex and Marital Therapy, 13,* 168–182.

Kinsey, A. C., Pomeroy, W. B., & Martin, C. E. (1948). *Sexual behavior in the human male.* Philadelphia: Saunders.

Krane, R. J., Goldstein, I., & Saenz de Tejada, I. (1989). Impotence. *New England Journal of Medicine, 321,* 1648–1659.

Krauss, D. J. (1987). Management of impotence. II: Selected surgical procedures: Penile prostheses. *Clinical Therapeutics, 9,* 149–156.

Krauss, D. J., Bogin, D., & Culebras, A. (1983). The failed penile prosthesis, despite technical success. *Journal of Urology, 129,* 969–971.

Krauss, D. J., Lantinga, L. J., Carey, M. P., Meisler, A. W., & Kelly, C. M. (1989). Use of the malleable penile prosthesis in the treatment of erectile dysfunction: A prospective study of post-surgical adjustment. *Journal of Urology, 142,* 988–991.

Krauss, D. J., Lantinga, L. J., & Kelly, C. M. (1990). In treating impotence, urology and sex therapy are complementary. *Urology, 36,* 467–470.

Krauss, D. J., Taub, H. A., Lantinga, L. J., Dunsky, M. H., & Kelly, C. M. (1991). Risk of blood volume changes in hypogonadal men treated with testosterone enanthate for erectile impotence. *Journal of Urology, 146,* 1566–1570.

Leiblum, S. R., & Rosen, R. C. (1991). Couples therapy for erectile disorders: Conceptual and clinical considerations. *Journal of Sex and Marital Therapy, 17,* 147–159.

Masters, W. H., & Johnson, V. E. (1970). *Human sexual inadequacy.* Boston: Little, Brown.

McKinlay, J. B. (1992). The prevalence and demographics of impotence. In the *Proceedings of the*

Consensus Development Conference on Impotence (p. 29). Bethesda, MD: National Institutes of Health.

Meisler, A. W., & Carey, M. P. (1990). A critical reevaluation of nocturnal penile tumescence monitoring in the diagnosis of erectile dysfunction. *Journal of Nervous and Mental Disease, 178,* 78–89.

Meisler, A. W., Carey, M. P., Krauss, D. J., & Lantinga, L. J. (1988). Success and failure in penile prosthesis surgery: Two cases highlighting the importance of psychosocial factors. *Journal of Sex and Marital Therapy, 14,* 108–119.

Melman, A., & Tiefer, L. (1992). Surgery for erectile disorders: Operative procedures and psychological issues. In R. C. Rosen & S. R. Leiblum (Eds.), *Erectile disorders: Assessment and treatment* (pp. 255–282). New York: Guilford.

Meyer, J. J. (1988). Impotence: Assessment in the private-practice office. *Postgraduate Medicine, 84,* 87–91.

Mohr, D. C., & Beutler, L. E. (1990). Erectile dysfunction: A review of diagnostic and treatment procedures. *Clinical Psychology Review, 10,* 123–150.

Morales, A., Condra, M., Owen, J. A., Surridge, D. H., Fenemore, J., & Harris, C. (1987). Is yohimbine effective in the treatment of organic impotence? Results of a controlled trial. *Journal of Urology, 137,* 1168–1172.

Regier, D. A., Myers, J. K., Kramer, M., Robins, L. N., Blazer, D. G., Hough, R. L., Eaton, W. W., & Locke, B. Z. (1984). The NIMH Epidemiologic Catchment Area program. *Archives of General Psychiatry, 41,* 934–941.

Renshaw, D. C. (1988). Profiles of 2376 patients treated at Loyola Sex Clinic between 1972 and 1987. *Sexual and Marital Therapy, 3,* 111–117.

Salaspuro, M. (1989). The organ pathogenesis of alcoholism: Liver and gastrointestinal tract. In H. W. Goedde & D. P. Agarwal (Eds.), *Alcoholism: Biomedical and genetic aspects* (pp. 133–166). Elmsford, NY: Pergamon.

Schover, L. R., & Jensen, S. B. (1988). *Sexuality and chronic illness: A comprehensive approach.* New York: Guilford.

Segraves, R. T., & Segraves, K. B. (1992). Aging and drug effects on male sexuality. In R. C. Rosen & S. R. Leiblum (Eds.), *Erectile disorders: Assessment and treatment* (pp. 96–140). New York: Guilford.

Shabsigh, R., Fishman, I. J., Schum, C., & Dunn, J. K. (1991). Cigarette smoking and other vascular risk factors in vasculogenic impotence. *Urology, 38,* 227–231.

Sidi, A., Pratap, R., & Chen, K. (1988). Patient acceptance of and satisfaction with vasoactive intracavernous pharmacotherapy for impotence. *Journal of Urology, 140,* 293–294.

Spanier, G. B. (1989). *Manual for the Dyadic Adjustment Scale.* North Tonawanda, NY: Multi-Health Systems.

Spark, R. F. (1991). *Male sexual health: A couple's guide.* Mount Vernon, NY: Consumer Reports Books.

Spector, I. P., & Carey, M. P. (1990). Incidence and prevalence of the sexual dysfunctions: A critical review of the literature. *Archives of Sexual Behavior, 19,* 389–408.

Susset, J., Tessier, C., Wincze, J., Bansal, S., Malhotra, C., & Schwacha, M. (1989). Effect of yohimbine hydrochloride on erectile impotence: A double-blind study. *Journal of Urology, 141,* 1360–1363.

Thase, M. E., Reynolds, C. F., Jennings, J. R., Frank, E., Howell, J. R., Hovck, P. R., Berman, S., & Kupfer, D. J. (1988). Nocturnal penile tumescence is diminished in depressed men. *Biological Psychiatry, 24,* 33–46.

Tiefer, L., & Melman, A. (1987). Adherence to recommendations and improvement over time in men with erectile dysfunction. *Archives of Sexual Behavior, 16,* 301–309.

Turner, L. A., Althof, S. E., Levine, S. B., Kursh, E., Bodner, D., & Resnick, M. (1990). Treating erectile dysfunction with external vacuum device: Impact upon sexual, psychological and marital functioning. *Journal of Urology, 144,* 79–82.

Weizman, R., & Hart, J. (1987). Sexual behavior in healthy married men. *Archives of Sexual Behavior, 16,* 39–44.

Wincze, J. P., & Carey, M. P. (1991). *Sexual dysfunctions: Guide for assessment and treatment.* New York: Guilford.

Wolpe, J. (1958). *Psychotherapy by reciprocal inhibition.* Stanford, CA: Stanford University Press.

Zilbergeld, B. (1992). *The new male sexuality: A guide to sexual fulfillment.* New York: Bantam.

Zilbergeld, B., & Evans, M. (1980, August). The inadequacy of Masters and Johnson. *Psychology Today,* 29–43.

18

Insomnia

Brant W. Riedel and Kenneth L. Lichstein

Description of the Disorder

Clinical Features

Insomnia complaints can be divided into two categories: (1) sleep-onset insomnia (difficulty in initiating sleep), and (2) sleep maintenance insomnia (difficulty in remaining asleep). The latter can be further divided into: (a) frequent and/or long-lasting awakenings during the night, and (b) early morning awakening with an inability to fall back to sleep (terminal insomnia). Insomniacs may present with only a single complaint or a combination of the above-mentioned categories. Because of the subjective nature of insomnia complaints, the actual degree of sleep onset or sleep maintenance disturbance varies greatly and is not necessarily correlated with the intensity of an insomniac's dissatisfaction. For example, among three sleepers who average identical 40-minute sleep latencies, one may complain of severe insomnia, another may report mild insomnia, and the third person may be unconcerned about his or her sleep pattern. The frequency of insomnia also varies. Some insomniacs report difficulty sleeping nearly every night; others complain of less frequent sleep disturbance.

Associated Features

Some insomniacs experience significant daytime impairment, but many do not. Researchers have generally found no significant difference between insomniacs and noninsomniacs on objective measures of daytime sleepiness (Mendelson, Garnett,

Brant W. Riedel and **Kenneth L. Lichstein** • Department of Psychology, Memphis State University, Memphis, Tennessee 38152.

Handbook of Prescriptive Treatments for Adults, edited by Michel Hersen and Robert T. Ammerman. Plenum Press, New York, 1994.

Gillin, & Weingartner, 1984; Seidel et al., 1984). Mendelson et al. (1984) also found that daytime measures of psychomotor functioning, attention, vigilance, and episodic memory did not reliably distinguish insomniacs from normal sleepers. However, insomniacs exhibited significantly poorer long-term semantic memory at each measurement point during the day. Also, there is evidence that insomniacs believe that their nocturnal sleep difficulties produce significant daytime impairment. Insomniacs score highly on the Insomnia Impact Scale, a self-report questionnaire that assesses subjects' perception of the effect of insomnia on physical, cognitive, emotional, social, and occupational aspects of daytime functioning (Hoelscher, Ware, & Bond, 1993).

Epidemiology

Epidemiologic studies have investigated the prevalence and severity of sleep disturbance in the general population. Insomnia is the most prevalent sleep disorder (Bixler, Kales, Soldatos, Kales, & Healey, 1979), and occasional insomnia has been estimated to afflict about 35% of the adult population (Mellinger, Balter, & Uhlenhuth, 1985). Surveys suggest that roughly 10 to 20% of adults suffer from severe or chronic insomnia (Buysse & Reynolds, 1990). Sleep maintenance problems are common among older insomniacs, whereas younger insomniacs more frequently complain of difficulty falling asleep. More women than men report insomnia, and the incidence of insomnia symptoms increases with age (Ford & Kamerow, 1989; Mellinger et al., 1985).

Etiology

Insomnia can emanate from several diverse sources including psychological or psychiatric determinants, poor sleep hygiene, and medical or drug-related factors.

Psychological.   Insomnia will often include a learning component. A transient insomnia (duration less than 1 month) resulting from a particular stressor (lifestyle changes, interpersonal difficulties) may evolve into chronic insomnia as a person begins to associate going to bed with insomnia rather than sleep. The bedroom, the bed itself, and rituals associated with going to bed may become conditioned stimuli that continue to elicit insomnia long after the original stressor is removed. In addition, a person who experiences transient insomnia may develop fears connected with his or her inability to sleep and may also begin to "try" to sleep, both of which tend to produce physiologic and cognitive arousal that is not conducive to sleep. A vicious cycle is established in which a person's fears concerning sleep and over-zealous attempts to sleep serve to maintain current sleep difficulties and threaten to engender chronic insomnia.

There is also evidence that cognitions unrelated to sleep can produce insomnia. Intrusive cognitions may include problem solving, planning future activities, and other thoughts that tend to arouse rather than relax. In two separate investigations, insomniacs have identified cognitive factors as a more frequent source of sleep disruption than somatic variables such as bodily tension or restlessness (Espie, Brooks, & Lindsay, 1989; Lichstein & Rosenthal, 1980). In addition, Gross and Borkovec (1982) demonstrated that an experimental manipulation intended to increase cognitive arousal led to lengthier sleep latencies in a sample of normal sleepers. Other studies of insomniac subjects, however, have failed to evince such a relationship between cognitive arousal and sleep initiation difficulties (Haynes, Adams, & Franzen, 1981; Sanavio, 1988).

Unrealistic sleep goals may also give birth to an insomnia complaint. People who require little sleep may covet superfluous sleep. Similarly, elderly sleepers may strive to sleep as well as they did when younger. In each case, dissatisfaction exists although no detrimental effects result directly from the individual's sleep pattern (Lichstein, 1988b).

Psychiatric. Insomnia is commonly associated with affective disorders, although it is still unclear whether affective disorders cause insomnia or are merely correlates of disturbed sleep. Researchers have detected a relationship between insomnia and depressive symptomatology (Levin, Bertelson, & Lacks, 1984; Mendelson et al., 1984). In addition, insomniacs tend to produce high scores on scales associated with anxiety such as the Psychasthenia Scale of the Minnesota Multiphasic Personality Inventory (MMPI) (Levin et al., 1984).

Sleep Hygiene–Related. Sleep hygiene is a general category that encompasses a diverse group of behaviors and environmental variables that tend to promote sleep. A lack of attention to any of these behavioral factors may produce or at least perpetuate insomnia. Examples of poor sleep hygiene include (a) lack of exercise, or exercise close to bedtime, (b) poor dietary habits (e.g., caffeine use), (c) an uncomfortable or noisy sleep environment, (d) napping, and (e) an irregular sleep schedule. A more detailed discussion of the relationship between sleep hygiene violations and poor sleep will be presented in the section on behavioral treatments for insomnia.

Medical. Certain medical conditions may underlie complaints of insomnia. Medical problems commonly associated with insomnia include neurologic disorders (e.g., dementia, parkinsonism), chronic obstructive pulmonary disease, asthma, gastroesophageal reflux, peptic ulcer disease, and pain syndromes such as fibrositis (see *International Classification of Sleep Disorders*, American Sleep Disorders Association [ASDA], 1990).

Drug–Related. Many prescribed medications, including analgesics that contain caffeine, bronchodilators, steroids, and some antihypertensive drugs, can produce insomnia as a side effect (Espie, 1991). In addition, although one drug may not cause insomnia by itself, an interaction among several drugs may lead to sleep disturbance. Ironically, sleeping pills can exacerbate insomnia. Withdrawal from benzodiazepines, the most widely used class of sleeping pills, can cause "rebound insomnia," which is often more severe than the original insomnia for which the pill was taken (Kales, Soldatos, Bixler, & Kales, 1983b). Insomnia is often associated with the use of alcohol, nicotine, and certain illegal drugs. Alcohol may decrease sleep latency but tends to increase wakefulness during the second half of the sleep period (Kay & Samiuddin, 1988). Nicotine can contribute to sleep disturbance (Soldatos, Kales, Scharf, Bixler, & Kales, 1980), and users of other stimulants such as cocaine and amphetamines may also find sleep elusive.

Brant W. Riedel and
Kenneth L.
Lichstein

Differential Diagnosis and Assessment

DSM-III-R Categorization

DSM-III-R (1987) divides insomnia into three categories. Insomnia related to another mental disorder includes insomnia that results from such mental disorders as major depression, generalized anxiety disorder, or adjustment disorder with anxious mood. The label insomnia related to a known organic factor is given to insomnia that is produced by physical disorders (e.g., pain syndromes, sleep apnea) or the use of medication or other drugs. Primary insomnia refers to insomnia complaints that are not encompassed by the first two categories. Primary insomnia is what is usually meant by the term *insomnia*, and it includes a wide range of psychological causes of poor sleep.

The International Classification of Sleep Disorders (ICSD) (ASDA, 1990) provides a more detailed description of sleep syndromes and divides primary insomnia into several categories (Table 18.1). Psychophysiological insomnia is the most prevalent ICSD diagnosis for patients presenting with insomnia. Disorders that would fall under the broad DSM-III-R categories insomnia related to a known organic factor (e.g., apnea) and insomnia related to another mental disorder are listed as distinct sleep disorders.

Differential Diagnosis

Because other sleep disorders may produce symptoms similar to those associated with primary insomnia, the process of differential diagnosis can prove challenging for the clinician. Many clues for differential diagnosis can be extracted from an interview, but referral of a patient for nocturnal polysomnography (PSG) may be imperative. This procedure involves all-night monitoring of brain activity with EEG, eye movement with electro-oculography (EOG), muscle tension with electromyography

---

TABLE 18.1. The International Classification of Sleep Disorders Categorization of Insomnia[a]

1. *Psychophysiological insomnia*: "Disorder of somatized tension and learned sleep-preventing associations that results in a complaint of insomnia and associated decreased functioning during wakefulness" (p. 28).
2. *Sleep state misperception*: "Disorder in which a complaint of insomnia or excessive sleepiness occurs without objective evidence of sleep disturbance" (p. 33).
3. *Idiopathic insomnia*: "A lifelong inability to obtain adequate sleep that is presumably due to an abnormality of the neurological control of the sleep-wake system" (p. 35).
4. *Inadequate sleep hygiene*: "A sleep disorder due to the performance of daily living activities that are inconsistent with the maintenance of good quality sleep and full daytime alertness" (p. 73).
5. *Environmental sleep disorder*: "A sleep disturbance due to a disturbing environmental factor that causes a complaint of either insomnia or excessive sleepiness" (p. 77). Examples of disruptive environmental factors include noise, uncomfortable room temperature, and bedpartner movements.
6. *Altitude insomnia*: "An acute insomnia, usually accompanied by headaches, loss of appetite, and fatigue, that occurs following ascent to high altitudes" (p. 80).
7. *Adjustment sleep disorders*: "Sleep disturbance temporally related to acute stress, conflict or environmental change causing emotional arousal" (p. 83).

[a]Insomnia types that are primarily associated with childhood were omitted from this table.
Quoted material from American Sleep Disorders Association (1990).

(EMG), respiration during sleep (and awake time), and other physiologic variables and is necessary for the definitive diagnosis of certain sleep disorders. A brief description of sleep disorders that may be confused with insomnia is provided below, and features that discriminate these disorders from insomnia are discussed.

Narcolepsy is characterized by excessive daytime sleepiness (EDS), which often results in an inability to stay awake during tasks requiring substantial vigilance (e.g., driving a car). In addition to such sleep attacks, narcoleptics may also report cataplexy (loss of muscle tone induced by strong emotions), hypnagogic hallucinations (vivid, dream-like images seen while falling asleep), and sleep paralysis (an inability to move while falling asleep or immediately after awakening). Insomnia and narcolepsy can initially be confused because nighttime sleep difficulties and EDS may be associated with both disorders. However, many insomniacs do not experience EDS (especially not to the degree found among narcoleptics), and some narcoleptics will not complain of nocturnal sleep disturbance. In addition, insomniacs will not report other symptoms associated with narcolepsy (i.e., cataplexy, sleep paralysis). PSG and multiple sleep latency tests (MSLTs) are essential for the diagnosis of narcolepsy. MSLTs consist of PSG monitoring during four 20-minute daytime nap opportunities and are used to document the presence of two narcoleptic earmarks, excessive daytime sleepiness and rapid eye movements (REMs) at sleep onset.

Circadian rhythm disorders may also be mistaken for insomnia. Many biological functions, including body temperature and the sleep-wake system, follow a rhythmic cycle that lasts about 25 hours (circadian rhythm). Circadian rhythm disorders result when a person's circadian rhythm does not match the demands of his or her environment. Two circadian disorders may be commonly confused with insomnia. A person with delayed sleep phase syndrome (DSPS) will be unable to fall asleep until much later than conventional times. Typically, such a person will not be able to fall asleep until sometime early in the morning (2:00 to 6:00 A.M.) yet will be forced to awaken only a few hours later in order to fulfill daytime responsibilities. Patients with advanced sleep phase syndrome (ASPS) fall asleep and awaken earlier than is desired. For example, an individual with ASPS may be unable to stay awake past 6:00 P.M. and will awaken for the last time the next morning at 1:00 A.M. Thus, DSPS mimics sleep-onset insomnia, while ASPS imitates terminal insomnia.

Certain characteristics of DSPS distinguish it from sleep-onset insomnia. A sleep history assessment with DSPS patients will often reveal a pattern of sleeping unusually late on weekends and holidays when early morning arising is not required. DSPS patients, unlike insomniacs, will tend to experience high-quality sleep of normal duration when environmental constraints on sleep time are removed. A consistent sleep onset time favors a diagnosis of DSPS, as it suggests a problem with the time that one is trying to fall asleep rather than a general inability to initiate sleep. Also, insomniacs may experience sleep onset difficulties only a few nights per week, whereas people with DSPS experience an inability to fall asleep nearly every night.

ASPS and insomnia differ in that individuals with ASPS are unable to stay awake past a very early hour in the evening. The timing of their sleep is awkward, but sleep length is not abbreviated. Terminal insomniacs, however, will be able to stay awake later in the evening, but their sleep period will be brief. As is the case with DSPS, ASPS is manifested nearly every night, whereas terminal insomnia may occur only a few times per week.

Short sleepers are individuals who sleep for only a short period each night but exhibit no consequent impairment of functioning during the day. Short sleepers may complain of insomnia because they view their sleep pattern as abnormal, have unsuccessfully attempted to increase sleep length, or fear that dire consequences may result from limited sleep. Some short sleepers attempt to solve their perceived problem by spending more time in bed. Rather than significantly increasing sleep time, this strategy frequently results in an increase in awake time, and a sleep pattern resembling insomnia is established. An assessment of sleep history will often distinguish a short sleeper from a sleep-maintenance insomniac. Short sleepers usually report a long history of obtaining a small amount of high-quality sleep (even on weekends and holidays when allowed to "sleep in") and experiencing no deleterious daytime effects. In contrast, insomniacs describe significantly lengthier sleep time prior to their insomnia complaint. The short sleeper who complains of insomnia should be assured that acquiring a limited amount of sleep is not necessarily dangerous or "abnormal," and the establishment of more realistic sleep goals should be pursued.

Sleep apneics will usually not report sleep initiation difficulties but may complain of sleep maintenance problems. Clues that suggest a diagnosis of apnea rather than primary insomnia include bed partner report of breathing irregularities or heavy snoring, obesity, morning headaches, and sleeping better when sitting upright.

Periodic limb movements during sleep (PLMS) may also be mistaken for primary insomnia. Patients with PLMS who complain of sleep maintenance difficulties are often unaware of the cause of their problem. Because of this lack of awareness, the observations of a bed partner can provide valuable information to the clinician during the process of differential diagnosis. Another indicator of PLMS is the presence of restless legs syndrome (RLS). RLS consists of uncomfortable, "crawling" sensations in one's legs that interfere with sleep onset, and nearly every RLS patient also suffers from PLMS (although the converse is not true). PSG is required to investigate the role of sleep apnea and PLMS in a patient's sleep concerns.

Primary insomnia may also be confused with insomnia resulting from an underlying mental disorder. Psychiatric testing and diagnostic interviews will provide important information to the clinician, and there is some evidence that PSG may be useful for diagnosing insomnia due to a psychiatric disorder. In one study, primary insomniacs, subjects with generalized anxiety disorder, and patients with major depression experienced similar sleep continuity problems, but depressed patients could be distinguished from the other two groups on the basis of shortened REM latency and increased eye movements during REM sleep (Reynolds et al., 1984).

Assessment Strategies

When presented with a sleep-related complaint, a clinician will first want to conduct a thorough interview with the patient. Communication with the bed partner of the patient is also recommended, as this may provide important supplementary information about nocturnal occurrences of which the patient is unaware (e.g., apnea, limb movements). An initial interview should investigate the following areas:

1. What is the nature of the difficulty (e.g., sleep-onset insomnia, daytime sleepiness) and its severity?
2. What is its frequency of occurrence?
3. When did the sleep-related problem begin, and what were the circumstances (e.g., social, economic) surrounding its commencement? If the problem is

sporadic rather than chronic, what circumstances (e.g., stress) are usually associated with its recurrence?

4. What are the details of sleep history preceding the current symptoms (e.g., number of hours slept, number of awakenings)?

5. Daytime sleepiness, fatigue, performance, and mood: Do these factors fluctuate with the quality of the previous night's sleep?

6. The patient's emotional and behavioral reactions during a bad night of sleep: What fears (possibly irrational) are associated with not being able to sleep? What does the patient do when unable to sleep?

7. What are details of sleep hygiene (e.g., regularity of sleep schedule, exercise, napping)?

8. Psychiatric factors: Is the patient experiencing depressive symptomatology or feeling anxious? (If psychiatric factors are uncovered during the initial interview, a more detailed psychiatric diagnostic interview is recommended.)

9. Medical factors: Are there breathing irregularities, limb twitches, pain?

10. Medication and other drugs: What medication is being taken, and does the patient smoke, drink alcohol, or use other drugs of abuse? What are frequency and quantity of use?

11. What have been past treatment attempts, treatment response, and compliance with treatment procedures?

12. What does the patient think might be the cause of his or her complaint? Also, what goal (possibly unrealistic) is the patient hoping to attain through treatment?

After the initial interview, several assessment options are available. PSG is indispensable for the assessment of sleep apnea and periodic limb movements, but its usefulness for primary insomnia assessment is questionable for several reasons. First, insomnia may be setting specific, and an overnight study in a sleep laboratory might not fairly represent a patient's insomnia. PSG assessment in a person's natural environment has been developed to compensate for this problem, but certainly the intrusiveness of the procedure is not totally removed. Second, multiple overnight studies are impractical due to the substantial expense associated with PSG. This is problematic, because a single overnight study may not detect insomnia that is not experienced every night. Third, a major contributor to some insomnias, trying too hard to sleep, could be eliminated because insomniacs may feel less pressure to sleep at the laboratory and may actually want to prove their inability to sleep. Finally, PSG does not measure subjective sleep perception (e.g., satisfaction, patient's estimates of sleep variables), an important aspect of any insomnia complaint.

Some investigators have advanced an alternate point of view on the utility of PSG with insomnia (Edinger et al., 1989). They point out that sleep apnea, PLMS, and other sleep disorders that may have a similar clinical presentation to insomnia occur at increasing rates with advancing age. For patients 40 years old and older, PSG assessments of "insomniacs" have a substantial likelihood of altering the initial diagnosis of insomnia.

Objective sleep measurement instruments less expensive and intrusive than PSG have been developed. The Sleep Assessment Device (SAD) monitors patients' responses to faint tones during the night and provides estimates of sleep latency, duration of awakenings, total sleep time, and sleep efficiency that closely match PSG measurements (Lichstein, Nickel, Hoelscher, & Kelley, 1982). Wrist actigraphy offers estimates of sleep and wake time but may exhibit substantial disagreement with PSG results (Hauri & Wisbey, 1992). In contrast to PSG, neither device provides information about sleep stages.

Sleep diaries are the most popular method of self-report. Figure 18.1 contains the sleep questionnaire that we use for clinical and research purposes. Diaries are completed daily and should include estimation of at least the following sleep parameters: (a) time entering and leaving bed, (b) latency to sleep, (c) number of awakenings and total awake time, (d) time of final awakening, (e) napping, (f) subjective sleep ratings (e.g., quality, satisfaction), (g) daytime sleepiness, and (h) medication/alcohol usage. From this self-report data additional variables such as total time in bed, total sleep time, and sleep efficiency percentage (100 × total sleep time/time in bed) can be calculated. The clinician will probably also want insomniacs to monitor other sleep-related variables such as caffeine consumption and exercise.

Certainly, self-report measures are subject to inaccuracy. Despite a lack of precision, however, insomniacs' self-reports tend to correlate significantly with PSG measures (Carskadon et al., 1976; Haynes, Fitzgerald, Shute, & Hall, 1985) and therefore can be useful for tracking treatment progress. In addition to assessment of subjective sleep perception, sleep diaries offer several advantages over objective measures, including reduced intrusiveness, greater availability, and lowered expense.

Treatment

Evidence for Prescriptive Treatments

The following section will concentrate on treatment of primary insomnia. When insomnia results from medical or psychiatric factors, the focus of treatment becomes the underlying disorder rather than the insomnia. Possible treatment approaches for medical or psychiatric contributors to insomnia are numerous and beyond the scope of the present discussion.

Behavior Therapy

Relaxation Techniques. Several relaxation strategies have been proposed as treatments for insomnia. Popular relaxation methods will be briefly depicted here, along with empirical evidence pertinent to their effectiveness. A more detailed discussion of various relaxation techniques is provided elsewhere (Lichstein, 1988a).

Progressive relaxation (PR) is the most widely researched treatment for insomnia (Lichstein & Fischer, 1985) and involves sequentially tensing and relaxing the body's major muscle groups while concentrating on and contrasting somatic sensations of tension and relaxation. About 16 muscle groups are tensed and released, and significantly less time is spent tensing muscles (7 seconds) than on the relaxation phase (45 seconds). Numerous studies have demonstrated the superiority of PR to no treatment for diminishing sleep onset latency (Lick & Heffler, 1977; Nicassio, Boylan, & McCabe, 1982; Turner & Ascher, 1979). The record of PR against placebo intervention is less impressive, with some studies showing greater sleep latency improvement for PR subjects (Freedman & Papsdorf, 1976; Lick & Heffler, 1977) and other researchers finding no significant outcome differences between PR and placebo (Lacks, Bertelson, Gans, & Kunkel, 1983; Nicassio et al., 1982).

Guided imagery may also offer some relief from insomnia. During guided

SLEEP QUESTIONNAIRE

Name _____

Please answer the following questionnaire **when you awake in the morning**.
Enter the date you are filling it out and provide the information to describe your
sleep the night before.
Definitions explaining each line of the questionnaire are given on the back side.

	Example							
This morning's date	10/16/93							
1. Nap (yesterday)	70 min.							
2. Bedtime (last night)	10:55							
3. Time to fall asleep (last night)	65 min. *or* 12:00 am							
4. Number of awakenings (last night)	4							
5. Total time spent awake (last night)	110 min. *or* 1:50							
6. Final wake-up time (this morning)	6:05							
7. Out of bed time (this morning)	7:10							
8. Quality rating (of last night's sleep)	2							
9. Sleepiness (yesterday afternoon)	6							
10. Medication (include amount and hour)	wine: 1 at 8pm Halcion: 0.25 mg at bedtime							

Figure 18.1a. Sample sleep diary used to collect one week's worth of data. (Adapted from the Department of Psychology, Memphis State University.)

Brant W. Riedel and
Kenneth L.
Lichstein

ITEM DEFINITIONS

1. If you napped yesterday, enter total time napping in minutes.
2. What time did you enter bed for the purpose of going to sleep; or, if you were reading or engaging in other activities in bed, at what time did you wish to fall asleep?
3. Counting from the time you wished to fall asleep, how many minutes did it take you to fall asleep?
4. How many times did you awaken during the night?
5. What is the total amount of time you were awake during the night? This does not include time to fall asleep at the beginning of the night or awake time in bed before the final morning arising.
6. What time did you wake up this morning?
7. What time did you actually get out of bed this morning?
8. Enter *one* of the numbers below to indicate your overall *quality rating*, or the general level of satisfaction of your sleep last night:

   1. Very poor
   2. Poor
   3. Fair
   4. Good
   5. Excellent

9. Enter *one* of the numbers below to indicate the greatest amount of sleepiness you felt yesterday afternoon (Stanford Sleepiness Scale).

   1. Feeling active and vital; alert; wide awake.
   2. Functioning at a high level, but not at peak; able to concentrate.
   3. Relaxed; awake; not at full alertness; responsive.
   4. A little foggy; not at peak; let down.
   5. Fogginess; beginning to lose interest in remaining awake; slowed down.
   6. Sleepiness; prefer to be lying down; fighting sleep; woozy.
   7. Almost in reverie; sleep onset soon; lost struggle to remain awake.

10. List any sleep medication, caffeine, or alcohol taken at or near bedtime.

Figure 18.1b. Sleep diary instructions that are printed on the reverse side of the form. (Adapted from the Department of Psychology, Memphis State University.)

imagery, patients are encouraged to focus their attention on an image such as a pleasant nature scene or a particular object. Retaining patients' attention on the image is essential, and this may be aided by having them concentrate on particular sensations associated with the nature scene or various details of a neutral object. The employment of imagery training as a method for combatting intrusive cognitions is intuitively appealing, and its usefulness is empirically supported (Woolfolk & McNulty, 1983).

There is evidence that traditional relaxation strategies are less effective for older insomniacs. Lick and Heffler (1977) observed a poorer treatment response to PR among older subjects, and Morin and Azrin (1988) found no significant outcome difference between imagery training (IT) and no treatment in a sample whose average

age was 67.4 years. Lichstein developed a hybrid relaxation procedure that is
designed to be less physically demanding and complex than traditional methods and
therefore may be better suited for older insomniacs. The procedure involves concentration on relaxed somatic sensations, but the muscle tension/release cycles of PR are
omitted. Breathing exercises and the repetition of an autogenic phrase are also
included. In a recent empirical investigation involving subjects 60 years and older, the
hybrid procedure led to significant sleep improvement for nonhypnotically medicated insomniacs and reduced hypnotic usage without sleep deterioration for medicated insomniacs (Lichstein & Johnson, 1993).

In addition to the type of relaxation procedure employed and the number of
practice opportunities provided by treatment sessions, the extent of practice between sessions may heavily influence outcome. Therapists should encourage daily
practice of relaxation techniques, monitor compliance with this assignment, and, if
necessary, investigate reasons for noncompliance.

Stimulus Control.   Stimulus control (SC) therapy emerged from the belief that
some insomnia may be due to the bedroom's becoming a poor discriminative stimulus
for sleep. Whereas the noninsomniac associates the bedroom with rapid sleep onset,
the bedroom elicits a wakeful response in insomniacs. With this philosophy in mind,
the following six instructions are given to the patient:

1. Do not use your bed or bedroom for anything (at any time of the day) except
   sleep (or sex). Activities that patients may have to avoid include eating,
   watching television, and working in the bedroom.
2. Go to bed only when sleepy.
3. If you do not fall asleep within about 15 to 20 minutes, leave the bed and do
   something in another room. Go back to bed only when you feel sleepy again.
   Clock watching to hold to the 15 to 20 minute rule is not recommended; this
   may put undue pressure on the insomniac.
4. If you do not fall asleep quickly upon returning to bed, repeat instruction 3 as
   many times as necessary. Also, if you do not fall asleep rapidly after an
   awakening, follow rule 3 again.
5. Use your alarm to leave bed at the same time every morning regardless of the
   amount of sleep obtained. This will aid your body in establishing a consistent
   sleep rhythm.
6. Do not nap.

Studies have consistently shown SC to be more effective than no treatment for
sleep latency reduction (Ladouceur & Gros-Louis, 1986; Puder, Lacks, Bertelson, &
Storandt, 1983; Turner & Ascher, 1979). In addition, most investigations that have
compared SC to placebo interventions have demonstrated superior sleep latency
curtailment for SC subjects (Espie, Lindsay, Brooks, Hood, & Turvey, 1989; Lacks et al.,
1983; Turner & Ascher, 1979). Researchers have also provided evidence that SC leads
to significantly greater improvement of sleep maintenance insomnia than no treatment or placebo interventions (Morin & Azrin, 1987, 1988; Turner & Ascher, 1979).

Bedtime Restriction.   A relatively new behavioral approach to insomnia involves limiting a patient's time in bed. Sleep restriction therapy (SRT) was developed
in response to the proposal that excessive time in bed perpetuates insomnia (Spielman, Saskin, & Thorpy, 1987). SRT consists of the following steps:

1. Patients complete 2 weeks of sleep diaries, and the therapist uses these questionnaires to calculate average total subjective sleep time (TST).
2. The amount of time patients are allowed to spend in bed is initially restricted to this average TST. However, no patient is asked to limit time in bed (TIB) to less than 4.5 hours, regardless of baseline TST. Napping or lying down during periods outside of the prescribed time limits is prohibited throughout treatment.
3. Patients choose fixed times to enter and leave bed. Thus, a patient prescribed 6 hours in bed may choose an 11:00 P.M. to 5:00 A.M. schedule or, perhaps, a 1:00 A.M. to 7:00 A.M. schedule. A consistent awakening time is emphasized.
4. When mean sleep efficiency ($100 \times$ TST/TIB) over a period of 5 days is at least 90%, a patient's TIB is increased by allowing the patient to enter bed 15 minutes earlier. Five days of unaltered sleep schedule always follow a TIB increase.
5. If sleep efficiency drops below an average of 85% for a period of 5 days, TIB is reduced to the mean TST for those 5 days. No curtailment of TIB occurs during the first 10 days of treatment or for 10 days following a sleep schedule change.
6. If mean sleep efficiency falls between 85% and 90% during a 5-day period, a patient's sleep schedule remains constant.

Spielman et al. (1987) tested the effectiveness of SRT with a group of 35 chronic insomniacs whose average age was 46. After an 8-week treatment program, subjects showed significant improvement in sleep latency, total wake time, sleep efficiency, and total sleep time. Lichstein (1988b) recognized the usefulness of bedtime restriction for "insomnoids," patients who experience nocturnal sleep disruption but no daytime sleepiness. Insomnoid states may be particularly prevalent among older patients, who frequently experience reduced TST and increased awake time but no daytime sleepiness. Lichstein's sleep compression therapy (SCT) differs from SRT in that SCT does not immediately reduce TIB to the baseline TST average. Instead, the patient's time in bed is reduced by gradually delaying the time entering bed and advancing morning arising time. Lichstein (1988b) treated a 59-year-old "insomnoid" with SCT and observed substantial improvement in sleep latency, total awake time, sleep efficiency, and sleep quality ratings. Hoelscher and Edinger (1988) successfully reduced sleep latency and wake time after sleep onset (WASO) in a small group of older insomniacs by using a treatment package that included bed-time restriction, stimulus control, and sleep education. Friedman, Bliwise, Yesavage, and Salom (1991) applied a modified version of SRT to a group of 10 geriatric insomniacs. Subjects experienced significant reductions in sleep latency and WASO after treatment, and sleep latency remained significantly shortened at 3-month follow-up. Unfortunately, none of the above-mentioned studies included a control group.

Sleep Hygiene Instruction. Sleep hygiene refers to behaviors and environmental conditions that promote sleep. General daytime activity level and exercise may influence sleep. A survey by Marchini, Coates, Magistad, and Waldum (1983) indicated that insomniacs were less active during the day than normal sleepers. It has also been suggested that exercise increases delta (deep) sleep. Torsvall (1981) reviewed 20 studies and concluded that the hypothesis of a relationship between deep sleep and exercise was usually supported in physically fit subjects but was less often upheld in untrained participants. Thus, long-term commitments to exercise that result in physical fitness are more likely to improve sleep quality than short-term increases in exercise. A few studies included in the review suggested additional benefits, such as extended sleep length and decreased sleep latencies, in response to increased exercise. However, Torsvall (1981) reports that exercise close to bedtime and increases in physical activity by untrained subjects appear to increase wakefulness and restless sleep.

Poor dietary habits may also contribute to insomnia. For example, caffeine is derived from several sources in one's diet, including coffee, tea, and soft drinks, and can produce insomnia. A recent study found that nocturnal sleep following caffeine consumption was characterized by significantly reduced total sleep time and less stages 2 and 4 sleep and significantly greater sleep latencies and total awake time than sleep preceded by caffeine-free days (Bonnet & Arand, 1992). However, tolerance to the effects of caffeine (with the exception of reduced stage 4 sleep) developed after a week, suggesting that regular users of caffeine may be less at risk for sleep disturbance than sporadic consumers. In addition, the effects of caffeine differed substantially across individuals. Because sensitivity to the effects of caffeine varies greatly, its role in perpetuating insomnia should be considered even in patients with low to moderate consumption rates.

Napping may also detract from nighttime sleep, but empirical investigations have produced mixed results. One group of researchers found that an afternoon nap was followed by significantly longer sleep latencies and reduced total sleep time at night (Feinberg et al., 1985). However, in another study, no significant nocturnal sleep impairment was observed after a short daytime nap (Aber & Webb, 1986). The effect of a daytime nap probably varies significantly across individuals, and differences in duration and timing of the naps may have contributed to discrepant results. Insomniacs should be advised to experiment with eliminating naps, and long naps late in the day should especially be discouraged.

A treatment study that compared sleep hygiene instruction, stimulus control, and a meditation technique showed improvement in all groups but no significant differences between groups on the outcome variables wake time after sleep onset, duration of awakenings, and number of awakenings. Self-reported compliance with treatment instructions, however, was significantly lower among stimulus control subjects than in the remaining two groups (Schoicket, Bertelson, & Lacks, 1988). Despite comparable sleep maintenance improvement, subjects who received sleep hygiene instruction were significantly more likely than stimulus control and mediation participants to still consider themselves insomniacs after treatment. A survey of noninsomniacs and insomniacs suggested that insomniacs possess more sleep hygiene knowledge but actually practice sleep hygiene less than noninsomniacs (Lacks & Rotert, 1986). Because knowledge and practice were generally high for both groups, the authors concluded that poor sleep hygiene is not likely to be a primary cause of insomnia but nevertheless should be addressed in treatment because of its potential for perpetuating poor sleep.

Pharmacotherapy. Benzodiazepines are the most popular pharmacologic intervention for insomnia. Although they tend to improve sleep latency and maintenance (Kay & Samiuddin, 1988), several problems are associated with their use. First, tolerance appears to develop after only a few weeks of nightly consumption which results in a return of the original insomnia symptoms (Gillin & Byerly, 1990). Second, adverse daytime effects, including performance deficits and increased sleepiness, may be observed (Roth, Roehrs, & Zorick, 1988). Benzodiazepines with a long elimination half-life, such as flurazepam (Dalmane), are particularly likely to produce "carry-over effects," and older patients may be especially prone to residual effects because of their tendency to eliminate drugs more slowly. Third, withdrawal from benzodiazepines may produce rebound insomnia and heightened anxiety (Kales et al., 1983b). Rapidly eliminated benzodiazepines such as triazolam (Halcion) appear to be more likely to cause rebound insomnia and may lead to increased morning wakefulness (Kales, Soldatos, Bixler, & Kales, 1983a; Kales et al., 1983b). Rebound insomnia and rebound anxiety can produce an additional problem by fostering psychological dependence on benzodiazepines as insomniacs attempt to avoid adverse withdrawal effects through the chronic use of sleeping pills. Finally, benzodiazepines are typically associated with increased stage 2 sleep and reduced stages 3 and 4 and REM sleep (Roth et al., 1988). Because of these undesirable effects associated with benzodiazepines, they are usually recommended only for short-term treatment of transient sleep difficulties and are unlikely to provide a permanent solution for chronic insomnia.

Alternative Treatments. Unlike most treatment strategies that require insomniacs to take specific steps to induce sleep, paradoxical intention (PI) therapy suggests that patients attempt to remain awake. Supporters of PI propose that sleep is an involuntary physiologic reaction and therefore cannot be fully controlled by conscious effort. Attempts to control the sleep process (i.e., trying to make oneself fall asleep) result in arousal that prevents sleep onset. PI is designed to relieve the sleep-incompatible performance anxiety that accompanies repeated failures to fall asleep rapidly by reframing wakefulness as a successful performance rather than failure. Specifically, patients are asked to assume a comfortable position in bed, turn out the lights, and attempt to stay awake as long as possible. Patients are encouraged to try to keep their eyes open, but more active methods for maintaining wakefulness such as physical activity, reading, or watching television should be avoided.

Despite the success of PI in early studies, Espie and Lindsay (1985) demonstrated that it may be a poor treatment choice for some insomniacs. In a study of 6 patients treated with PI, 3 subjects exhibited favorable sleep latency changes but 2 participants experienced sleep latency exacerbation to such a degree that PI treatment was discontinued. The average sleep latency of a sixth subject increased during the first 3 weeks of treatment but dropped below baseline levels for weeks 4 through 8.

Selecting Optimal Treatment Strategies

When choosing an optimal treatment strategy, two approaches are appropriate. First, a clinician can select an intervention that has proven to be more effective in treatment comparison studies. Second, a treatment package could be tailored to meet the perceived needs of a particular client. Although numerous treatment comparison studies exist, little empirical guidance is available to the clinician who adopts the second alternative.

A recent review of insomnia treatment studies suggests that bed-time restriction strategies and stimulus control (SC) will lead to greater improvement by the end of treatment than paradoxical intention (PI) and progressive relaxation (PR) (Lacks & Morin, 1992). However, the differences between treatment approaches were less substantial at follow-up (2 months posttreatment). Three studies have directly compared PR, SC, and PI. Turner and Ascher (1979) found that PR, SC, and PI were equally effective for sleep latency and number of awakenings and performed significantly better than no treatment or placebo on the same measures. Conflicting results were reported by Lacks et al. (1983), who observed that SC led to significantly greater sleep latency reduction at posttreatment and follow-up than PR, PI, and placebo, which were comparably potent. In a third investigation, SC and PI subjects showed more substantial sleep latency amelioration than PR, placebo, and no-treatment groups (Espie, Lindsay, et al., 1989). Sleep latency reduction was comparable for SC and PI, but latency diminution occurred more quickly with SC. However, in comparison to SC and PI, PR produced superlative increases in sleep quality variables such as "restedness after sleep" and "enjoyment of sleep." In summary, these studies suggest that SC, PR, and PI are useful treatments for insomnia, and SC appears to be the quickest route to sleep latency curtailment, but PR may produce greater qualitative improvement.

Another research group conducted two studies that compared SC to IT. The first study included subjects with an average age of 57, and sleep maintenance difficulties were the focus of treatment (Morin & Azrin, 1987). Stimulus control therapy reduced nocturnal awake time 65%, significantly more than IT (16%), at posttreatment. By 3-month follow-up, IT subjects had significantly reduced awake time but still lagged significantly behind SC subjects. By one-year follow-up no significant differences for awake time existed between the two groups. A second investigation treated subjects with an average age of 67 and found significant improvement in duration of awakenings for both SC and IT groups posttreatment, but only SC was significantly more effective than no treatment (Morin & Azrin, 1988). No significant differences in duration of awakenings were observed between the SC and IT groups at one-year follow-up. A significantly greater increase in total sleep time from baseline to posttreatment was produced by SC than by IT and no treatment. In addition, SC subjects reported being more satisfied with treatment progress than IT subjects.

Friedman et al. (1991) compared sleep restriction therapy (SRT) to relaxation training (RT) in a group of older insomniacs. The RT protocol consisted of a slightly modified form of progressive relaxation and unspecified visualization exercises. Subjects in RT and SRT groups exhibited significant paring of sleep latency and WASO by posttreatment, and significant latency gains were maintained for both groups at 3-month follow-up. Although no significant differences in WASO or sleep latency were observed between groups, the percentage decrease of WASO in SRT subjects (32.7%) was twice that of RT participants (15.9%).

Two studies have explored the efficacy of tailored treatments. Sanavio (1988) hypothesized that patients demonstrating high cognitive arousal when trying to fall asleep would respond more favorably to a cognitively based intervention than to biofeedback. However, the cognitive treatment, which included cognitive restructuring, thought stopping, and paradoxical intention, proved to be no more effective than biofeedback for shortening sleep latency.

Espie, Brooks, and Lindsay (1989) compared the progress of insomniacs receiving tailored treatment (TT) to those randomly assigned to either PI, PR, or SC. Assignment to a particular treatment in the TT group was based on a questionnaire that attempted to identify significant causal factors. Ironically, posttreatment sleep latency improvement was greater for random therapy (49%) than for TT (35%). These researchers reanalyzed their results from the perspective of clinical significance. Two criteria defined clinically significant improvement: 50% sleep latency reduction, and final sleep latency of no more than 30 minutes. Tailored treatment was compared on both criteria to random assignment to PR, PI, or SC. By both criteria, SC was the best treatment, with 64% of SC subjects abbreviating sleep latency by 50% or more and 71% ending treatment with mean latencies of 30 minutes or less. Tailored treatment finished second in both categories (50%, 43%), PI was a close third (47%, 40%), and PR was last (21%, 7%). Although the results of this particular study offer strong support for SC's being an optimal treatment strategy, it must be remembered that sleep latency reduction does necessarily correlate with subjective sleep quality.

Some matches between treatment strategies and insomnia complaints are intuitively appealing and should be given consideration despite a lack of empirical evidence. For example, relaxation strategies seem appropriate for the insomniac who complains of significant anxiety or muscle tension during the day or while attempting to fall asleep. Similarly, bed-time restriction strategies appear especially suited for the insomniac who complains of disrupted sleep but little daytime impairment.

Problems in Carrying Out Interventions

Difficulties with pharmacotherapy have been detailed in a previous section. Administration of behavioral interventions can also prove problematic. Regardless of the potency of a chosen treatment plan, the behavior therapist's efforts can be thwarted by poor patient compliance. Those prescribed SC may find it difficult to use their bedrooms only for sleeping, and relaxation patients may not faithfully practice between sessions. Compliance with SC and bed-time restriction approaches requires discipline and resourcefulness; patients must carefully regulate entering and leaving bed and develop strategies for filling additional out-of-bed time.

Patient compliance may also be impeded by exacerbation of sleep-related difficulties during initial phases of behavioral treatment. Higher levels of exercise may increase wakefulness in the unfit subject, and PI could produce greater sleep latencies. Decreases in total sleep time and daytime fatigue may accompany the early stages of therapies that restrict time in bed (Spielman et al., 1987). Friedman et al. (1991) altered the standard protocol of SRT in an effort to increase compliance. Although the modified intervention allowed for greater tolerance of patient sleep schedule preferences, the dropout rate for the sleep restriction group was greater than that for a relaxation condition. Education about possible negative treatment side effects and an emphasis on long-term benefits that should result form short-term sacrifices may combat discouragement on the part of patients.

Relapse Prevention

Although to our knowledge there are no empirical investigations of methods for preventing insomnia relapse, clues can be drawn form work in other health psychology domains. Marlatt and George (1990) propose a relapse prevention model that was originally developed for addictive behaviors (e.g., smoking, alcoholism) but can be applied to any therapeutic program that requires behavior change. First, the patient is provided with skills to recognize and effectively cope with "high-risk situations." Weekends and holidays would be high-risk situations for the insomniac whose sleeping difficulties stem mainly from excessive time in bed. Successfully coping with the situation might involve scheduling early morning activities to motivate a timely departure from bed. Second, the patient is encouraged to cognitively reframe initial relapses as "lapses," or isolated slips that do not necessarily imply a full-blown relapse to baseline levels of a disorder. Such an intervention is particularly appropriate for insomniacs, because they may overreact to a single night of poor sleep. Disputing the importance of one bad night should dampen fears that might impair future efforts to sleep. In addition to the suggestions of Marlatt and George (1990), therapists may employ other relapse prevention strategies such as enlisting the aid of the patient's social support system and establishing a reward system contingent on sleep-enhancing behavior.

Case Illustration

Case Description

Mr. C., a 66-year-old patient, presented at a sleep disorders center with complaints of difficulty initiating and maintaining sleep nearly every night. A thorough interview revealed the following background information:

1. The patient's sleep difficulties had begun shortly after his retirement and had persisted for about 18 months.
2. He reported satisfactory sleep latencies (about 10 minutes) prior to retirement but noted that frequency and duration of awakenings had increased significantly a few years before his retirement.
3. The patient complained of mild daytime sleepiness.
4. After his retirement, the patient had begun taking naps late in the afternoon, and he admitted to a lack of exercise.
5. He had recently stopped drinking caffeine-containing beverages because of his sleeping difficulties. He also did not consume alcohol or use other drugs of abuse.
6. The patient had been taking 0.125 mg of triazolam (Halcion) every night for about 6 months. It initially reduced sleep latency but lost its effectiveness after a few weeks. He experienced severe insomnia when attempting abrupt withdrawal from the medication and consequently resumed nightly triazolam usage.
7. His goals for therapy included reducing sleep latency to 20 minutes or less, limiting awakenings to no more than one per night, and sleeping later in the morning.

Differential Diagnosis and Assessment

The information gathered suggested a diagnosis of primary insomnia. Psychiatric factors were investigated during the interview, but the patient denied depressive symptoms and reported minimal anxiety outside of sleep-related concerns. Neither the patient nor his wife had noticed nocturnal breathing irregularities or limb twitches, and the patient did not report chronic pain. A circadian rhythm disorder was doubtful because the patient's sleep complaints persisted despite a lack of pressure to sleep at a particular time.

Before being asked to return a week later, the patient was given a week's worth of sleep diaries, and he was also asked to monitor frequency, timing, and quantity of caffeine use, and frequency, timing, and duration of exercise. The Stanford Sleepiness Scale (Hoddes, Dement, & Zarcone, 1972) was used to monitor daytime sleepiness.

The initial portion of the second session was spent reviewing the patient's sleep diaries. The diaries revealed an average sleep latency of 45 minutes and an average of five awakenings per night that lasted about 15 minutes each. Consistent with his previous global report, Mr. C. took a 30-minute nap every afternoon, did not consume caffeinated beverages, and engaged in minimal exercise. The patient usually entered bed at about 10:15 P.M., and the time he left bed ranged from 7:30 to 9:00 A.M., although his last awakening usually occurred at about 5:30 A.M.. He had stated earlier that prior to retirement, he went to bed about 11:00 P.M. and consistently left bed at 5:45 A.M.. At this point in the session I inquired as to why he was spending more time in bed since retirement. His response was enlightening, and it heavily influenced the treatment plan. Mr. C. explained that he was an avid fan of many prime time television shows and therefore watched television until 10:00 P.M. every night. Before his retirement, he would afterward spend about an hour every night preparing for work the next day. After several preparatory activities, including selecting his clothes for the following day, preparing his lunch, and making a list of goals he wanted to accomplish, he would enter bed shortly after 11:00 P.M. Since his retirement, preparing for the following day was not necessary, and he began entering bed around 10:00 P.M. He stayed in bed later in the morning because he had always looked forward to being able to "sleep in" rather than getting up early for work. He also stated that there was "nothing to do" once he left bed. In fact, Mr. C. admitted to a lack of recreational interests and described his current lifestyle as "pretty boring."

Treatment Selection

At this juncture in the treatment process, several potential problem areas had been identified. Triazolam initially had shortened sleep latency but at this point was only maintaining poor sleep. The physician who prescribed the triazolam was contacted shortly after the patient's initial session. She agreed that withdrawal from the medication was advisable and suggested reducing the patient's dosage by one dose per week. Napping might be exacerbating the patient's sleeping difficulties. Mr. C. believed that he must nap because night after night of poor sleep left him sleepy the following afternoon. An alternative viewpoint, which I promoted in my sessions with the patient, is that daytime napping causes nighttime sleep disruption, which in turn creates an urge to nap the following day. Also, Mr. C.'s general activity level during the day was low, and he did not have a regular exercise routine. In addition, his sleep goals appeared unrealistic. Although he was more than 60 years old, he expected to initiate sleep early, sleep late in the morning, and experience few awakenings.

With these potential problem areas in mind, the following treatment plan was selected:

1. *Medication withdrawal and relaxation*: The patient will gradually withdraw from triazolam by reducing his dosage by one dose per week while continuing to practice relaxation.
2. *Sleep hygiene*: Napping will be eliminated, and an attempt will be made to increase the activity level during the day and establish a regular exercise routine.

3. *Education*: Mr. C. will be educated about sleep changes associated with advancing age.
4. *Bedtime restriction*: Compression of the patient's sleep schedule is recommended. Consequently, strategies for filling up spare time created by bedtime curtailment will need to be discussed.

Treatment Course and Problems in Carrying Out Interventions

The remainder of the second session was devoted to training the patient to use a hybrid relaxation procedure described earlier (Lichstein & Johnson, 1993). I explained to the patient that part of the treatment plan was to gradually reduce his triazolam use, having already solicited the consent of his physician. Relaxation would serve as a substitute for sleep medication in order to minimize possible withdrawal effects. The patient was provided with a handout that summarized the relaxation procedures and was encouraged to practice at least once during each day of the following week and once every night before retiring. He was also asked to record the date and time of each practice session and, on a scale from 1 to 10, how relaxed he felt before and after each session.

At the start of our third session, the patient admitted to extreme anxiety over the prospect of withdrawing from triazolam. When he had abruptly withdrawn from triazolam 4 months prior, he had experienced severe sleep onset difficulties and nightmares for 3 nights before resuming consumption of the medication. He also revealed that he had expected me to provide him with an alternative sleep medication because triazolam was no longer effective, and he expressed dismay at the fact that we had already met for two sessions and his sleep had not improved. I was informed that the current session might very well be his last. In my experience, such impatience on the part of insomniacs is not uncommon. For many medical problems, patients are able to visit a doctor one time and receive a prescription that begins to provide immediate relief of their symptoms. Those who envision such a treatment process for insomnia will no doubt experience frustration with a careful, lengthy assessment procedure.

I wanted to avoid being overly defensive of my treatment plan and instead assured the patient that I understood his legitimate concerns about the progress of treatment. I acknowledged that previous sessions had focused mainly on assessment rather than treatment and, unfortunately, this had resulted in a temporary persistence of his insomnia complaints. It was emphasized, however, that a long assessment period before treatment began was in his best interest because insomnia could result from a great variety of factors, and proper treatment selection depended on careful assessment. We also discussed disadvantages of sleep medication usage, including tolerance, carry-over effects, and withdrawal side effects.

Near the end of our session, the patient's confidence in my treatment approach appeared to be increasing. He was developing more realistic expectations regarding the pace of treatment progress and was no longer focusing on medication as his only treatment alternative. A quick review of the patient's relaxation log revealed consistent improvement in relaxation after practice sessions. Consequently, a brief review of the relaxation procedure was conducted, and the patient was asked to continue daily relaxation practice. In addition, the patient agreed to avoid napping and instead would engage in a brisk walk during the time when he was most tempted to nap.

Mr. C. arrived for his fourth treatment session in an upbeat mood. He reported that he was experiencing fewer awakenings during the night and more "restful" sleep since he discontinued napping. However, he was still not satisfied with an average of three awakenings per night and was looking forward to further improvement. I seized the opportunity to address age-related sleep changes by mentioning that increased sleep fragmentation was common among older sleepers, and therefore his goal of only one awakening per night might be difficult to attain. We continued to discuss sleep changes associated with advancing age and eventually arrived at the topic of sleep compression. An excerpt from our fourth session follows.

THERAPIST: There is evidence that reducing time in bed will often result in improvements in measures such as sleeping latency and awake time during the night.

PATIENT: It seems that spending less time in bed would decrease my chances of obtaining more sleep.

T: Why do you need more sleep?

P: Well, I don't seem to get much sleep. I take so long to fall asleep, and I wake up so much.

T: It's true that you take longer to fall asleep and wake up more often than you used to, but I think you are obtaining about the same amount of sleep as you did before your retirement, only in a less efficient manner.

P: I'm an older man, and I need more sleep to keep me rested and healthy.

T: Do you feel sleepy or fatigued during the day?

P: Well, I used to take a nap every day, but I think I proved this week that I didn't really need it. I guess I feel pretty good most of the time.

T: I'm afraid that you are wanting more sleep than you need. Sleep needs vary from individual to individual and therefore the amount of time slept is a poor gauge to sleep adequacy. A better measurement of sleep adequacy is how you feel the next day.

P: So lying around in bed longer probably isn't going to increase the amount of sleep I get, and that's fine because I probably don't need more sleep.

T: Exactly! Staying in bed longer is probably just increasing awake time, not sleep time.

Mr. C. agreed to enter bed later (11:00 P.M.) and to get out of bed earlier (7:00 A.M.). He decided that the extra time created before he went to bed would be filled by reading, and additional time early in the morning would be spent watching movies he had taped. He was also ready to begin withdrawing from triazolam by not taking it one night the following week. In addition, he was to continue practicing relaxation, resist napping, and exercise daily.

Our fifth session opened with a review of the past week. Predictably, Mr. C. experienced a poor night's sleep when he did not take triazolam. An hour was required to fall asleep, and his sleep was disrupted by frequent awakenings. Because he was previously warned about withdrawal side effects, Mr. C. did not seem discouraged by one night of poor sleep. Sleep onset latencies for the other six nights appeared to significantly improve in response to a later bedtime: sleep latency dropped from a baseline average of 45 minutes to 20 minutes. Despite reduction in bed time, total sleep time remained stable and daytime sleepiness was not evident. Mr. C. reported compliance with all the treatment components except for leaving bed early and exercising daily. I spent most of the remaining session exploring reasons behind noncompliance with an early morning arising time.

T: Why did you find it difficult to get out of bed early?

P: Well, I guess I'm just lazy (*laughs*).

T: Maybe I should rephrase my question. What would motivate you to get out of bed earlier?

P: My job used to motivate me, but now I really don't have any responsibilities. I never thought I would say this, but it seems that I have too much time. Staying in bed is one way to use it up.

T: I think we need to find more things you can do during the day, for two important reasons. First, lying in bed later than necessary may be negatively affecting your sleep the following evening. Second, having more interesting things to do would raise your general activity level during the day, which may improve your sleep.

P: Not long ago I would have been resistant to that advice. I thought retirement was for sitting around and doing nothing. Frankly, I can't stand it. I want to become more active, and if it improves my sleep, then that's just an added bonus.

The patient's wife agreed to help him comply with an early arising time, and they decided to walk at a nearby park each morning shortly after arising. Mr. C. also planned to become involved in some volunteer work.

During our next session, Mr. C. reported that an early arising time and exercising were made easier by his wife's support, and time in bed had been reduced to about 7.5 hours. Also, he had decided to work during weekday afternoons as a volunteer at a local hospital. His sleep latency appeared to be stabilizing at about 15 to 20 minutes, but he still experienced some difficulty on the 2 nights per week he did not take triazolam. We decided to meet again in about 3 weeks. During the time between sessions, he would concentrate on maintaining a high activity level during the day and would continue to gradually withdraw from triazolam while practicing relaxation.

Outcome and Termination

Three weeks later we met for our last session. The patient had further restricted time in bed to about 7 hours, was taking triazolam only 2 nights per week, and was experiencing satisfactory sleep latencies of about 20 minutes. He was still averaging about three awakenings per night but was exhibiting no daytime fatigue or sleepiness. Because of his significantly increased satisfaction with his sleep, we mutually consented to discontinue our sessions, and he agreed to contact me if his sleep deteriorated. A phone call 2 weeks later confirmed that he had discontinued triazolam use entirely and was still experiencing satisfactory sleep.

In summary, Mr. C.'s insomnia complaint stemmed mainly from unrealistic sleep goals and naiveté concerning the effect of his lifestyle on sleep. He initially turned to medication to cope with his sleep difficulties, but this strategy proved ineffective. Relaxation was used to facilitate withdrawal from the sleep medication with minimal side effects. Education about age-associated sleep alterations and an emphasis on his lack of sleepiness during the day resulted in the establishment of more feasible sleep expectations and greater sleep satisfaction. This case illustrates the necessity of carefully assessing lifestyle variables rather than just narrowly focusing on a patient's nighttime sleep experience. A major lifestyle change (retirement) was directly responsible for two important contributors to the patient's insomnia complaint, excessive time in bed and reduced activity level.

Mr. C.'s case also underscores the importance of the therapeutic relationship itself. The patient's initial impatience with me as a therapist threatened to cause him to prematurely terminate treatment. It was essential first to effectively communicate my understanding of his concerns and later to offer a convincing rationale for my treatment approach. An interest in establishing a better therapeutic relationship with the patient also motivated a change in my treatment plan. Triazolam withdrawal, with which the patient was uncomfortable, was delayed, and instead a simple behavioral intervention (no napping) was implemented. Fortunately, this resulted in immediate sleep improvement and increased the patient's confidence in both my therapeutic skills and his ability to improve sleep by means other than sleep medication.

Follow-Up and Maintenance

I spoke with the patient 6 months later in order to assess maintenance of treatment gains. He reported average sleep latencies of 15 minutes and about three awakenings per night. Mr. C. stated that he had not used sleep medication during the prior 6 months, and his work at the hospital prevented his previous habit of afternoon napping. His wife played a crucial role in the patient's long-term compliance by continuing to support his efforts to maintain a compressed sleep schedule and to exercise regularly.

Summary

Insomnia is a prevalent disorder that is particularly common among females and older individuals. The use of a single, descriptive term to describe sleeplessness is deceptive, because insomnia is a heterogeneous disorder with etiology and symptoms that vary significantly across individual patients. Such diversity demands careful differential diagnosis and assessment before treatment implementation. Objective assessment procedures provide greater assurance of accuracy but ignore the insomniac's subjective sleep perception. Self-report measures appear to sacrifice precision, but subjective sleep evaluation is usually what prompts an insomnia complaint and therefore should not be dismissed lightly. Similarly, objective improvement after treatment does not necessarily imply increased sleep satisfaction.

Pharmacotherapy may provide short-term relief of insomnia but is contraindicated for the treatment of chronic insomnia. Several behavioral treatments effectively reduce insomnia symptoms, but patient compliance is essential for therapeutic results. Despite the existence of these helpful interventions, further research is required on strategies for designing treatments that fit a particular patient's need. Information on tailoring interventions would be a valuable source of assistance to therapists attempting to maximize the probability of a successful treatment outcome.

References

Aber, R., & Webb, W. B. (1986). Effects of a limited nap on night sleep in older subjects. *Psychology and Aging, 1,* 300–302.

American Psychiatric Association (1987). *Diagnostic and statistical manual of mental disorders* (3rd ed., rev.). Washington, DC: Author.

American Sleep Disorders Association (1990). *International classification of sleep disorders: Diagnostic and coding manual.* Rochester, MN: Author.

Bixler, E. O., Kales, A., Soldatos, C. R., Kales, J. D., & Healey, S. (1979). Prevalence of sleep disorders in the Los Angeles metropolitan area. *American Journal of Psychiatry, 136,* 1257–1262.

Bonnet, M. H., & Arand, D. L. (1992). Caffeine use as a model of acute and chronic insomnia. *Sleep, 15,* 526–536.

Buysse, D. J., & Reynolds, C. F. (1990). Insomnia. In M. J. Thorpy (Ed.), *Handbook of sleep disorders* (pp. 375–433). New York: Marcel Dekker.

Carskadon, M. A., Dement, W. C., Mitler, M. M., Guilleminault, C., Zarcone, V. P., & Spiegel, R. (1976). Self-reports versus sleep laboratory findings in 122 drug-free subjects with complaints of chronic insomnia. *American Journal of Psychiatry, 133*, 1382–1388.

Edinger, J. D., Hoelscher, T. J., Webb, M. D., Marsh, G. R., Radtke, R. A., & Erwin, C. W. (1989). Polysom-nographic assessment of DIMS: Empirical evaluation of its diagnostic value. *Sleep, 12*, 315–322.

Espie, C. A. (1991). *The psychological treatment of insomnia.* Chichester, United Kingdom: Wiley.

Espie, C. A., Brooks, D. N., & Lindsay, W. R. (1989). An evaluation of tailored psychological treatment of insomnia. *Journal of Behavior Therapy and Experimental Psychiatry, 20*, 143–153.

Espie, C. A., & Lindsay, W. R. (1985). Paradoxical intention in the treatment of chronic insomnia: Six case studies illustrating variability in therapeutic response. *Behaviour Research and Therapy, 23*, 703–709.

Espie, C. A., Lindsay, W. R., Brooks, D. N., Hood, E. M., & Turvey, T. (1989). A controlled comparative investigation of psychological treatments for chronic sleep-onset insomnia. *Behaviour Research and Therapy, 27*, 79–88.

Feinberg, I., March, J. D., Floyd, T. C., Jimison, R., Bossom-Demitrack, L., & Katz, P. H. (1985). Homeostatic changes during post-nap sleep maintain baseline levels of delta EEG. *Electroencephalography and Clinical Neurophysiology, 61*, 134–137.

Ford, D. E., & Kamerow, D. B. (1989). Epidemiologic study of sleep disturbances and psychiatric disorders. *Journal of the American Medical Association, 262*, 1479–1484.

Freedman, R., & Papsdorf, J. D. (1976). Biofeedback and progressive relaxation treatment of sleep-onset insomnia: A controlled all-night investigation. *Biofeedback and Self-Regulation, 1*, 253–271.

Friedman, L., Bliwise, D. L., Yesavage, J. A., & Salom, S. R. (1991). A preliminary study comparing sleep restriction and relaxation treatments for insomnia in older adults. *Journal of Gerontology, 46*, 1–8.

Gillin, J. C., & Byerly, W. F. (1990). The diagnosis and management of insomnia. *New England Journal of Medicine, 322*, 239–248.

Gross, R. T., & Borkovec, T. D. (1982). Effects of a cognitive intrusion manipulation on the sleep-onset latency of good sleepers. *Behavior Therapy, 13*, 112–116.

Hauri, P. J., & Wisbey, J. (1992). Wrist actigraphy in insomnia. *Sleep, 15*, 293–301.

Haynes, S. N., Adams, A., & Franzen, M. (1981). The effects of presleep stress on sleep-onset insomnia. *Journal of Abnormal Psychology, 90*, 601–606.

Haynes, S. N., Fitzgerald, S. G., Shute, G. E., & Hall, M. (1985). The utility and validity of daytime naps in the assessment of sleep-onset insomnia. *Journal of Behavioral Medicine, 8*, 237–247.

Hoddes, E., Dement, W. C., & Zarcone, V. (1972). The development and use of the Stanford Sleepiness Scale. *Psychophysiology, 9*, 150.

Hoelscher, T. J., & Edinger, J. D. (1988). Treatment of sleep-maintenance insomnia in older adults: Sleep period reduction, sleep education, and modified stimulus control. *Psychology and Aging, 3*, 258–263.

Hoelscher, T. J., Ware, J. C., & Bond, T. (1993, June). *Initial validation of the Insomnia Impact Scale.* Paper presented at the annual meeting of the Association of Professional Sleep Societies, Los Angeles.

Kales, A., Soldatos, C. R., Bixler, E. O., & Kales, J. D. (1983a). Early morning insomnia with rapidly eliminated benzodiazepines. *Science, 220*, 95–97.

Kales, A., Soldatos, C. R., Bixler, E. O., & Kales, J. D. (1983b). Rebound insomnia and rebound anxiety: A review. *Pharmacology, 26*, 121–137.

Kay, D. C., & Samiuddin, Z. (1988). Sleep disorders associated with drug abuse and drugs of abuse. In R. L. Williams, I. Karacan, & C. A. Moore (Eds.), *Sleep disorders: Diagnosis and treatment* (pp. 315–371). New York: Wiley.

Lacks, P., Bertelson, A. D., Gans, L., & Kunkel, J. (1983). The effectiveness of three behavioral treatments for different degrees of sleep onset insomnia. *Behavior Therapy, 14*, 593–605.

Lacks, P., & Morin, C. M. (1992). Recent advances in the assessment and treatment of insomnia. *Journal of Consulting and Clinical Psychology, 60*, 586–594.

Lacks, P., & Rotert, M. (1986). Knowledge and practice of sleep hygiene techniques in insomniacs and good sleepers. *Behaviour Research and Therapy, 24*, 365–368.

Ladouceur, R., & Gros-Louis, Y. (1986). Paradoxical intention vs. stimulus control in the treatment of severe insomnia. *Journal of Behavior Therapy and Experimental Psychiatry, 17*, 267–269.

Levin, D., Bertelson, A. D., & Lacks, P. (1984). MMPI differences among mild and severe insomniacs and good sleepers. *Journal of Personality Assessment, 48*, 126–129.

Lichstein, K. L. (1988a). *Clinical relaxation strategies.* New York: Wiley.

Lichstein, K. L. (1988b). Sleep compression treatment of an insomnoid. *Behavior Therapy, 19,* 625–632.

Lichstein, K. L., & Fischer, S. M. (1985). Insomnia. In M. Hersen & A. S. Bellack (Eds.), *Handbook of clinical behavior therapy with adults* (pp. 319–352). New York: Plenum.

Lichstein, K. L., & Johnson, R. S. (1993). Relaxation for insomnia and hypnotic medication use in older women. *Psychology and Aging, 8,* 103–111.

Lichstein, K. L., Nickel, R., Hoelscher, T. J., & Kelley, J. E. (1982). Clinical validation of a sleep assessment device. *Behaviour Research and Therapy, 20,* 292–297.

Lichstein, K. L., & Rosenthal, T. L. (1980). Insomniacs' perceptions of cognitive versus somatic determinants of sleep disturbance. *Journal of Abnormal Psychology, 89,* 105–107.

Lick, J. R., & Heffler, D. (1977). Relaxation training and attention placebo in the treatment of severe insomnia. *Journal of Consulting and Clinical Psychology, 45,* 153–161.

Marchini, E. J., Coates, T. J., Magistad, J. G., & Waldum, S. J. (1983). What do insomniacs do, think, and feel during the day? A preliminary study. *Sleep, 6,* 147–155.

Marlatt, G. A., & George, W. H. (1990). Relapse prevention and the maintenance of optimal health. In S. Shumaker, E. B. Schron, & J. Ockene (Eds.), *The handbook of health behavior change* (pp. 44–63). New York: Springer.

Mellinger, G. D., Balter, M. B., & Uhlenhuth, E. H. (1985). Insomnia and its treatment. *Archives of General Psychiatry, 42,* 225–232.

Mendelson, W. B., Garnett, D., Gillin, J. C., & Weingartner, H. (1984). The experience of insomnia and daytime and nighttime functioning. *Psychiatry Research, 12,* 235–250.

Morin, C. M., & Azrin, N. H. (1987). Stimulus control and imagery training in treating sleep-maintenance insomnia. *Journal of Consulting and Clinical Psychology, 55,* 260–262.

Morin, C. M., & Azrin, N. H. (1988). Behavioral and cognitive treatments of geriatric insomnia. *Journal of Consulting and Clinical Psychology, 56,* 748–753.

Nicassio, P. M., Boylan, M. B., & McCabe, T. G. (1982). Progressive relaxation, EMG biofeedback and biofeedback placebo in the treatment of sleep-onset insomnia. *British Journal of Medical Psychology, 55,* 159–166.

Puder, R., Lacks, P., Bertelson, A. D., & Storandt, M. (1983). Short-term stimulus control treatment of insomnia in older adults. *Behavior Therapy, 14,* 424–429.

Reynolds, C. F., Taska, L. S., Sewitch, D. E., Restifo, K., Coble, P. A., & Kupfer, D. J. (1984). Persistent psychophysiologic insomnia: Preliminary research diagnostic criteria and EEG sleep data. *American Journal of Psychiatry, 141,* 804–805.

Roth, T., Roehrs, T., & Zorick, F. (1988). Pharmacological treatment of sleep disorders. In R. L. Williams, I. Karacan, & C. A. Moore (Eds.), *Sleep disorders: Diagnosis and treatment* (pp. 373–395). New York: Wiley.

Sanavio, E. (1988). Pre-sleep cognitive intrusions and treatment of onset-insomnia. *Behaviour Research and Therapy, 26,* 451–459.

Schoicket, S. L., Bertelson, A. D., & Lacks, P. (1988). Is sleep hygiene a sufficient treatment for sleep-maintenance insomnia? *Behavior Therapy, 19,* 183–190.

Seidel, W. F., Ball, S., Cohen, S., Patterson, N., Yost, D., & Dement, W. C. (1984). Daytime alertness in relation to mood, performance, and nocturnal sleep in chronic insomniacs and noncomplaining sleepers. *Sleep, 7,* 230–238.

Soldatos, C. R., Kales, J. D., Scharf, M. B., Bixler, E. O., & Kales, A. (1980). Cigarette smoking associated with sleep difficulty. *Science, 207,* 551–553.

Spielman, A. J., Saskin, P., & Thorpy, M. J. (1987). Treatment of chronic insomnia by restriction of time in bed. *Sleep, 10,* 45–56.

Torsvall, L. (1981). Sleep after exercise: A literature review. *Journal of Sports Medicine and Physical Fitness, 21,* 218–225.

Turner, R. M., & Ascher, L. M. (1979). Controlled comparison of progressive relaxation, stimulus control and paradoxical intention therapies for insomnia. *Journal of Consulting and Clinical Psychology, 47,* 500–508.

Woolfolk, R. L., & McNulty, T. F. (1983). Relaxation treatment for insomnia: A component analysis. *Journal of Consulting and Clinical Psychology, 51,* 495–503.

19

Borderline, Narcissistic, and Histrionic Personality Disorders

Ralph M. Turner

Description of the Disorders

This chapter focuses on three of the four personality disorders included in the dramatic, emotional, and impulsive cluster defined by DSM-III-R (American Psychiatric Association, 1987). The personality disorders we will discuss are borderline (BPD), histrionic (HPD), and narcissistic personality disorders (NPD). These disorders appear to have many common features and often co-occur in patients. These are the disorders of the self. Antisocial personality disorder has been eliminated from this review of the dramatic-impulsive cluster disorders; it deserves its own distinct review because it has a long history and extensive literature. In contrast to the extensive empirical literature on antisocial personality disorder, we are just beginning to examine the disorders of the self.

Clinical Features

Persons with HPD are self-dramatizing, attention seeking, superfluously gregarious, seductive, exhibitionistic, shallow, vain, and demanding of attention. Their interpersonal interactions are marked by excitability and high levels of emotional display. Characteristically, there is a driven quality to the emotional displays. Histrionic persons show a desperate need to be conspicuous and attract attention and

Ralph M. Turner • Department of Psychiatry, Temple University School of Medicine, Philadelphia, Pennsylvania 19140.

Handbook of Prescriptive Treatments for Adults, edited by Michel Hersen and Robert T. Ammerman. Plenum Press, New York, 1994.

affection. Yet the experience of others is that the histrionic's desire for affection is shallow and manipulative. There is an urgent need for dependency and guidance, cloaked in glamour.

Patients with NPD are grandiose, lack empathy, and are hypersensitive to evaluation by others. Entitlement and exploitation are characteristic of this pattern. Evaluation leads to shame, rage, anger, humiliation, or massive denial of personal faults. Such persons look inward for reinforcement and gratification. Weakness and dependency are threatening. The diagnostic term conveys that these individuals magnify their personal worth, orient their affections toward themselves, and expect others to recognize and cater to them in light of this self-characterization.

Borderline personality disorder can be described from two orthogonal but interlocking viewpoints. First, BPD may be viewed as a clinical entity with characteristic features. Second, it may be seen as a level of psychopathology that is serious and involves repeated, brief psychotic episodes and deficits in social competence. An implication of the second perspective is that the borderline syndrome represents a more disturbed variant of the histrionic and narcissistic conditions (Millon, 1981).

Impulsivity is the central feature of BPD. An erratic and unreflective quality characterizes borderlines' tempers and actions. Emotional instability is also a striking feature of borderlines. Their emotions change rapidly and often. Third, BPD patients have difficulty in maintaining a stable, cohesive sense of their identity. Developmentally, BPD patients have failed to form a coherent and integrated set of self schemata. Behaviorally, this is evidenced in rapidly changing presentations of the self. In addition, because the self system is deficient, they cling to others for centering. Mild paranoia, in the sense that they are constantly predicting that a significant other will abandon them, is characteristic. Patients also display anxiety, guilt, depression, and hostility. Often there is self-destructive and self-damaging behavior. Parasuicidal behavior is frequently present.

Despite the apparent distinctness of these clinical descriptions, recent research suggests that several distinct subgroups may make up the broader diagnostic groups. Hurt, Clarkin, Munroe-Blum, and Marziali (1992) have identified three clusters of BPD patients. Each cluster is defined by a specific constellation of BPD criteria. The first cluster is called the identity cluster. The definitional criteria for the identity cluster include identity disturbance, intolerance of being alone, and chronic feelings of emptiness and boredom. The second BPD subgroup is termed the affect cluster. The defining criteria for cluster two include unstable affect, unstable interpersonal relationships, and inappropriate anger. The third subgroup is referred to as the impulsive cluster. Self-damaging behavior and impulsive behavior are the primary defining criteria for the impulsive subgroup. Hurt et al. (1992) argue that treatment strategies will be prescriptively different for the different clusters of borderline patients.

Current research in our clinic at Temple University Medical School supports Hurt et al.'s (1992) contention that specific subgroups of BPD patients exist. Using hierarchical cluster analysis to cluster BPD patients into homogenous subgroups, we have identified both a three group and a four group model. Our findings are quite similar to those of Hurt et al. (1992). Our first cluster is an affect cluster. The defining criteria consist of unstable affect and unstable interpersonal relationships. The second cluster we obtained is termed impulsive-angry. Unlike Hurt et al.'s (1992) impulsive cluster, this subgroup does not meet the criteria for self-harm. The third subgroup we detected is defined by identity disturbance, feelings of emptiness, and self-harm. We have termed this the identity-parasuicide cluster. Our fourth group is another self-harm subgroup. The defining criteria for this cluster include self-harm, emptiness, unstable interpersonal relationships, and anger. This subgroup we have called the unstable relationship-anger-self-harm cluster. Although slightly different, these results support Hurt et al.'s view that BPD patients can be classified into clusters based upon their prototypical clinical presentations. We also agree that the prescriptive treatment for one cluster will not necessarily be the treatment of choice for one of the other clusters.

Following up on this work, we have also used hierarchical cluster analysis to identify subgroups of histrionic and narcissistic personality disorder patients. The analyses for the HPD patients have yielded three clusters. The first cluster is the seductive cluster. The criteria defining this cluster include being overly seductive, self-centered, and overly concerned with attractiveness. The second HPD cluster appears to be an emotionally unstable cluster. Exaggerated shifting emotions define this subgroup. The third HPD subgroup is defined primarily by an excessive need for attention and approval, excessively colorful speech, and exaggerated emotions. This subgroup can be thought of as the attention and approval cluster. Our analysis of subgroups in the NPD category currently suggest two main groups need to be taken into account when thinking about the clinical features of these patients. Thus far, we have identified an ideal fantasy-entitled cluster and an exploitive-non-empathetic cluster. The ideal fantasy-entitled cluster is defined by the title criteria plus feelings of envy, feeling special, and the experience of uniqueness. The exploitive-non-empathetic subgroup is marked by the criteria exploitive, lack of empathy, needing to be the center of attention, and difficulty in tolerating criticism. Future research will focus on cross validating these subgroups of dramatic-impulsive patients, but the point to be made is that the clinical features of these patients can and do vary. Consequently, so will the etiological factors contributing to these subgroups and the types of treatment they are likely to respond to. It is not sufficient to speak of *the* borderline, or *the* histrionic, or *the* narcissistic patient.

Associated Features

The most significant associated feature of these disorders is the vulnerability to Axis I disorders. Dysthymia and depression often co-occur with these disorders. Anxiety surrounding separation issues can be distressing for histrionic and borderline patients. Interpersonal problems regularly are features of these disorders. Self-mutilation has been reported to occur in both BPD and HPD patients (Fruensgaard & Flindt-Hansen, 1988). Comorbidity of organic disorders may also occur in patients with BPD. About 6 to 27% of BPD patients have a history of neurologic disorders (Buysse, Nathan, & Soloff, 1990). Alcohol and substance abuse disorders are also common among these patients (Buysse et al., 1990; Fruensgaard & Flindt-Hansen, 1988; Stone, 1990).

Epidemiology

The prevalence rates for histrionic, narcissistic, and borderline personality disorders, as defined according to DSM-III-R criteria, have only just begun to be investigated. This is primarily the result of changing definitions of these disorders with the coming of DSM-III. There are several studies, however, that provide rough estimates from which to work.

In the Stirling County Study (Leighton, 1963), the rate of emotionally unstable personality disorder was estimated to be 1.7 per 100 persons. This estimate has been taken by various authors to represent an approximation of the prevalence of BPD, because the emotionally unstable diagnosis is similar to that of BPD. This personality disorder was found to be more common in women than in men. The same study found a prevalence of 2.2% for an older diagnostic entity, "emotionally unstable character disorder," which provides an approximation for the incidence of HPD (Marmar, 1988).

A more recent epidemiological study of HPD has been reported by Nestadt, Romanoski, Chahal, and Merchant (1990). The information was extracted from a two-stage population survey conducted as a part of the NIMH Epidemiological Catchment Area Program. Using DSM-III-R criteria, HPD showed a prevalence of 2.1% in the general population. Importantly, this study found that males and females were equally affected with the disorder.

Using Schedule for Affective Disorders and Schizophrenia- Research Diagnostic Criteria (SADS-RDC) criteria, Weissman and Meyers (1980) reported BPD to be very rare in the New Haven Community Survey. The rate was 0.2 per 100 persons. Borderline personality disorder was twice as prevalent in women as in men. Contrasting with these data, a survey conducted by the Institute of Medicine (1985) suggested that approximately 4% of the general population may suffer from BPD. The ratio of women to men diagnosed with BPD has ranged from 2 : 1 (Gunderson, 1984; Leighton, 1963; Weissman & Meyers, 1980) to 4 : 1 (Stiver, 1988). It is generally believed that HPD occurs more frequently among women and that NPD occurs more frequently among men (Perry & Vaillant, 1989). The report of Nestadt, Romanoski, Chahal, and Merchant (1990) would appear to challenge the general wisdom regarding the gender ratio for HPD.

Etiology

Speculation about the etiology of the histrionic, narcissistic, and borderline personality disorders abounds, but few empirical data exist. The empirical studies that have been conducted have addressed the borderline syndrome. Regardless of theoretical orientation, most contributors to the literature on the etiology of these disorders have proposed a disturbed early relationship between the child and the parents. Specifically, the various theories purport that ruptures in the separation-individuation process account for the personality pathology seen in later life. Harsh and abusive family environments have been associated with the borderline disorder; ambivalent family interaction styles have been postulated for histrionics. Both harsh and overenriched early family environments are theorized for narcissistic individuals.

The empirical literature appears to support the notion that disturbed early child–parent experiences are crucial to the development of BPD, at least. Bradley (1979) found that adolescent BPD patients suffered significantly more early caregiver separations than matched groups of psychotic, nonpsychotic, and delinquent control subjects. Related to this finding, Soloff and Millward (1983) found that borderline patients show a significantly higher rate of early parental loss and subsequent pathological sensitivity to separation experiences than do depressed patients. Father absence because of divorce or death was the most prominent factor. Similarly, Akiskal, Chen, Davis, Puzantian, Kashgarian, and Bolinger (1985) found that BPD patients were significantly more likely than subjects with an affective disorder to have a history of childhood caretaker loss and parental assortive mating (i.e., both parents had psychiatric illnesses). Troubled home environments with frequent separations, foster care, or adoption are also associated with BPD. Ogata, Silk, and Goodrich (1990) found that families of BPD patients have more hostile conflict and are less cohesive than are families of depressed patients. When BPD patients do grow up in an intact family environment they appear to receive less parental care and bonding experiences than non-BPD psychiatric patients (Paris & Frank, 1989; Goldberg, Mann, Wise & Segall, 1985). Additionally, Zanarini, Gunderson, Marino, Schwartz, and Frankenburg (1989), Herman, Perry, and van der Kolk (1989), Ogata et al. (1990), Stone, Unwin, Beachman, and Swenson (1988), and van der Kolk, Perry, and Herman (1991) have documented high levels of sexual and physical abuse in the developmental backgrounds of BPD patients. The study by Herman et al. (1989) showed 81% of BPD patients had suffered serious childhood trauma, with 67% reporting sexual abuse, 17% reporting physical abuse, and 62% reporting witnessing domestic violence. Corroborating these findings, van der Kolk, Perry, and Herman (1991) related that 77% of BPD patients who had made a recent suicide attempt reported histories of abuse and 79% of patients engaging in self-cutting had a history of child abuse. However, despite the consensus of findings relating physical and sexual abuse and early loss of caregivers to BPD psychopathology, there are major methodological problems with all of these studies. Each of these studies has relied on retrospective, historical techniques to obtain the data about early life experiences also; research on the development of autobiographical memory suggests that many recollections adults make about events during childhood suffer from distortions (Nelson, 1993). Therefore, the validity of these studies has been seriously questioned by Marziali (1992). In addition, as Marziali (1992) has pointed out, not all BPD patients have histories of abuse and neglect. Furthermore, all persons who go through severe childhood trauma do not develop BPD.

Another line of etiological theorizing and research has centered on the neurobehavioral model (Andrulonis, Glueck, Stroebel, Vogel, Shapiro, & Aldrige, 1981; Andrulonis & Vogel, 1984). This model suggests that BPD symptoms are the result of the pernicious developmental effects of childhood brain dysfunction. Supporting this model, Andrulonis et al. (1981) found that 38% of a group of 91 BPD patients showed a history of Minimal Brain Dysfunction (MBD) or some other form of organic deficit. They were able to form three distinct subgroups of BPD patients based on these findings. One subgroup showed MBD with no organic involvement, a second with a history of attention deficits and learning disabilities, and a third with organic brain dysfunction due to traumatic brain injury. In a follow-up study, Andrulonis and Vogel (1984) reported discovering four groups of BPD patients, two of which were defined by organic dysfunction. These two organic subgroups were again MBD and general organic. Importantly, their findings indicated that male BPD patients showed greatly higher rates of neurological disorder than female BPD patients. Fifty-two percent of the males, compared to 28% of the females, showed a past history of head trauma, while 40% of the males, compared to 14% of the females, were diagnosed with attention deficit disorder or learning disability. Thus, research on the neurobehavioral model, to date, has more bearing on the development of BPD in males than in females. Organically impaired BPD patients are primarily male. They also appear to have an earlier onset of emotional instability and impulsiveness due to constitutional factors. Again, however, not all BPD males show organic dysfunction, and not all organically impaired persons develop BPD.

Genetic hypotheses have also been promulgated. Several studies document high

397

Borderline,
Narcissistic, and
Histrionic
Personality
Disorders

frequencies of familial aggregation of substance abuse and antisocial behavior among BPD probands (Soloff & Millward, 1983; Zanarini, Gunderson, Marino, Schwartz, & Frankenburg, 1989). Loranger, Oldham, and Tulis (1982) found that relatives of BPD patients showed two to three times higher rates of alcoholism than relatives of bipolar and schizophrenic patients. Alcoholism was most common in the fathers. Akiskal (1981) and Akiskal, Chen, Davis, Puzantian, Kashgarian, and Bolinger (1985) have argued from data that BPD is a variant of affective illness, and consequently, is due to the same factors predisposing persons to depression and bipolar disorder. However, an extensive review of this issue by Gunderson and Phillips (1991) suggests there is no causal linkage between affective illness and BPD.

Etiology Revisited: Multidimensional Causality and Developmental Psychopathology

The discussion of the etiology of BPD, NPD, and HPD has primarily centered on BPD because no empirical work has been conducted on NPD and HPD. Yet, even with BPD, no clear picture of etiology has emerged. There appear to be several paths through development to the status of borderline functioning adult. In light of this complex picture, Marziali (1992) has argued that a multidimensional model is required to adequately explain the etiology of BPD. I am in agreement with the multidimensional position. With regard to the etiology of HPD, NPD, as well as BPD, our view is that a multidetermined, interactional, developmental psychopathology model is required to understand and eventually explain the development of the dramatic-impulsive personality disorders.

An interactional-developmental interpretation of these findings suggests that both hereditary and environmental factors result in the pattern of impulsive emotional instability seen in these patients. Interactional-developmental models of psychopathology consider mental illness to eventuate from additive and multiplicative interactions of persons' biological and environmental circumstances (Lewis, 1990). When characteristics of the person interact with the environment in a multiplicative causal fashion, the interactional model becomes a transactional model.

There are at least three critical theoretical implications of viewing the development of dramatic-impulsive personality disorders from this multidimensional transactional model. From this perspective, both the child and the environment are active in determining an individual's course of development whether it be a pattern of normal development or results in adult psychopathology. Transactional-developmental models of psychopathology focus the search for causes of stability and change in human behavior on the characteristics of the person and his or her environment. Individual behavior is adaptive, but one's ability to behave adaptively is connected to the environment. Consequently, persons may act in maladaptive ways because maladaptive environments demand it of them. From this perspective, maladaptive behavior shown by dramatic-impulsive persons is conceived as adaptive to their maladaptive environments. Altering the dramatic-impulsive patients' will consequently involves modifying the social systems within which the patients are embedded, as well as modifying individuals' coping behaviors.

A second implication is that transactional-developmental models do not permit personal regression to earlier modes of adaptation, nor environmental regression. Since changes are not simply additive, there can be no return to a former state of affairs. Thus, changes, either toward increased pathological functioning or increased normalized functioning, involve evolution to a new level, or character, of functioning. It is not simply returning to some idealized homeostatic state in which the dramatic-impulsive patient is stabilized and functioning adaptively. Breakdowns in functioning, or crises involving micropsychotic episodes, cutting, or suicidal threats, occur as evolving developmental responses to increasing strain between the person and the environment. Likewise, therapeutic change will involve an evolution in the patient–environment interactional pattern to a more adaptive level.

The third implication arises from the multideterminant causal processes proposed in this model. This proposition argues that there are many developmental routes to generating a dramatic-impulsive personality disorder. There is no one royal etiological road. Consequently, instead of looking for one primary etiological factor, progress will be made by looking for causal interactions among multiple risk factors. Furthermore, it would be expected that diagnostic subgroups of BPD, HPD, and NPD patients exist. Different etiological mechanisms might likely be relevant as causal processes for these subgroups.

In summary, the implications of our multideterminant, transactional-developmental model for the etiology of the dramatic-impulsive personality disorders are as follows. Constitutional factors can and do set the stage for the development of these disorders. There is not just one constitutional factor predisposing a person to develop a dramatic-impulsive disorder, however. Hereditary factors, constitutional factors, and temperament factors are interactively at work. Early environmental factors such as the quality of attachment and bonding experiences can transact with the child to heighten the probability of the development of a dramatic-impulsive disorder. Later, harsh environmental factors (such as sexual or physical abuse) or family pathology (such as drug abuse and alcoholism) can impact on the system of development. Ongoing disturbance is maintained through transactional interactions between the person and the environment. Levels of disturbance, or health, are evolved into by way of transactions between the person and the environment. Dramatic-impulsive persons act in maladaptive ways because maladaptive environments demand it of them; maladaptive environments become increasingly disturbing because the dramatic-impulsive person pushes them to be so. From this perspective, maladaptive behavior shown by dramatic-impulsive persons is conceived as adaptive to their maladaptive environments. Some research already supports this perspective. For instance, van der Kolk, Perry, and Herman (1991) suggest that, although severe childhood trauma contributes heavily to the onset of some of the characteristics of BPD (i.e., self-destructive behavior), it is the lack of secure attachments or a stable home environment throughout childhood and adolescence, which maintains it. Future research on the etiology of dramatic-impulsive disorders from the multideterminant, transactional-developmental model is certain to produce a more coherent picture of the etiology of these disorders.

Differential Diagnosis and Assessment

DSM-IV Categorization

Histrionic, narcissistic, and borderline personality disorders are diagnosed on Axis II according to a prototype diagnostic system. This means that patients need meet only a subset of the total collection of criteria outlined in DSM-III-R (American Psychiatric Association, 1987) and the DSM-IV Draft Criteria (American Psychiatric Association, 1994). In addition, a given patient may meet the criteria for several Axis II diagnoses. Complicating matters still further, patients meeting criteria for an Axis-II disorder can be diagnosed with an Axis-I disorder.

The DSM-IV Draft Criteria (American Psychiatric Association, 1993) criteria for histrionic personality disorder concentrate on the extent to which persons are excessively attention-seeking and overly emotional. It is important to note that while many persons show histrionic traits, the disorder is diagnosed when these traits are inflexible, maladaptive, and persistent. To be diagnosed with HPD an individual must meet five of the following eight criteria: (1) discomfort in situations in which he or she is not the center of attention; (2) interaction with others that is often characterized by inappropriate sexually seductive or provocative behavior; (3) rapidly shifting and shallow expression of emotions; (4) consistent use of physical appearance to draw attention to him- or herself; (5) style of speech that is excessively impressionistic and lacking in detail; (6) self-dramatization, theatricality, and exaggerated expression of emotion; (7) suggestibility or being easily influenced by others or circumstances; and (8) considering relationships to be more important than they are.

The DSM-IV Draft Criteria (American Psychiatric Association, 1993) criteria for narcissistic personality disorder emphasize a pervasive pattern involving grandiosity in fantasy or behavior, a need for admiration, and a lack of empathetic capacity. Five of the following criteria are necessary to make the diagnosis: (1) a grandiose sense of self-importance; (2) preoccupation with fantasies of unlimited success, power, brilliance, beauty, or ideal love; (3) the belief that he or she is special and unique and can only be understood by, or should only associate with, other special or high-status people; (4) need for excessive admiration; (5) a sense of entitlement; (6) being interpersonally exploitive; (7) lack of empathy; (8) being envious of others or the belief that others are envious of him or her; and (9) arrogant or haughty behaviors or attitudes.

Borderline personality disorder is defined by DSM-IV Draft Criteria (American Psychiatric Association, 1993) instability of interpersonal relationships, self-image, and affects, as well as marked impulsivity. Five of the following nine criteria are required to make the diagnosis: (1) frantic efforts to avoid real or imagined abandonment; (2) a pattern of unstable and intense interpersonal relationships characterized by alternating between extremes of idealization and devaluation; (3) identity disturbance or unstable self-image; (4) impulsivity in at least two areas that are potentially self-damaging; (5) recurrent suicidal behavior, gestures, or threats, or self-mutilating behavior; (6) affective instability due to a marked reactivity of mood; (7) chronic feelings of emptiness; (8) inappropriate, intense anger or difficulty controlling anger; and (9) transient, stress-related paranoid ideation or severe dissociative symptoms.

Currently DSM-IV is in the final stages of development. The Axis-II work group is attempting to refine the classification scheme so that there will be less overlap among the specific disorders and more specificity for each of the individual items (Hirschfeld, 1993). Researchers and practitioners can expect the meanings of the dramatic-impulsive disorders to remain consistent with DSM-III-R. However, it appears likely that there will be modifications of individual items for each of these disorders as suggested by the most recent set of draft criteria listed above. For instance, for BPD a proposed new criterion is transient, stress-related paranoid ideation (Gunderson, Zanarini, & Cassandra, 1991). For the final version of the criteria the DSM-IV should be consulted.

Differential Diagnosis

401

Borderline,
Narcissistic, and
Histrionic
Personality
Disorders

Differential diagnosis of histrionic, narcissistic, and borderline personality disorders involves discrimination along the domains of affective illness, schizophrenia, anxiety disorders, and other personality disorders. The relevant dimensions of differential diagnosis vary for these three disorders.

A need to make a diagnostic distinction between the dramatic-impulsive disorders and major depression is common to all three. Dramatic cluster patients seldom come to the clinic because of the personality disorder. More often a depressive episode caused by an environmental stressor, particularly interpersonal stresses, will be the presenting problem. The crucial distinction to be made is that the problems the personality-disordered patient reports will have a long history. In other words, there will be a significant trait-versus-state component to the depression. A vital distinction can be made according to whether the depression is based on guilt themes and connected to loss, or is associated with conflicts over identity, dependency–independence needs, and self-destructive behavior. Typical depression is based on guilt and loss. The depression of these impulsive personality styles is typically based upon identity problems and dependency–independence conflicts.

Although less common than once thought, when BPD was considered to mean borderline schizophrenia, the discrimination between BPD and schizophrenia is an additional diagnostic consideration. Causing the confusion are the brief psychotic episodes frequenty shown by borderline patients. However, these episodes are of short duration. The wide gap between the socially awkward and distant relationships of schizophrenic patients and the needy, affectively charged relationships of borderline patients should make them readily distinguishable to clinicians.

Posttraumatic stress disorder, panic disorder, and generalized anxiety disorder are relevant discriminations for histrionic patients. However, the most difficult discrimination is among the various Axis II disorders. The DSM-III-R criteria for these disorders are based upon a prototypic definition. In a prototypic diagnostic system, no one of the criteria is either necessary or sufficient to the diagnosis or the clinical description of the disorder. The clinical pictures of the patients included in the classification are heterogeneous, and the boundaries between diagnostic groups are permeable and overlapping. Consequently, multiple clinical pictures will present within a given diagnostic class. Patients are likely to fit several categories on Axis II. This potential is increased because these three disorders have several criteria in common.

Another factor regarding differential diagnosis of the dramatic-impulsive disorders involves the consideration of the subgroup to which a given patient belongs. As the research base develops on the issue of patient subgroups, it will become increasingly important to specify which type of BPD, HPD, or NPD patient one is dealing with.

Assessment Strategies

Currently, the optimal Axis II assessment is accomplished with semistructured clinical interviews. There are two structured interviews that assess the full range of Axis II disorders worthy of consideration. The first is the Personality Disorder Examination (PDE) (Loranger, 1988). The PDE has 128 items and is designed for use by an experienced clinician. It takes approximately 90 minutes to administer. Between-rater agreement across two raters has been reported as 0.98 for BPD and

0.87 for HPD (Loranger, Sussman, Oldham, & Russakoff, 1987). The other useful interview format is the Structured Interview for the DSM-III-R Personality Disorders (SIDP) (Pfohl, Stangl, & Zimmerman, 1982) and its revision the *SIDP-R* (Pfohl, 1989). The SIDP-R contains 160 interview items and covers 11 Axis II disorders. The SIDP joint interview kappas for the presence or absence of a personality disorder have been established as 0.71. Individual kappas for BPD and HPD are 0.85 and 0.75, respectively.

Additional reliability and validity work is being conducted on each of these interview formats. There are several drawbacks to these assessment strategies. First, both the PDE and SIDP-R are essentially self-report instruments and consequently are vulnerable to all the problems associated with this methodology. They assume that individuals can provide valid portraits of their personality. However, patients may be unaware of aspects of their personality or fail to acknowledge personality traits that are socially undesirable.

Treatment

Evidence for Prescriptive Treatments

Behavior Therapy. Several cognitive and behavioral models have been developed for therapeutic work with the dramatic-impulsive cluster (Beck, Freeman, & Associates, 1990; Bux, 1992; Davis, 1990; Flemming, 1990; Freeman & Leaf, 1989; Linehan & Wasson, 1990; Pretzer, 1990; Turner, 1988, 1992a, 1992b, 1993). Most of this work has focused on BPD (Linehan, 1987a, 1987b, 1987c; Linehan, Armstrong, Suarez, & Allmon, 1987; Linehan, Armstrong, Suarez, Allmon, & Heard, 1991; Linehan & Wasson, 1990; Pretzer, 1990; Turner, 1983, 1988, 1989, 1992a, 1992b, 1992c, 1993). However, Beck et al. (1990) have developed a general cognitive paradigm for the histrionic and narcissistic disorders.

Dialectical Behavior Therapy. In contrast to Beck et al.'s general approach, Linehan's Dialectical Behavior Therapy (DBT) model has been created for intervention with multiple parasuicidal, female BPD patients and Turner's Dynamic-Cognitive Behavior Therapy (DCBT) model is geared toward patients who fall into the impulsive-anger subgroup. Linehan's dialectical behavior therapy (DBT) model is the behavioral approach most rigorously evaluated to date (Linehan et al., 1987; Linehan et al., 1991; Linehan, Heard, & Armstrong, 1993). Linehan designed the DBT approach as an outpatient treatment for chronically parasuicidal persons with conditions diagnosed as BPD. The DBT treatment plan hierarchically arranges therapy goals into three categories: first, reduction of parasuicide and life-threatening behavior; second, reduction of behavior that interferes with the process of therapy; and third, reduction of behavior that seriously interferes with the quality of life.

DBT emphasizes three central aspects of intervention. The first is a problem-solving focus. The second is an emphasis on dialectical processes. Observation and management of the contingencies operating in the client–therapist relationship are the third characteristic that defines the DBT method. The dialectical thrust, which links the various treatment components, involves accepting BPD clients as they are while engaging in a process of change. Linehan's use of the term *dialectical* in her treatment approach has more important implications, however. It serves as a core philosophy for the form of thinking the therapist uses during treatment. It is also the form of thinking BPD patients must adopt to normalize their thinking, feelings, and behavior.

Linehan's DBT treatment model is composed of an individual treatment component plus four sequential group models. The group models include core skills (observing, describing, spontaneously participating, being mindful, being nonjudgmental, and focusing on effectiveness), interpersonal skills, emotion-regulation skills, and distress-tolerance skills.

Specific treatment strategies involved in the DBT approach include dialectical strategies, problem-solving strategies, irreverent communication strategies, the therapist's acting as a consultant, validation strategies, capability enhancement strategies, relationship strategies, contingency management strategies, and the provision of supervision and support for the therapist. Individual therapy is typically scheduled as a 1-hour session once per week. The group sessions are scheduled once per week and are 2 hours in duration. In addition, telephone contact between the therapist and client is a usual part of DBT procedures.

Linehan and her colleagues (Linehan et al., 1987, 1991, 1993) have reported the results of a long-term, randomized, clinical trial comparing DBT with a control condition consisting of treatment as usual in the community. The results show substantial evidence for the efficacy of DBT in the treatment of borderline parasuicidal behavior. Patients in the studies were women with recent, multiple parasuicidal episodes who also met the criteria for BPD. Treatment lasted for one year. Assessments were conducted at 4, 8, and 12 months. The patients who received DBT had fewer parasuicidal events, fewer medically serious parasuicides, and fewer inpatient hospitalization days. Perhaps the most important finding, patients assigned to DBT stayed in treatment with their original therapists at a significantly higher rate than did the community controls. The 83% retention rate reported by Linehan et al. (1987, 1991) is extraordinarily good given the conventional wisdom that out of every 5 BPD patients, only 3 remain in treatment longer than 6 months, and of those 3 who remain, 2 show marked improvement at one year.

Dynamic-Cognitive-Behavior Therapy. Turner (1983, 1988, 1989, 1992a, 1992b, 1992c, 1993) has also proposed a cognitive-behavioral treatment plan for BPD. This CBT-based treatment model is designated dynamic-cognitive-behavior therapy (DCBT). DCBT has been developed to focus primarily on the impulsive-anger components of BPD.

DCBT derives from principles of developmental psychopathology. The approach draws on an transactional model of development (Lewis, 1990). In this model, it is assumed that relatively stable personal characteristics and the environment interact in additive and multiplicative ways to cause personality patterns. Bowlby's (1988) attachment and bonding theory forms the core motivational component of this transactional developmental model.

This approach to cognitive-behavioral therapy integrates dynamic therapeutic strategies to clarify and modify clients' tacit and feedforward schemata. The DCBT clinician interprets conflicts and uses cognitive and behavioral strategies to modify conflicted distortions, and uses interpretive techniques to break down barriers to change. DCBT stresses the significance of interpersonal relationships in human functioning. The therapeutic relationship is viewed as the primary vehicle through which treatment works.

The DCBT treatment plan covers one year, although treatment can continue in a supportive mode following the intensive phase. The treatment schedule is intense during the first 6 months of treatment. Three sessions per week are scheduled during the first 10 weeks. For the next 16 weeks the sessions occur twice weekly. If treatment has progressed well, the schedule is then changed to once per week. The sessions are structured around an agenda, as is typical of cognitive therapy.

Six phases characterize the treatment program: (1) Crisis management, (2) therapeutic contracting, (3) problem assessment, (4) cognitive-dynamic case formulation, (5) intensive intervention, (6) supportive therapy booster sessions, and (7) termination.

The crisis management phase is necessary when chronic self-harm behavior and crisis bring patients into treatment. The provision of an intensive, structured therapeutic environment and the development of a treatment contract are the cornerstones of containment. Three sessions per week provide the patient with enough contact to allow thoughtful reflection to begin to inhibit impulsiveness. Therapists also make use of the telephone to impose reflection in the midst of impulsive chaos.

The therapeutic tasks of the problem assessment stage involve identifying the patient's primary presenting problems and other areas of concern. In addition, the DCBT clinician attempts to provide a basis for hope that the therapeutic process can cause mutually agreed upon change. During this stage a contract for the session schedule and for handling emergencies is developed collaboratively. Phone contact is an integral component of therapy, but contractual limits are placed on it. Finally, the patient and the therapist establish the goals for therapy through a collaborative effort.

The next task is to conduct the formal structured interviews for DSM-III-R Axis I and Axis II disorders. The Personality Disorder Examination is used to determine the presence of personality disorders. The SADS-L (Spitzer & Endicott, 1979) or SCID I (Spitzer, Williams, Gibbons, & First, 1990) can be used to determine the presence of any Axis I disorders. These interviews usually take several hours each.

There are several caveats to keep in mind. In cases of severe disturbance, expect that the crisis propelling the patient into therapy will continue to exhaust the patient's energy and concentration for developing a long-term plan for psychological change. A part of these early sessions is devoted to problem solving and crisis resolution with the patient.

The case formulation phase focuses on specifying an idiographic cognitive-dynamic assessment for the BPD patient. Cognitive-dynamic assessment focuses on defining four key components of cognitive processing: the patient's (1) cognitive-dynamic triad, (2) triangle of restraints, (3), self and other schemata, and (4) habitual patterns of responding to interpersonal stress.

It is helpful to imagine a triangle when conceptualizing the cognitive-dynamic triad. The apex of the triangle defines the patient's reinforcement agenda. The reinforcement agenda consist of schemata for needs, wishes, or intentions (pursuit of gain or avoidance of aversive circumstances) that consciously and tacitly motivate the patient.

The lower left corner of the triangle represents the schemata, beliefs, automatic assumptions, and expectancies the person holds, consciously and tacitly, about what will happen (the responses of others and the environment) when she attempts to pursue her motivational goals. These schemata act as barriers or restraints on the individual's quest for reinforcement. These schemata are composed of cognitive, emotional, and behavioral barriers and are formulated in terms of the triangle of restraints, to be discussed below.

The base of the cognitive-dynamic triad represents emotional responses to the

405

**Borderline,
Narcissistic, and
Histrionic
Personality
Disorders**

match or mismatch of reinforcement goals and restraints. The lower right corner of the triad represents the behavioral reaction to the match or mismatch of the previous components. Persons have two typical responses to blocked goal seeking: (a) problematic, or symptom, solutions; and (b) compensatory solutions. These problematic and compensatory solutions make up the individual's habitual patterns of responding to interpersonal and general environmental stress. Clients use these problematic and compromise solutions to handle different environmental pressures. They are learned problem-solving strategies. The cognitive sets are stored in hierarchically arranged supraordinate schemata. These schemata contain the templates for self and other scripts and role scenarios.

The triangle of restraints consist of the cognitive, emotional, and behavioral barriers which block the individual's attainment of reinforcement. In the cognitive domain, dysfunction may exist in problem solving; automatic thoughts, assumptions, beliefs, and schema; unrealistic expectations; faulty attributions; inappropriate standards; and misperceptions. All these problems impede the person's ability to manage both cognitive and emotional information. Emotional barriers and restraints to reinforcement attainment include faulty emotional decoding skills and excessive or insufficient emotional responsivity. Behavioral deficits or barriers include social skills deficits, inability to inhibit behavioral responses, inability to delay gratification, and lack of self-control skills. The cognitive, emotional, and behavioral domains of functioning reciprocally affect one another. Consequently, clinicians need to assess patients' deficits in each of these domains and develop a formulation of the problem with these deficits in mind.

Self and significant-other schema are constructed from the data obtained from the previous analyses and include a collection of self and other scripts and role scenarios. An additional assumption of the "cognitive-dynamic pattern" is made in this step. The concept of dynamic pattern assumes that patients develop a complex symptomatic response to the conflict between their goals and dysfunctional schemata and beliefs. Clients dynamically use either their problematic or compromise solutions, described above, to reduce the immediate distress. The pattern of response which includes both the compromise and problematic response types and expectations about significant others' behavior, as well as the client's own behavior, are prepotent cognitive sets which guide behavior. Thus, the cognitive sets are like cognitive maps which apriori determine the client's beliefs, emotional reactions, and behavior. The supraordinate schemata contain the templates for self and other role scenarios and scripts. These cognitive maps for self and significant others' role and scenario interactions dictate what the patient will experience in future interpersonal interactions, regardless of the reality of what really transpires during those interactions. These cognitive sets are stored in hierarchically arranged supraordinate schemata.

The final case formulation consists of a cumulation of the data from the two triangles and the role and script scenarios. The focus is on determining what cognitive, emotional, and behavioral barriers and deficits lead to symptoms when patients' pursue particular goals or reinforcement. The formulation provides the clinician and patient with a cognitive map, or model, for intervention. The most important use of the formulation consists of the patient's learning to use it as a cognitive map guiding self-control and identity regulation.

The strategies of intervention are categorized according to Bruner's (1964) notion of the three differing modes of mental representation or of encoding information: the enactive mode (involves action on objects or behavior), the imaginal mode, and the mode of lexical thought (involves various forms of linguistic encoding and processing).

Enactive treatment strategies include (a) homework, particularly personal experimenting and practicing new modes of thinking, acting, and feeling; (b) role play and role reversal; (c) self-monitoring; (d) communication skill training; (e) contracting; (f) exposure and response prevention; (g) practicing problem-solving skills; and (h) the emotional and behavioral experience of transference interpretations.

Imaginal strategies include interventions such as covert self-modeling, guided imagery, and implosive therapy, or evocative imaginal exposure.

The lexical strategies involve conceptualization, abstraction, and reasoning. Interpretation and questioning of common cognitive distortions are a main technique. Confrontation, defined as questioning current emotional and behavioral reactions and querying for alternative coping processes, is another important lexical DCBT technique. Other lexical interventions include actively educating clients about their cognitive-dynamic structure, dysfunctional beliefs and cognitive distortions, and motivations; teaching problem-solving skills; correcting cognitive distortions and dysfunctional beliefs; and enhancing clients' capacity to control and regulate their information-processing style.

During the supportive therapy and termination stages, patients learn that individuals do not function autonomously. The essential lesson from attachment theory is that people are healthiest when they can function interdependently. This phase essentially involves teaching patients to adopt a new set of beliefs that include: (a) reality is to be accepted as it is; (b) meaningful work provides the greatest chance of creating personal meaning; (c) balance can be achieved through the selective use of play and a positive attributional outlook; and (d) being honest with ourselves and others is integral to mental well-being. Continued problem-solving training and use of the therapeutic alliance are the primary tools used during the supportive therapy phase.

The DCBT approach is multidimensional in terms of the format of treatment. Individual therapy is the primary mode of intervention. However, both family and group intervention modes are used. The emphasis is on attempting to work with patients in the context of their natural environment and the systems within which they are embedded. Thus, family therapy sessions might be accomplished in the patient's home. Group therapy, from the DCBT perspective, does not imply a group of BPD patients seen in the clinic. Rather, it is conceived as a group of relevant persons (both extended family and friends) making up the subsystems in the patient's life. Both the family and group interventions are psychoeducational. The focus of the work is on teaching communication skills and problem-solving skills. In addition to the systems focus, the DCBT model emphasizes a team approach to treatment in the outpatient setting. The team most often consists of a psychologist, social worker, psychiatrist, and an internist. The aim of the team approach is to provide comprehensive care in order to increase patients' functioning in the domains of global mental health, physical health, family functioning, social functioning, leisure functioning, and work functioning.

Two studies (Turner, 1989, 1993) show that DCBT positively influences the symptom status of BPD patients. The first study consisted of an intensive, multiple case study (Turner, 1989). Four patients, all meeting DSM-III-R criteria for borderline personality disorder, were treated by a psychiatric resident trained in the DCBT model. Three of four patients were much improved at the end of the one year follow-up. They were engaging in virtually no self-harm ideation and were functioning much better at work and school. None of these patients were rehospitalized at the one year follow-up assessment.

More recently Turner (1992c) conducted a naturalistic experiment comparing the effectiveness of DCBT with a Supportive Psychotherapy condition (SP) in the treatment of patients diagnosed with borderline personality disorder. Outcome analyses at 6 months and one year showed the DCBT group was significantly more improved than the supportive psychotherapy group. The DCBT group was more improved on self-harm ideation, depression, anxiety, anger, impulsivity, and global mental health functioning. From the results of this study it appears that DCBT is more effective than supportive psychotherapy. However, the results showed that supportive psychotherapy was also beneficial. Since the study did not include a no-treatment control condition, no conclusive statements can be made about either treatment's efficacy. However, when the results of Linehan's studies are combined with the results of this study, I believe we can infer that cognitive behavioral based models are the treatment of choice for most BPD patients.

Pharmacotherapy. Histrionic and narcissistic personality disorders have generally been assumed to belong in the domain of exclusively psychosocial intervention. Borderline personality disorder, however, has an extensive history of attempts at pharmacological therapy.

Pharmacotherapy can be targeted at either the dramatic-impulsive aspects of BPD or at the symptoms associated with the comorbid Axis I disorders that bring the patient to treatment. It is with this second domain of state symptoms that pharmacotherapy has had its most favorable impact.

Virtually every class of psychotropic drug has been tested with BPD patients. Buysse et al. (1990) suggest that there is an emerging body of evidence showing specificity of action for the following drugs: haloperidol, thiothixene, perphenazine, chlorpromazine, imipramine, amitriptyline, tranylcypromine, phenelzine, and carbamazepine. However, Buysse et al. (1990) report that, in practice, psychiatrists recurrently have to go through several medication trials, at a variety of dosages, before finding the best strategy for a given patient. Unfortunately, dramatic-impulsive patients experience a high rate of side effects and frequently fail to comply with the prescribed regimen. In addition, the abuse and suicide potential of many pharmacological agents makes drug treatment a risky venture at best (Gunderson & Phillips, 1991). In fact, Zanarini, Gunderson, and Frankenburg (1988) retrospectively studied the charts of 50 BPD patients and compared their response to "adequate" trials of pharmacotherapy with the responses of dysthymic and antisocial-personality-disordered cohorts, respectively. Zanarini et al. (1988) found that, although the BPD cohort received more adequate trials of pharmacotherapy, they showed significantly less improvement of target symptoms. Related to this finding, Waldenger and Frank (1989) studied the prescribing practices of psychiatrists involved in treating BPD patients. The results showed that the physicians prescribed medications when they felt patients could not benefit from psychotherapy. However, they did not prescribe medication in 47% of the cases because these patients had a history of substance abuse or attempted suicide.

Alternative Treatments. Psychodynamically oriented psychotherapy has been the primary mode of treatment for dramatic-impulsive cluster patients. Two psychodynamic treatment orientations have been suggested for this patient population. The two strategies include the provision of a supportive therapy regimen or an intensive explorative-interpretive treatment plan. Comprehensive models for explorative-interpretive treatment plans have been put forward by Kernberg (1975, 1982, 1984). Adler and Buie (Adler, 1985; Adler & Buie, 1972, 1979; Buie & Adler, 1982) have argued for a supportive model of treatment.

Currently, no experimental studies of the psychodynamic treatment of borderline or other dramatic-impulsive patients have been conducted. However, two short-term and six long-term uncontrolled, longitudinal, follow-up studies have been carried out (Akiskal, 1981; Kroll, Carey, & Sines, 1985; McGlashen, 1985; Paris, Brown, & Nowlis, 1987; Plakun, Burkhardt, & Muller, 1985; Pope, Jonas, & Hudson, 1983; Stone, 1990; Wallerstein, 1986). This group of studies focused on assessing the impact of long-term psychodynamic psychotherapy and pharmacotherapy provided in the context of inpatient hospitalization. The research strategy has been to reinterview patients at periodic intervals over 3 years, in the case of short-term assessment, or over 5 years, in the case of long-term follow-up. Outcome measures have usually consisted of patients' scores on the Health Sickness Rating Scale (HSRS; Luborsky, 1963) and the Global Assessment Scale (GAS), the number of rehospitalizations, job functioning, marital functioning, and the number of suicides. These longitudinal follow-up studies lack the controls that allow unequivocal statements about treatment efficacy. In addition, the impact of psychodynamic psychotherapy has been confounded with pharmacotherapy. Yet the studies do have the strength of describing the life trajectory of borderline patients following treatment over an extensive period. They also have the advantage of telling us what happens in real clinical contexts, unlike true experiments.

Unfortunately, the results of the studies have produced equivocal conclusions. Four of the studies report relatively good outcomes for borderline patients (McGlashen, 1985; Paris et al., 1987; Plakun et al., 1985; Stone, 1990). In contrast, four studies report poor outcomes for BPD patients (Akiskal, 1981; Kroll et al., 1985; Pope et al., 1983; Wallerstein, 1986). When BPD patients have improved, it appears that the full impact of treatment has been delayed by several years (McGlashen, 1985). Most BPD patients show continued problems through their twenties and thirties but then show a marked improvement in functioning during their forties and fifties (Stone, 1990). Of course, this type of improvement may not be due to treatment at all but, rather, reflect a life-span developmental mechanism at work. In addition, an infinite number of propitious life events may account for the improvement in functioning.

Perhaps the most thoughtful study of the inpatient psychodynamic treatment of borderline patients has been reported by Stone (1990). Stone reported that 73 of 193 borderline patients (38%) were completely recovered in 5 to 15 years. When Stone combined the number of patients whose outcomes were fair to recovered, 153 (79%) had good results. Approximately 60% of the patients showed complete alleviation of parasuicide and other impulsive behavior. Stone indicated that supportive psychodynamic treatment was associated with the positive response.

Selecting Optimal Treatment Strategies

Currently, there is no empirical basis for selecting the optimal treatment strategies for the narcissistic or histrionic personality disorders. However, with regard to BPD patients, it seems possible to infer that cognitive behavior therapy is the

409

Borderline,
Narcissistic, and
Histrionic
Personality
Disorders

treatment of choice. Indeed, when parasuicide symptoms predominate the clinical picture, the DBT treatment model is clearly the treatment of choice. When anger, impulsiveness, and unstable interpersonal relationships constitute the primary symptom picture, then DCBT would be preferred. For cases in which impulsive behavior and anger dominate the clinical presentation, the clinician might use either DBT or DCBT. Finally, when patients do not show blatant crisis behavior, such as parasuicide or impulsive self-harm, but are characterized by brief psychotic episodes or paranoia and chronic identity disturbance, then psychodynamically-oriented or cognitively-oriented supportive psychotherapy should be considered.

Additionally, treatment plan decisions are necessary for two aspects of comprehensive treatment. These decisions involve when hospitalization is necessary and whether or not medication is warranted.

Our perspective is that hospitalization should be avoided whenever possible. The goal of psychosocial treatment for dramatic-impulsive patients is to increase their capacity to cope and function with the tasks of everyday living. Outpatient treatment focuses on this goal, whereas inpatient treatment does not. In addition, extensive research by Kiesler (1993) indicates that outpatient care is very much more cost effective than hospitalization for all forms of mental illness. The important point of Kiesler's argument is that outpatient treatment is more efficacious than inpatient treatment. The primary reason that hospitalization is the most often used treatment for mental illness, including the dramatic-impulsive disorders, is that the United States health care system is driven by the hospital mentality and economic politics. The hospital model works for the physical health care system, but it is not an appropriate model for the mental health care system (Kiesler, 1993; VandenBoss, 1993).

Yet when dramatic-impulsive patients are imminently suicidal or are suffering from a comorbid major depressive episode, inpatient hospitalization is necessary. The goal of this treatment option must be containment and termination of the acute episode. A return to outpatient treatment and functioning in the real world environment should be accomplished as quickly as possible.

For which dramatic-impulsive patients and under what circumstances medication should be provided is another treatment strategy option clinicians have to deal with. As noted in the section on pharmacotherapy, there is no pharmacological treatment of choice for BPD, NPD, or HPD. Some rules of thumb can probably be applied, however. When patients are actively suicidal, medication should probably be avoided. When patients show a definitive major depressive or anxiety disorder episode, the appropriate agent for the comorbid disorder should be considered. In any event, because of the great variability of clinical states seen among these patients, careful analysis of each individual patient will be necessary in making medication treatment decisions.

Problems in Carrying Out Interventions

The major problem is the high rate of early termination of therapy. In particular, NPD and HPD patients will seldom recognize that they have a need for mental health care. Typically, they will enter treatment only when they have been faced with interpersonal or work role loss which results in a depressive episode. As soon as they have experienced enough of the supportive relationship elements of therapy and their sense of self-esteem is restored, or they find a replacement person or activity, they will terminate treatment. BPD patients, on the other hand, will show an ambivalent attitude about psychotherapy. This ambivalence will tend to reproduce the same unstable relationship properties in the therapist–patient dyad as it does in patients' real world interpersonal relationships. Alliance ruptures then occur, and BPD patients abandon treatment.

It is often possible to hold these patients in therapy by allowing dramatic-impulsive patients to focus attention upon themselves. Direction the content of these sessions toward discussions of past successes and strengths will act as a catalyst for rebuilding patients' self esteem. After patients' interest is caught therapists can use the psychoeducational format of cognitive behavior therapy as a nonthreatening method to begin to increase self-control, strengthen problem-solving skills, and improve communication skills. At this point, the therapist might have gathered enough good will with the patient to pursue a directive approach to the dysfunctions in the personality organization.

As pointed out above, major ruptures in the therapeutic alliance are likely to occur at any time, especially with narcissistic and borderline patients. The therapist's skill in working through alliance ruptures is the intervention strategy that best attends to these problems. Readers are referred to Safran and Segal (1990) for a thorough discussion of handling alliance ruptures in cognitive therapy. The aspect of Linehan's model which prescribes validation versus invalidation interventions at key points in treatment attends to fostering the therapeutic alliance and retaining BPD patients in treatment. As previously observed, Linehan's model has been extraordinarily successful in this regard.

Another factor influencing the course of treatment is the almost constant state of crisis among the more severely disturbed patients. The full range of crisis events is limited only by life itself. However, the types of crises most often seen include self-harm behavior and suicidal ideation and intent. These crises are associated with both the presentation of the dramatic-impulsive disorders and as response patterns to normal life stressors. Normal, predictable life events can overwhelm dramatic-impulsive patients because of their rigid and limited repertoire for shouldering stresses, vulnerability to attachment and abandonment challenges, and susceptibility to induced and reactive brief psychotic episodes. More severe life stressors, which precipitate crisis, include divorce or the loss of an important relationship, interpersonal demands of the workplace or educational setting, death of a parent or loved one, job loss, serious illness, relocation, or excessive demands involved in parenting.

Faulty coping skills leave dramatic-impulsive patients reeling from the aforementioned stressors. Relief from anxiety and depression is sought through parasuicidal behavior, including self-mutilation, drug and alcohol intoxication and poisoning, gravely dangerous acts such as driving with eyes closed or driving recklessly or while intoxicated, and unprotected, promiscuous sexual behaviors. Under these conditions, dramatic-impulsive patients' mental health status may suggest psychosis. Throughout such episodes, they are especially unstable and distressed.

To adequately respond to patients' crisis episodes, clinicians need to be flexible enough to move from a change-oriented mode of treatment into a supportive mode. However, clinical responsiveness must be calibrated to the type of crisis. We (Turner, Becker, & Delaoch, in press) have suggested that intervention intensity and intrusiveness vary on a continuum depending on the type of crisis. The ends of the continuum are defined by two classes of crisis: suicidal ideation and self-harm episodes. In the case of high levels of suicidal ideation, clinician's responses must be rapid and vigorous. Intervention for self-harm behavior entails viewing the problem in the context of the longer-term goals of the treatment plan and lessening therapist's activity.

Relapse Prevention

411

**Borderline,
Narcissistic, and
Histrionic
Personality
Disorders**

Currently, long-term supportive psychotherapy is the optimal solution for the problem of relapse with the dramatic-impulsive patients. Turner's concept of supportive cognitive therapy sessions following the intensive phase of treatment attempts to attend to this problem.

The supportive psychotherapy model has a long history in the psychoanalytic literature (Luborsky, 1984). Cognitive-behavioral practitioners, in contrast, have emphasized comprehensive short-term treatment plans and have not considered a long-term supportive cognitive-behavioral model. Whereas long-term supportive models have not been necessary for the Axis I disorders for which cognitive-behavioral therapy has been so effective, the severe developmental deficits evident among dramatic-impulsive patients argue for the provision of long-term care and relapse prevention. Long-term supportive cognitive-behavioral care involves providing patients with a therapeutic relationship in which the therapist acts as a coach and independent arbiter of reality. The therapist aids patients in applying the cognitive-behavioral lessons they learned during intensive treatment to current life problems in order to prevent relapse.

A common criticism of long-term supportive models of treatment, and mental health treatment in general, is that often mental disorders are not cured. However, in physical medicine there are certain disorders that are chronic and not amenable to cure. Rather, disorders such as diabetes and multiple sclerosis are treated and managed for patients' lifetimes. Unequivocally, however, the level of functioning and quality of life of patients with chronic disorders are markedly improved. It is our position that patients with mental disorders such as schizophrenia and many cases of dramatic-impulsive personality disorder will show an increased level of functioning and quality of life through the provision of supportive cognitive-behavioral therapy. We hope that future research validates this belief. For now, it is our best advice toward preventing relapses among dramatic-impulsive patients.

Case Illustration

Case Description

Cathy was first seen in the psychiatry emergency service. Rex, her boyfriend, brought her to the hospital because she had overdosed on alprazolam (Xanax) and alcohol. Rex reported that she had threatened to commit suicide earlier in the evening. The emergency room staff judged that Cathy had made a serious suicide attempt. They pumped her stomach and held her overnight for observation. The staff reported that Cathy and Rex were hostile toward each other. Cathy had consistently denied any suicidal ideation or intent, and she appeared stable after 8 hours of observation. The psychiatric emergency room nurse reported that he believed Cathy was depressed and while not imminently suicidal, was still at risk for another overdose. She was referred for outpatient care. Cathy was 17 and at the time living with her boyfriend.

Differential Diagnosis and Assessment

Following Cathy's initial presentation, during which she described her immediate problems, I conducted a formal analysis of her depressive symptoms. She acknowledged sleep disturbance, depressed mood, loss of interest in sex, loss of interest in activities, and feelings of worthlessness. She did not experience crying spells often, but described herself as constantly on the verge of tears. I then had Cathy take the Beck Depression Inventory to assess her level of depression. Cathy scored a 28, suggesting a moderate to high level of depression. She said that this was always the way she felt.

I then turned the interview toward assessing her suicide potential. In particular, I needed to learn where she was obtaining the Xanax and if she was already in treatment. She had wanted to get high, fall asleep, and avoid interacting with Rex that night. She had told Rex that she would kill herself that night if he did not leave her alone. Cathy said she was not serious in her threats and had wanted to frighten him. Further inquiry revealed that Cathy had threatened to harm herself often. In addition she scratched her wrist with the edge of bent aluminum foil about 15 times per week. When I questioned Cathy about her previous mental health care, she said that her mother had taken her to a therapist when she was 14 years old for nervousness and depression. Cathy had not wanted to go to therapy, but her mother had insisted. After 6 months of talking and getting nowhere, Cathy had quit treatment. Her mother and father then arranged for Cathy to see their family physician. The family doctor prescribed the Xanax. Cathy had been taking the medication for approximately two years.

Cathy's presentation warranted investigating the possibility that a personality disorder was present. I conducted the Personality Disorder Examination and SADS-L during the next three sessions. Cathy met seven criteria for BPD and seven criteria for HPD. She also met criteria for major depression. The evaluation suggested the depressive episode might be secondary to the personality disorder. The working diagnosis was histrionic and borderline personality disorder with a concurrent major depressive episode.

Treatment Selection, Course, and Problems in Carrying Out Interventions

Containment Phase.   Over the next 4 weeks, Cathy reported powerful suicidal ideation six times. This problem was managed by contracting for telephone contacts between sessions. Cathy called the therapist in the morning and evening to talk about her emotions and thoughts. In addition, the therapist instructed her to call whenever she felt she would act on her ideas. The therapeutic strategy was to challenge the distorted cognitions and propose alternative coping strategies. After this phase, Cathy's suicidal ideation slowed to once per week. This permitted the therapist to turn the therapy sessions toward the next stages of treatment.

Case Conceptualization.   During the following sessions, I had Cathy tell me of important events that had occurred between her and significant others in her life. These sessions were audiotaped. I then reviewed the portions of the tapes in which Cathy discussed her parents, Rex, and her brother. As I reviewed these interpersonal episodes, I scored them according to the procedure of the dynamic cognitive formulation that was based on Luborsky's (1984) psychodynamically oriented core conflictual relationship theme method. Cathy wanted to be loved, taken care of, and directed. She also had an opposing desire to be independent and respected. This set of conflictual needs reflected her psychological development stage. Cathy was attempting to individuate from her family, but she was doubtful of her ability to function as an independent adult.

Cathy was blocked in the growth process by tacit schemata that predicted that if she acted autonomously, her parents and her lover would rebuke and abandon her. The pattern of behavior control exercised in her family caused Cathy to form this schema. The schema Cathy learned was that to obtain love one must be compliant, feminine, and emotionally needy; being self-reliant and authentic leads to being reproached and abandoned. Yet she found herself aspiring to make her own life decisions and become self-reliant. However, taking control of her life frightened her because she was not completely sure of the direction she wanted to take. She retained a strong need for guidance. Consequently, she vacillated between submission and depression, on the one hand, and defiance and anger, on the other. The struggle produced severe anxiety. To cope with the anxiety, she often wished for life to return to the period of tranquility she associated with her childhood. To realize this feeling Cathy often abused alcohol and drugs, or pretended that everything was all right. Thus, Cathy had two types of reactions to these tacit schemata: anger, histrionic acting out, and self-harm, or histrionic resignation, submission, and depression. Because acting on her hostility and anger threatened her relationships, she often suppressed these reactions by abusing alcohol and drugs and acting seductively. However, she could also behave rebelliously.

The audiotapes were also evaluated to find out Cathy's self and significant-other schemata. This analysis revealed Cathy's expectations about significant others' actions toward her. These schemata begat many of her cognitive distortions. Cathy experienced herself as trapped in two omnibus roles in life. Sometimes she experienced herself as an "Angry, Incapable, and Unlovable Adult." When Cathy's significant others threatened to abandon her, Cathy's anxiety would increase. The elevated anxiety caused Cathy's self-perception to switch to the "Downtrodden but Capable and Lovable-Adorable Child." She was unable to consolidate her self-image because she interminably vacillated between these conflictual perceptions.

Optimal Treatment Selection. A guiding principle of DCBT is that to ensure that patients master the model, the knowledge is presented in the multiple encoding domains of the enactive, imaginal, and lexical categories. Repetition and overlearning are the key to comprehension. Consequently, the full range of cognitive and behavioral strategies was employed with Cathy. She showed significant deficits in self-monitoring, problem solving, identifying her needs, communication, and impulse control. Her schemata for self and significant others and her role relationship models were rigidly construed as the only possibilities for guiding her behavior. Behavioral, imaginal, and verbal techniques that could be used to target these domains were strategically applied. Because of the rigidity in her cognitive map of interpersonal relations, we used more evocative techniques in the hope of producing more change. This clinical perspective led to the selection of the treatment strategies listed below.

In addition, it was evident that she needed to learn about her psychological history and the dynamic triggers that led to her impulsive behavior. To accomplish these goals, both historical interpretations and here-and-now interpretations were used. In a break with traditional psychodynamic psychotherapy, however, Cathy's personality patterns were interpreted as learned patterns, not immutable traits. Given that they were learned patterns, they could be changed through self-observation, prompting, and cognitive restructuring.

Medication was not considered an optimal strategy for Cathy because of her drug and alcohol abuse history and her potential for suicide. In addition, since the assessment determined that her depression was secondary to her personality disorder and life circumstances, it was felt that psychosocial treatment was more appropriate than antidepressants.

Homework (particularly personal experimenting and practicing new modes of thinking, acting, and feeling), role play, self-monitoring, communication skill training, contracting, practicing problem-solving skills, and the emotional and behavioral experience of transference interpretations were used. The imaginal strategies used with Cathy included guided imagery and evocative imaginal exposure. Lexical strategies used included interpretation, confrontation, and questioning of common cognitive distortions. Much of the time in therapy was spent actively educating Cathy about her cognitive-dynamic structure, dysfunctional beliefs and cognitive distortions, and motivations and defensive styles. We also used a problem-solving approach to enable her to think through problems rather than act impulsively.

Treatment lasted for 53 sessions. There were two periods during treatment when Cathy threatened to stop and missed sessions for 3 weeks in a row. These alliance ruptures were worked through by focusing on her cognitions and emotions about feeling controlled and the potential for abandonment.

She successfully ceased taking the medication, although she went through a period of resistance to giving up alcohol and sedatives. This caused one break in the treatment protocol. After some initial resistance she began to do the homework assignments. To end her resistance to the homework, we reviewed the pros and cons of doing the homework, and we examined how her resistance was similar to some of her other patterns of behavior. Cathy eventually became adept at recognizing her implicit schemata about relationships and her cognitive distortions, and developing alternatives to them.

Assertiveness training plus five family sessions, conducted at home, focused on improving family communications enabled her to make her needs known to her parents. We examined her motivations for, and the pros and cons of, staying in the relationship with Rex. Six conjoint sessions were held with the two of them. Eventually, she broke off the relationship with Rex and moved back in with her parents for a month. Five months later, she obtained an apartment of her own. The following fall, she started her first year of college at a local university. She is progressing well and pursuing a degree in economics.

After breaking up with Rex, she contracted with the therapist to avoid romantical involvement with a man for the duration of treatment. This proved to be particularly painful for her, because, as she said, "I have to really do it on my own now." The negative emotions and desires to act impulsively with men were discussed and interpreted continually during this period of treatment. We worked together to increase her tolerance of these emotions through using evocative imagery, teaching her that emotions do not dictate behavior, experiential balancing, and using problem solving to prevent impulsive acting out.

Relapse Prevention. The last 3 months of therapy consisted of providing Cathy with a supportive cognitive therapy environment. In addition, she returned to supportive treatment for four brief intervals following the termination of formal treatment. Two occasions consisted of one visit only; the other two supportive periods consisted of five and eight sessions, respectively. In the supportive mode we focused

415

Borderline,
Narcissistic, and
Histrionic
Personality
Disorders

on helping her to cope with day-to-day problems and to practice problem-solving strategies for crises. The goal was to reduce Cathy's anxiety and help her solve the new problems facing her. Supportive cognitive-behavioral therapy accomplished these goals by providing Cathy with a comfortable environment and reinforcing her ability to problem solve. The therapist took a nondirective stance and acted as a sounding board for Cathy as she actively solved problems on her own. During the supportive phase, sessions were scheduled once every other week, and as needed.

A crisis that brought Cathy back to supportive treatment involved her parents. About a year after termination, her parents came close to divorcing. Although Cathy knew her parents both experienced discontent with their marriage, and that this had been going on for many years, she nonetheless felt depressed about the possibility of their divorce. She described her thinking about the possibility as feeling the ground was being removed from under her. Her concern and worry led her to actively try to intervene with them. Arguments, taking sides, and recriminations ensued. Because of the increasing hostility and her sense of loss of her family, she went on several drinking binges and sexual escapades. After 3 weeks of feeling more and more depressed and acting impulsively, she finally scrutinized her cognitive, behavioral, and emotional pattern and decided to get supportive help to put the brakes on it. During the five sessions she examined her thoughts about the meaning of her parents' divorcing. She felt she was being abandoned by her parents. At one level, she was amazed to discover that her concern was not with her parents' experience, but with her own. At another level, she worked through her automatic thoughts and beliefs and became confident that she would not disintegrate if they divorced, that their problems as a couple were not hers, and that is they divorced it did not mean that either one of them would abandon her. She decided that her best plan of action would be to provide both of her parents with support and care but not become involved with their decisions.

Problems in Carrying Out Treatment.   Despite a reasonably rapid course of treatment, there were many difficult moments in working with Cathy. Her reliance on drugs and alcohol for anxiety reduction and soothing proved to be the major obstacle to treatment. This was due not only to the problem of addiction itself, but because the substances markedly increased her impulsive acting out.

In retrospect, it was not a cognitive or behavioral technique that caused her to give up substance abuse. Numerous sessions were spent with Cathy discussing the pros and cons of her extensive drinking and sedative use. It was frustrating to Cathy and the therapist, because they both wanted to focus on her self-image and identity problems. However, as long as she continued to abuse substances, she would not be able to consolidate any learnings and she was vulnerable to episodes of losing control and suicidal ideation. In addition, Cathy refused to attend Alcoholics Anonymous meetings even though they would have provided a supplement to therapy. The event which caused her to discontinue substance use was deciding to lose weight and start an exercise program. She decided that drinking and drugs were causing her to gain weight.

There were also many times when Cathy directed her anger and rageful emotions toward the therapist. This was a common mode in which she interacted with others, not just the therapist. On several occasions early in treatment, she would respond to the therapist's spending time on the phone at night with her by disparaging his level of concern for her. Although therapists who work consistently with BPD patients know to expect this type of reaction, it does heighten the tension in the relationship.

Managing the tension and providing the resources to keep the therapeutic relationship at an active working level constitute a constant difficulty in working with dramatic-impulsive patients.

Another difficulty in Cathy's case was the emotional response of her parents toward Cathy. At times they were intrusive and overcontrolling; at other times they were rejecting and hostile. This vacillating pattern made it difficult to conduct the family sessions and make lasting improvements in family communication. Although Cathy's parents did provide her with the emotional space to develop her independence following the family sessions, occasionally the high level of expressed emotion in the family did resurface. When it did, Cathy lost ground, as was described in the relapse prevention section.

Outcome and Termination

During our final sessions, Cathy told me she felt changing her tacit distortions about her self-image was her most important accomplishment in treatment. She felt that obtaining a stable sense of identity and defining a meaning for her life was crucial to her improved sense of balance and control over her emotions. She described herself as no longer a slave to her emotions.

As we approached termination, Cathy expressed concern, stating that she did not know if she could cope independently. We focused on the relationship of this theme to the one that brought her into treatment. Her fear of leaving treatment and managing life on her own was similar to her previous need to depend on lovers for guidance. In addition, her tendency to avoid the anxiety of separation was made explicit to Cathy. These learnings aided Cathy in developing a cognitive structure that eased her leaving treatment. Additionally, the knowledge that she could return at any time for supportive counseling provided her with a sense of continuation of the therapeutic relationship that was extremely helpful to Cathy.

Summary

Dramatic-impulsive personality disorders are the most frequently encountered personality disorders in both outpatient and inpatient practice. Histrionic, narcissistic, and borderline patients also give clinicians some of their most difficult clinical challenges. Seldom do these patients see that what is required is change within them. They view others as the problem. This factor, coupled with their dramatic and impulsive style, constantly creates a tension during treatment unlike that experienced with any other type of patient.

Despite the extensive psychoanalytic literature on these disorders, it has only been during the last decade that a substantial empirical database has developed. Yet we still know little about the dramatic-impulsive cluster patients. Most of the work that has been done has centered on borderline personality disorder. As the 1990s progress, we will see increasing attention paid to the histrionic and narcissistic conditions.

Treatment outcome data currently suggest that there are potentially efficacious treatments for borderline personality disorder. Stone (1990) has made a convincing case for the utility of psychodynamically oriented psychotherapy in the inpatient setting. A powerful case for the efficacy of Linehan's DBT treatment model has been

417

Borderline,
Narcissistic, and
Histrionic
Personality
Disorders

made through a long-term randomized controlled clinical trial (Linehan et al. 1987, 1991). Work by Turner (1989, 1993) suggests that the DCBT treatment protocol may be effective in reducing self-harm behavior and other symptoms of BPD. However, these steps are only the beginning of efforts directed at deriving prescriptive treatment for dramatic-impulsive personality disorders.

ACKNOWLEDGMENT.   Support for the preparation of this chapter was provided by NIDA grant #1 P5O DA07697-01.

References

Adler, G. (1985). *Borderline psychopathology and its treatment*. New York: Jason Aronson.

Adler, G., & Buie, D. (1972), The misuse of confrontation with borderline patients. *International Journal of Psychoanalytic Psychotherapy, 1*, 109–120.

Adler, G., & Buie, D. (1979). Aloneness and borderline psychopathology: The possible relevance of child develop issues. *International Journal of Psychoanalysis, 60*, 83–96.

Akiskal, H. S. (1981). Subaffective disorders: Dysthymic, cyclothymic, and bipolar II disorders in the borderline realm. *Psychiatric Clinics of North America, 4*, 25–46.

Akiskal, H. S., Chen, S. E., Davis, G. C., Puzantian, V. R., Kashgarian, M., & Bolinger, J. M. (1985). Borderline: An adjective in search of a noun. *Journal of Clinical Psychiatry, 46*, 41–48.

American Psychiatric Association (1987). *Diagnostic and statistical manual of mental disorders* (3rd. ed., rev.). Washington, DC: Author.

American Psychiatric Association (1993). *DSM-IV-Draft Criteria*. Washington, DC: Author.

Andrulonis, P. A., Glueck, B. C., Stroebel, C. F., Vogel, N. G., Shapiro, A. L., & Aldridge, D. (1981). Organic brain dysfunction and the borderline syndrome. *Psychiatric Clinics of North America, 4*, 47–66.

Andrulonis, P. A., & Vogel, N. G. (1984). Comparison of borderline personality subcategories to schizophrenic and affective disorders. *British Journal of Psychiatry, 144*, 358–363.

Beck, A. T., Freeman, A., & Associates (1990). *Cognitive therapy of personality disorders*. New York: Guilford.

Bowlby, J. (1988). *A secure base*. New York: Basic Books.

Bradley, S. J. (1979). The relationship of early maternal separation to borderline personality in children and adolescents: A pilot study. *American Journal of Psychiatry, 136*, 424–426.

Bruner, J. S. (1964). The course of cognitive growth. *American Psychologist, 19*, 1–19.

Buie, D., & Adler, G. (1982). The definitive treatment of the borderline personality. *International Journal of Psychoanalytic Psychotherapy, 9*, 51–87.

Bux, D. A. (1992). Narcissistic personality disorder. In A. Freeman & F. M. Dattillio (Eds.), *Comprehensive casebook of cognitive therapy* (pp. 223–230). New York: Plenum.

Buysse, D. J., Nathan, R. S., & Soloff, P. H. (1990). Borderline personality disorder: Pharmacotherapy. In A. S. Bellack & M. Hersen (Eds.), *Handbook of comparative treatments for adult disorders* (pp. 436–458). New York: Wiley.

Davis, D. (1990). Narcissistic personality disorder. In A. T. Beck & A. Freeman (Eds.). *Cognitive therapy of personality disorders* (pp. 233–256). New York: Guilford.

Flemming, B. (1990). Histrionic personality disorder. In A. T. Beck & A. Freeman (Eds.) *Cognitive therapy of personality disorders* (pp. 208–232). New York: Guilford.

Freeman, A., & Leaf, R. C. (1989). Cognitive therapy applied to personality disorders. In A. Freeman, K. Simon, L. E. Beutler, & H. Arkowitz (Eds.), *Comprehensive handbook of cognitive therapy* (pp. 403–434). New York: Plenum.

Fruensgaard, K., & Flindt-Hansen, H. (1988). Disease patterns seen in self-mutilating patients. *Nordisk-Psykiatrisk-Tidsskrift, 42*, 281–288.

Goldberg, R. L., Mann, L. S., Wise, T. N., & Segall, E. A. (1985). Parental qualities as perceived by borderline personality disorders. *Hillside Journal of Clinical Psychiatry, 7*, 134–140.

Gunderson, J. (1984). *Borderline personality disorder*. Washington, DC: American Psychiatric Press.

Gunderson, J. G., & Phillips, K. A. (1991). A current view of the interface between borderline personality disorder and depression. *American Journal of Psychiatry, 148*, 967–975.

Gunderson, J. G., Zanarini, M. C., & Cassandra, L. K. (1991). Borderline personality disorder: A review of data on DSM-III-R descriptions. *Journal of Personality Disorders, 5*, 340–352.

Herman, J. L., Perry, J. D., & van der Kolk, B. A. (1989). Childhood trauma in borderline personality disorder. *American Journal of Psychiatry, 146,* 490–495.

Hirschfeld, R. M. A. (1993). Personality disorders: Definition and diagnosis. *Supplement to Journal of Personality Disorders: The NIMH Williamsburg Conference on Personality Disorders,* 7, 9–17.

Hurt, S. W., Clarkin, J. F., Munroe-Blum, H., & Marziali, E. (1992). Borderline behavioral clusters and different treatment approaches. In J. F. Clarkin, E. Marziali, & H. Munroe-Blum (Eds.), *Borderline personality disorder: Clinical and empirical perspectives.* New York: Guilford.

Institute of Medicine (1985). A report of the Board on Mental Health and Behavioral Medicine: Research on mental illness and addictive disorders: Progress and prospects. *American Journal of Psychiatry, 142,* 627–630.

Kernberg, O. (1975). *Borderline conditions and pathological narcissism.* New York: Jason Aronson.

Kernberg, O. (1982). Supportive psychotherapy with borderline conditions. In J. Cavenar & H. Brodie (Eds.), *Critical problems in psychiatry* (pp. 180–202). Philadelphia: Lippincott.

Kernberg, O. (1984). *Severe personality disorders: Psychotherapeutic strategies.* New Haven: Yale University Press.

Kiesler, C. A. (1993). Mental health policy and mental hospitalization. *Current Directions in Psychological Science, 2,* 93–95.

Kroll, J. L., Carey, K. S., & Sines, L. K. (1985). Twenty-five year follow-up of borderline personality disorder: A pilot study. In C. Shagass (Ed.), *Fourth world congress of biological psychiatry* (Vol. 7, pp. 577–579). Philadelphia: Elsevier.

Leighton, D. H. (1963). *The Stirling County study of psychiatric disorder and sociocultural environment.* New York: Basic Books.

Lewis, M. (1990). Models of developmental psychopathology. In M. Lewis & S. Miller (Eds.), *Handbook of developmental psychopathology* (pp. 15–28). New York: Plenum.

Linehan, M. M. (1987a). Dialectical behavior therapy: A cognitive-behavioral approach to parasuicide. *Journal of Personality Disorder, 1,* 328–333.

Linehan, M. M. (1987b). Dialectical behavior therapy for borderline personality disorder: Theory and method. *Bulletin of the Menninger Clinic, 51,* 261–276.

Linehan, M. M. (1987c). Dialectical behavior therapy in groups: Treating borderline personality disorders and suicidal behavior. In C. M. Brody (Ed.), *Women's therapy groups: Paradigms of feminist treatment.* New York: Springer.

Linehan, M. M., Armstrong, H. E., Suarez, A., & Allmon, D. J. (1987, November). *Comprehensive behavioral treatment for suicidal behaviors and borderline personality disorder.* Paper presented at the 21st meeting of the Association for Advancement of Behavior Therapy, Boston, MA.

Linehan, M. M., Armstrong, H. E., Suarez, A., Allmon, D. J., & Heard, H. L. (1991). Cognitive-behavioral treatment of chronically parasuicidal borderline patients. *Archives of General Psychiatry, 48,* 1060–1064.

Linehan, M. M., & Wasson, E. J. (1990). Borderline personality disorder: Behavior Therapy. In A. S. Bellack & M. Hersen (Eds.), *Handbook of comparative treatments for adult disorders* (pp. 420–462). New York: Wiley.

Linehan, M. M., Heard, H. L., & Armstrong, H. E. (1993). Naturalistic follow-up of a behavioral treatment for chronically parasuicidal borderline patients. *Archives of General Psychiatry, 50,* 971–974.

Loranger, A. (1988). *Personality disorder examination manual.* Yonkers, NY: DV Communications.

Loranger, A., Oldham, J., & Tulis, E. (1982). Familial transmission of DSM-III borderline personality disorder. *Archives of General Psychiatry, 39,* 795.

Loranger, A., Sussman, V. L., Oldham, J. M., & Russakoff, L. M. (1987). The Personality Disorder Examination (PDE): A preliminary report. *Journal of Personality Disorders, 1,* 1–13.

Luborsky, L. (1984). *Principles of psychoanalytic psychotherapy.* New York: Basic Books.

Luborsky, L. (1963). Clinicians' judgement of mental health. *Archives of General Psychiatry, 9,* 407–417.

Marmar, C. R. (1988). Personality disorders. In H. H. Goldman (Ed.), *Review of General Psychiatry* (pp. 401–424). Norwalk, CT: Appleton & Lange.

Marziali, E. (1992). The etiology of borderline personality disorders: Developmental factors. In J. F. Clarkin, E. Marziali, & H. Munroe-Blum (Eds.), *Borderline personality disorder: Clinical and empirical perspectives.* New York: Guilford.

McGlashen, T. H. (1985). The prediction of outcome in borderline personality disorder: Part V of the Chestnut Lodge follow-up study. In T. H. McGlashen (Ed.), *The borderline: Current empirical research* (pp. 63–98). Washington, DC: American Psychiatric Press.

419

Borderline,
Narcissistic, and
Histrionic
Personality
Disorders

Millon, T. (1981). *Disorders of personality: DSM-III: Axis-II*. New York: Wiley.

Nelson, K. (1993). The psychological and social origins of autobiographical memory. *Psychological Science, 4*, 7–14.

Nestadt, G., Romanoski, A. J., Chahal, R., & Merchant, A. (1990). An epidemiological study of histrionic personality disorder. *Psychological Medicine, 20*, 413–422.

Ogata, S. N., Silk, K. R., & Goodrich, S. (1990). Childhood experiences and borderline personality disorder. In P. Links (Ed.), *The family environment and borderline personality disorder*. Washington, DC: American Psychiatric Association.

Paris, J., Brown, R., & Nowlis, D. (1987). Long-term follow-up of borderline patients in a general hospital. *Comprehensive Psychiatry, 28*, 530–535.

Perry, J. C., & Vaillant, G. E. (1989). Personality disorders. In H. I. Kaplan & B. J. Sadock (Eds.), *Comprehensive textbook of psychiatry* (pp. 1352–1387). Baltimore: Williams & Wilkins.

Pfohl, B. (1989). *Structured Interview for DSM-III (R) personality disorders-Revised (SIDP-R)*. Iowa City: Department of Psychiatry, University of Iowa Hospitals and Clinics.

Pfohl, B., Stangl, D., & Zimmerman, M. (1982). *The Structured Interview for DSM-III personality disorders (SID-P)*. Iowa City: University of Iowa Hospitals and Clinics.

Plakun, E. M., Burkhardt, P. E., & Muller, J. P. (1985). Fourteen year follow-up of borderline and schizotypal personality disorders. *Comprehensive Psychiatry, 26*, 448–455.

Pope, H. G., Jonas, J. M., & Hudson, J. (1983). The validity of DSM-III borderline personality disorder. *Archives of General Psychiatry, 40*, 23–30.

Pretzer, J. (1990). Borderline personality disorder. In A. T. Beck & A. Freeman (Eds.), *Cognitive therapy of personality disorders* (pp. 176–207). New York: Guilford.

Safran, J. D., & Segal, Z. V. (1990). *Interpersonal processes in cognitive therapy*. New York: Basic Books.

Soloff, P. H., & Millward, J. W. (1983). Psychiatric disorders in the families of borderline patients. *Archives of General Psychiatry, 39*, 686–692.

Spitzer, R. L., & Endicott, J. E. (1979). *Schedule for Affective Disorders and Schizophrenia—Lifetime Version*. New York: Department of Research Assessment and Training, New York State Psychiatric Institute.

Spitzer, R. L., & Williams, J. B. W., Gibbon, M., & First, M. B. (1990). *SCID users guide for the structured clinical interview for DSM-III-R*. Washington, DC: American Psychiatric Association.

Stiver, I. (1988). Developmental psychopathology: Introducing a consultant in the treatment of borderline patients. *McLean Hospital Journal, 13*, 89–113.

Stone, M. H. (1990). *The fate of borderline patients*. New York: Guilford.

Stone, M. H., Unwin, A., Beachman, B., & Swenson, C. (1988). Incest in female borderlines: Its frequency and impact. *International Journal of Family Psychiatry, 9*, 277–293.

Turner, R. M. (1983). Behavioral therapy with borderline patients. *Carrier Foundation Journal, 88*, 1–4.

Turner, R. M. (1988). The cognitive-behavioral approach to the treatment of borderline personality disorders. *International Journal of Partial Hospitalization, 5*, 279–289.

Turner, R. M. (1989). Case study evaluation of a bio-cognitive-behavioral approach for the treatment of borderline personality disorder. *Behavior Therapy, 20*, 477–489.

Turner, R. M. (1992a). Borderline personality disorder. In A. Freeman & F. M. Dattilio (Eds.), *Comprehensive casebook of cognitive therapy* (pp. 215–222). New York: Plenum.

Turner, R. M. (1992b). Launching cognitive-behavioral therapy for adolescent depression and drug abuse. In S. H. Budman, M. F. Hoyt, & S. Friedman (Eds.), *The first session of brief therapy* (pp. 135–155). New York: Guilford.

Turner, R. M. (1992c, November). *An empirical investigation of the utility of psychodynamic techniques in the practice of cognitive behavior therapy*. Paper presented at the 26th Annual Meeting of the Association for the Advancement of Behavior Therapy, Boston, MA.

Turner, R. M. (1993). Dynamic-cognitive-behavior therapy. In T. Giles (Ed.), *Handbook of effective psychotherapy* (pp. 437–454). New York: Plenum.

Turner, R. M., Becker, L., & Delaoch, C. (in press). Clinical management of the borderline personality patient in crisis. In A. Freeman & F. Dattilio (Eds.), *Handbook of cognitive behavior therapy and crisis intervention*. New York: Plenum.

VandenBoss, G. R. (1993). U.S. mental health policy: Proactive evolution in the midst of health care reform. *American Psychologist, 48*, 283–290.

van der Kolk, B. A., Perry, J. C., & Herman, J. L. (1991). Childhood origins of self-destructive behavior. *American Journal of Psychiatry, 148*, 1665–1671.

Waldenger, R. J., & Frank, A. F. (1989). Clinicians' experiences in combining medication and psychotherapy in the treatment of borderline patients. *Hospital and Community Psychiatry, 40,* 712–718.

Wallerstein, R. (1986). *Forty-two lives in treatment.* New York: Guilford.

Weissman, M. M., & Meyers, J. K. (1980). Psychiatric disorders in a U.S. community. *Acta Psychiatrica Scandinavia, 62,* 69–111.

Zanarini, M. C., Frankenburg, F. R., & Gunderson, J. G. (1988). Pharmacotherapy of borderline outpatients. *Comprehensive Psychiatry, 29,* 372–378.

Zanarini, M. C., Gunderson, J. G., Marino, M. F., Schwartz, E. O., & Frankenburg, F. R. (1989). Childhood experiences of borderline patients. *Comprehensive Psychiatry, 30,* 18–25.

III

SPECIAL ISSUES

20

Psychophysiologic Disorders

Donald A. Williamson and Shannon B. Sebastian

Introduction

Psychophysiologic disorders are medical conditions that are influenced by psychological factors such as stress or behavioral habits (American Psychiatric Association, 1987). Earlier these disorders were referred to as psychosomatic disorders. Many medical conditions have been considered to be psychophysiologic disorders, including headaches, essential hypertension, insomnia, asthma, and various dermatologic and gastrointestinal disorders (Williamson, Barker, & Lapour, in press). Prescriptive treatments for these disorders have been advanced by research in behavioral medicine over the past 20 years. We have selected three psychophysiologic disorders for review in this chapter: headaches, irritable bowel syndrome, and cardiovascular disease. These three disorders were selected because prescriptive treatment interventions with a strong research base have been developed for all three.

Headache

Description of the Problem

Migraine Headache. It has been estimated that 16% of adults experience migraine headaches (Diamond & Dalessio, 1982). Migraine often begins as a dull ache that progressively worsens into throbbing or pulsating pain. About 70% of migraine headaches are unilateral and are located in the frontal, temporal, or occipital regions of the head. In severe cases, attacks may occur daily. In most cases, migraines occur once or twice per year with a duration of 4 to 48 hours. About 15% of migraine

Donald A. Williamson and **Shannon B. Sebastian** • Department of Psychology, Louisiana State University, Baton Rouge, Louisiana 70803.

Handbook of Prescriptive Treatments for Adults, edited by Michel Hersen and Robert T. Ammerman. Plenum Press, New York, 1994.

patients are diagnosed with "classic" migraine. Classic migraine is distinguished from common migraine by the experience of warning signs, or prodromal symptoms, that precede the headache. Common prodromes are visual disturbances (e.g., flashing lights, or blind spots in the visual field) and somatosensory disturbances (e.g., numbness or tingling in one arm or leg). During or before the attack, migraine sufferers may also experience nausea, vomiting, or sensitivity to bright lights and noises. In cases diagnosed as "common" migraine, headaches are not preceded by prodromal symptoms. Both classic and common migraines are believed to be caused by vasoconstriction. Vasoconstriction of intracranial arteries has been associated with prodromal symptoms, whereas vasodilation of extracranial arteries results in throbbing pain (Diamond & Dalessio, 1982).

Muscle Contraction Headache. Muscle contraction, or tension, headache is characterized by a dull, steady, bilateral ache located in the muscles of the forehead, scalp, or neck. Muscle contraction headache is presumed to develop slowly in response to stress and results from chronic muscle contraction of the head, neck, shoulders, or face. Prodromal symptoms, sensitivity to bright lights, and nausea (all symptoms of migraine headache) generally do not occur with muscle contraction headache (Williamson et al., in press). Approximately 70% of adults have suffered at least one muscle contraction headache (Olesen, 1978).

Combined Headache. Patients may be diagnosed as experiencing combined, or mixed, headache. In these cases, both migraine and muscle contraction headaches occur in the same patient. Symptoms from the two types of headache may co-occur, or the patient may suffer from migraine and muscle contraction headaches on separate occasions (Blanchard & Andrasik, 1985).

Assessment Strategies

The first step in diagnosis of headache involves interviewing the patient in order to identify intensity, duration, frequency, and disability associated with headache. Patient report of the pattern of headache occurrence over a distinct period offers information about frequency of headache and common antecedents or consequences of headaches. The diagnostic interview delineates symptom clusters in order to identify headache type (Williamson et al., in press). Individual and family history of previous treatments for headache and other medical problems should be considered. Blanchard and Andrasik (1985) have developed a structured interview for assessment of headache, which has been found to concur reliably with diagnosis by an independent evaluation by a neurologist.

Following the initial diagnostic interview, it is often necessary to refer the patient for examination by a physician. The medical examination typically investigates possible physiologic causes of headache, such as subdural hematomas, recent spinal tap, low spinal fluid pressure, seizure activity, aneurysm, and angina.

For comprehensive headache assessment, it is suggested that headache questionnaires as well as self-monitoring data instruments be completed by the patient. Two headache questionnaires have been developed (Arena, Blanchard, Andrasik, & Dudek, 1982; Williamson, Ruggiero, & Davis, 1985). Self-monitoring, such as keeping a daily diary of headache antecedents, duration, intensity, frequency, and consequences, assists patients in accurate recall of headache episodes and can be used as an outcome measure to evaluate the effectiveness of treatment (Williamson et al., 1985).

Evidence for Prescriptive Treatments

Relaxation and Biofeedback Training. Although various forms of relaxation training have been employed in the treatment of migraine and muscle contraction headaches, progressive muscle relaxation has become the relaxation technique of choice. Various manuals offer step-by-step instructions for learning progressive muscle relaxation (e.g., Bernstein & Borkovec, 1973). Training includes systematically tensing and relaxing each of the major muscle groups of the body.

Biofeedback has also been found to be effective for reducing the pain associated with migraine and muscle contraction headaches. Through practice in biofeedback, headache patients learn to control skin temperature and reduce electromyographic (EMG) activity in the muscles of the forehead or frontal region of the head. Skin temperature biofeedback training has been found to be associated with improvement of migraine. Skin temperature biofeedback has been used to produce increased blood flow to the hand and generalized relaxation. Training in temperature biofeedback usually consists of at least 4 to 5 weeks of intensive training, home practice, and supplementary monthly follow-up visits. EMG biofeedback to reduce muscle tension of the frontal region of the head has been found to be an effective treatment for tension headache (Diamond & Dalessio, 1982).

In recent years, headache researchers have tested the effectiveness of more cost-effective means for training headache patients to relax or use biofeedback. Home-based relaxation and biofeedback programs have been evaluated most thoroughly (Blanchard, 1992). Most home-based treatment programs use audiotapes and treatment manuals to guide home training. When biofeedback training is prescribed, subjects receive portable biofeedback systems for home practice. Most of the home-based treatment programs that have been reported in the scientific literature require headache patients to attend three to five clinic sessions.

Biofeedback and progressive muscle relaxation training have been the focus of many empirical investigations of headache treatment and are now well accepted by health care providers who specialize in headache treatment (Blanchard, 1992). There is no strong evidence that biofeedback is more or less effective than relaxation training for the treatment of migraine or muscle contraction headaches (Andrasik & Blanchard, 1987). Although biofeedback alone may not be necessary, it often improves treatment outcome when combined with relaxation training (Blanchard, 1992).

Cognitive Therapy. Cognitive therapy has also been found effective for reduction of headaches. This approach emphasizes that affective and behavioral responses are a direct function of maladaptive cognitions. Headache results from psychological stress, which is dictated by an individual's thoughts. Patients are taught to monitor thoughts and feelings associated with stressful situations and are encouraged to attribute headache to internal processes rather than to external causes.

Treatment outcome studies suggest that cognitive therapy may be useful for treating tension headache, but this technique has not been found to be particularly effective for treating migraines. For example, cognitive therapy has been found to result in greater reduction in headache frequency than EMG biofeedback or self-monitoring at posttreatment and at 2-year follow-up in a study of tension headache (Holroyd & Andrasik, 1982; Holroyd, Andrasik, & Westbrook, 1977). However, several comparisons of cognitive therapy with biofeedback, relaxation training, or both have failed to find cognitive therapy to be more effective for treating migraine headache (Blanchard, 1992).

A recent placebo-controlled study of tension headache found that both treatments used were superior to a credible placebo condition and that cognitive therapy combined with relaxation yielded significantly more headache relief than relaxation alone (Blanchard, Appelbaum, Radnitz, Michultka, et al., 1990). A similar investigation of migraine headache failed to find an advantage for a combination of biofeedback and cognitive therapy over biofeedback alone (Blanchard, Appelbaum, Radnitz, Morrill, et al., 1990).

Pharmacotherapy. Pharmacotherapy is the most frequently used method of headache management and may be either abortive or prophylactic. Ergotamine tartrate (a vasoconstrictor agent) is a commonly used abortive pharmacologic agent for migraine attacks. To be effective, ergotamine must be administered during prodromes or soon after headache onset. Clonidine (an antihypertensive drug), flunarizine (a calcium antagonist), and propranolol (a beta-blocking agent) have been used as drugs for prevention of migraine. Antidepressant drugs have been successful in the prophylaxis of migraine and muscle contraction headaches. Amitriptyline hydrochloride (Elavil), imipramine hydrochloride (Tofranil), and desipramine hydrochloride (Pertofrane or Norpramin) have all been found to be effective in reducing headaches (Diamond & Dalessio, 1982).

Several studies have compared psychological and pharmacologic headache treatment outcome studies. Mathew (1981) compared biofeedback, relaxation, amitriptyline, and propranolol as treatments for migraine headache. He found the propranolol treatment to be more effective than biofeedback or relaxation. Amitriptyline was not significantly more effective than biofeedback, however. Biofeedback and relaxation combined with propranolol did not differ in effect from propranolol alone. A combination of biofeedback and relaxation has also been compared to ergotamine tartrate in migraine and combined headache patients (Holroyd et al., 1988). This study found no difference between conditions at posttreatment or at 4-month follow-up. In a second study, amitriptyline was compared to cognitive stress coping plus relaxation (Holroyd, Nash, Pingel, Cordingley, & Jerome, 1991). The cognitive treatment was found to be more effective than amitriptyline for reducing migraine headache symptoms. In summary, published research suggests that pharmacologic interventions produce improvements in migraine and tension headache, with success rates ranging from 40 to 60% (Blanchard, 1992). Evidence for the efficacy of propranolol for migraine and amitriptyline for tension headache is quite strong. Nonpharmacologic treatments for headache have generally been found to be more or less equivalent in efficacy to pharmacologic interventions (Blanchard, 1992).

Selecting Optimal Intervention Strategies. Figure 20.1 illustrates the decision-making process for selecting an optimal treatment plan for headache patients. The first step is diagnosis. If the patient is diagnosed as having migraine or combined headache, a medication trial (e.g., propranolol, clonidine, or ergotamine tartrate) should be prescribed as a first step. These medications have been found to be effective in many cases and are relatively easy to administer. Most headache patients referred to nonphysicians will have already attempted medication without success. If pharmacotherapy is unsuccessful or side effects are too severe, the second step should be a trial of home-based relaxation for 6 to 10 weeks. If this relatively low intensity intervention is unsuccessful, we recommend a trial of clinic-based skin temperature biofeedback with home practice for 6 to 10 weeks. If this intervention is unsuccessful, referral to a specialized pain clinic is probably warranted as a last alternative for treatment-resistant cases.

For cases diagnosed as muscle contraction headache, a similar decision-making process is recommended (see Figure 20.1). A medication trial (e.g., analgesics or antidepressants)is recommended as a first step. If pharmacotherapy is unsuccessful, home-based relaxation should be prescribed for 6 to 10 weeks. If home-based relaxation is unsuccessful, a trial of clinic-based EMG biofeedback is warranted. If success is not achieved after 6 to 10 weeks of biofeedback training, a program of cognitive therapy should be added. Cognitive therapy should emphasize coping with stress and emotion as a primary goal (Holroyd & Andrasik, 1982). In the rare

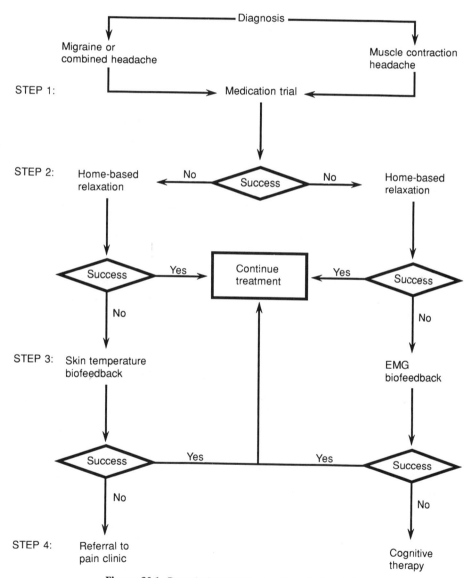

Figure 20.1. Prescriptive treatment options for headache.

individuals who do not respond positively to these first four steps, a referral to a pain clinic should be made or the diagnosis should be reconsidered (e.g., another psychiatric diagnosis may be more appropriate).

Problems in Carrying Out Interventions. Blanchard (1992) has noted three types of headache patients who often show a poor response to the types of treatment interventions mapped in Figure 20.1. These refractory subgroups are those with geriatric headache, high medication consumption headache, and chronic daily high-intensity headache. Headache patients more than 60 years of age have been found to respond better when a variety of psychological interventions are used over a longer treatment period (Blanchard, 1992). Headache patients who consume large amounts of analgesic medications often experience rebound headaches when medications are abruptly withdrawn. A more gradual withdrawal of medication combined with psychological treatment may be required for such patients. Chronic daily headache patients may require more extensive psychological therapy, as illustrated in the case history at the end of this chapter.

Failure to comply with home-based practice assignments may limit treatment effectiveness. Patients should become active participants in treatment in order to promote symptomatic improvement. The importance of home practice of relaxation for long-term management of headache is somewhat unclear. Current data suggest that regular home practice of relaxation may be more important for successful treatment of tension headache than for migraine.

The therapist must be attentive to possible analgesic medication abuse while emphasizing lifestyle changes as a means of headache reduction. Subjects who use excessive amounts of opiate medications are especially vulnerable to addiction.

Relapse Prevention. A combination of headache treatment strategies may assist in relapse prevention. Patients who participate in more than one type of treatment report greater and more rapid headache relief (Blanchard, Appelbaum, Radnitz, Michultka, et al., 1990). For example, effectiveness of progressive muscle relaxation may be enhanced by the addition of cognitive therapy and biofeedback training.

The majority of treatment regimens emphasize regular home practice of relaxation in the natural environment in order to promote generalization of treatment effects. In addition, home-based practice of a broad range of headache reduction strategies lowers relapse potential and improves cost effectiveness (Blanchard et al., 1991). In general, if patients report relapse, it is imperative that they return to the treatment program that was effective previously.

Irritable Bowel Syndrome

Description of the Problem

Irritable bowel syndrome (IBS) is characterized by abdominal pain and disturbed intestinal motility (constipation, diarrhea, or both) for which no organic cause can be identified. Concomitant symptoms may include decreased food consumption, nausea, headache, weakness, and insomnia. Irritable bowel syndrome sufferers often experience visible distention of the stomach, relief of abdominal pain by a bowel movement, more frequent bowel movements, looser stools with the onset of pain, mucus in the stool, and a sensation of incomplete evacuation (Whitehead & Schuster, 1985).

Irritable bowel syndrome afflicts between 8 and 17% of the adult population (Radnitz & Blanchard, 1988). A majority of IBS sufferers are women between the ages of 30 and 40 years who typically present for nonpharmacologic prescriptive treatment after suffering from gastrointestinal distress for at least 5 years (Ford, 1986). Irritable bowel syndrome is usually considered a functional disorder, with more than 50% of IBS sufferers reporting worsening of abdominal pain with increases in environmental stressors. Psychological factors, including anxiety, depression, and psychosomatic concerns, have been associated with onset and maintenance of IBS. Irritable bowel syndrome patients are often described as compulsive, overconscientious, dependent, sensitive, guilty,and unassertive, although patients who consult doctors for treatment of IBS may be most psychologically distressed (Whitehead, 1992). Current research suggests that IBS patients may be highly sensitive to painful sensations from the viscera (Whitehead, 1992).

Assessment Strategies

A multidimensional framework has been found useful in assessing IBS. The impact of physiologic, emotional, cognitive, and behavioral components on etiology and maintenance of IBS should be considered. Initially, the patient should be interviewed for symptom severity and frequency. The interview serves to evaluate dietary habits, neurotic personality characteristics, dysfunctional beliefs related to IBS, and recent behavioral changes. Secondary gain, such as attention from family members or avoidance of unpleasant activities, should also be investigated (Williamson et al., in press).

Medical evaluation is necessary to assess medication side effects as well as physiologic abnormalities, such as distal colon hyperreactivity. Physiologic symptoms must be differentiated from gastrointestinal disease, ulcer, inflammatory bowel disease, esophageal motility disorders, medication side effects, and lactose or food intolerance. Further physiologic testing may be indicated if family history of gastrointestinal difficulties implies biological disposition to related problems. It is recommended that medical records be requested from prior evaluations in order to verify validity of patient report.

Self-report questionnaires and self-monitoring can assist in assessment of IBS by alleviating embarrassment experienced by some patients during interview inquiries. Self-report questionnaires evaluate emotional disturbance as well as symptom onset, frequency, and severity. Irritable bowel syndrome symptom diaries are important in performing a thorough functional analysis (evaluation of antecedents and consequences associated with IBS symptom reports). Symptom diaries assist in gathering information concerning a patient's bowel movement schedule, pain severity, and dietary intake over a period of 1 to 6 weeks. Environmental events and mood fluctuations can also be monitored as potential antecedents for an IBS episode (Williamson et al., in press).

Intervention Strategies

Evidence for Prescriptive Treatments
Relaxation and Biofeedback Training. The symptoms of IBS may become conditioned so that episodes of IBS are triggered by specific situations. Systematic

desensitization attempts to modify the gastrointestinal response to events associated with IBS attacks. The patient is initially guided through relaxation exercises by the therapist. Once skilled at relaxation, the patient is instructed to remain relaxed while imagining a situation that often elicits IBS symptoms. The goal of treatment is for the patient to enter the identified situation, become relaxed, and remain free of IBS symptoms.

Biofeedback of colon motility teaches IBS sufferers to directly control motility of the bowel. Bowel sound biofeedback involves placement of an electronic stethoscope on the abdomen of the patient in order to provide feedback on bowel sounds (Furman, 1973). With practice, patients learn to decrease their bowel sounds, which results in symptomatic improvement. Pressure biofeedback involves insertion of a balloon-tipped tube into the colon to provide pressure measurements. Significant decreases in motility may be experienced as quickly as in 2 to 5 hours.

Empirical evidence in support of bowel sound and pressure biofeedback in the treatment of IBS is lacking. Early reports of the effectiveness of this treatment technique (e.g., Bueno-Miranda, Cerulli, & Schuster, 1976; Furman, 1973) have not been replicated. In addition, Radnitz and Blanchard (1988) found a variable degree of treatment success investigating bowel sound biofeedback using a multiple baseline design across subjects. Whitehead (1985) compared pressure biofeedback, systematic desensitization, and stress management in the treatment of IBS. Findings suggested that stress management was more effective than pressure biofeedback or systematic desensitization. Based on these negative findings, biofeedback training may be contraindicated in the treatment of IBS (Whitehead, 1992).

Stress Management Training. Stress management training is based on the assumption that IBS is triggered by environmental stressors. Arousal reduction training and self-control training are the most commonly employed stress management strategies. Arousal reduction training instructs the patient in relaxation methods (e.g., progressive muscle relaxation) to reduce sympathetic arousal. It is assumed that cognitive control of physiologic arousal will result in decreased abdominal distress when environmental stressors are encountered. Arousal reduction training is usually combined with self-control training, which promotes physiologic arousal recognition.

Evidence in support of the role of emotional factors in the exacerbation of IBS symptoms has led to the implementation of behavioral intervention strategies. Stress management training is the most often investigated and best validated of the behavioral treatment approaches for IBS. However, the research evidence consists mostly of uncontrolled single case descriptions without evidence of long-term treatment effectiveness of stress management training (Whitehead & Schuster, 1985).

Cognitive-Behavioral Therapy. Cognitive-behavioral treatment is individualized according to the hypothesized factors in the development and maintenance of IBS for a particular patient. For example, a patient who suffers from social anxiety may receive social skills training, whereas, a patient with negative thoughts and a sense of hopelessness may require cognitive restructuring. Cognitive-behavioral therapy attempts to distract IBS patients from their symptoms by suggesting behavioral homework assignments. These assignments serve to increase interpersonal contact and reinforcement for healthy behavior. Patients are also reinforced for symptom reduction, and expectations for improvement are emphasized (Whitehead & Schuster, 1985).

The efficacy of multicomponent cognitive-behavioral therapy has been investigated by Blanchard et al. (1992). They have developed a program that includes education about psychological stress, progressive muscle relaxation, biofeedback, skin temperature biofeedback, and cognitive skills training. A recent placebo-controlled investigation of this multicomponent treatment program found that the placebo group improved to the same degree as the active treatment group. Thus, it is possible that expectancy effects may contribute substantially to treatment outcome (Whitehead, 1992).

Pharmacotherapy. Medical treatment of IBS has included dietary modification and pharmacotherapy. The most common medical treatment (Ritchie & Truelove, 1980) includes antidepressant/anxiolytic medication, smooth muscle relaxants, and bulking agents. Bennett and Wilkinson (1985) compared the effectiveness of this standard pharmacotherapy regimen to stress management training. Results indicated that stress management raining, as opposed to pharmacotherapy, decreased both IBS and anxiety symptoms. The authors recommended cognitive therapy as the treatment of choice for IBS, but suggested that psychological intervention should be employed in combination with pharmacotherapy in severe cases.

Selecting Optimal Intervention Strategies. No universally accepted treatment has been found for IBS. Psychological treatment for IBS patients is often the modality of choice, because a majority of medical patients with IBS have significant psychological problems (Whitehead, Enck, Anthony, & Schuster, 1989).

As shown in Figure 20.2, dietary modification is the first step in the treatment of IBS. If IBS symptoms continue following the addition of fiber supplements, a drug trial (e.g., anxiolytic medication) is recommended. Adding systematic desensitization and relaxation training often enhances effectiveness. If IBS symptoms are not alleviated by clinical treatment, cognitive-behavioral therapy may be indicated, because somatization disorder, depression, and anxiety are often concomitant problems in IBS patients (Whitehead, 1992).

Problems in Carrying Out Interventions. When treatment progress is impaired by noncompliance, the possibility of secondary gain for IBS symptomatology must be considered. Patients may sabotage treatment outcome if symptoms are reinforced by sympathy from significant others or result in the opportunity to avoid aversive activities. In such cases, instruction in the use of distraction techniques may decrease thoughts related to IBS as well as curtail discussion of symptoms with others (Whitehead & Schuster, 1985). If distraction techniques are ineffective, it may be necessary to involve significant others in treatment.

In the interest of cost effectiveness, researchers have adapted individual multicomponent treatment of IBS to a group format (Blanchard & Schwarz, 1987). In general, group therapy for IBS is as effective as individual treatment. However, some patients may find the group format difficult or embarrassing and, subsequently, withdraw from treatment. Also, a group format may hinder the effectiveness of cognitive treatment because individual attention is reduced.

Relapse Prevention. Irritable bowel syndrome is a chronic problem that can persist throughout adulthood with fluctuations in symptom severity. Approximately two-thirds of IBS sufferers report symptom remission within 2 months without medical or psychological treatment. However, a majority of these patients experience relapses.

Patients who participate in treatment also frequently relapse. Therefore, clinicians must choose interventions that patients are most likely to continue practicing after treatment termination. The research literature suggests that progressive muscle relaxation and stress management training not only are preferred by patients, but also are most readily incorporated into the patient's lifestyle.

Successful treatment of IBS not only consists of rapid symptomatic improvement, but also results in reductions in concomitant depression, anxiety, and psychosomatic complaints (Blanchard, Radnitz, Schwarz, Neff, & Gerardi, 1987). If treatment fails to address these emotional components of IBS, the possibility of relapse is enhanced.

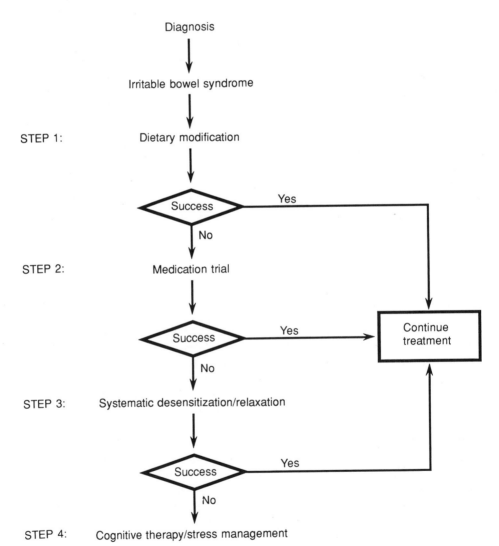

Figure 20.2. Prescriptive treatment options for irritable bowel syndrome.

Description of the Problem

Prescriptive treatments for cardiovascular disease have focused on the development of nonpharmacologic therapies to modify coronary risk factors (e.g., hypertension, obesity, smoking, inactivity, and Type A behavior pattern). Cardiovascular disease refers to diseases affecting the heart or vascular system. Hypertension, or elevated blood pressure, has been established as a primary risk factor for increased morbidity and mortality. Hypertension affects 15 to 24% of the United States population (Polefrone, Manuck, Larkin, & Francis, 1987). Coronary heart disease and stroke are generally caused by atherosclerosis (or fatty lesions of the inner lining of coronary arteries). Hypertension and atherosclerosis are "silent" medical disorders in that they produce no significant symptoms for many years. Often, a thrombosis (blood clot) eventually develops, resulting in obstruction (embolism) of the artery. Complete obstruction of an artery can cause an infarction (death of tissue), which is experienced as a heart attack or stroke. Most cases (90 to 95%) of hypertension are of unknown cause and are diagnosed as "essential hypertension." Recent research has shown that most cardiovascular disease results from various lifestyle and medical variables that have been referred to as cardiovascular risk factors. Lifestyle behaviors that significantly increase the risk of heart attacks and strokes are cigarette smoking, Type A behavior pattern, sedentary behavior, overeating, and consuming excessive amounts of dietary fat. Medical factors that increase the risk of infarction are obesity, hypertension, and insulin resistance. Recent biomedical research has identified a possible link between obesity, insulin resistance, and cardiovascular disease. This research has found that obesity, non-insulin-dependent diabetes, hypertension, atherosclerosis, dyslipidemia, and hyperinsulinemia may be symptomatic of a single metabolic syndrome. The underlying cause of this syndrome may be insulin resistance (DeFronzo & Ferrannini, 1991; Reaven, 1988). Thus, interventions that reduce insulin resistance (e.g., certain drugs, weight loss programs, or exercise programs) may be useful in modifying multiple cardiovascular risk factors.

Assessment Strategies

Assessment of hypertension requires measurement of blood pressure. The most common method for measuring blood pressure uses an inflatable cuff, a sphygmomanometer, and a stethoscope to determine the highest (systolic) and lowest (diastolic) blood pressures. Normal blood pressure is 120 mm of mercury (Hg) for systolic and 80 mmHg for diastolic. Hypertension is generally defined as systolic blood pressure above 160 mmHg, diastolic pressure above 95 mmHg, or both.

There is considerable controversy concerning the methods for assessing Type A behavior pattern (Thoresen & Powell, 1992). The most widely accepted method is the structured interview developed by Friedman and Rosenman (1974). The most widely used self-report inventory is the Jenkins Activity Survey (Jenkins, Zyzanski, & Rosenman, 1979).

Obesity, eating behavior, nutrition, and activity are very much interrelated. Obesity is defined as excessive adiposity or fat tissue. The best measures of obesity involve estimation of body fat, which requires special skills and equipment (Henningfield & Obarzanek, 1992). Definitions of obesity that are based on body weight include percent overweight from actuarial tables of normal weight and the body mass index (weight/height^2). Eating behavior, nutrition, and activity are typically assessed via self-report, either by interview or by self-monitoring. It is very likely that obese subjects tend to underestimate their eating (Brownell & Wadden, 1992), which has led some to question the validity of self-report methods in obesity research and treatment.

Cigarette smoking is typically assessed via interviews, self-monitoring, or biochemical assays for the metabolites of nicotine or other biological indicators of smoking. Measurement of cotinine is probably the best measure, unless nicotine replacement therapies are used; then carbon monoxide is a better choice (Lichtenstein & Glasgow, 1992).

Intervention Strategies

Evidence for Prescriptive Treatments

Pharmacological Approaches.   The standard pharmacological treatment regimen for essential hypertension is called the stepped-care approach (Hutchins, 1981). The first step for reducing blood pressure is prescription of a diuretic for reduction of fluid. If blood pressure is not thereby normalized, the second step is to prescribe either an alpha- or beta-blocker or a centrally acting agent (e.g., clonidine). These drugs reduce sympathetic activity, cardiac output, and peripheral vascular resistance (Ganguly, 1977). If blood pressure remains elevated, the third step is to use a more potent vasodilator. A fourth step, which is used in only the most resistant cases, is prescription of a drug for inhibiting the release of norepinephrine. The stepped-care approach for treating essential hypertension is very effective in most cases. There are, however, many side effects of these medications, including sexual dysfunction, depression, and postural hypotension. Because of these side effects, it is desirable to use nonpharmacological interventions that result in normalization of blood pressure with the lowest dosages and fewest types of antihypertensive medications.

Biofeedback/Relaxation Training.   Reduction of sympathetic arousal via relaxation or biofeedback training has been evaluated as a treatment for essential hypertension. Controlled research studies have found that these strategies lower blood pressure by 5 to 20 mmHg systolic and 3 to 15 mmHg diastolic. This line of research began in the early 1970s with attempts to treat hypertension via direct blood pressure biofeedback (Blanchard, 1990). After this approach resulted in only limited success, researchers turned to various relaxation approaches, ranging from progressive muscle relaxation to autogenic training and meditation. More recently, skin temperature biofeedback has been added to relaxation training, resulting in some improvement in outcome (Blanchard, 1990). These studies have also shown that relaxation strategies, in addition to lowering blood pressure, allow antihypertensive medications to be lowered in dosage or discontinued without an increase in blood pressure (Hatch et al., 1985). Given such findings, we believe that relaxation and biofeedback approaches are best regarded as adjunctive therapies for traditional pharmacotherapy strategies (Williamson & Waggoner, 1988).

Weight Reduction Strategies.   As noted earlier, there is a growing consensus that insulin resistance, which is highly associated with obesity, may be a primary determinant of hypertension and atherosclerosis (Reaven, 1988). Based on this formulation, weight loss strategies that reduce insulin resistance may become a very important intervention in a multicomponent treatment approach for cardiovascular disease. Behavioral approaches to modifying eating and exercise habits have yielded short-term success (Brownell & Wadden, 1992). Recent studies (Guy-Grand, 1992; Weintraub, 1992) have found that long-term use of new appetite suppressant medications (e.g., fenfluramine, phentermine, and fluoxetine) may enhance the weight loss and weight maintenance effects of behavior therapy. For example, Weintraub (1992) found that behavior therapy combined with fenfluramine and phentermine yielded weight losses of about 17 kg, which were maintained for up to 4 years if the medication regimen was continued.

Very low calorie diets in combination with behavior therapy have yielded average weight losses of 15 to 20 kg (Wadden & Van Itallie, 1992), but problems with long-term weight maintenance have recently been reported (Wadden, Stunkard, & Liebschutz, 1988). Promotion of low-fat diets and exercise enhancement may be especially important for achieving long-term success in weight management (Brownell & Wadden, 1992). Also, modification of binge eating via pharmacological (Marcus et al., 1990) and behavioral (Marcus, Wing, & Hopkins, 1988) interventions may be especially important for a substantial subset of obese patients.

Based on these considerations, Brownell and Wadden (1991, 1992) have proposed a stepped-care approach for treating obesity. Depending on the patient's initial weight status and presence or absence of complicating factors (e.g., depression, binge eating, metabolic complications), the patient may be prescribed treatment programs ranging from self-help to surgery. If a less intensive intervention is unsuccessful, then the next most intensive intervention is prescribed. Inclusion of weight strategies in multicomponent treatment programs for cardiovascular disease can be valuable, as evident by the substantial reduction in blood pressure associated with weight loss (Hovell, 1982).

Type A Behavior Pattern. Treatment of Type A behavior pattern (TABP) has focused primarily on cognitive-behavioral therapy approaches. The targets of these treatment programs include reducing hostility, improving interpersonal relationships, and coping with stress. Recent controlled outcome studies have validated the efficacy of cognitive-behavioral therapy for TABP, finding improvement in cardiovascular health, reduction of coronary recurrences, and reduction of mortality over long-term follow-up (Thoresen & Powell, 1992).

Cigarette Smoking. For smokers diagnosed with a cardiovascular illness, it is best to provide a clinic-based outpatient program to assist them in smoking cessation (Lichtenstein & Glasgow, 1992). For persons without cardiovascular illness, self-help and brief, low-cost interventions are probably the most reasonable prescriptions, because most people want to "quit on their own" (Gallup, 1974).

Clinical interventions generally combine cognitive-behavioral therapy, release prevention strategies, and nicotine replacement therapy. Nicotine replacement therapies have developed from nicotine gum to nicotine patches in recent years because of the better administration of nicotine via transdermal patches. The combination of these approaches allows gradual withdrawal from nicotine and the acquisition of alternate habits to replace cigarette smoking. Outcome research shows an average quit rate of about 20 to 40% over 1 year when these approaches are used (Lichtenstein & Glasgow, 1992). Treatment research has suggested that it is best to think of smoking cessation as a process whereby the person begins by contemplating change, then tries to quit smoking, and then maintains abstinence for a considerable period of time (DiClemente et al., 1991). Many smokers must go through this process several times before finally quitting smoking. It is important for health care providers to keep this concept in mind when helping a patient deal with relapse.

Exercise. Patients diagnosed with cardiovascular illness are often very sedentary. Programs to enhance exercise habits (e.g., walking, jogging, tennis) have been found to reduce mortality by 20% (Dubbert, 1992) when combined with a multicomponent treatment such as we have described. Exercise programs have also been found to be effective for prevention of coronary heart disease and reduction of risk factors (Blair et al., 1989). Adherence to exercise programs is often problematic, with about 50% attrition reported after one year in most studies (Dubbert, 1992).

Selecting Optimal Intervention Strategies. Figure 20.3 illustrates a decision chart for selecting the best treatment strategy for a specific patient. The first step is to identify cardiovascular risk factors that are treatable and relevant to the case. We have reviewed prescriptive treatment strategies for five risk factors: essential hypertension, obesity, TABP, cigarette smoking, and sedentary lifestyle. The next step is

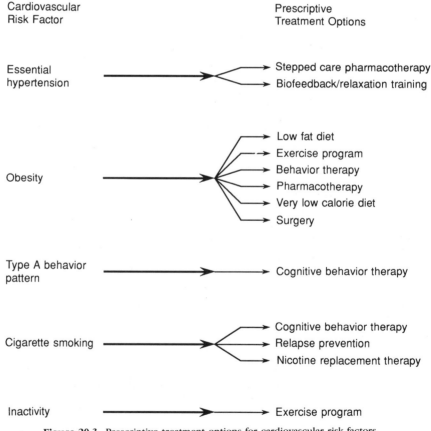

Figure 20.3. Prescriptive treatment options for cardiovascular risk factors.

to set a priority for each risk factor based on the probability that it is a contributor to this patient's cardiovascular illness. The healthcare provider then prescribes one or more of the treatment strategies for each risk factor. For risk factors that have more than treatment strategy (e.g., obesity), it is best to assess probable adherence and prescribe first, on that basis.

Problems in Carrying Out Interventions. Compliance with treatment recommendations is the primary problem in successfully treating cardiovascular disease. Because hypertension and coronary heart disease are "silent," or asymptomatic, disorders, patients are often unmotivated to take medicines as prescribed, alter diets, or practice relaxation. Unlike headaches or IBS, the symptoms of cardiovascular disease are not terribly painful and generally go undetected until the advanced stages of the disease (e.g., thrombosis or infarction). For this reason, it is best to develop structured programs for modifying a particular risk factor so that patients can form a social support system to enhance motivation for behavior change. Use of group therapy and involvement of family members in therapy can be very helpful, especially when one is trying to modify behaviors that are inherently reinforcing, such as eating, smoking, TABP, or inactivity.

Relapse Prevention. Progress in changing cardiovascular risk factors is usually interspersed with periods of relapse. This is especially true of obesity and cigarette smoking. Therefore, it is very important to include relapse prevention strategies in a structured program for these problems. Relapse prevention should target situations that place the individual at risk for relapse. These situations can be avoided in some instances, but in most cases the person will require training in strategies to prevent a return to previous habits (e.g., smoking the first cigarette during a period of stress or while at a party). Finally, it is very important that the healthcare provider maintain a compassionate view of the struggle to achieve a healthier lifestyle in order to avoid expressing frustration to a patient who is already feeling guilty.

Case Illustration

Case Description

Joan was a 35-year-old married woman referred for treatment of headaches. She had two adolescent daughters from a previous marriage. Her husband was a professional in the community and she was employed as a legal secretary. She reported almost daily headaches and severe, incapacitating headaches two to three times per week. These headaches were described as unilateral at onset, with severe throbbing pain. She reported seeing black spots in her visual field before the headaches began and feeling nauseated before and during the headaches. She sometimes vomited, which relieved the nausea. During a headache she usually left work and went to bed. She noted that bright lights and loud noises were very disturbing when she had a headache. These headaches were diagnosed as classic migraine. On other days she often had dull aching headaches in the frontal and occipital regions of the head. These headaches were diagnosed as muscle contraction headaches, and some were probably residual effects of the migraines. Joan's headaches were best described as combined headache, because she experienced both migraine and tension headaches.

Assessment

Further assessment found that Joan was very anxious and perfectionistic. She had experienced recurrent episodes of depression and was currently dysthymic. She also reported many obsessions and compulsions. She was very concerned about order and cleanliness and spent much of her time cleaning and straightening her home and office. She demanded perfectionism in her work, which had been strongly reinforced by the lawyers for whom she worked. Self-monitoring of headache suggested that the stress of her work compounded with her perfectionism were probable determinants of a substantial proportion of her headaches. Based on this information she was given three psychiatric diagnoses: obsessive-compulsive disorder, dysthymia, and psychological factors affecting a physical condition (combined headache). Joan had been treated pharmacologically with antidepressant medication and prescription analgesics without success. She had never sought psychological or psychiatric treatment. She and her family had just accepted the fact that she was "high strung" and had tried to live with her condition. They sought psychological treatment at the recommendation of her physician after he became concerned about the increasing consumption of analgesic medication.

Intervention Selection

The treatment program illustrated in Figure 20.1 was followed, with a few modifications. Since a trial of medications had been attempted but had been unsuccessful, the treatment plan was initiated at Step 2 and involved home-based relaxation. Also, a separate treatment program for obsessive-compulsive disorder and dysthymia was planned, including exposure with response prevention, cognitive therapy, and anxiety management.

Intervention Course and Problems in Carrying Out Interventions

During the first 6 weeks of treatment, Joan was trained in progressive muscle relaxation. She attended the clinic for three sessions, during which she was relaxed by the therapist. Also, headache monitoring records were reviewed to assess progress. She was assigned daily practice of relaxation at home using an audiotape of the instructions for progressive muscle relaxation. She reported very good compliance with the home-based relaxation program. Next, she was instructed to use relaxation when she felt the first signs of a headache. Review of her headache monitoring records showed no significant improvement.

Based on the lack of response to home-based relaxation, a 6-week trial of skin temperature biofeedback was prescribed. During this period, she attended the clinic twice per week and was provided with a portable biofeedback trainer for home practice. We also introduced the treatment program for obsessive-compulsive disorder and dysthymia during this time period. Joan found the exposure with response prevention treatment to be very distressing. This intervention required her to leave her home environment in progressively greater disorder without cleaning and straightening. The result of combining the two modes of therapy was a dramatic worsening of migraine headaches, resulting in several visits to the emergency room. After continuing this treatment plan for 2 months, we decided that headache treatment and treatment of obsessive-compulsive disorder could not be conducted simultaneously.

A decision was made to refer Joan to an inpatient pain clinic, where she could learn the skills for managing headaches in a relatively low stress environment. She reluctantly agreed to this plan. In the pain clinic, she received more intensive biofeedback therapy and learned the techniques of applying relaxation to prevent the occurrence of headaches. Also, her medication was changed to fluoxetine, 40 mg a day, and propoxyphene napsylate (Darvocet) or oxycodone (Tylox) to be used if a headache became very severe. Propranolol and clonidine were prescribed, but the patient could not tolerate the hypotension which resulted from these antihypertensive drugs. After 1 month her headaches were reduced to one per week and after 3 months, she was experiencing about two headaches per month. After headaches were improved for a 5-month period, another trial of exposure with response prevention and cognitive therapy was prescribed. Six months later obsessive-compulsive habits were very much improved and she was placed on a follow-up schedule.

Outcome and Termination

Over the next year, Joan experienced a few relapses during which headaches, obsessive-compulsive habits and depression worsened. In each instance, she returned for a series of booster sessions and remission of these problems occurred. Each relapse was associated with a new stressor: serious illnesses of both parents and the start of a new job with a very demanding boss. She eventually decided to leave this job because the boss activated her perfectionism to an extent that she could never control. On each occasion, she had to be reminded to utilize the headache management program that had been learned in the pain clinic.

Follow-Up and Maintenance

Joan was followed for 2 more years and maintained contact over the next 5 years. She continues to experience about one or two headaches per month. She has not visited the emergency room in 2 years. She continues to take fluoxetine, 20 mg a day, and must manage the tendency to become perfectionistic, especially during times of stress. She reports feeling very happy, enjoying the company of her family and grandchild.

Summary

Prescriptive treatments for psychophysiologic disorders have advanced considerably in the last 20 years. This chapter presented a step-by-step approach for treating three psychophysiologic disorders: headache, irritable bowel syndrome, and cardiovascular disease. A case history of one headache patient was presented in order to illustrate how the practitioner must approach such cases. Many persons with these disorders present with multiple problems, which requires a degree of flexibility in administering the prescriptive treatments. Because of the combination of medical and psychological factors that maintain psychophysiologic disorders, it is best to develop a multidisciplinary team that can assist in the management of all facets of the patient's problem.

References

American Psychiatric Association (1987). *Diagnostic and statistical manual of mental disorders* (3rd ed., rev.). Washington, DC: Author.

Andrasik, F., & Blanchard, E. B. (1987). Task force report on the biofeedback treatment of tension headache. In J. P. Hatch, J. D. Rugh, & J. G. Fisher (Eds.), *Biofeedback studies in clinical efficacy*. New York: Plenum.

Arena, J. G., Blanchard, E. B., Andrasik, F., & Dudek, B. C. (1982). The headache symptom questionnaire: Discriminant classificatory ability and headache syndromes suggested by factor analysis. *Journal of Behavioral Assessment, 4*, 55–69.

Bennett, P., & Wilkinson, S. (1985). A comparison of psychological and medical treatment of the irritable bowel syndrome. *British Journal of Clinical Psychology, 24*, 215–216.

Bernstein, D. A., & Borkovec, T. D. (1973). *Progressive muscle relaxation training*. Champaign, IL: Research Press.

Blair, S. N., Kohl, H. W., III, Paffenbarger, R. S., Clark, D. G., Cooper, K. H., & Gibbons, L. W. (1989). Physical fitness and all-cause mortality. *Journal of the American Medical Association, 262*, 2395–2401.

Blanchard, E. B. (1990). Biofeedback treatments of essential hypertension. *Biofeedback and Self-Regulation, 15*, 209–228.

Blanchard, E. B. (1992). Psychological treatment of benign headache disorders. *Journal of Consulting and Clinical Psychology, 4*, 537–551.

Blanchard, E. B., & Andrasik, F. (1985). *Management of chronic headaches: A psychological approach*. Elmsford, NY: Pergamon.

Blanchard, E. B., Appelbaum, K. A., Radnitz, C. L., Michultka, D., Morrill, B., Kirsch, C., Hillhouse, J., Evans, D. D., Guarnieri, P., Attanasio, V., Andrasik, F., Jaccard, J., & Dentinger, M. P. (1990). Placebo-controlled evaluation of abbreviated progressive muscle relaxation and of relaxation combined with cognitive therapy in the treatment of tension headache. *Journal of Consulting and Clinical Psychology, 58*, 210–215.

Blanchard, E. B., Appelbaum, K. A., Radnitz, C. L., Morrill, B., Michultka, D., Kirsch, C., Guarnieri, P., Hillhouse, J., Evans, D. D., Jaccard, J., & Barron, K. D. (1990). A controlled evaluation of thermal biofeedback and thermal biofeedback combined with cognitive therapy in the treatment of vascular headache. *Journal of Consulting and Clinical Psychology, 58*, 216–224.

Blanchard, E. B., Nicholson, N. L., Taylor, A. E., Steffek, B. D., Radnitz, C. L., & Appelbaum, K. A. (1991). The role of regular home practice in the relaxation treatment of tension headache. *Journal of Consulting and Clinical Psychology, 59*, 467–470.

Blanchard, E. B., Radnitz, C. L., Schwarz, S. P., Neff, D. F., & Gerardi, M. A. (1987). Psychological changes associated with the self-regulatory treatments of irritable bowel syndrome. *Biofeedback and Self-Regulation, 12*, 31–37.

Blanchard, E. B., & Schwarz, S. P. (1987). Adaptation of a multicomponent treatment for irritable bowel syndrome to a small-group format. *Biofeedback and Self-Regulation, 12*, 63–69.

Blanchard, E. B., Schwarz, S. P., Suls, J. M., Gerard, M. A., Scharf, L., Greene, B., Taylor, A. E., Berreman, C., & Malamood, H. S. (1992). Two controlled evaluations of a multicomponents psychological treatment of irritable bowel syndrome. *Behaviour Research and Therapy, 30*, 175–189.

Brownell, K. D., & Wadden, T. A. (1991). The heterogeneity of obesity: Fitting treatments to individuals. *Behavior Therapy, 22*, 153–177.

Brownell, K. D., & Wadden, T. A. (1992). Etiology and treatment of obesity: Understanding a serious, prevalent, and refractory disorder. *Journal of Consulting and Clinical Psychology, 60*, 505–517.

Bueno-Miranda, F., Cerulli, M., & Schuster, M. M. (1976). Operant conditioning of colonic motility in irritable bowel syndrome (IBS). *Gastroenterology, 70*, 867.

DeFronzo, R. A., & Ferrannini, E. (1991). Insulin resistance: A multifaceted syndrome responsible for NIDDM, obesity, hypertension, dyslipidemia, and atherosclerotic cardiovascular disease. *Diabetes Care, 14*, 173–194.

Diamond, S., & Dalessio, D. J. (1982). *The practicing physician's approach to headache*. Baltimore: Williams & Wilkins.

DiClemente, C. C., Prochaska, J. O., Fairhurst, S. K., Velicer, W. F., Velasquez, M. M., & Rossi, J. S. (1991). The process of smoking cessation: An analysis of precontemplation, contemplation, and preparation stages of change. *Journal of Consulting and Clinical Psychology, 59*, 295–304.

Dubbert, P. M. (1992). Exercise in behavioral medicine. *Journal of Consulting and Clinical Psychology, 60*, 613–618.

Ford, M. J. (1986). Invited review: The irritable bowel syndrome. *Journal of Psychosomatic Research, 30*, 399–410.

Friedman, M., & Rosenman, R. H. (1974). *Type A behavior and your heart*. New York: Knopf.

Furman, S. (1973). Intestinal biofeedback in functional diarrhea: A preliminary report. *Journal of Behavior Therapy and Experimental Psychiatry, 4*, 317–321.

Gallup, G. (1974, June). Public puffs on after 10 years of warnings. In *Gallup Opinion Index* (Report No. 108, pp. 20–21). Princeton, NJ: Gallup Organization.

Ganguly, A. (1977, November). Drugs in the treatment of hypertension: Pharmacology and interactions. *Journal of the Indiana Medical Association*, 879–881.

Guy-Grand, B. (1992). Clinical studies with d-fenfluramine. *American Journal of Clinical Nutrition, 55*, 1735–1765.

Hatch, J. P., Klatt, K. D., Supik, J. D., Rios, N., Fisher, J. G., Bauer, R. L., & Shimotsu, G. W. (1985). Combined behavior and pharmacological treatment of essential hypertension. *Biofeedback and Self-Regulation, 10*, 119–138.

Henningfield, J. E., & Obarzanek, E. (1992). Task Force 2: Methods of assessment, strategies for research. *Health Psychology, 11*, 10–16.

Holroyd, K. A., & Andrasik, F. (1982). Do the effects of cognitive therapy endure? A two year follow-up of tension headache sufferers treated with cognitive therapy or biofeedback. *Cognitive Therapy and Research, 6*, 325–333.

Holroyd, K. A., Andrasik, F., & Westbrook, T. (1977). Cognitive control of tension headache. *Cognitive Therapy and Research, 1*, 121–123.

Holroyd, K. A., Holm, J. E., Hursey, K. G., Penzien, D. B., Cordingley, G. E., Theofanous, A. G., Richardson, S. C., & Tobin, D. L. (1988). Recurrent vascular headache: Home-based behavioral treatment versus abortive pharmacological treatment. *Journal of Consulting and Clinical Psychology, 56*, 218–223.

Holroyd, K. A., Nash, J. M., Pingel, J. D., Cordingley, G. E., & Jerome, A. (1991). A comparison of pharmacological (amitriptyline HCl) and nonpharmacological (cognitive-behavioral) therapies for chronic tension headaches. *Journal of Consulting and Clinical Psychology, 59*, 387–393.

Hovell, M. F. (1982). The experimental evidence for weight-loss treatment of essential hypertension: A critical review. *American Journal of Public Health., 72*, 359–368.

Hutchins, L. H. (1981). Drug treatment of high blood pressure. *Nursing Clinics of North America, 16*, 365–376.

Jenkins, C. D., Zyzanski, S. J., & Rosenman, R. H. (1979). *The Jenkins Activity Survey*. New York: Psychological Corporation.

Lichtenstein, E., & Glasgow, R. E. (1992). Smoking cessation: What have we learned over the past decade? *Journal of Consulting and Clinical Psychology, 60*, 518–527.

Marcus, M. D., Wing, R. R., Ewing, L., Kern, E., Gooding, W., & McDermott, M. (1990). Psychiatric disorders among obese binge eaters. *International Journal of Eating Disorders, 9*, 69–77.

Marcus, M. D., Wing, R. R., & Hopkins, J. (1988). Obese binge eaters: Affect, cognitions, and response to behavioral weight control. *Journal of Consulting and Clinical Psychology, 56*, 433–439.

Mathew, N. T. (1981). Prophylaxis of migraine and mixed headache: A randomized controlled study. *Headache, 21*, 105–109.

Olesen, J. (1978). Some clinical features of the acute migraine attack: An analysis of 750 patients. *Headache, 18*, 268–271.

Polefrone, J. M., Manuck, S. B., Larkin, K. T., & Francis, M. E. (1987). Behavioral aspects of arterial hypertension and its treatment. In R. L. Morrison & A. S. Bellack (Eds.), *Medical factors and psychological disorders* (pp. 203–229). New York: Plenum.

Radnitz, C. L., & Blanchard, E. B. (1988). Bowel sound biofeedback as a treatment for irritable bowel syndrome. *Biofeedback and Self-Regulation, 13*, 169–179.

Reaven, G. M. (1988). Role of insulin resistance in human disease. *Diabetes, 37*, 1595–1607.

Ritchie, J. A., & Truelove, S. C. (1980). Comparison of various treatments for irritable bowel syndrome. *British Medical Journal, 281*, 1317–1319.

Thoresen, C. E., & Powell, L. H. (1992). Type A behavior pattern: New perspectives on theory, assessment, and intervention. *Journal of Consulting and Clinical Psychology, 60*, 595–604.

Wadden, T. A., Stunkard, A. J., & Liebschutz, J. (1988). Three-year follow-up of the treatment of obesity by very low calorie diet, behavior therapy, and their combination. *Journal of Consulting and Clinical Psychology, 56*, 925–928.

Wadden, T. A., & Van Itallie, T. B. (Eds.). (1992). *Treatment of the seriously obese patient*. New York: Guilford.

Weintraub, M. (1992). Long-term weight control: The National Heart, Lung, and Blood Institute funded multimodal intervention study. *Clinical Pharmacological Therapy, 13,* 581–645.

Whitehead, W. E. (1985). Psychotherapy and biofeedback in the treatment of irritable bowel syndrome. In N. E. Read (Ed.), *Irritable bowel syndrome.* London: Grune & Stratton.

Whitehead, W. E. (1992). Biofeedback treatment of gastrointestinal disorders. *Biofeedback and Self-Regulation, 17,* 59–76.

Whitehead, W. E., Enck, P., Anthony, J. C., & Schuster, M. M. (1989). Psychopathology in patients with irritable bowel syndrome. In M. V. Singer & H. Goebell (Eds.), *Nerves and the gastrointestinal tract.* Lancaster, UK: Falk Symposium 50.

Whitehead, W. E., & Schuster, M. M. (1985). *Gastrointestinal disorders: Behavioral and physiological basis for treatment.* New York: Academic.

Williamson, D. A., Barker, S. E., & Lapour, K. J. (in press). Psychophysiological disorders. In M. Hersen & S. M. Turner (Eds.), *Diagnostic interviewing* (2nd ed.). New York: Plenum.

Williamson, D. A., Ruggiero, L., & Davis, C. J. (1985). Headache, In M. Hersen & A. S. Bellack (Eds.), *Handbook of clinical behavior therapy with adults* (pp. 417–442). New York: Plenum.

Williamson, D. A., & Waggoner, C. D. (1988). Psychophysiological disorders. In M. Hersen (Ed.), *Pharmacological and behavioral treatment* (pp. 312–341). New York: Wiley.

21

Pain Management

Robert D. Kerns

Description of the Problem

There is no greater source of stress and human suffering than the experience of chronic pain. Defined most simply as an experience of pain of at least 6 months duration, chronic pain affects millions of Americans and is a significant contributor to the increasing economic burden experienced by society as a function of growing healthcare costs. In a recent survey of subscribers to a large community health maintenance organization, Von Korff and his colleagues reported that 41% had suffered from low back pain in the prior 6 months. In the same sample, 26% had recurrent headaches, 18% reported abdominal pain, 12% had chest pain, and 12% had facial pain (Von Korff, Dworkin, LeResche, & Kruger, 1988). In a review of the literature, Steinberg (1982) found that in industrialized countries the lifetime prevalence of low back pain is between 50 and 80%. Evidence suggests that among those who experience significant back pain, 7% will have pain persisting beyond six months.

The economic costs of chronic pain are equally staggering. Direct costs include those associated with use of healthcare services as well as prescribed and over-the-counter medications. Indirect costs include the financial burden of unemployment and underemployment, lost productivity, and disability compensation. Low back pain alone costs the United States an estimated $14 billion per year (Dworkin, Handlin, Richlin, Brand, & Vannucci, 1985). As another example, the lifetime economic costs of rheumatoid arthritis have been estimated to be more than $20,000 per case—in 1977 dollars (Stone, 1984).

Contributing to the severity of the problem is a continued lack of agreement on such central issues as what pain is or how it should be measured, let alone how to treat

Robert D. Kerns • Psychology Service, West Haven VA Medical Center, West Haven, CT 06516, and Departments of Psychiatry, Neurology, and Psychology, Yale University, New Haven, CT 06520.

Handbook of Prescriptive Treatments for Adults, edited by Michel Hersen and Robert T. Ammerman. Plenum Press, New York, 1994.

or manage it effectively. "Somatic" or "peripheralist" models of pain that hypothesize a relatively linear, one-to-one relationship between structural pathology and pain intensity remain as the primary neurophysiologic theories of pain (Campbell et al., 1989). These models, although important in outlining basic somatosensory processes, are readily criticized in terms of the layman's phenomenology of pain and common anecdotes that acknowledge the apparent influence of a range of psychological and environmental variables (e.g., distraction). The lack of empirical evidence that supports a significant relationship between extent of peripheral nociception and the experience of pain or impairment further undermines the credibility of these models (Boden, Davis, Dina, Patronis, & Wiesel, 1990). Ultimately, dissatisfaction with these models rests in the dramatic failure of purely somatic treatment efforts to relieve chronic pain (Flor & Turk, 1984).

More comprehensive "centralist" perspectives on chronic pain emphasize the roles that central nervous system and psychological factors play in the modulation or perpetuation of peripheral nociception. Central models range from those that are primarily neurophysiologic or neurochemical to those that are distinctly psychological or behavioral.

One particularly comprehensive model is the gate control theory of pain (Melzack & Wall, 1965). This model has been particularly important in fostering a multidimensional perspective of pain and pain treatment. From a psychological perspective the model has been important in emphasizing the integration of sensory-discriminative, cognitive-evaluative, and motivational-affective dimensions in determining the individual's perception of pain. Although postulated physiologic and anatomic bases for the gate control theory have been challenged, the multidimensional perspective has received substantial support, thus opening the door for psychologists to investigate the relevance of a broad range of psychosocial variables in the perpetuation of pain, disability, and distress.

As early as 1968, Wilbert Fordyce (Fordyce, Fowler, & DeLateur, 1968) at the University of Washington proposed that chronic pain could be viewed as a behavioral disorder identified by a set of observable "pain behaviors." These behaviors include excessive time spent reclining, excessive pain medication use, verbal complaints of pain, and protective behaviors such as limping and bracing. Fordyce (1976) suggested that, although these behaviors may initially be expressed in direct relationship to peripheral nociception or acute pain, over time, as a function of social contingencies (e.g., attention from doctors and family members, escape from aversive work situations), these behaviors may be maintained by their environmental consequences rather than by some structural pathology and continued nociceptive stimulation. Fordyce and his colleagues provided initial demonstrations of the efficacy of an intervention that applied behavioral strategies to alter environmental consequences of pain (Fordyce et al., 1968, 1973). These reports document dramatic recoveries in previously treatment-refractory chronic pain patients.

A more recent innovation in the field of pain control has been the extension and elaboration of Fordyce's operant conditioning model by the incorporation of cognitive-social learning theory and cognitive-behavioral intervention perspectives (Turk, Meichenbaum, & Genest, 1983). Turk and his colleagues have emphasized the crucial role of chronic pain patients' idiosyncratic beliefs, attitudes, and coping resources in optimal pain management. In addition to modifying of maladaptive behaviors and encouraging a return to an improved functional status, proponents of a cognitive-behavioral perspective emphasize the importance of fostering the development of a perception of self-control and personal mastery in relation to pain to replace the common perceptions of helplessness, hopelessness, and uncontrollability.

Additional integrative models have been proposed that further explicate possible mechanisms or processes that may mediate the development of chronic pain. Flor, Birbaumer, and Turk (1990) have proposed a biobehavioral model of chronic pain that emphasizes the interaction among four components: (1) a predisposition to respond with a specific bodily system; (2) external or internal aversive stimulation; (3) maladaptive information processing of and coping with pain-related social and/or physiological stimuli; and (4) operant, respondent, and observational learning processes.

Kerns and Jacob (1993; in press) have recently proposed an integrative diathesis–stress model of chronic pain that hypothesizes important prior vulnerabilities in neurobiological and psychosocial domains that may become activated in the face of acute nociception and associated challenges. Important domains include brain neurochemical systems relevant to the regulation of pain, mood, activity, and sleep such as the serotonin system, the instrumental skill and cognitive coping skills of the individual, and social support. To the extent that prior areas of vulnerability are challenged in the face of acute pain—for example, via declines in activity that foster muscle deconditioning, tax coping resources, or reduce levels of already limited social rewards—persistent pain, disability, and distress may be likely to evolve.

Consistent with these important psychological models of chronic pain are data that document significant relationships between the experience of pain and associated disability, and relevant psychological and social variables. Among these variables are attention and distraction (McCaul & Malott, 1984), beliefs about pain, styles of thinking, and ways of coping (Jensen, Turner, Romano, & Karoly, 1991), and mood (Haythornthwaite, Sieber, & Kerns, 1991; Letham, Slade, Troup, & Bentley, 1983). Recently, evidence has been accumulating to support an important role of pain-relevant social interaction in the maintenance, if not the development, of chronic pain (Kerns et al., 1991; Romano et al., 1992; Turk, Kerns, & Rosenberg, 1992).

These contemporary models of chronic pain have been important in encouraging the multidimensional assessment of the chronic pain experience and the development of multimodal, and frequently interdisciplinary, plans for intervention. Attention to the *patient* with chronic pain has displaced a more unidimensional focus on the relief of pain only. Although the field of chronic pain management remains in its infancy and is far from being "prescriptive" in its approach, a multidimensional approach to assessment, conceptualization, treatment planning, intervention, and follow-up holds substantial promise in clinical efforts to aid the chronic pain sufferer.

Assessment Strategies

Psychological Evaluation

Comprehensive psychological assessment is increasingly viewed as a crucial component of the evaluation of the chronic pain patient. The context in which such an assessment occurs varies greatly. Patients may be referred for psychological evaluation by primary care physicians or pain specialists who are interested in the opinion of the psychologist to assist in their own treatment planning, to consider the need for referral for adjunctive psychological intervention, or both. Alternately, psychologists frequently serve as members of multidisciplinary teams that offer comprehensive pain management services to chronic pain patients. Across these settings the relative focus on psychosocial factors in treatment planning varies widely; these factors can be viewed as of secondary importance, or psychological interventions can serve a primary integrating role in a comprehensive treatment or rehabilitation program.

The breadth and extent of the psychological evaluation of the chronic pain patient similarly varies widely depending on the setting and purpose of the evaluation. The following discussions emphasize the role of psychological evaluation and intervention in the context of more comprehensive and interdisciplinary efforts. The intent is to encourage the development of collaborative networks of healthcare providers with specific expertises in the management of chronic pain either in private practice community settings or in institutionally based programs. Such interdisciplinary collaboration is clearly indicated given the complexity of the problem, the demonstrated relevance of both medical and psychosocial variables, and the viability of multiple treatment approaches.

There are several important goals of the psychological evaluation (Kerns & Jacob, 1992; Turk & Kerns, 1983, 1985). Psychologists rely on standardized methods to obtain information relevant to the comprehensive evaluation of the individual's experience of pain. The information is used to identify potential problems and intervention targets, to identify contributors to the development and perpetuation of the problems, and to provide a baseline for comparison following treatment and at follow-up. The comprehensive psychological pain evaluation also serves an important role by reinforcing a multidimensional perspective on pain. The psychologist demonstrates a broad interest in and concern for the impact of chronic pain on the patient's life and acknowledges the multiple concurrent problems commonly experienced by the patient, such as depression, unemployment, and family distress. Ultimately, the comprehensive evaluation process serves a crucial role in engaging the patient in more specific evaluation, treatment planning, and intervention efforts.

Hypothesis Generation and Evaluation

The psychological evaluation should follow a hypothesis-generating and testing approach. Multidimensional models of chronic pain emphasize the possible role of multiple contributing factors that may interact with one another over time in the development and maintenance of pain, disability, and distress. Given this perspective it is important to begin the assessment process with a broad approach that scans for current problem areas and their possible contributors. As problems are identified, contributors to the concern are hypothesized, as are the mechanisms by which these variables may exert their effects. These hypotheses are subsequently examined by an assessment process that is increasingly focused and behaviorally specific. Ultimate tests of the validity of the hypothesized mechanisms may be based in the treatment efforts prescribed for the patient.

An example may help develop an appreciation for this approach to assessment and treatment planning. A commonly hypothesized contributor to significant functional disability is anxiety, specifically fear of pain and further injury (McCracken, Zayfert, & Gross, 1992). Additional links between such fears and perpetuation of peripheral nociception have been proposed and include negative or distorted cognition about possible adverse effects of activity, behavioral inhibition and avoidance, muscle deconditioning secondary to declining activity, and site-specific muscle hyperreactivity to stress. Identification of significant disability and anxiety during broad-based screening of the patient should be an indication for subsequent assessment of these additional psychological, behavioral, and psychophysiologic variables. The goal of the process is the development of an integrative model to explain the patient's idiosyncratic experience of pain and the development of a treatment plan that is equally specific to the individual patient. To the extent that the treatment recommendations and their rationale are understandable and relatively consistent with the patient's beliefs about the pain experience, there is a greater likelihood that the patient will approve the plan and be prepared to enter treatment.

Specific Assessment Methods

Multiple methods are used by the psychologist to converge on the nature and extent of the patient's pain, disability, and distress. Behavioral interviewing, observation, paper-and-pencil measures, and diary methods are commonly used to explore the cognitive, affective, behavioral, and interpersonal domains of the experience of the patient (Bradley, Haile, & Jaworski, 1992). The use of standardized methods and more than one measure of important variables increases the reliability and validity of the information obtained.

The most frequently used method is the behavioral interview. The skilled interviewer obtains a broad array of relevant information and also engages the patient in collaborative discussions about important variables. Interviews are enhanced by the inclusion of family members. The interviewer often begins by obtaining relevant demographic information that places the patient in a broader social and historical context. Attention to the specific details of the patient's current pain experience and its history generally follows. The patient and family members' attributions for the pain and their beliefs about variables that contribute to fluctuations in intensity are also relevant. Details about past treatment and rehabilitation efforts are also obtained. The remainder of the interview typically focuses on the perceived impact of pain across the multiple domains of the patient's life, including marital and family functioning, employment and work-related activities, and social and recreational activities. The presence of significant psychopathology and emotional distress is also assessed. Given the high incidence of alcohol and substance abuse and dependence and major depression, these disorders should be routinely and thoroughly evaluated.

Questionnaires, inventories, and behavioral diaries are also commonly employed. These methods provide quantifiable indices of relevant variables that are helpful in specifying goals for treatment and evaluating outcome. The past decade has seen the emergence of a host of measures that owe their theoretical foundations to the evolving chronic pain literature and that have been developed and standardized on groups of chronic pain patients. Measures include those designed to assess single constructs of interest such as coping with pain (Coping Strategies Inventory; Rosenstiel & Keefe, 1983) or pain-related anxiety (McCracken, Zayfert, & Gross, 1992). Others are more comprehensive in their scope (West Haven–Yale Multidimensional Pain Inventory; Kerns, Turk, & Rudy, 1985). The recently published *Handbook of Pain Assessment* by Turk and Melzack (1992) provides a detailed examination of a broad array of the most commonly used self-report measures in the assessment of the chronic pain patient. These measures are typically supplemented by the inclusion of widely accepted measures of more general constructs of interest such as measures of depressive symptom severity, anxiety, and marital and family functioning.

A recent advance in the assessment of chronic pain is the development of observational methods for the quantification of demonstrations of pain (e.g., Keefe &

Block, 1982). The domain of pain behaviors includes verbal complaints of pain as well as nonverbal behaviors such as grimacing, bracing and guarding, using pain medications, and visiting doctors. Several observational coding systems have been developed and validated with a broadening array of specific patient samples.

Psychophysiological assessment is also common (Flor, Miltner, & Birbaumer, 1992; Flor & Turk, 1989). Recent technological advances permit concurrent dynamic electromyographic evaluation of multiple muscle sites and other psychophysiologic parameters. Examination of reactivity to mental or physical challenge appears to provide the most relevant information. Psychophysiologic assessment and feedback to the patient can be particularly useful in offering credibility to the psychological assessment in the eyes of the patient, and may offer support for an integrative biobehavioral rationale for the treatment and rehabilitation plan. Results may have specific implications for biofeedback and muscle relaxation exercises, physical conditioning recommendations, efforts designed to increase work tolerance and endurance, and stress management training.

Intervention Strategies

Evidence for Prescriptive Interventions

Over the past decade there have been multiple published reports on the efficacy of various "nontraditional" approaches to the management of chronic nonmalignant pain. A substantial literature is now available that reports on the efficacy of multidimensional and multidisciplinary inpatient and outpatient treatment programs. An important subset of this literature reports more specifically on the efficacy of outpatient operant-behavioral and cognitive-behavioral treatment approaches. In addition, a much larger literature has evaluated the efficacy of tricyclic antidepressants, the most frequent pharmacologic alternative to narcotic analgesics in the management of chronic nonmalignant pain. A brief review of these literatures follows.

Multidisciplinary Treatment Programs.   Numerous reports have been published on the efficacy of both inpatient and outpatient multidisciplinary pain treatment programs. Common among these programs is an emphasis on the assessment and management of psychosocial factors presumed to contribute to the experience of chronic pain. Most frequently a cognitive-behavioral, self-management, and rehabilitative perspective serves an integrating role in the organization and conceptualization of the overall treatment program.

A recent meta-analytic review of this literature by Flor, Fydrich, and Turk (1992) considered 65 studies that evaluated the efficacy of multidisciplinary treatments for chronic back pain. Results of their analysis revealed that multidisciplinary treatments are superior to no treatment, waiting list controls, and single-discipline interventions such as medication or physical therapy. Improvements are commonly reported in pain, mood and depressive symptoms, and disability, including return to work. Decreases in use of healthcare system and of pain medication are also noted. The authors temper their enthusiasm for their conclusions by noting the relatively poor quality of the study designs. Limitations are also highlighted regarding the failure to evaluate the contributions of individual components of these programs to their overall efficacy.

Psychological Treatment Approaches.   Several studies have evaluated the efficacy of outpatient behavioral or cognitive-behavioral approaches to the management of chronic pain (Heinrich, Cohen, Naliboff, Collins, & Bonnebakker, 1985; Keefe et al., 1990a, 1990b; Kerns, Turk, Holzman, & Rudy, 1986; Moore & Chaney, 1985; Nicholas, Wilson, & Goyen, 1991; Phillips, 1987; Pilowsky & Barrow, 1990; Turner, 1982; Turner & Clancy, 1988; Turner, Clancy, McQuade, & Cardenas, 1990). The best of these studies have included relevant control conditions (e.g., waiting list, educational programs, alternative treatment comparisons, placebo medications), reasonable sample sizes, multiple outcome measures, and moderate (6- to 12-month) follow-up periods. Results of controlled studies support the short-term and longer-term effectiveness of either outpatient behavioral or cognitive-behavioral treatments. There is no consistent evidence to support one approach over the other, either in terms of breadth of effectiveness on important dimensions of the chronic pain experience or in terms of long-term efficacy.

Pharmacotherapy.   The rationale for the use of tricyclic antidepressant medications in the treatment of chronic pain is based in the clinical observation of the prevalence of depression symptoms, including sleep disturbances, anergia, and a decline in activity level among chronic pain patients. At least 60 published studies have examined the efficacy of tricyclics in the treatment of chronic pain of varying etiologies. A recent meta-analytic review of 39 well-controlled studies found substantial benefits of the antidepressants compared to placebo medications (Onghena & Van Houdenhove, 1992). Studies have reported improvement in pain among depressed as well as nondepressed patients. Head pain patients appear to be the most likely to benefit from antidepressants. The mechanism by which these medications exert their analgesic effect is unclear, although evidence suggests a relatively direct analgesic action as opposed to an indirect psychological mediation. Several weaknesses in the literature remain, including use of self-report measures of pain and pain-related variables of questionable reliability and the failure to provide follow-up data. Comparison with alternative pharmacologic or psychological approaches is lacking.

Evidence for prescriptive interventions in the field of chronic pain is sorely lacking. The few efforts that have been made to evaluate possible predictors of treatment outcome have generally failed to identify reliable predictors. Variables that have face validity and considerable support from clinicians, such as employment status, disability compensation status, and pending litigation, fail to be reliable predictors of either participation in treatment or success. Other psychological or psychiatric variables such as personality style and depression, and demographic and descriptive variables, are inconsistently cited as being predictive of outcome.

In the absence of specific indications for different treatments, clinicians are encouraged to base treatment planning decisions on a multidimensional assessment and conceptualization of the individual patient such as the process described earlier. An integrative multimodal plan for intervention that is individually tailored to meet the needs of each patient remains the state of the art.

Selecting Optimal Intervention Strategies

An important strength of the cognitive-behavioral perspective on chronic pain management (Turk et al., 1983) is its emphasis on the development of individually tailored treatment plans. The approach accommodates a variety of specific cognitive, behavioral, and psychophysiologically based treatment strategies. While describing an integrative approach to the management of chronic pain and associated disability and distress, proponents of cognitive-behavioral therapy emphasize an inherent flexibility in the approach that encourages choices among multiple possible treatment targets and cognitive and behavioral intervention strategies (Hanson & Gerber, 1990; Kerns & Jacob, 1993, in press; Turk et al., 1983). Clinicians are encouraged to base decisions about specific intervention techniques or strategies on the hypotheses and goals for the patient developed through the comprehensive assessment process. In this manner, an active treatment phase serves as a test of the hypotheses regarding contributors to and mediating mechanisms of the patient's pain, disability, distress, and other associated problems. A few examples may help clarify this perspective.

When considering options for attempting to reduce the experience of pain per se, a number of specific strategies can be applied. Selection among these strategies or decisions about relative emphases can be based on specific assessment findings. For example, several strategies can be emphasized for patients who manifest particularly heightened anxiety, stress-related, site-specific muscle reactivity, and behavioral avoidance. These include progressive muscle relaxation, stress management training, and behavioral contracting for increased activity.

For patients who are particularly disabled and who evidence physical deconditioning, a graded exercise program, behavioral contracting for increased productive and pleasurable activity, and education about activity–rest cycling may prove particularly beneficial. A high frequency of observed pain behaviors in the context of a highly solicitous marital or family environment may be an indication for couples or family therapy that specifically attempts to alter patterns of pain-relevant communication.

In the face of evidence of concurrent depression, one may prescribe a trial of an antidepressant as well as psychological treatments that target negative cognitions, especially problem-solving and coping deficits and perceptions of low self-control, interpersonal distress, and declines in pleasurable activity. Patients may be encouraged to examine pain–mood relationships and their ability to moderate these effects. Sleep disturbances are frequently targeted as well.

It is crucial to identify and develop plans for targeting additional clinically significant problems such as marital or family dysfunction, alcohol or substance abuse, and specific anxiety disorders. Depending on the nature and extent of the concern, these problems may take precedence over pain management therapy, for example, in the case of active alcohol and substance abuse. Plans for addressing other concerns can be developed that call for concurrent or sequential treatment.

Problems in Carrying Out Interventions

Difficulty in engaging the pain patient in psychological treatment efforts is the primary factor that has been identified as limiting the overall effectiveness of these clinical efforts. This problem is perhaps understandable from within a cognitive-behavioral perspective when one considers that patients are likely to adhere strongly to a unidimensional, biomedical, and sensory model of pain that encourages continued search for medical or surgical treatment. Such beliefs are quite discordant from a multidimensional perspective on chronic pain. Stigma associated with psychologists and psychological treatments further obstructs engagement of many patients.

Acceptance of this problem has contributed to specific attention to the engagement process and establishment of a therapeutic relationship within a cognitive-behavioral approach. In fact, the cornerstone of such an approach is the process of "reconceptualization" that emphasizes acceptance of the idiosyncratic beliefs of the patient (and his or her family members) and implementation of strategies designed to gradually shape the patient's beliefs to accommodate to a multidimensional perspective on pain and concepts of self-control and personal mastery. Nevertheless, failure to engage referred patients in the evaluation process and a high frequency of treatment dropouts continue to plague pain management efforts (Turk & Rudy, 1991).

Lack of adherence to treatment recommendations, particularly failure to practice prescribed relaxation and coping skills exercises, is an additional problem that appears to interfere with optimal treatment effectiveness. Collaborative establishment of short-term goals for treatment and skills practice that are judged to be almost certain to be accomplished, discussion of specific rationales for their production, ongoing refinement of goals and expectations that match the patient's efforts, and delivery of social reward contingent on the accomplishment of these goals are emphasized within a cognitive-behavioral framework. Use of diaries and other self-monitoring forms, and charting of progress, are additionally useful.

Relapse Prevention

Consolidation and review of treatment gains are particularly addressed in most cognitive-behavioral pain management programs. Specific attention is paid to developing an overall problem-solving perspective and plans for "high-risk" situations previously believed by the patient to be associated with increased pain. Prevention of pain exacerbation and relapse is emphasized. At the same time, the patient is encouraged to accept the likelihood of periods of pain exacerbation despite substantial treatment gains and to develop plans for minimizing the duration and intensity of these episodes.

Empirical tests of application of models of relapse prevention have not systematically made their way into the chronic pain management literature. This is unfortunate, given repeated demonstrations of reversal or declines in treatment gains over periods of follow-up. Studies designed to identify patients at risk for relapse and the development and evaluation of relapse prevention efforts are clearly indicated in order to advance the field.

Case Illustration

Case Description

Mr. C., a 49-year-old married man, was referred to the Comprehensive Pain Management Center at the West Haven VA Medical Center by the Neurosurgery Clinic at the same hospital for evaluation and possible rehabilitation. The patient was known to have moderate disc herniation with two lesser disc protrusions in the lumbar spine, as evidenced on a recent radiologic workup. He was free of neurologic deficits (e.g., sensory loss or motor weakness). He described a progression of pain in his low back, with intermittent exacerbations for the past 10 years and increasing functional limitations, particularly over the past year. He had been treated conservatively with narcotics and nonnarcotic analgesics and anti-inflammatory agents, as well as physical therapy and transcutaneous nerve stimulation. Surgery had been inconsistently recommended. He continued to view narcotics as "essential" for "taking the edge off" his experience of pain but expressed a passive interest in a self-management, rehabilitation program.

Receipt of the referral led to a brief discussion with the referring physician, who emphasized her frustration with Mr. C. and his frequent visits to the emergency room and outpatient clinic, his demands for narcotics, and his expressions of irritation and anger. She expressed little optimism for his active participation in the Pain Center. Review of the available medical record generally corroborated the physician's impressions about his extensive use of the healthcare system and medical history. The patient was subsequently scheduled for an initial outpatient screening appointment with a primary clinician (a psychologist) from the center. Mr. C. proceeded through the outpatient screening phase and agreed with little reluctance to admission to the Pain Center for a comprehensive interdisciplinary evaluation.

Assessment

Immediately noted during the initial interviews was Mr. C.'s somewhat angry, cynical, and hopeless affective state, a high frequency of pain behaviors (e.g., intermittent standing during the interview, frequent grimacing and rubbing and holding his lower back), and his extensive history of "doctor shopping" and narcotic use. Although he continued to work as a draftsman, he reported extensive absenteeism. His second wife, of 8 years, attended the screening meeting with him and reported a high level of frustration and conflict in the relationship. She acknowledged that she was considering separation or divorce if her husband "didn't get his act together." However, she reinforced her husband's frustration at doctors who "take your money but don't do a thing to help."

Information about the patient's experience of pain, obtained via a semistructured pain interview, was supplemented by several questionnaires and inventories including subscales from the West Haven–Yale Multidimensional Pain Inventory (Kerns et al., 1985), the McGill Pain Questionnaire (Melzack, 1975), and the Pain Behavior Check List (Kerns et al., 1991). Videotaped observation of his attempts at five simple activities following a modified version of the Keefe and Block (1982) protocol revealed a high frequency of overt pain behaviors. The patient was also trained in the use of the Self-Monitored Pain Intensity procedure (Kerns, Finn, & Haythornthwaite, 1988), from which hourly pain intensity ratings for the week of evaluation were obtained. The patient consistently rated his experience of pain as "excruciating" and "incapacitating" with little fluctuation in intensity. Records of pain medication use in conjunction with the pain intensity ratings failed to document analgesic effectiveness. Nursing and other staff observations of the patient on the unit revealed a generally withdrawn and solemn individual who interacted with staff infrequently other than to request medications or to respond briefly to others' efforts to engage him in conversation.

During the inpatient evaluation, several additional clinically significant problems were noted. The Schedule for Affective Disorders and Schizophrenia (SADS; Endicott & Spitzer, 1979) was administered, from which the diagnosis of current major depressive disorder was made manifest by pervasive dysphoria and irritation; sleep-onset, middle, and terminal insomnia; anergia; pervasive loss of interest and satisfaction with activities; and complaints of difficulty in concentrating. Several standardized self-report measures of depression and anxiety were used to quantify his level of depressive symptoms and affective distress. Careful interviewing also documented clear evidence of prescription substance abuse, including abuse of narcotic analgesics and benzodiazepines. A high level of marital and family distress was noted during interview and on a standardized marital satisfaction inventory. Additional concerns of the patient included financial worries related to extensive medical bills and the possible loss of his job. Mr. C. appeared to be extremely limited in his social and recreational interests and activities, and reported spending most of his time in bed or lying on the couch when not at work. These reports were generally corroborated by the interview, questionnaire, diary, and pain behavior observation studies, and by the casual observation of the staff. The psychophysiologic evaluation revealed heightened site-specific electromyographic stress reactivity in the lumbar region. The physical therapy evaluation confirmed a general deconditioned state and a pattern of complaints and mobility limitations that were grossly exaggerated and somewhat inconsistent with the radiographic evidence of traumatic lumbar disc disease.

Intervention Selection

The assessment process should lead to an increasingly specific conceptualization of the patient's problems, factors contributing to their development and maintenance, and hypothesized mechanisms by which these factors exert their influence on pain, disability, and distress. Interdisciplinary discussions that focus on integration of professional perspectives on the patient in pain serve as the cornerstone of this process. Disagreements about the etiology of the patient's pain and associated problems are almost inevitable given the multiple perspectives represented among pain specialists. Broad or inclusive conceptual frameworks such as Flor's biobehavioral perspective or Kerns and Jacob's diathesis–stress model of chronic pain are potentially useful in resolving differences and finding consensus. Development of a clear conceptualization of the patient in pain is a necessary step in the development of an integrative and viable treatment plan.

In the case of Mr. C., the diathesis–stress framework was used to develop a detailed explanatory model for the patient's problems. The process of conceptualization began with a labeling of the multiple overlapping problems experienced by Mr. C. Primary among these were a high level of pain intensity, a high level of depressive symptoms, overreliance on the healthcare system (including prescription substance abuse), a high rate of absenteeism from work and a generally low level of functional activity, and chronic marital distress.

These problems were viewed as highly interrelated, that is, each problem domain was viewed as both a contributor to and a result of interactions with other problem domains. For example, consistent with a cognitive-behavioral mediation model of depression among chronic pain patients (Kerns & Haythornthwaite, 1988; Rudy, Kerns, & Turk, 1988), the experience of pain was viewed as a likely contributor to declines in activity and associated rewards for productive activity as well as declines in perceptions of self-control and self-efficacy. These behavioral and cognitive deficits are viewed as important contributors to the development of depressed mood and other symptoms of depression. Conversely, depression can further reinforce the experience of pain.

Specific pathogenic components of each domain were also specified in terms of their possible contributions to deficits or excesses in functioning in other domains. For example, declines in functioning and overall levels of activity were hypothesized to contribute to decreased conditioning, further exacerbating muscular vulnerabilities in the lower back and increasing baseline and stress-mediated muscle reactivity and associated nociception. Chronic marital dysfunction and specific maladaptive patterns of communication within the marriage almost certainly played an important role in the evolution of Mr. C.'s complex of problems. Noted during the evaluation was a generally high level of negative interactions between the couple. Such a pattern has specifically been documented to be associated with depressive symptom severity among chronic pain patients (Kerns, Haythornthwaite, Southwick, & Giller, 1990). In addition, there was evidence during the evaluation that Mrs. C. shared her husband's view of his pain as a medical problem. She consistently reinforced his anger and resentment toward healthcare providers, his continued efforts to find "the right doctor," and his use of pain medications. In the absence of other "positive" attention from his spouse for more adaptive cognition and coping efforts, these maladaptive responses on the part of Mr. C. were strongly reinforced by her attention and shared affective response.

From a neurobiological perspective it has been hypothesized that persistence of the experience of peripheral nociception may deplete stores of serotonin in the central nervous system that are important in the regulation of mood, sleep, and pain. It can be hypothesized that Mr. C., given a family history of depression, had an underlying neurobiological vulnerability that was activated by chronic pain and its deleterious effects on monoamine, specifically serotonin, regulation. This model, although highly speculative, may help explain the high coprevalence of chronic pain and depression (Romano & Turner, 1985), as is apparent in the case of Mr. C.

Finally, Mr. C.'s overuse of narcotics and benzodiazepines almost certainly had adverse effects on the patient's sleep, mental status, and mood. Although controversial, there is also reason to hypothesize that these medications, rather than promoting pain relief, contribute to the perpetuation of pain as a function of changes in brain monoamine regulation. Certainly the intermittent dispensing of medications by healthcare providers can be viewed as an effective reinforcer of use of the healthcare system and escalating efforts to obtain prescription medication. Interdisciplinary team discussions led to a consensus rehabilitation plan. The plan consisted of four primary components, to be completed on an outpatient basis: pharmacologic treatment by the team psychiatrist, structured cognitive-behavioral treatment by a team psychologist, couples therapy with a separate team psychologist, and a graded physical exercise and conditioning program to be developed and monitored by the physical therapy department. The plan was reviewed with Mr. and Mrs. C. and found to be consistent with their stated interests and specific goals.

Intervention Course and Problems in Carrying Out Interventions

Mr. C.'s treatment began on an outpatient basis within one week of discharge from the inpatient evaluation phase. Treatment was coordinated by the cognitive-behavioral pain management therapist, who was identified to Mr. and Mrs. C. as their "case manager and primary clinician." The plan called for multiple appointments with the psychiatrist, the two psychologists, and the physical therapist on a single day in order to minimize the inconvenience to the couple of coming to the medical center for appointments. Generally, the couple met briefly with the case manager/primary clinician upon their arrival at the medical center to plan for their other scheduled meetings. Following were appointments with each of the other three professionals. The last appointment of the day was again with the primary clinician, who reviewed the day's events, conducted a pain management session, and collaborated with the couple in the planning of the week's homework assignments.

Goals of pharmacologic intervention were: (a) treatment of major depressive disorder, including insomnia; (b) nonnarcotic pain relief; (c) reduced dependency on prescription medications; (d) education about the neurochemistry of pain and depression; and (e) overall consolidation and control of medical management efforts. The specific plan called for weekly, progressing to biweekly, sessions with the psychiatrist involving educational discussions, monitoring of symptoms and side effects, and prescription of medication use for the next intersession interval. Simultaneously, narcotic (oxycodone [Percocet]) and benzodiazepine (diazepam [Valium]) use was tapered until eliminated, and treatment with doxepin, a tricyclic antidepressant, was rapidly begun. The analgesic, antidepressant, and sleep-enhancing qualities of doxepin were emphasized.

Weekly outpatient cognitive-behavioral treatment followed the outline presented in Table 21.1. Considerable time was spent initially addressing Mr. C.'s unidimensional and somatic view of his pain. His fears about being without "painkillers" and about becoming an invalid were particularly targeted. Progress was made within the first 2 weeks in association with the successful tapering of Percocet use, and with the initial improvements in his sleep and activity level. Mr. C.'s skepticism and passive cooperation was replaced by a measure of excitement and investment in "taking charge of his life." Success in progressive muscle relaxation and the use of pleasurable imagery reinforced a developing positive self-management perspective. By week 5, Mr. C. reported a high level of satisfaction with his newfound coping skills and used the therapy session to review successful application of these skills over the last week. The final weeks emphasized constructive problem-solving during acute exacerbations of his chronic pain experience, and application of the same principles in managing stressful work, family, and social situations. Throughout the therapy program, progress toward social, recreational, and household goals was monitored, and weekly contracts for short-term steps were negotiated. Emphasis was placed on realistic goal setting and on the development of a constructive problem-solving perspective that took into account his back problem and associated pain.

Therapist goals for couples therapy were: (a) recommitment to the marriage; (b) improved communication, particularly listening skills; (c) increased participation in pleasurable activities together; and (d) active renegotiation of household responsibilities. With specific reference to pain, the therapist attempted to target coercive and aversive communication around pain and pain behaviors (e.g., withdrawal from household responsibilities). The process drew heavily on Jacobson's model of behavioral marital therapy (Jacobson & Margolin, 1979). As with the pain management therapy, couples therapy started slowly and, in fact, remained conflictual and difficult throughout.

Mr. C. began to participate more actively in household management, and the couple began to plan social activities that had declined in frequency. The couple's pattern of coercive and aggressive communication presented a particularly difficult challenge. Reevaluation after 10 weeks of treatment resulted in a decision to continue couples counseling with similar goals for another 3 months.

Dramatic gains in physical conditioning and exercise capacity are common outcomes of an active graded exercise program monitored by a physical therapist. Although Mr. C. was found to be grossly limited by pain complaints prior to treatment, implementation of a walking and isotonic exercise program, in addition to an aerobic

TABLE 21.1. Cognitive-Behavioral Treatment Protocol

Session 1
Introduction—rationale for program
   1. Concomitants of pain experince
   2. Focus on self-control and coping
Discussion of previous pain experience
   1. Set expectations for points of intervention
Review of assessment phase
   1. Begin reconceptualization—multiple factors affect pain experience
   2. Review existing coping strategies
Review treatment goals
   1. Behavioral contracting—short-term behavioral goal for upcoming week; rationale for "small steps"

Session 2
Review progress toward behavioral goal for week
   1. Focus on progress (positive), review problems
   2. Negotiate appropriate goal for next week
Rationale for relaxation training
   1. Discuss relationship between muscle tension and pain
   2. Review psychophysiologic data, when appropriate
   3. Learned behavior requiring practice
Relaxation training
   1. Sixteen-muscle-group progressive muscle relaxation
Home practice of relaxation
   1. Daily practice—duration, amount, ratings
   2. Ideal conditions

Session 3
Review progress toward behavioral goal for week
   1. Focus on progress (positive), review problems
   2. Negotiate appropriate goal for next week
Review home practice of relaxation
   1. Adherence—reinforce practice, not success
   2. Appropriate practice and time
   3. Problem solving around difficulties
Discussion of alternative modes of relaxation
   1. Multiple functions—decrease tension, distraction
Relaxation exercise
   1. Sixteen-muscle-group progressive muscle relaxation
Home practice of relaxation
   1. Review solutions from review of home practice

Session 4
Review progress toward goal for week
   1. Focus on progress (positive), review problems
   2. Negotiate appropriate goal for next week
   3. Discuss importance of planning activities around limitations and incorporating periods of rest/ relaxation
Review home practice of relaxation
Brief discussion of gate control theory
   1. Distraction/relaxation as ways of "closing gate"
   2. Situations that "open gate"
Concept of cognitive control—distractions
   1. Activities and thoughts as examples
Relaxation incorporating imagery
   1. Seven-muscle-group progressive muscle relaxation
   2. Patient-generated example of relaxing image
Home practice—generate ideas for "opening/closing gate"

(continued)

TABLE 21.1. *(Continued)* 457

Pain Management

Session 5

Review progress toward goal for week
   1. Discuss importance of working within limitations
Review home practice of relaxation with imagery
Discuss ideas on "opening/closing gate"
Expand on discussion of relationship among thoughts, emotions, activities, and pain experience
   1. Incorporate items from Pain Experience Scale
   2. Discuss coping self-statements
Rehearsal/application of coping self-statements
Relaxation exercise with imagery (seven-muscle-group progressive muscle relaxation)
Home application of coping self-statements at lower levels of pain

Session 6

Review progress toward treatment goals
   1. Focus on positives; problem solving around difficulties
   2. Set goal for coming week
Review use of coping self-statements at home
Incorporation of different strategies at different levels of pain—begin problem solving
Relaxation exercise with imagery
Home application of coping strategies at varying levels of pain
   1. Relaxation/distraction
   2. Imagery
   3. Coping self-statements
   4. Mental activities for attentional control

Session 7

Review progress toward behavioral goal for week
Review home use of coping strategies
Further problem solving around use of various coping strategies at varying levels of pain
Discussion of reinforcers of pain behaviors
   1. Medications
   2. Careful discussion of attention-eliciting behaviors and involvement of family members

Session 8

Review of conceptualization
   1. Incorporating of concrete examples from patient's experience
   2. Use of coping strategies as means of gaining or maintaining control
Problem-solving discussion around continuing problems
Review of progress to goals; formation of future goals
Review of follow-up
   1. Bimonthly "booster" sessions
   2. Posttreatment questionnaires and follow-up questionnaires
   3. Whom to contact, if necessary

fitness program, resulted in immediate and continued gains. Implementation of a self-monitoring procedure for recording progress further reinforced these efforts. Feedback regarding posture, body mechanics, and energy conservation, and proper means of lifting, bending, and similar movements, complemented the activity program.

Outcome and Termination

Reevaluation after the initial treatment phase documented significant gains in most of the targeted areas. Evaluation included extensive interviewing, including detailed assessment of behavioral goal accomplishment, completion of many of the questionnaires and inventories administered pretreatment, and completion of 2 weeks of self-monitored pain intensity ratings. The patient was videotaped completing the pain behavior observation protocol; both Mr. and Mrs. C. subsequently reviewed the tape with the primary clinician and physical therapist.

Besides pain reduction and improved functional capacity, Mr. C. no longer met criteria for a major depressive episode, had been free of narcotic and benzodiazepine use for 4 weeks, and had not been absent from work for the duration of treatment. Questionnaire data corroborated these clinical impressions and reports. They also documented increases in perceptions of self-control, declines in perceived interference of pain, and improvements in activity. No change in global marital satisfaction was noted, although both partners acknowledged a decrease in Mrs. C.'s frequency of negative responding to Mr. C.'s expressions of pain.

A new schedule of outpatient treatment was established that included weekly couples therapy, participation in a weekly outpatient pain support group, and 2-month follow-up appointments with the psychiatrist, the case manager/primary clinician, and the physical therapist.

Follow-Up and Maintenance

At one-year follow-up, Mr. and Mrs. C. participated in a thorough reevaluation that is a routine component of the Comprehensive Pain Management Center program. The assessment protocol generally included the same procedures as the pretreatment and posttreatment evaluations. Despite termination of formal contact with any of the therapists 3 months prior to the reevaluation appointments, Mr. C. continued to maintain treatment gains, including abstinence from narcotics, minimal depressive symptoms, low absenteeism, and substantial gains in social, recreational, and household activities. The couple reported a moderate improvement in global marital satisfaction. Mr. C. denied seeking alternate means of pain management for the prior year.

Mr. C. reported continued regular practice of stretching exercises and frequent walking for exercise. He also reported practicing muscle relaxation at least once per week. In addition, he stated that he used relaxation and his "coping plan" to deal with difficult situations on a routine basis. He attributed his improvements in his pain to a combination of factors, but emphasized the relaxation exercise and his improved physical conditioning. No further treatment or follow-up was planned.

Summary

Multidimensional models of chronic pain have displaced unidimensional somatosensory models that have failed in their efforts to foster effective treatment approaches. These contemporary models have encouraged attention to the broad experience of the *patient* in pain, including functional disability, affective distress, and associated clinical and social concerns. In particular, a wide range of psychological variables have been identified as contributors to the maintenance, if not the development, of the chronic pain experience. Assessment and treatment efforts that target these variables have proven useful in improving outcomes for an increasing proportion of chronic pain sufferers.

This chapter encouraged a theory-driven, hypothesis-testing approach to assessment of the patient that leads to the development of an integrative plan for intervention. A broad range of assessment strategies available to the pain management clinician were described. In the absence of a substantial empirical literature that can inform clinical decisions regarding treatment choices, clinicians were encouraged to base treatment decisions on assessment data and their evolving conceptualization of the patient's problems. Additional issues related to the engagement of patients, improving adherence and outcomes, and reducing relapse were discussed. A case example was offered in an effort to clarify the clinical process.

References

Boden, S. D., Davis, D. O., Dina, T. S., Patronis, N. J., & Wiesel, S. W. (1990). Abnormal magnetic-resonance scans of the lumbar spine in asymptomatic subjects. *Journal of Bone and Joint Surgery, 77-A,* 403–408.

Bradley, L. A., Haile, J. M., & Jaworski, T. M. (1992). Assessment of psychological status: Using interviews and self-report instruments. In D. C. Turk & R. Melzack (Eds.), *Handbook of pain assessment* (pp. 193–213). New York: Guilford.

Campbell, J. N., Raja, S. N., Cohen, R. H., Manning, D. C., Khan, A. A., & Meyer, R. A. (1989). Peripheral neural mechanisms of nociception. In P. D. Wall & R. Melzack (Eds.), *Textbook of pain* (pp. 22–45). New York: Churchill Livingstone.

Dworkin, R. H., Handlin, D. S., Richlin, D. M., Brand, L., & Vannucci, C. (1985). Unraveling the effects of compensation, litigation, employment on treatment response in chronic pain. *Pain, 23,* 49–59.

Endicott, J., & Spitzer, R. (1979). Use of the research diagnostic criteria and the schedule for affective disorders and schizophrenia to study affective disorders. *American Journal of Psychiatry, 136,* 52–56.

Flor, H., Birbaumer, N., & Turk, D. C. (1990). The psychobiology of chronic pain. *Advances in Behavior Research and Therapy, 12,* 47–84.

Flor, H., Fydrich, T., & Turk, D. C. (1992). Efficacy of multidisciplinary pain treatment centers: A meta-analytic review. *Pain, 49,* 221–230.

Flor, H., Miltner, W., & Birbaumer, N. (1992). Psychophysiological recording methods. In D. C. Turk & R. Melzack (Eds.), *Handbook of pain assessment* (pp. 169–190). New York: Guilford.

Flor, H., & Turk, D. C. (1984). Etiological theories and treatments for chronic low back pain. I: Somatic models and interventions. *Pain, 19,* 105–121.

Flor, H., & Turk, D. C. (1989). Psychophysiology of chronic pain: Do chronic pain patients exhibit symptom-specific psychophysiological responses? *Psychological Bulletin, 105,* 215–259.

Fordyce, W. E. (1976). *Behavioral methods for chronic pain and illness.* St. Louis: Mosby.

Fordyce, W. E., Fowler, R. S., & DeLateur, B. (1968). An application of behavior modification technique to a problem of chronic pain. *Behaviour Research and Therapy, 6,* 105–107.

Fordyce, W. E., Fowler, R. S., Lehmann, J. F., DeLateur, B. J., Sand, P. L., & Trieschmann, R. B. (1973). Operant conditioning in the treatment of chronic pain. *Archives of Physical Medicine and Rehabilitation, 54,* 399–408.

Hanson, R. W., & Gerber, K. E. (1990). *Coping with chronic pain: A guide to patient self-management.* New York: Guilford.

Haythornthwaite, J. A., Sieber, W. J., & Kerns, R. D. (1991). Depression and the chronic pain experience. *Pain, 46,* 177–184.

Heinrich, R. L., Cohen, M. J., Naliboff, B. D., Collins, G. A., & Bonnebakker, A. D. (1985). Comparing physical and behavior therapy for chronic low back pain on physical abilities, psychological distress, and patient perceptions. *Journal of Behavioral Medicine, 8,* 61–78.

Jacobson, N. S., & Margolin, G. (1979). *Marital therapy: Strategies based on social learning and behavior exchange principles.* New York: Brunner/Mazel.

Jensen, M. P., Turner, J. A., Romano, J. M., & Karoly, P. (1991). Coping with chronic pain: A critical review of the literature. *Pain, 47,* 249–284.

Keefe, F. J., & Block, A. R. (1982). Development of an observational method for assessing pain behavior in chronic low back pain patients. *Behavior Therapy, 13,* 363–375.

Keefe, F. J., Caldwell, D. S., Williams, D. A., Gil, K. M., Mitchell, D., Robertson, D., Robertson, C., Martinez, S., Nunley, J., Beckham, J. C., & Helms, M. (1990a). Pain coping skills training in the management of osteoarthritic knee pain: A comparative study. *Behavior Therapy, 21,* 49–62.

Keefe, F. J., Caldwell, D. S., Williams, D. A., Gil, K. M., Mitchell, D., Robertson, D., Robertson, C., Martinez, S., Nunley, J., Beckham, J. C., & Helms, M. (1990a). Pain coping skills training in the management of osteoarthritic knee pain. II: Follow-up results. *Behavior Therapy, 21,* 435–447.

Kerns, R. D., Finn, P., & Haythornthwaite, J. (1988). Self-monitored pain intensity: Psychometric properties and clinical utility. *Journal of Behavioral Medicine, 11,* 71–82.

Kerns, R. D., & Haythornthwaite, J. (1988). Depression among chronic pain patients: Cognitive-behavioral analysis and effect on rehabilitation outcome. *Journal of Consulting and Clinical Psychology, 56,* 870–876.

Kerns, R. D., Haythornthwaite, J., Rosenberg, R., Southwick, S., Giller, E. L., & Jacob, M. C. (1991). The Pain Behavior Check List (PBCL): Factor structure and psychometric properties. *Journal of Behavioral Medicine, 14,* 155–167.

Kerns, R. D., Haythornthwaite, J., Southwick, S., & Giller, E. L., Jr. (1990). The role of marital interaction in chronic pain and depressive symptom severity. *Journal of Psychosomatic Research, 34,* 401–408.

Kerns, R. D., & Jacob, M. C.(1992). Assessment of the psychosocial context of the experience of chronic pain. In D. C. Turk & R. Melzack (Eds.), *Handbook of pain assessment* (pp. 235–253). New York: Guilford.

Kerns, R. D., & Jacob, M. C. (1993). Psychological aspects of back pain. In S. Newman & M. Shipley (Eds.), *Psychological aspects of rheumatic disease* (pp. 337–356). London: Bailliere Tindall.

Kerns, R. D., & Jacob, M. C. (in press). Toward an integrative diathesis–stress model of chronic pin. In A. J. Goreczny & M. Hersen (Eds.), *Handbook of health and rehabilitation psychology.* New York: Plenum.

Kerns, R. D., Southwick, S., Giller, E. L., Jr., Haythornthwaite, J. A., Jacob, M. C., & Rosenberg, R. (1991). The relationship between reports of pain-related social interactions and expressions of pain and affective distress. *Behavior Therapy, 22,* 101–111.

Kerns, R. D., Turk, D. C., Holzman, A. D., & Rudy, T. E. (1986). Comparison of cognitive-behavioral and behavioral approaches to the outpatient treatment of chronic pain. *Clinical Journal of Pain, 1,* 195–203.

Kerns, R. D., Turk, D. C., & Rudy, T. E. (1985). The West Haven–Yale Multidimensional Pain Inventory (WHYMPI). *Pain, 23,* 345–356.

Letham, J., Slade, P. D., Troup, J. D. G., & Bentley, G. (1983). Outline of a fear-avoidance model of exaggerated pain perception. I. *Behaviour Research and Therapy, 21,* 401–408.

McCaul, K. D., & Malott, J. M. (1984). Distraction and coping with pain. *Psychological Bulletin, 95,* 516–533.

McCracken, L. M., Zayfert, C., & Gross, R. T. (1992). The Pain Anxiety Symptoms Scale: Development and validation of a scale to measure fear of pain. *Pain, 50,* 379–381.

Melzack, R. (1975). The McGill Pain Questionnaire: Major properties and scoring methods. *Pain, 1,* 277–299.

Melzack, R., & Wall, P. (1965). Pain mechanisms: A new theory. *Science, 50,* 971–979.

Moore, J. E., & Chaney, E. F. (1985). Outpatient group treatment of chronic pain: Effects of spouse involvement. *Journal of Consulting and Clinical Psychology, 53,* 326–334.

Nicholas, M. K., Wilson, P. H., & Goyen, J. (1991). Comparison of operant-behavioural and cognitive-behavioural group treatment with and without relaxation training, for chronic low back pain. *Behaviour Research and Therapy, 29,* 225–238.

Onghena, P., & Van Houdenhove, B. (1992). Antidepressant-induced analgesia in chronic non-malignant pain: A meta-analysis of 39 placebo-controlled studies. *Pain, 49,* 205–221.

Phillips, H. C. (1987). The effects of behavioural treatment on chronic pain. *Behaviour Research and Therapy, 25,* 365–377.

Pilowsky, I., & Barrow, C. G. (1990). A controlled study of psychotherapy and amitriptyline used individually and in combination in the treatment of chronic intractable, "psychogenic" pain. *Pain, 40,* 3–19.

Romano, J., & Turner, J. (1985). Chronic pain and depression: Does the evidence support a relationship? *Psychological Bulletin, 97,* 18–34.

Romano, J. M., Turner, J. A., Friedman, L. S., Bulcroft, R. A., Jensen, M. P., Hops, H., & Wright, S. F. (1992). Sequential criterion analysis of chronic pain behaviors and spouse responses. *Journal of Consulting and Clinical Psychology, 60,* 777–782.

Rosenstiel, A. K., & Keefe, F. J. (1983). The use of coping strategies in low back pain patients: Relationship to patient characteristics and current adjustment. *Pain, 17,* 33–40.

Rudy, T. E., Kerns, R. D., & Turk, D. C. (1988). Chronic pain and depression: Toward a cognitive-behavioral mediation model. *Pain, 35,* 129–140.

Steinberg, G. G. (1982). Epidemiology of low back pain. In M. Stanton-Hicks & R. A. Bogs (Eds.), *Chronic low back pain* (pp. 1–13). New York: Raven Press.

Stone, C. E. (1984). The lifetime economic costs of rheumatoid arthritis. *Journal of Rheumatology, 11,* 819–827.

Turk, D. C., & Kerns, R. D. (1983). Conceptual issues in the assessment of clinical pain. *International Journal of Psychiatry in Medicine, 13,* 52–68.

Turk, D. C., & Kerns, R. D. (1985). Assessment in health psychology: A cognitive-behavioral perspective. In P. Karoly (Ed.), *Measurement strategies in health psychology* (pp. 335–372). New York: Wiley.

Turk, D. C., Kerns, R. D., & Rosenberg, R. (1992). Effects of marital interaction on chronic pain and disability: Examining the down side of social support. *Rehabilitation Psychology, 37,* 259–274.

Turk, D.C., & Melzack, R. (1992). *Handbook of pain assessment.* New York: Guilford.

Turk, D. C., Meichenbaum, D. H., & Genest, M. (1983). *Pain and behavioral medicine: A cognitive-behavioral perspective.* New York: Guilford.

Turk, D. C., & Rudy, T. E. (1991). Neglected topics in the treatment of chronic pain patients—relapse, noncompliance, and adherence enhancement. *Pain, 44,* 5–28.

Turner, J. A. (1982). Comparison of group progressive-relaxation training and cognitive-behavioral group therapy for chronic low back pain. *Journal of Consulting and Clinical Psychology, 50,* 757–765.

Turner, J. A., & Clancy, S. (1988). Comparison of operant-behavioral and cognitive-behavioral group treatment for chronic low back pain. *Journal of Consulting and Clinical Psychology, 56,* 261–266.

Turner, J. A., Clancy, S., McQuade, K. J., & Cardenas, D. D. (1990). Effectiveness of behavior therapy for chronic low back pain: A component analysis. *Journal of Consulting and Clinical Psychology, 58,* 573–579.

Von Korff, M., Dworkin, S. F., LeResche, L., & Kruger, A. (1988). An epidemiologic comparison of pain complaints. *Pain, 32,* 173–183.

22

The Violent Patient

Grant T. Harris and Marnie E. Rice

Description of the Problem

One of the most worrisome parts of any mental health clinician's job is the fear that a client will be violent. Clinicians often bear special legal responsibility and authority to detect those people (among their clientele) who present a risk of imminent violence and to prevent it through treatment or incapacitation. There is also often public outrage when psychiatric patients or ex-patients commit seriously violent acts, and a large share of that outrage is often directed toward clinicians who treated the client. The outrage is based on an assumption that if a client hurts some innocent person, the clinician must have been negligent in failing to notice the danger, failing to provide treatment, or failing to have or keep the dangerous client locked up.

Is this public outrage over violence committed by clients justified? Until very recently, there has been little evidence that clinicians possess the expertise to identify violent clients. The literature shows that clinicians' unaided judgments under such circumstances are insensitive to differences in base rates, do not agree with one another, do not make use of special technical information, and are not different from judgments made by laypeople (Quinsey & Ambtman, 1979). Such findings have led to the widespread belief that violence is fundamentally unpredictable (except for age and sex, perhaps) and that clinicians should never describe anyone as violent or likely to be violent (Melton, Petrila, Poythress, & Slobogin, 1987; Simon, 1987). There is also little evidence that any form of treatment can reduce the likelihood of violence, a situation that led to a belief that "nothing works" and that violent persons (e.g., sex offenders, psychopaths) are untreatable. Finally, almost nothing is known about specifiable immediate dynamic precursors to violence, either in the environment or in the individual (Quinsey & Walker, 1992). Thus, those who treat and

Grant T. Harris and **Marnie E. Rice** • Mental Health Centre, Penetanguishene, Ontario, L0K 1P0 Canada.

Handbook of Prescriptive Treatments for Adults, edited by Michel Hersen and Robert T. Ammerman. Plenum Press, New York, 1994.

supervise potentially violent individuals have had little other than intuition to guide them. In such a situation, a high error rate is inevitable, and the human cost of errors is very high.

Despite the lack of expertise in identification and treatment, violent clients must be managed. We argue that there are sufficient data to inform rational assessment and treatment decisions about such persons, and that clinicians can play an important role in making society a safer place. The purpose of this chapter is to provide a system to guide clinicians in identifying, assessing, treating, and supervising that small group of individuals who present a significant danger in the community. We believe our system applies to clients of private practitioners as well as to people being released by mental health facilities, by correctional institutions, and by institutions for the mentally handicapped. As much as possible, our advice is grounded in the available empirical literature, but that literature is admittedly incomplete. Consequently, we propose a system that is fairly comprehensive but not always as empirically based as we would like.

The low base rate of violent behavior in almost all clinical groups means that a clinician who predicts that individual clients will be violent will necessarily make more errors than a clinician who never makes such a prediction (Monahan, 1981; Quinsey, 1980). There are, however, exceptions to this general rule. There are some clients who exhibit violent behavior that is sufficiently frequent and serious that they can be regarded as characteristically violent. Most such individuals are institutionalized, either in prison after being convicted of criminal offenses or in psychiatric hospitals subject to civil commitment. The task of providing prescriptive treatment for violent institutionalized clients is a daunting one. We have described methods to deal with persons who are violent in institutions in detail elsewhere (Harris & Rice, 1992; Rice, Harris, & Quinsey, 1994; Rice, Harris, Varney, & Quinsey, 1989; Rice, Helzel, Varney, & Quinsey, 1985; see also Wong, Slama, & Liberman, 1987). There exist a variety of pharmacologic, behavioral, and organizational techniques with effectiveness that is empirically established. The empirical literature supports a multifaceted approach to minimizing violence in institutions.

First, behavioral and pharmacologic interventions can be prescribed for the small minority of persons who exhibit frequent violent behavior inside institutions. Behavior therapy procedures that provide predetermined consequences both for aggressive acts and for prosocial, cooperative behavior are strongly indicated. Behavioral techniques should be supported by cognitive-behavioral therapy to teach anger management techniques, and by ward-wide token economies. Pharmacologic treatments prescribed to treat clients' psychiatric disorders as described in other chapters of this book will sometimes be effective in reducing violent behavior. In addition, other drugs may be effective in reducing violence. The client characteristics that predict a positive drug response are largely unknown (Eichelman, 1988), however, and long observation periods are necessary to determine whether a drug has been effective (Harris, 1989). Second, institutional staff members require training in verbal strategies when dealing with upset clients and in other methods used to prevent and control violence. Third, administrators must arrange contingencies for staff and clients that promote the generalization of skills acquired in training and therapy to the ward environment. In the rest of this chapter we concern ourselves with the identification and treatment of clients whose violence occurs (or might occur) in the community.

Many individuals whose violence in the community may be sufficiently frequent and serious to be predictable are those persons who exhibit chronic violence toward their spouses, parents, or children. Many clinicians may have such persons among their clientele. The chapter following this one covers this issue specifically and at length. In this chapter we will consider those clients who have already committed at least one violent act, usually against a non–family member, and for whom there is concern about the potential for serious future violence. For purposes of this chapter, we will consider as violence serious criminal acts against persons: for example, assault, sexual assault, armed robbery, and homicide. The issue of which individuals are likely to be violent has long been of considerable concern in the area of clinical decision making. The issue most commonly arises when releasing offenders on parole or from indeterminate sentences, or when releasing persons from forensic psychiatric facilities.

Statistical approaches to the prediction of violence are more accurate than unaided clinical judgments (Faust & Ziskin, 1988), but at this time few statistical approaches have achieved practical utility in predicting violence even among incarcerated offenders after release (Nuffield, 1982). This failure is due partly to the relatively low base rate of violent recidivism even among released felons. We have reported, however, some promising findings among mentally disordered male offenders with long follow-up periods. Among such men, all of whom had already committed at least one serious offense, the base rate of violent recidivism exceeded 30% (Harris, Rice, & Quinsey, 1993).

Assessment Strategies

Actuarial Risk Appraisal

We propose a three-step system to identify, treat, and supervise dangerous clients. According to this system, judgments about the likelihood of violence are "anchored" by a statistical estimate, which may be adjusted at the second stage using clinical judgment. This anchoring/adjustment process has been termed "structured discretion" (Gottfredson, Wilkins, & Hoffman, 1978). The first step is a statistical appraisal of risk. As discussed above, research on the prediction of violence supports the use of an actuarial method with individuals who already have committed at least one serious offense. Our own research (Harris, Rice, & Quinsey,1993) on male mentally disordered offenders identified 12 variables that, when combined, bore a strong and clinically useful relationship to violent reoffense. The variables and their individual correlations with violent recidivism are listed in Table 22.1 (all coefficients, $p < .05$). The variables, as used in the instrument, are all static inasmuch as they were all scored from historical data available just after the violent offense that resulted in the patient's admission to a secure hospital.

Most variables are straightforward, but a few require some careful evaluation: diagnosis, assessment of alcohol problems, severity of school maladjustment, and degree of psychopathy. As used in our research, diagnosis was relatively straightforward: merely deciding whether, based on clinical records, the client met the DSM-III criteria for any form of schizophrenia or any personality disorder. Alcohol problem was the sum of several dichotomous variables: whether the client had an adolescent or adult drinking problem, whether alcohol was involved in the current or a prior offense, and whether he had a drinking problem at the time of the index offense. The most difficult component was the 20-item revised Psychopathy Checklist (Hare, 1991), which in our study was scored exclusively from detailed psychosocial histo-

**TABLE 22.1. Univariate Correlations
Between Each Predictor Variable and
Violent Recidivism**[a]

Variable	r
1. Psychopathy Checklist score	.330
2. Elementary school maladjustment	.313
3. Never married	.181
4. Schizophrenia (DSM-III)	−.174
5. Separation from parents before age 16	.252
6. Victim injury in index offense	−.163
7. Criminal history—property offenses	.200
8. Female victim-index offense(s)	−.107
9. Age at index offense	−.258
10. Personality disorder (DSM-III)	.258
11. Failure on prior conditional release	.241
12. Alcohol abuse score	.126

[a]Missing data deleted pairwise.

ries, although it is often scored based on information gained from both an interview and the client's clinical record.

The relationship between scores on the instrument and violence is shown in Figure 22.1. By far the best single predictor was the Psychopathy Checklist—a finding replicated by others (Hare & McPherson, 1984; Rice, Harris, Lang, & Bell, 1990; Rice, Harris, & Cormier, 1992; Serin, Peters, & Barbaree, 1990). The variables included in the actuarial prediction instrument were selected from a larger set using multiple regression and cross-validation on a sample of 618 serious offenders from a maximum security psychiatric institution. Variable weights, however, were not those computed

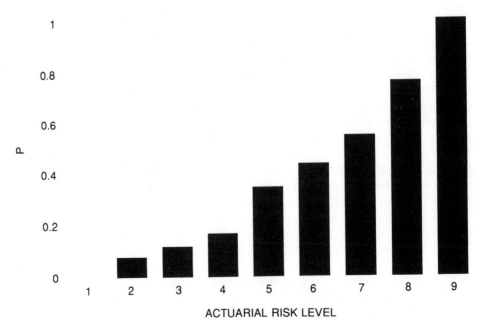

Figure 22.1. Probability of violent recidivism as a function of nine levels of actuarially determined risk.

by multiple regression analyses. Rather, to minimize shrinkage, weights were based on a univariate method described by Nuffield (Harris, Rice, & Quinsey, 1993). The nine categories on the abscissa of Figure 22.1 were made by dividing the range of possible scores on the instrument into nine equal-size bins. Steps were taken in the development of the actuarial tool to ensure its validity upon further cross-validation. Its value lies in the nearly monotonic increase, as a function of actuarial score, in the proportion of subjects who committed another violent act upon release. The probability of violent recidivism ranged from zero to unity. The value of such an instrument lies in its application to new cases: offenders of high risk can be identified for intensive treatment and supervision (or, in the worst cases, for long-term detention); offenders of low risk can be identified for release and less intensive supervision; and the intensity of service can reflect the degree of risk.

There are several implications of these results. First, using only these static factors it was possible to identify individuals whose risk of violence was high. The probability of violence, in a 7-year follow-up, exceeded 50% among the three subgroups with the highest scores. Second, some of the violent recidivism occurred long after release. This means that an intervention (or its effects) must persist over many years. It also means that a clinician usually need not worry that the treatment have an instant effect. Treatment that takes a long time or the teaching of skills that improve gradually with in vivo practice are viable options. Third, there are a few individuals whose risk of violence is so great that it would be unrealistic to expect any intervention to lower it to an acceptable level. Such persons may be candidates for incapacitation. Fourth, there are also some individuals whose risk of further violence is so low that no intervention can realistically be expected to lower it further. Thus, in a world of limited treatment resources, it is sensible to incapacitate the highest-risk individuals if possible and then to apportion intervention (treatment and supervision) resources in direct relation to the level of risk of violence.

Although this advice may seem pessimistic, we suggest, along with others (e.g, Simon, 1987) that all reasonable efforts be made to incapacitate very high risk individuals through civil commitment, interderminant dangerous offender/predator legislation, or denial of conditional release. When all these avenues are closed and a clinician becomes responsible for such a person in the community, considerable resources should be spent on developing and monitoring a treatment/supervision plan. In our experience, clients at the highest risk levels quickly violate supervision conditions, sometimes by committing relatively minor offenses (which may permit reincarceration), or abandon therapy completely by moving away.

How should assessment proceed? First, it must be stressed that no evidence exists to suggest that serious criminal violence can be predicted among individuals who have not already committed at least one violent act. There are also no data pertaining to women. However, among men who have committed at least one violent offense, the first step in prediction involves a consideration of static risk predictors. Although we have obtained good results with the actuarial risk prediction instrument described here, we present it primarily to show the potential value in such an approach. Until the instrument has been shown to yield useful prediction results with other populations, it could be directly applied only to populations very similar to those on which it was validated. However, because the Psychopathy Checklist and certain other variables (most notably, past offense history, age, alcohol problems, and marital status) have been found to predict violent recidivism in studies of other groups of offenders, they should certainly be given consideration as a starting point for any assessment of dangerousness.

Grant T. Harris and
Marnie E. Rice

Dynamic Risk Appraisal

The second stage of the three-step procedure used to manage violent clients is the identification of dynamic (changeable or potentially changeable) clinical factors related to the risk of future violence. In making any judgment about the likelihood of violence, the clinician should use relevant dynamic factors to adjust the previously derived actuarial anchor point. Because of their demonstrated relationship to violent recidivism, those factors that indicate high actuarially determined risk and that are changeable should be the first factors to consider again in assessment at the second stage. Thus, a change in diagnosis, marital status, or alcohol use since the commission of previous violent acts might indicate a change in risk of future violence. Some of these issues are addressed in the subsections that follow. As discussed in the next section, however, the treatments suggested by noting these factors are limited, and evidence of their efficacy in preventing violence is nonexistent.

The dearth of empirical work on other personal characteristics that predict violence and on the personal characteristics that, when altered, lead to reductions in violence means that clinicians' choices of assessment and treatment methods cannot be guided completely by empiricism. We propose that assessment and treatment be guided by a theory constructed for each client. There are several personal characteristics one might employ in such a theory. Several have at least some empirical support and might be changeable with treatment; we will now discuss these.

Substance Abuse. As mentioned above, there is evidence linking substance (especially alcohol) abuse to violence (Bushman & Cooper, 1990; Hillbrand, Foster, & Hirt, 1991; Lewis, Robins, & Rice, 1985; Lindqvist, 1986; Rice, Harris, Lang, & Bell, 1990; Ross & Lightfoot, 1985; Swanson, Holzer, Ganju, & Jono, 1990). The best approach to assessment is a self-report method that evaluates the amount of drinking in a wide variety of social and affective contexts (Annis & Davis, 1986; Morey, Skinner, & Blashfield, 1984). There is evidence that those alcoholics who confine their drinking to a subset of contexts are significantly better treatment candidates than are those who drink in all contexts (Annis & Davis, 1986). Clinicians also recognize the problems inherent in relying exclusively on self-reported drinking and sometimes use urine alcohol testing as an adjunct measure.

Criminal Lifestyle or Personality. Although their relationship to violent crime has rarely been investigated, some personal characteristics are associated with criminal conduct in general, and may be related to violent offenses in some clients. Some of these characteristics are attitudes and values: procriminal values and attitudes unfavorable toward convention (Rice, Harris, Lang, & Bell, 1990; Rice, Harris, & Cormier, 1992). Some characteristics appear to reflect an antisocial or criminal lifestyle such as sensation seeking, irresponsibility, insincerity, manipulativeness, having criminal associates (Weiner & Wolfgang, 1989; Wolfgang, Thornberry, & Figlio, 1987), avoiding gainful employment, having a parasitic lifestyle, and lacking realistic goals. Some seem to be skill deficits, including immature moral reasoning, poor relationships with spouse and family, and poor social problem-solving skills. Finally, some appear to reflect criminal personality: callousness (lack of empathy), lack of remorse, selfishness, impulsivity, affective shallowness, poor behavioral controls, and insensitivity to aversive consequences. Many of these qualities or characteristics are those identified by Hare (1991) and Cleckley (1976) as psychopathic. On closer examination, it is not always clear whether these characteristics are best regarded as reflecting an antisocial lifestyle or an underlying personality. Regardless, they may represent sensible assessment and treatment targets for violent clients.

Our advice, therefore, is that a clinician working with a violent client consider which of the characteristics mentioned above appear to be involved in the particular case and employ relevant assessments. Candidate assessment targets are antisocial values and attitudes (see Andrews, 1980); vocational adjustment (see Ethridge, 1968; Manuele, 1983); social problem solving (see Arbuthnot & Gordon, 1986; Platt, Scura, & Hannon, 1973; Ross & Fabiano, 1985; Spivak, Platt, & Shure, 1976); moral reasoning (see Arbuthnot & Gordon, 1983; Colby & Kohlberg, 1987; Goldstein & Glick, 1987); empathy (see Hogan, 1969; Lomis & Baker, 1985); insensitivity to punishment (see Newman, 1987; Newman & Kosson, 1986; Newman, Patterson, & Kosson, 1987); and sensation seeking. In addition to Hare's (1991) Psychopathy Checklist, the 55-item Level of Supervision Inventory (LSI; Andrews, Kiessling, & Kominos, 1983) identifies offender aspects important for both risk appraisal and identification of clinical needs. The LSI comprises items in several categories including criminal history, interpersonal adjustment, vocational and recreational activities, substance abuse, and education. It has demonstrated considerable predictive validity for general criminal behavior (Bonta & Motiuk, 1985), but not for violence.

Deviant Sexuality. Violent offenses, especially offenses against women and children, are frequently sexual in nature. There is substantial evidence that extra-familial child molesters (Harris, Rice, Quinsey, Chaplin, & Earls, 1992; Quinsey, 1986) and rapists (Harris et al., 1992; Quinsey, 1984) tend to have sexual preferences different from those of non–sex offenders. Rapists, when compared to nonrapists, prefer violent and coercive sex to consenting sex. Men who molest children, compared to other men, show higher sexual arousal to stories of sex with children, even when physical violence is used to gain the child's compliance (Harris et al., 1992). In addition, deviant sexual preferences are related to sexual and violent recidivism among sex offenders (Rice, Harris, & Quinsey, 1990; Rice, Quinsey, & Harris, 1991). Phallometric assessment produces the best measure of sexual preferences in offender populations (Harris et al., 1992).

Anger. In several studies of the problems exhibited by mentally disordered offenders and other psychiatric patients (Harris, Hilton, & Rice, 1993; Harris & Rice, 1990; Rice & Harris, 1988), anger was among the most commonly endorsed problems. Anger has been reported to contribute to aggression (Rule & Nesdale, 1976), problematic personal relationships (Deffenbacher, Demm, & Brandon, 1986; Novaco, 1975, 1983), and domestic violence (Patterson, 1985). Methods for measuring anger are of two sorts: behavioral coding and self-report. Systems for coding naturalistic observations have been combined with diaries for recording affect and attributions made about the behavior of others (Biaggio, 1987; Novaco, 1975; Patterson, 1985). More commonly, paper and pencil questionnaires have been used to evaluate the frequency and severity of self-reported angry behaviors (Buss & Durkee, 1957; Siegel, 1985, 1986; Spielberger et al., 1985; see also Novaco & Welsh, 1989).

Positive Schizophrenic Symptoms. Recent large epidemiologic studies have suggested a causal link between mental illness and violent behavior (Lindqvist &

Allebeck, 1990; Link, Andrews, & Cullen, 1992; Monahan, 1992; Swanson, Holzer, Ganju, & Jono, 1990). In those studies, persons at that time experiencing positive schizophrenic symptoms (hallucinations and, especially, delusions) reported significantly more violent conduct than persons not reporting such symptoms. In the Link et al. (1992) study, it is also noteworthy that, although significant, the effect sizes were small compared to the effects of self-reported alcohol abuse on violent behavior. It is clear, therefore, that clinicians need more than diagnostic tools. Rather, measures of symptom type and severity that are sensitive to treatment are required. Fortunately, an expanded version of the Brief Psychiatric Rating Scale (Overall & Gorham, 1962; see also Lukoff, Liberman, & Nuechterlein, 1986) can be used to generate an index of psychosis that is easily administered, has acceptable psychometric properties, and is sensitive to treatment. In addition, clinicians should attend carefully to paranoid statements in which a client blames a particular individual for his troubles. However (and consistent with studies showing the importance of *current* symptomatology), our research (Rice & Harris, 1992) has shown that schizophrenics exhibited lower recidivism than other offenders (most of whom qualified for a diagnosis of personality disorder), and those schizophrenics who had committed violent offenses in response to paranoid delusions were no more violent upon release years later than those who had committed offenses for other reasons.

Physical Conditions. Although the evidence is limited, it has been suggested that paroxysmal disorders (assessed by EEG; Devinsky & Bear, 1984) or other brain anomalies (measured by computed tomographic scan; Langevin et al., 1985; see also Adams, Meloy, & Moritz, 1990) contribute to the etiology of some violent behavior. In addition, there is suggestive evidence that violent behavior is mediated by an imbalance in any of several neurotransmitters including serotonin, norepinephrine, and gamma-aminobutyric acid (GABA) (Eichelman, 1987, 1988, 1992; Virkkunen & Linnoila, 1993). It is unclear, however, whether such imbalances could be detected with blood or cerebrospinal fluid assays. Finally, there is a very wide array of other medical conditions, ranging from heart disease to genetic disorders (e.g., Huntington's disease) to hypoglycemia, that are thought to contribute to aggression in some cases (Tardiff, 1992). It is sensible to arrange a medical examination for any violent client.

Other Considerations. Many of the assessment strategies discussed have depended primarily on self-report. Clinical experience and common sense lead to the conclusion that many violent individuals underreport and in other ways minimize the severity of their own violent and aggressive behavior. It is clinically sound to elicit collateral sources of information about past and current aggression, and a wise clinician would doubt the truthfulness of any client who would refuse permission for the collection of such information. We will return to this point in our discussion of supervision of violent clients.

Many clinicians who work with offenders regard ongoing denial and minimization as important treatment targets (e.g., Marshall & Barrett, 1990), based on the theory that an offender who refuses to acknowledge violent crimes or who excuses and rationalizes them is more likely to repeat them. Unfortunately, however, good general measures of denial and minimization do not exist (Hanson, Cox, & Woszczyra, 1991). The use of validity scales from standardized personality tests has been reported to detect denial in child abusers (Lanyon, Dannenbaum, & Brown, 1991). There are some assessments for attitudes about sexual aggression (Burt, 1980; Pollock & Hashmall, 1991), but as yet none of these has yielded evidence of predictive validity for violent offenses.

Once the dynamic factors have been considered, the clinician (and client) possess a theory to guide intervention. Thus, for example, the identification of poor anger control, alcohol abuse, and EEG abnormalities as the only previously listed dynamic factors relevant to violence present in a given case essentially constitutes a theory that these factors *caused* the past violence (perhaps triggered by situational factors outside the individual's control) and, without intervention, could cause violence again. These factors, then, are the appropriate targets for treatment. Resources allocated to intervention should be related to the client's estimated (anchored with actuarial prediction and adjusted based on dynamic factors) level of risk.

The actuarial instrument described in Table 22.1 and Figure 22.1 used exclusively static predictor variables. As empirical evidence accumulates, it is to be expected that dynamic variables will be incorporated into actuarial predictions. Under such circumstances, actuarial risk would not be fixed and dynamic variables would be high-priority treatment targets or targets for supervision.

Intervention Strategies

Evidence for Prescriptive Interventions

As the foregoing implies, violence is not a disorder, a syndrome, or a disease, and there is no reason to suppose that all aggressive behaviors have common etiologies, pathways, or prognoses. Consequently, it cannot be expected that any particular treatment will reduce or eliminate violent behavior in general. Rather, interventions must be selected prescriptively. Unfortunately, however, there is little evidence to indicate which interventions provided for dangerous clients in the community, regardless of their characteristics, reduce violent behavior. Indeed, there is evidence that clinicians do not even agree about what treatments are indicated for violent clients (Quinsey & Maguire, 1983).

Eichelman (1987, 1988, 1992) reviewed mostly uncontrolled reports that some benzodiazepines (which enhance activity in the GABA neurotransmitter system), neuroleptics (which block activity in the dopamine system), lithium and beta-adrenergic drugs (which block activity in the norepinephrine system) and serotonergic drugs (which enhance activity in the serotonin system) all decrease aggressive behavior in violent clients with a wide variety of diagnoses. There are a few reports that anticonvulsant drugs (Eichelman, 1992) may reduce aggression in some violent clients. Antiandrogens are used to reduce sexual drive in sex offenders (Berlin, 1983).

Unfortunately, however, this literature does not provide a complete basis for prescriptive treatment. The evidence is far from conclusive that drugs were causally related to reductions in violence; there is little evidence that the clients whose violence was decreased after taking the drugs described had abnormal neurotransmitter levels, electroencephalographic findings, or testosterone levels in the first place. The reported effectiveness of the drugs was often unrelated to diagnosis: the drugs were often reported to be effective for diagnoses for which they would not otherwise be prescribed (for example, lithium for conduct disorder; propranolol for organic impairment; haloperidol for conduct disorder, dementia, and mental retardation). A sensible strategy would be to follow the prescriptive course described in earlier chapters of this book in providing pharmacologic treatment for identified disorders. Deteriorating mood, worsening symptoms, increasing hostility, and decreasing social contact may all indicate greater likelihood of violence—and, as indicated in earlier chapters, they may be cues for changing medication or improving compliance. Beyond that, however, it would be extremely difficult to determine what drugs, if any, would be effective in decreasing aggression of clients who remain dangerous.

The empirical evidence for nondrug treatment is, unfortunately, no better. For example, although there is strong evidence supporting a link between violence and alcohol abuse, there is little evidence that any treatments for alcohol abuse are effective in reducing alcohol intake (see Rice, Harris, Quinsey, & Cyr, 1990) and no evidence that treatment for alcohol abuse reduces violence. Similarly, there are some reports that cognitive-behavioral treatment of child molesters reduces recidivism (Marshall & Barbaree, 1988), but just as many report that the same treatment failed to reduce sexual recidivism (Furby, Weinrott, & Blackshaw, 1989; Quinsey, Harris, Rice, & Lalumière, 1993; Rice, Quinsey, & Harris, 1991). Finally, there are reports that social skills training and cognitive-behavioral training in social problem solving are associated with reductions in criminal recidivism (Goldstein & Glick, 1987; Ross & Fabiano 1985), but no demonstration that violent recidivism is affected.

The reader should not conclude that it is pointless to treat violent clients. Rather, one should conclude that the field is insufficiently developed to provide much empirical support for any particular form of drug or nondrug treatment. One hopes that this is a temporary situation and that powerfully effective treatment effects will soon be demonstrated. In the interim, however, the field does have some sensible advice to offer based on meta-analytic studies of the effects of intervention on criminal recidivism in general.

Andrews et al. (1990; see also Gendreau & Ross, 1987) reviewed a large number of controlled studies of treatment for criminal offenders and identified important principles of effective treatment:

1. *Risk.* More intensive service should be provided to higher-risk cases. (We would qualify this statement by noting that there are a few individuals whose histories of violence are so serious and whose risk of violent recidivism is so high that preventive detention should be the goal).
2. *Needs.* Service should target *criminogenic* needs: that is, personal characteristics that contribute to the commission of crime. Known criminogenic targets include changing antisocial attitudes, promoting familial affection and supervision, increasing self-control, replacing lying and aggression with prosocial skills, reducing substance abuse, and improving interpersonal and vocational skills. Inappropriate targets include self-esteem, increasing the cohesiveness of antisocial peer groups, and focusing on intrapsychic forces not empirically linked with criminality.
3. *Style of treatment.* Behavioral or cognitive-behavioral treatments consistently produced larger treatment effects than other styles of treatment (nondirective, punitive, insight-oriented, psychodynamic, evocative and relationship-dependent therapies). There is no guarantee that these same principles apply to treatment for violent (as opposed to general criminal) behavior. However, in the absence of evidence to the contrary, we propose that these principles be applied in selecting treatments for violent clients.

Suggestive evidence supporting these principles in treating violent individuals comes from our study of the effects of an evocative, insight-oriented therapeutic community program on the violent recidivism in a group of mentally disordered offenders (Rice, Harris, & Cormier, 1992). In this study we compared the violent recidivism of violent offenders who participated for an average of 5 years in a therapeutic community program to that of matched offenders who were imprisoned. Overall, participation in the treatment program had little effect. For psychopaths, however, participation in the program was associated with significantly *more* violent recidivism, whereas for nonpsychopaths treatment was associated with significantly *less* violent recidivism. Psychopathy was operationally defined as a score of at least 25 on the revised Psychopathy Checklist (Hare, 1991). Our study showed that treatment effectiveness can be powerfully affected by some risk or needs factors; we speculate that, for offenders who were initially antisocial and represented relatively high risks, insight-oriented, peer-operated therapy was strongly contraindicated. The human cost of inappropriate service might be worse than complete ineffectiveness: violence might be made more likely.

Selecting Optimal Intervention Strategies

As described above, those factors identified as having caused past violence or as contributing to the likelihood of future violence will be the targets of prescriptive treatment. Candidate factors include poor anger control, social skill/problem-solving deficits, antisocial values, substance abuse, lack of empathy, irresponsibility, impulsivity, immature moral reasoning, minimization of past and present difficulties, deviant sexual preferences, neurotransmitter imbalance, and paroxysmal disorders. In addition to treatment, supervision should be provided for those changeable environmental factors that, in the clinician's theory about the individual case, contribute to violence. Such environmental factors include availability of weapons, large amounts of unstructured time, criminal or violent friends, access to potential victims, and use of alcohol or other drugs.

The therapist should arrange community supervision for all but very low risk cases. As much as possible, the therapist should negotiate an agreement with the client proscribing certain behaviors and prescribing others. For example, a man with a history of violent sexual assaults on children might be expected to agree to stay away from schoolyards, avoid being alone with any child, and refrain from possessing child pornography—and furthermore, to contract to volunteer at a senior citizen's center, maintain steady employment, and take antiandrogen medication. In addition to making such agreements, the therapist should verify they are being kept by obtaining independent confirmation. Consequences should be applied for both meeting and failing to meet the conditions. We will discuss some of the difficulties in supervising high-risk clients in the later section on relapse prevention.

We suggest that the prescriptive approach to treatment for violent clients rarely depends on diagnosis; rather, prescriptions target criminogenic factors regardless of diagnosis. There may, however, be instances in which the treatment that is delivered to address a criminogenic need must be tailored according to the diagnosis of the client. For example, there is good reason to believe that confrontational techniques frequently used in the treatment of substance abusers would be countertherapeutic for schizophrenic substance abusers (Mueser, Bellack, & Blanchard, 1992). Future research may reveal additional instances of differential responses to treatment.

However, for now, clinicians who treat violent clients (of any diagnosis) are on the most solid empirical ground if they employ a behavioral or cognitive-behavioral approach. Insofar as they use behavioral methods and nonpunitive authority and seek to promote generalization, the treatments recommended to reduce the risk of violence in the community are similar to those indicated for the reduction of violence in institutions discussed briefly at the start of this chapter.

We will now describe three programs that exemplify the desirable therapeutic characteristics. These examples were chosen because the programs were shown to reduce antisocial behavior, had an articulated theoretical rationale, have been shown to yield proximal changes in theoretically relevant measures, and have been described in sufficient detail that a clinician could determine that the treatment is being delivered with integrity (see Quinsey, 1990).

Andrews (1980) described experimental tests of differential association theory, which asserts that criminal conduct is learned through exposure to criminal thought and behavior patterns in intimate personal relationships. Andrews manipulated the social environment of offenders by exposing them to anticriminal, prosocial models in long-term discussion groups. Groups were composed of offenders and volunteers. Group leaders were instructed to encourage open, warm, and frank communication during discussions about the functions of rules, rationalizations for law breaking, and a social learning view of self-control. Andrews (1980) showed that, compared with controls, offenders who participated in the treatment showed large attitude changes and reductions in recidivism.

The Sex Offender Treatment and Evaluation Project (Marques, Day, Nelson, Miner, & West, 1989; Marques, Day, Nelson, Miner, & West, 1993) is an ambitious evaluation of intensive cognitive-behavioral treatment for sex offenders. Inmate volunteers are randomly assigned either to treatment or no treatment, and there is also an untreated nonvolunteer group. The treatment, an intensive two-year relapse prevention program, is a prescriptive approach in which clients learn to anticipate and cope with relapse (see Laws, 1989). In both assessment and treatment, the steps in the chain of events that leads to sexual assault are identified and changed. Lifestyle factors (e.g., substance abuse), cognitive distortions, skill and knowledge deficits (e.g., relaxation skills, sexual knowledge, social skills), and deviant sexual arousal are considered. Offenders in the program have shown improvement on pre-post measures of these factors. There is also evidence that these measures are related to recidivism. Unfortunately, there are as yet no data to show that these in-treatment changes result in lower rates of sexual offending. Preliminary data do suggest that completing treatment indicates a favorable prognosis: men who complete treatment seem to have lower rates of sexual recidivism than untreated controls, whereas men who drop out of treatment show higher rates (Marques et al., 1993).

Ross, Fabiano, and Ewles (1988) tested a theory that criminal offenders exhibit deficits in a variety of cognitive skills, especially those associated with social adaptation. According to such a view, crime is a maladaptive response to ordinary situations that is characterized by concreteness, egocentricity, and impulsiveness. An extensive training program (Ross & Fabiano, 1985) that used behavioral techniques to teach social skills, problem solving, logical reasoning, prosocial values, assertiveness, negotiation skills, perspective taking, and interpersonal problem solving was evaluated using an experimental design in which offenders were randomly assigned to conditions. Compared to an alternative treatment (and to no treatment), participation in the intensive training program was associated with reductions in criminal recidivism.

There are several problems that often arise in working with violent clients. The most evident issue is the safety of the therapist and, if the therapy is done in a group setting, other clients. Therapists must consider the possibility that the client will be violent during a session or will, under exceptional circumstances, seek out the therapist outside of the therapy sessions. The latter may be more likely if the therapist has applied negative consequences (e.g., reporting a parole violation) for noncompliance with agreed-upon terms of supervision. Although the probability of a client's stalking the therapist is remote, therapists should recognize the possibility and be clear that visits or calls to the therapist's home and unscheduled visits are unwelcome (Carmel, Dietz, & Eichelman, 1991). The therapist should consider safety in arranging the office and should ensure that assistance is nearby and that someone is close enough to hear if a client becomes loud and threatening. Use of a personal alarm device should also be considered, especially if the therapist is alone with the client.

Another difficulty is that antisocial clients tend to benefit least from treatment (Gertsley et al., 1989; Shea, Widiger, & Klein, 1992; Woody, McLellan, Luborsky, & O'Brien, 1985) and are likely to resist it. It is rare in our experience that persons who have behaved violently in the community participate in treatment without some coercion. The person attends because he believes it will hasten his release from an institution, or, if he is already in the community, because he has a probation order requiring him to attend. Although there is some evidence that treatment is no less effective when clients do not volunteer (Maletzky, 1980), there are some distinct differences between those who volunteer and those who are under coercion. Whereas volunteers for treatment are often grateful, many coerced clients see themselves as unjustly treated and complain that therapy is a waste of time. Indeed, it is common for these clients to see themselves as victims of a corrupt justice system. It is not surprising, therefore, that dropout rates tend to be high. There is evidence that the highest-risk cases are most likely to drop out (Abel, Mittelman, Becker, Rathner, & Rouleau, 1988) and that those who drop out of treatment have rates of recidivism higher than either treated clients or untreated controls (Marques et al., 1993).

The therapist should collect information to ascertain whether treatment is received as delivered. Thus, blood levels of prescribed drugs should be determined. Similarly, objective measures of skills, attitudes, personality, or knowledge should be obtained for therapies intended to alter these constructs. A variety of administrative, interpersonal, educational, and behavioral methods to improve treatment adherence have been described (Meichenbaum & Turk, 1987). The available research suggests that, without the use of such methods, antisocial clients will exhibit the lowest levels of treatment adherence (Meichenbaum & Turk, 1987).

A related problem concerns the aforementioned strong tendency of violent clients to minimize and deny responsibility for their offenses. As mentioned, there are no good measures of denial and there are no treatments known to be effective in reducing denial and minimization. Also, however, there is certainly no evidence that reductions in denial are followed by reductions in violence. In the face of continued and complete denial, however, cognitive therapies have little to offer, and the therapist may have to use behavioral treatments that do not rely on the client's admitting a problem.

Another hurdle that sometimes appears in the treatment of violent persons, especially those who deny responsibility, is anger on the part of the therapist (Dubin, 1989). Although such feelings, often said to be the result of countertransference reactions, can arise in any therapeutic encounter, they are more common and less easily resolved with antisocial clients. When there is more than one therapist present when such a situation occurs, the co-therapist can take control of the group to allow the angry therapist time to cool down and consider the next response. When he or she is working alone, the therapist who repeatedly becomes angry may have no choice but to terminate and possibly to refer the client elsewhere.

Lying is a defining characteristic of antisocial personality. The idea that a therapist cannot trust what the client says is a difficult one for those used to working with most other client groups. The therapist must keep in mind the need to corroborate what the client says with collateral information.

Group therapists sometimes have a difficult task ensuring that prosocial rather than antisocial values are promoted. Sometimes the client with the most antisocial attitudes is also the most assertive and vocal, and there is a danger that he may gather considerable support for his views among the others. Unless the therapist (or, preferably, therapists) intervenes quickly when other clients support rather than refute antisocial views expressed by a dominant client, there is a real possibility of doing harm (Andrews, 1980). Group leaders can present prosocial models, but when they are outnumbered by those espousing antisocial beliefs, they must be active if they are to keep group consensus on their side.

Therapists must be clear from the outset about the limits of confidentiality. Most clinicians are aware of their legal obligation to report specific threats to a third party (see Simon, 1987). Therapists will have to explain the local reporting laws but should also try to obtain the clients' consent to share additional information with parole officers, family members, peers, and workers with other agencies involved. As mentioned, it is often sensible and justifiable to make treatment contingent on clients' giving such consent. Regardless of any agreement made regarding confidentiality, judgment frequently must be exercised in determining whether there is sufficient risk to someone to warrant warning the police or potential victim. Consulting with colleagues on such matters is vital.

Finally, working with dangerous persons is stressful. Regardless of how well a therapist assesses risk and treats dangerous persons, some clients will commit violent acts, and when they do, the actions of the therapist will be called into question. Therapists must be prepared for such eventualities by keeping adequate records showing that they exercised competent judgment and provided treatment that would be judged reasonable by their peers.

Relapse Prevention

The key to preventing relapse (violent behavior) lies in effective communication among all involved in a particular case. This requires that the client's consent be obtained early in treatment permitting the therapist to discuss the client's behavior during follow-up not only with the client, but also with others. Usually, follow-up contact will be arranged at a gradually deceasing frequency as the client and the therapist accumulate evidence that the client is using skills gained in treatment to avoid high-risk behaviors and situations. Such sessions should focus on how the client has been spending his time and determining whether the client has successfully avoided those high-risk situations that could have been avoided, what techniques have been used to cope with unavoidable high-risk situations, and how similar situations might be better handled. Family members or the client's peers (with prior agreement) should be contacted to report on the client's behavior. Contact with probation officers or other agencies involved can reveal that the client, perhaps unwittingly, may be headed down a path leading to relapse.

Case Illustration

Case Description

Mr. Michaels is a 25-year-old white man. His parents separated when he was 2, his mother remarried soon after, and Mr. Michaels was raised as an only child. Nothing is known about his natural father. Both the mother and the stepfather had substance abuse and other psychological problems, and his stepfather has an extensive criminal history. Mr. Michaels was both beaten and neglected by his parents, and between the ages of 6 and 9, he claims, he was sexually abused by a male relative. He has always had a good relationship with his maternal grandmother. At age 11 he became a ward of the Children's Aid Society after a series of break-ins and attempts to run away from home. Until he was 20 he lived in more than 30 foster homes and psychiatric and correctional institutions. He was a mediocre student but he finished grade 9, quitting school at 16. He reported having been a binge beer drinker, a regular user of cannabis, and an occasional user of amphetamines. He also reported a short series of glue-sniffing episodes in his late teens. His longest job lasted 6 months. As an adult, the longest period he spent outside institutions was 10 months, during which he reported that he engaged in some criminal activity (to be described) for which he was not apprehended.

He had numerous admissions to psychiatric facilities. Typically, these followed episodes of slashing his wrists or arms, and his stays were short. Diagnoses included antisocial personality disorder, borderline personality disorder, schizophrenia, obsessive-compulsive disorder, and substance abuse. Psychological testing showed him to be of average intelligence. He presented symptoms of anxiety, depression, paranoia, obsessions, compulsions, and panic. His criminal history involved acquisitive crimes. In correctional institutions he typically sought placement in segregation or dissociation because of psychological difficulties.

At the time of his referral to us, he was nearing completion of a 4-year sentence for two break-ins and one count of arson. With the alleged intention of destroying evidence of a theft, he had set a fire in a school. Although damage was extensive, no one was hurt. Toward the end of his incarceration, he asked for psychological help and was reported to have shown a strong motivation to change and went along willingly with treatment. He received training in anger management, problem-solving skills, and relaxation, as well as individual psychotherapy. It was noted that he had made progress in each program in which he participated. However, in the course of treatment, he revealed disturbing information and his therapists referred him to us.

Mr. Michaels revealed that, although he had been caught only once, he had actually set several other fires (including fires in other schools). He also revealed that, during the most recent episode, he had masturbated shortly before setting the fire, although he denied being sexually aroused by the fire itself. He also stated that one of his two recent break-in convictions had been sexually motivated. Mr. Michaels had considered a young woman to be his girlfriend, although she had repeatedly rejected his advances. He said that he was obsessed with violent sexual fantasies about her and that in his fantasy he broke into her home, tied up her family members, and forced them to perform sadistic sexual acts on one another. When he did break into the woman's home, it was unoccupied and he took only a picture of her. He also reported violent fantasies of raping and, sometimes, killing her. He said he was worried that, without help, he might actually do so. Studies of sexual murderers, showing that they are often obsessed with their sadistic sexual fantasies over a long time before carrying them out (Quinsey, 1988), suggested to us that his concerns were valid.

Assessment

Mr. Michaels was transferred from the penitentiary to a locked ward of our psychiatric facility with 2 months left in his sentence. Upon his referral we reviewed his history and completed an actuarial appraisal of risk. Mr. Michaels scored in the fourth-highest category (see Figure 22.1). When dynamic risk factors were considered (to be outlined), we saw no reason to adjust the risk score downward. Mr. Michaels was a person for whom intensive treatment and supervision were indicated. Those treatment components specific to sexual deviance would be provided by us, and any others were to be obtained from other clinicians in our community.

On the basis of his self-admission that the breaking and entering at the home of his supposed girlfriend was sexually motivated, and the report of antecedent autoerotic activity involved in the firesetting, we offered Mr. Michaels a phallometric assessment of his sexual preferences. Mr. Michaels's assessment revealed a significant arousal to rape descriptions compared with descriptions of consenting sex. His responses were clearly deviant. Mr. Michaels also received an experimental arson assessment in which penile responses are monitored to audiotaped descriptions of consenting heterosexual activity, neutral scenes (involving neither sex nor arson), and various firesetting stories. These data showed that, in comparison with nonoffenders and other firesetters, Mr. Michaels showed an elevated response to stories that described fire as sexually arousing.

Intervention Selection

The first component of Mr. Michaels's treatment was a "Problem Identification" group. The purpose of this group was to identify those factors that contributed to his most recent offenses: the breaking and entering at the home of his "girlfriend," and the fire. The result was an explanation or theory of the offenses that was agreed on by all group members, especially by Mr. Michaels himself, and an intervention plan to address those changeable contributing factors that had not yet been resolved.

The following explanation or theory of Mr. Michaels's offenses was developed:

1. *Prior victimization.* Mr. Michaels attributed some of his sexual difficulties to having been sexually assaulted several times by male family members when he was a child. He also reported that he committed sexual assaults on younger boys in his family. More generally, Mr. Michaels attributed some of his anger and resentment toward society to physical and emotional abuse he suffered from his mother and stepfather.
2. *Attitudes toward others.* Mr. Michaels described a very antisocial background and lifestyle. He reported a childhood with negligent parents who engaged

heavily in crime and substance abuse. Mr. Michaels's own adolescence was marked by many property offenses and particularly antisocial values and attitudes.

3. *Negative feelings*. Mr. Michaels described himself as generally angry and frustrated at the time of his offenses. He reported considerable resentment toward his girlfriend and her family because of their rejection of him. He also reported that he was angry at society for restricting his freedom and "always telling me what to do." During the group discussions it also became clear that, at the time of the offenses, Mr. Michaels had no job and engaged in little constructive activity; he reported that the offenses also occurred because he was bored.

4. *Substance abuse*. Mr. Michaels reported abusing alcohol and street drugs heavily around the time of the offenses. The role, however, of such substance abuse in explaining the offenses was unclear.

5. *Opportunity*. As mentioned, Mr. Michaels had opportunity to commit the offenses because he had very little to occupy his time. In addition, he habitually kept track of the movements of his girlfriend's family (by calling them frequently on the phone). He also was checking the doors of the school late at night. These two patterns of behavior presented him with the specific opportunities to commit the offenses.

6. *Planning*. Mr. Michaels readily agreed that he planned both offenses.

7. *Lack of alternative partners and social deficits*. Mr. Michaels described himself as sexually frustrated and socially isolated at the time of the offenses. An examination of Mr. Michaels's recent history lent support to this idea; it appeared that he was less likely, and less tempted, to engage in some forms of antisocial behavior when he was in a mutually consenting sexual relationship.

8. *Sexual preferences*. Mr. Michaels exhibited sexual arousal to firesetting themes in his laboratory assessment. Although he reported having set other fires, Mr. Michaels strongly denied that these acts had any sexual component. He attributed them rather to anger and boredom. Mr. Michaels also exhibited high sexual arousal to rape scenarios. With regard to this assessment, Mr. Michaels agreed that he was sexually aroused in response to themes in which he exerted physical and emotional power over women. Examination of his recent behavior (which involved writing anonymous suggestive notes to a female staff member and making sexual advances to female clients) suggested to all group members (including Mr. Michaels) that interest in power and control continued to dominate his sexuality.

After developing this theory or explanation, the group members also examined which factors were still a problem for Mr. Michaels. The group agreed that, by participating in several skills-oriented therapy programs while in prison (as described), he had made progress toward resolving his anger toward society, his social skills deficits, and his antisocial values and attitudes. In addition to these strengths, the therapists noted that Mr. Michaels had been remarkably honest. He revealed several criminal offenses for which he had never been caught: sexual assaults on young boys, other fires, and burglaries. He was also honest in admitting his deviant sexual fantasies, and in saying that he had no intention of refraining from property offenses, although he intended to avoid arrest. All agreed, however, that Mr. Michaels still had further to go in reducing his level of anger, building social skills, and reducing antisocial attitudes and values, and, more important, that all the other crucial explanatory problems remained unresolved. The therapists (the present authors) and members of the group expressed concern that Mr. Michaels was at risk of violence while these problems were unresolved. Mr. Michaels agreed to a clinical plan that included the following components:

1. Attend school or a job full time. Mr. Michaels described two possibilities he was pursuing with local agencies with the help of his case manager.
2. Reduce intake of drugs and alcohol. Mr. Michaels did not agree to abstain absolutely but he did agree that heavy abuse would likely result in criminal behavior. He agreed to attend Alcoholics Anonymous meetings and to seriously consider entering a nearby residential substance abuse treatment program.
3. Avoid criminal associates. Mr. Michaels reported that he recognized the danger of "hanging around" with many of his criminal friends. Unfortunately, because of her own serious substance abuse problems, it was agreed that Mr. Michaels's mother represented a risk for him. Mr. Michaels reported that he planned not to live with her, and he and his case manager began a search for suitable housing. Also, it was generally agreed that continued contact with a group program offered by the institution's outpatient department would provide prosocial models and noncriminal associates.
4. Change deviant sexual preferences. Mr. Michaels agreed to enter a behavior therapy program to alter his sexual preferences.
5. Attend relapse prevention groups. Mr. Michaels agreed to attend our relapse prevention groups designed to further reduce the likelihood of reoffense.
6. Accept supervision. Mr. Michaels agreed to have this plan energetically supervised by a case manager from our institution's outpatient services department.

Intervention Course and Problems in Carrying Out Interventions

By the end of the series of Problem Identification groups, Mr. Michaels was just days away from his release date. Nevertheless, he agreed to stay as a voluntary patient until the treatment was completed. He remained an inpatient for 2 more months until he and his case manager located an apartment in a cooperative housing development, where Mr. Michaels was to assist with landscaping in summer and snow removal in winter. After discharge he continued treatment on an outpatient basis. At the time of his release, Mr. Michaels agreed that he would not initiate any contact with the woman whose home he had broken into. He gave consent for us to let her know that he was being released (in a small community such as ours, it was no surprise to find that she had already heard this). With his permission, we also obtained her agreement to let us know should he initiate any contact.

The first few sessions of individual treatment to alter Mr. Michaels's sexual preferences were devoted to developing a series of audiotapes representative of his deviant fantasies. Several scenes were created relating violent rape fantasies and scenes of sexual arousal in response to firesetting. These stimuli were then used in a course of aversion therapy designed to decrease arousal to deviant stimuli while maintaining or enhancing arousal to appropriate stimuli (in Mr. Michaels's case, stimuli describing consenting sexual acts with women). As in the usual course of aversion sessions, we began with covert sensitization, in which aversive imagery was paired with the deviant fantasies (Abel, Blanchard, & Becker, 1978). Because Mr.

Michaels was unsuccessful in altering his relative arousal levels using the covert sensitization paradigm, we proceeded to an aversion paradigm using his choice of a noxious odor (Earls & Castonguay, 1989). The therapy continued until his preferences were within the normal range. If Mr. Michaels's actuarial risk had been higher, we would also have proposed the use of an antiandrogen drug, at least temporarily to help control intrusive sadistic sexual fantasy.

Another treatment offered Mr. Michaels to reduce the likelihood of sexual offending was a relapse prevention group (Laws, 1989). Although there is as yet no evidence of its efficacy for sexual behavior, there is at least suggestive evidence in support of such an approach when applied to alcohol problems, and the techniques as applied to sexual offending are basically similar. Following this approach, the group members (including Mr. Michaels) conducted an in-depth examination of Mr. Michaels's high-risk situations, the emotional and situational triggers likely to initiate a lapse, how lapses would lead to relapse, and how to break the chain at each step (Pithers, Marques, Gibat, & Marlatt, 1983). In Mr. Michaels's case, the triggers included feelings of boredom, anger, and rejection. Mr. Michaels rehearsed appropriate ways to react to female rejection. Mr. Michaels's problem-solving and anger management skills were enhanced and practiced in specific situations relevant to his relapse process. Mr. Michaels was also enrolled in recreational floor hockey and basketball programs at the local YMCA to encourage constructive use of his leisure time and to increase the likelihood that he would find suitable prosocial friends. Social skills training techniques were also used to teach Mr. Michaels how to handle meetings with previous criminal associates.

Mr. Michaels was enrolled in a chef's course at a local community college. Because his alcohol intake was drastically reduced without further intervention, he did not enroll in the treatment program, but it was noted that this option could be pursued at a later date.

Outcome and Termination

To our knowledge, Mr. Michaels has not behaved violently in his 10 months of freedom. We will not, however, regard him as a treatment success until he has maintained a lifestyle free of violent offenses for many more years. Although he completed the formal part of our program when he finished the 20 sessions of relapse prevention, he has gone on to a follow-up and maintenance schedule, and we regard him as still in treatment.

Follow-Up and Maintenance

In this phase, Mr. Michaels's appointments are on a diminishing schedule, beginning weekly for 3 months and decreasing to monthly during the following year. We obtained Mr. Michaels's permission to contact his grandmother, with whom he has promised to have regular contact. We also have permission to contact his grandmother and case manager to monitor his substance abuse. For as long as the resources are available, Mr. Michaels has been assigned a case manager who visits him regularly at his residence and is helping him to work out any difficulties he has regarding school and employment, as well as gathering more accurate information about how he spends his time than is possible to ascertain by simply telephoning him. With assertive case management, a case worker will continue to visit him or be available for crisis situations until Mr. Michaels and the worker are confident that it is no longer necessary. Both private practitioners and those working for government agencies would be well advised to provide such assertive case management, arrange for its provision by another agency involved in the case, or at least spend some effort lobbying for its provision in cases such as that of Mr. Michaels.

Although treatment apparently has been successful so far, Mr. Michaels's risk of violence (as determined by static predictors) was only moderately high. His Psychopathy Checklist (Revised) score was a moderate 19. If his risk level (and Psychopathy Checklist score) had been much higher (in the highest category shown in Figure 22.1, for example), no treatment and supervision plan could have been expected to reduce the risk to a safe level. In such rare cases, we advocate the use of preventive detention—even, if there are no better alternatives, through civil commitment.

Summary

In this chapter we reviewed how clinicians assess the risk of violence clients present in the community, identify potential dynamic antecedents to violent offending, and select promising treatments to reduce the likelihood of violence. We reviewed the very limited literature on the effectiveness of prescriptive interventions for adults in reducing the risk of violence. Because that literature is so sparse, we broadened our scope to consider interventions that have shown promise for antisocial, but not necessarily violent, behavior in general. We suggested how clinicians can arrive at a theory that identifies the factors that contributed to a given violent act by a client, and which treatments can be used to address each contributing factor. Problems that frequently arise in carrying out interventions with violent persons include clients' resistance, denial, minimization, and lying. Assuring comprehensive supervision, adequate information about client behaviors, safety of the therapist, and peer support for the therapist are also important. Relapse can best be prevented by constructing a plan that includes identification of likely high-risk situations, training and practice in methods to avoid them, and supervision to ensure that the plan is followed. The principles described here were illustrated in the case of Mr. Michaels, a man whose history suggested he was at considerable risk for committing a violent offense in the community.

ACKNOWLEDGMENT. The authors thank V.L. Quinsey for helpful comments on an earlier version of this chapter.

References

Abel, G. G., Blanchard, E. B., & Becker, J. V. (1978). An integrated treatment program for rapists. In R. T. Rada (Ed.), *Clinical aspects of the rapist* (pp. 161–214). New York: Grune & Stratton.

Abel, G. G., Mittelman, M. S., Becker, J. V., Rathner, J., & Rouleau, J. L. (1988). Predicting child molesters' response to treatment. *Annals of the New York Academy of Sciences, 528,* 223–234.

Adams, J. J., Meloy, J. R., & Moritz, M. S. (1990). Neuropsychological deficits and violent behavior in incarcerated schizophrenics. *Journal of Nervous and Mental Disease, 178,* 253–256.

Andrews, D. A. (1980). Some experimental investigations of the principles of differential association through deliberate manipulations of the structure of service systems. *American Sociological Review, 45,* 448–462.

Andrews, D. A., Kiessling, J. J., & Kominos, S. (1983). *The Level of Supervision Inventory (LSI-6): Interview and scoring guide.* Toronto: Ontario Ministry of Correctional Services.

Andrews, D. A., Zinger, I., Hoge, R. D., Bonta, J., Gendreau, P., & Cullen, F. T. (1990). Does correctional treatment work? A clinically relevant and psychologically informed meta-analysis. *Criminology, 28*, 369–404.

Annis, H. M., & Davis, C. S. (1986). Self-efficacy and prevention of alcoholic relapse: Initial findings from a treatment trial. In J. B. Baker & D. Cannon (Eds.), *Addictive disorders: Psychological research on assessment and treatment* (pp. 88–112). New York: Praeger.

Arbuthnot, J., & Gordon, D. A. (1983). Moral reasoning development in correctional intervention. *Journal of Correctional Education, 34*, 133–138.

Arbuthnot, J., & Gordon, D. A. (1986). Behavioral and cognitive effects of a moral reasoning development intervention for high-risk behavior-disordered adolescents. *Journal of Consulting and Clinical Psychology, 54*, 208–216.

Berlin, F. S. (1983). A biomedical perspective and a status report on biomedical treatment. In J. G. Greer & I. R. Stuart (Eds.), *The sexual aggressor: Current perspectives on treatment* (pp. 83–123). New York: Van Nostrand Reinhold.

Biaggio, M. K. (1987). Therapeutic management of anger. *Clinical Psychology Review, 7*, 663–675.

Bonta, J., & Motiuk, L. L. (1985). Utilization of an interview-based classification instrument: A study of correctional halfway houses. *Criminal Justice and Behavior, 12*, 333–352.

Burt, M. R. (1980). Cultural myths and supports for rape. *Journal of Personality and Social Psychology, 38*, 131–150.

Bushman, B. J., & Cooper, H. M. (1990). Effects of alcohol on human aggression: An integrative research review. *Psychological Bulletin, 107*(3), 341–354.

Buss, A. H., & Durkee, A. (1957). An inventory for assessing different kinds of hostility. *Journal of Consulting Psychology, 21*, 343–349.

Carmel, H., Dietz, P., & Eichelman, B. (1991). Dangerous patients and your safety. *Audio-Digest Psychiatry, 20*.

Cleckley, H. (1976). *The mask of sanity.* St. Louis: Mosby.

Colby, A., & Kohlberg, L. (1987). *The measurement of moral judgment, Vol. 1: Theoretical foundations and research validation.* Cambridge, UK: Cambridge University Press.

Deffenbacher, J. L., Demm, P. M., & Brandon, A. D. (1986). High general anger: Correlates and treatment. *Behaviour Research and Therapy, 24*, 481–489.

Devinksy, O., & Bear, J. (1984). Varieties of aggressive behavior in temporal lobe epilepsy. *American Journal of Psychiatry, 141*, 561–566.

Dubin, W. R. (1989). The role of fantasies, countertransference, and psychological defenses in patient violence. *Hospital and Community Psychiatry, 40*, 1280–1283.

Earls, C. M., & Castonguay, L. G. (1989). The evaluation of olfactory aversion for a bisexual pedophile with a single-case multiple baseline design. *Behavior Therapy, 20*, 137–146.

Eichelman, B. (1987). Neurochemical bases of aggressive behavior. *Psychiatric Annual Report, 17*, 371–374.

Eichelman, B. (1988). Toward a rational pharmacotherapy for aggressive and violent behavior. *Hospital and Community Psychiatry, 39*, 31–39.

Eichelman, B. (1992). Aggressive behavior: From laboratory to clinic. *Archives of General Psychiatry, 49*, 488–489.

Ethridge, D. A. (1968). Pre-vocational assessment of rehabilitation potential of psychiatric patients. *American Journal of Occupational Therapy, 22*, 161–167.

Faust, D., & Ziskin, J. (1988). The expert witness in psychology and psychiatry. *Science, 241*, 501–511.

Furby, L., Weinrott, M. R., & Blackshaw, L. (1989). Sex offender recidivism: A review. *Psychological Bulletin, 105*, 3–30.

Gendreau, P., & Ross, R. R. (1987). Revivification of rehabilitation: Evidence from the 1980s. *Justice Quarterly, 4*, 349–407.

Gertsley, L., McLellan, A. T., Alterman, A. I., Woody, G. E., Luborsky, L., & Prout, M. (1989). Ability to form an alliance with the therapist: A possible marker of prognosis for patients with antisocial personality disorder. *American Journal of Psychiatry, 146*, 508–512.

Goldstein, A. P., & Glick, B. (1987). *Aggression replacement training: A comprehensive intervention for aggressive youth.* Champaign, IL: Research Press.

Gottfredson, D. M., Wilkins, L. T., & Hoffman, P. B. (1978). *Guidelines for parole and sentencing.* Toronto: Lexington.

Hanson, R. K., Cox, B., & Woszczyna, C. (1991). Assessing treatment outcome for sexual offenders. *Annals of Sex Research, 4*, 177–208.

Hare, R. D. (1991). *The Hare Psychopathy Checklist—Revised.* Toronto: Multi-Health Systems.

Hare, R. D., & McPherson, L. M. (1984). Violent and aggressive behavior by criminal psychopaths. *International Journal of Law and Psychiatry, 7*, 35–50.

Harris, G. T. (1989). The relationship between neuroleptic drug dose and the performance of psychiatric patients in a maximum security token economy program. *Journal of Behavior Therapy and Experimental Psychiatry, 20*, 57–67.

Harris, G. T., Hilton, N. Z., & Rice, M. E. (1993). Patients admitted to psychiatric hospital: Presenting problems and resolution at discharge. *Canadian Journal of Behavioural Science, 25*, 267–285.

Harris, G. T., & Rice, M. E. (1990). An empirical approach to classification and treatment planning for psychiatric inpatients. *Journal of Clinical Psychology, 46*, 3–14.

Harris, G. T., & Rice, M. E. (1992). Reducing violence in institutions: Maintaining behavior change. In R. D. Peters, R. J. McMahon, & V. L. Quinsey (Eds.), *Aggression and violence throughout the lifespan* (p. 263–284). Newbury Park, CA: Sage.

Harris, G. T., Rice, M. E., & Quinsey, V. L. (1993). Violent recidivism of mentally disordered offenders: The development of a statistical prediction instrument. *Criminal Justice and Behavior, 20*, 315–335.

Harris, G. T., Rice, M. E., Quinsey, V. L., Chaplin, T. C., & Earls, C. (1992). Maximizing the discriminant validity of phallometric assessment data. *Psychological Assessment, 4*, 502–511.

Hillbrand, M., Foster, H. G., & Hirt, M. (1991). Alcohol abuse, violence, and neurological impairment. *Journal of Interpersonal Violence, 6*, 411–422.

Hogan, R. (1969). Development of an empathy scale. *Journal of Consulting and Clinical Psychology, 33*, 307–316.

Langevin, R., Bain, J., Ben-Aron, M. H., Coulthard, R., Day, D., Handy, L., Heasman, G., Hucker, S. J., Purins, J. E., Roper, V., Russon, A. E., Webster, C. W., & Wortzman, G. (1985). Sexual aggression: Constructing a predictive equation. In R. Langevin (Ed.), *Erotic preference, gender identity, and aggression in men: New research studies* (pp. 39–62). Hillsdale, NJ: Erlbaum.

Lanyon, R. I., Dannenbaum, S. E., & Brown, A. R. (1991). Detection of deliberate denial in child abusers. *Journal of Interpersonal Violence, 6*, 301–309.

Laws, D. R. (Ed.). (1989). *Relapse prevention with sex offenders*. New York: Guilford.

Lewis, C. E., Robins, L., & Rice, J. (1985). Association of alcoholism with antisocial personality in urban men. *Journal of Nervous and Mental Disease, 173*, 166–174.

Lindqvist, P. (1986). Criminal homicide in Northern Sweden 1970–1981: Alcohol intoxication, alcohol abuse and mental disease. *International Journal of Law and Psychiatry, 8*, 19–37.

Lindqvist, P., & Allebeck, P. (1990). Schizophrenia and crime: A longitudinal followup of 644 schizophrenics in Stockholm. *British Journal of Psychiatry, 157*, 345–350.

Link, B. G., Andrews, H., & Cullen, F. T. (1992). Reconsidering the violent and illegal behavior of mental patients. *American Sociological Review, 57*, 275–292.

Lomis, M. J., & Baker, L. L. (1985). Micro-training of forensic psychiatric patients for empathic counseling skills. *Journal of Counseling Psychology, 32*, 84–93.

Lukoff, D., Liberman, R. P., & Nuechterlein, K. H. (1986). Symptom monitoring in the rehabilitation of schizophrenic patients. *Schizophrenia Bulletin, 12*, 578–602.

Maletzky, B. M. (1980). Self-referred versus court-referred sexually deviant patients: Success with assisted covert sensitization. *Behavior Therapy, 11*, 306–314.

Manuele, C. A. (1983). The development of a measure to assess vocational maturity in adults with delayed career development. *Journal of Vocational Behavior, 23*, 45–63.

Marques, J. K., Day, D. M., Nelson, C., Miner, M. H., & West, M. A. (1989). *The sex offender treatment and evaluation project: Third report to the Legislature in response to PC 1365*. Sacramento: California State Department of Mental Health.

Marques, J. K., Day, D. M., Nelson, C., & West, M. A. (1993). Findings and recommendations from California's experimental treatment program. In G. C. N. Hall & R. Hirschman (Eds.), *Sexual aggression: Issues in etiology and assessment, treatment, and policy*. Washington, DC: Hemisphere.

Marshall, W. L., & Barbaree, H. E. (1988). The long-term evaluation of a behavioral treatment program for child molesters. *Behaviour Research and Therapy, 26*, 499–511.

Marshall, W. L., & Barrett, S. (1990). *Criminal neglect: Why sex offenders go free*. Toronto: Doubleday.

Meichenbaum, D., & Turk, D. C. (1987). *Facilitating treatment adherence: A practitioner's guidebook*. New York: Plenum.

Melton, G. B., Petrila, J., Poythress, N. G., & Slobogin, C. (1987). *Psychological evaluations for the courts: A handbook for mental health professionals and lawyers* New York: Guilford.

Monahan, J. (1981). *The clinical prediction of violent behavior*. Beverly Hills, CA: Sage.

Monahan, J. (1992). Mental disorder and violent behavior: Perceptions and evidence. *American Psychologist, 47,* 511–521.

Morey, L. C., Skinner, H. A., & Blashfield, R. K. (1984). A typology of alcohol abusers: Correlates and implications. *Journal of Abnormal Psychology, 93,* 408–417.

Mueser, K. T., Bellack, A. S., & Blanchard, J. J. (1992). Comorbidity of schizophrenia and substance abuse: Implications for treatment. *Journal of Consulting and Clinical Psychology, 60,* 845–856.

Newman, J. P. (1987). Reaction to punishment in extraverts and psychopaths: Implications for the impulsive behavior of disinhibited individuals. *Journal of Research in Personality, 21,* 464–480.

Newman, J. P., & Kosson, D. S. (1986). Passive avoidance learning in psychopathic and nonpsychopathic offenders. *Journal of Abnormal Psychology, 95,* 252–256.

Newman, J. P., Patterson, C. M., & Kosson, D. S. (1987). Response perseveration in psychopaths. *Journal of Abnormal Psychology, 96,* 145–148.

Novaco, R. W. (1975). *Anger control.* Toronto: D. C. Heath.

Novaco, R. W. (1983). Stress inoculation therapy for anger control. In P. A. Keller & L. G. Ritt (Eds.), *Innovations in clinical practice: A source book* (Vol. 2). Sarasota, FL: Professional Resource Exchange.

Novaco, R. W., & Welsh, W. N. (1989). Anger disturbances: Cognitive mediation and clinical prescriptions. In K. Howells and C. R. Hollin (Eds.), *Clinical approaches to violence* (pp. 39–87). New York: Wiley.

Nuffield, J. (1982). *Parole decision-making in Canada: Research towards decision guidelines.* Ottawa: Supply and Services Canada.

Overall, J. E., & Gorham, D. R. (1962). The Brief Psychiatric Rating Scale. *Psychological Reports, 19,* 799–812.

Patterson, G. R. (1985). A microsocial analysis of anger and irritable behavior. In M. A. Chesney & R. H. Rosenman (Eds.), *Anger and hostility in cardiovascular and behavioral disorders* (pp. 63–79). New York: Hemisphere.

Pithers, W. D., Marques, J. K., Gibat, C. C., & Marlatt, G. A. (1983). Relapse prevention with sexual aggressives: A self control model of treatment and maintenance of change. In J. Greer & I. R. Stuart (Eds.), *The sexual aggressor: Current perspectives on treatment* (pp. 214–239). New York: Van Nostrand Reinhold.

Platt, J. J., Scura, W., & Hannon, J. R. (1973). Problem-solving thinking of youthful incarcerated heroin addicts. *Journal of Community Psychology, 1,* 278–281.

Pollock, N. L., & Hashmall, J. M. (1991). The excuses of child molesters. *Behavioral Sciences and the Law, 9,* 53–59.

Quinsey, V. L. (1980). The baserate problem and the prediction of dangerousness: A reappraisal. *Journal of Psychiatry and Law, 8,* 329–340.

Quinsey, V. L. (1984). Sexual aggression: Studies of offenders against women. In D. Weisstub (Ed.), *Law and mental health: International perspectives* (Vol. 1; pp. 84–121). New York: Pergamon.

Quinsey, V. L. (1986). Men who have sex with children. In D. Weisstub (Ed.), *Law and mental health: International perspectives* (Vol. 2; pp. 140–172). New York: Pergamon.

Quinsey, V. L. (1988). Sexual deviancy. *Current Opinion in Psychiatry, 1,* 688–690.

Quinsey, V. L. (1990). Sexual violence. In R. Bluglass and P. Bowden (Eds.), *Principles and practice of forensic psychiatry* (pp. 563–572). London: Churchill/Livingstone.

Quinsey, V. L., & Ambtman, R. (1979). Variables affecting psychiatrists' and teachers' assessments of the dangerousness of mentally ill offenders. *Journal of Consulting and Clinical Psychology, 47,* 353–362.

Quinsey, V. L., Harris, G. T., Rice, M. E., & Lalumière, M. L. (1993). Assessing treatment efficacy in outcome studies of sex offenders. *Journal of Interpersonal Violence, 8,* 512–523.

Quinsey, V. L., & Maguire, A. (1983). Offenders remanded for a psychiatric examination: Perceived treatability and disposition. *International Journal of Law and Psychiatry, 6,* 193–205.

Quinsey, V. L., & Walker, W. D. (1992). Dealing with dangerousness: Community risk management strategies with violent offenders. In R. DeV. Peters, R. J. McMahon, & V. L. Quinsey (Eds.), *Aggression and violence throughout the life span* (pp. 244–262). Newbury Park, CA: Sage.

Rice, M. E., & Harris, G. T. (1988). An empirical approach to the classification and treatment of maximum security psychiatric patients. *Behavioral Sciences and the Law, 6,* 497–514.

Rice, M. E., & Harris, G. T. (1992). A comparison of criminal recidivism among schizophrenic and nonschizophrenic offenders. *International Journal of Law and Psychiatry, 15,* 397–408.

Rice, M. E., Harris, G. T., & Cormier, C. (1992). Evaluation of a maximum security therapeutic community for psychopaths and other mentally disordered offenders. *Law and Human Behavior, 16,* 399–412.

Rice, M. E., Harris, G. T., Lang, C., & Bell, V. (1990). Recidivism among male insanity acquitees. *Journal of Psychiatry and Law, 18,* 379–403.

Rice, M. E., Harris, G. T., & Quinsey, V. L. (1990). A followup of rapists assessed in a maximum-security psychiatric facility. *Journal of Interpersonal Violence, 5,* 435–448.

Rice, M. E., Harris, G. T., & Quinsey, V. L. (1993). Evaluating treatment programs for child molesters. In J. V. Roberts & J. Hudson (Eds.), *Evaluating justice: Canadian policies and programs* (pp. 189–204). Toronto: Thompson.

Rice, M. E., Harris, G. T., & Quinsey, V. L. (1994). Control in the psychiatric setting-adults. In M. Hersen, R. T. Ammerman, & L. A. Sisson (Eds.), *Handbook of aggressive and destructive behavior in psychiatric patients* (pp. 125–139). New York: Plenum.

Rice, M. E., Harris, G. T., Quinsey, V. L., & Cyr, M. (1990). Planning treatment programs in secure psychiatric facilities. In D. Weisstub (Ed.), *Law and mental health: International perspectives* (Vol. 5; pp. 162–230). New York: Pergamon.

Rice, M. E., Harris, G. T., Varney, G. W., & Quinsey, V. L. (1989). *Violence in institutions: Understanding, prevention, and control.* Toronto: Hans Huber.

Rice, M. E., Helzel, M. F., Varney, G. W., & Quinsey, V. L. (1985). Crisis prevention and intervention training for psychiatric hospital staff. *American Journal of Community Psychology, 13,* 289–304.

Rice, M. E., Quinsey, V. L., & Harris, G. T. (1991). Sexual recidivism among child molesters released from a maximum security psychiatric institution. *Journal of Consulting and Clinical Psychology, 59,* 381–386.

Ross, R. R., & Fabiano, E. A. (1985). *Time to think: A cognitive model of delinquency prevention and offender rehabilitation.* Johnson City, TN: Institute of Social Science and Arts.

Ross, R. R., Fabiano, E. A., & Ewles, C. D. (1988). Reasoning and rehabilitation. *International Journal of Offender Therapy and Comparative Criminology, 32,* 29–35.

Ross, R. R., & Lightfoot, L. O. (1985). *Treatment of the alcohol-abusing offender.* Springfield, IL: Thomas.

Rule, B. G., & Nesdale, A. R. (1976). Emotional arousal and aggressive behavior. *Psychological Bulletin, 83,* 851–863.

Serin, R. C., Peters, R. DeV., & Barbaree, H. E. (1990). Predictors of psychopathy and release outcome in a criminal population. *Psychological Assessment, 2,* 419–422.

Shea, M. T., Widiger, T. A., & Klein, M. H. (1992). Comorbidity of personality disorders and depression: Implications for treatment. *Journal of Consulting and Clinical Psychology, 60,* 857–868.

Siegel, J. M. (1985). The measurement of anger as a multidimensional construct. In M. A. Chesney & R. H. Rosenman (Eds.), *Anger and hostility in cardiovascular and behavioral disorders* (pp. 59–82). New York: Hemisphere.

Siegel, J. M. (1986). The Multidimensional Anger Inventory. *Journal of Personality and Social Psychology, 51,* 191–200.

Simon, R. I. (1987). *Clinical psychiatry and the law.* Washington, DC: American Psychiatric Press.

Spielberger, C. D., Johnson, E. H., Russell, S. F., Crane, R. J., Jacobs, G. A., & Worden, T. J. (1985). The experience and expression of anger: Construction and validation of an anger expression scale. In M. A. Chesney & R. H. Rosenman (Eds.), *Anger and hostility in cardiovascular and behavioral disorders.* New York: Hemisphere.

Spivak, G., Platt, J. J., & Shure, M. B. (1976). *The problem-solving approach to adjustment: A guide to research and intervention.* San Francisco: Jossey-Bass.

Swanson, J., Holzer C., Ganju, V., & Jono, R. (1990). Violence and psychiatric disorder in the community: Evidence from the Epidemiologic Catchment Area Surveys. *Hospital and Community Psychiatry, 41,* 761–770.

Tardiff, K. (1992). The current state of psychiatry in the treatment of violent patients. *Archives of General Psychiatry, 49,* 493–499.

Virkkunen, M., & Linnoila, M. (1993). Serotonin in personality disorders with habitual violence and impulsivity. In S. Hodgins (Ed.), *Mental disorder and crime* (pp. 227–243). Newbury Park, CA: Sage.

Weiner, N. A., & Wolfgang, M. E. (1989). *Pathways to criminal violence.* Newbury Park, CA: Sage.

Wolfgang, M. E., Thornberry, T. P., & Figlio, R. M. (1987). *From boy to man, from delinquency to crime.* Chicago: University of Chicago Press.

Wong, S. E., Slama, K. M., & Liberman, R. P. (1987). Behavioral analysis and therapy for aggressive psychiatric and developmentally handicapped patients. In L. H. Roth (Ed.), *Clinical treatment of the violent person* (pp. 20–53). New York: Guilford.

Woody, G. E, McLellan, A. T., Luborsky, L., & O'Brien, C. P. (1985). Sociopathy and psychotherapy outcome. *Archives of General Psychiatry, 42,* 1081–1086.

23

Battering Men

Diane R. Follingstad and Heather Breiter

Description of the Problem

After many years of little recognition as a phenomenon worthy of empirical study, marital violence finally began to be investigated in the 1970s. Initially, incidence and prevalence estimates were reported. According to Straus's (1977) data, 28% of couples in a nationally representative sample reported at least one episode of physical force over the course of their relationship. However, based on the idea that individuals underreport socially undesirable behavior, Straus (1980) estimated the true incidence of marital violence to be about 50 or 60% in the general population. Although it is undetermined how many battering men there actually are in the United States, it is generally accepted that most severe injuries and severe battering episodes are caused by male partners (Saunders, 1989). Even a conservative estimate would yield large numbers of men in need of intervention to prevent further violent episodes in their relationships.

For a long time, information about battering men was elicited primarily from battered women's descriptions of their abusive partners (Gondolf, 1985; Ponzetti, Cate, & Koval, 1982), and especially from battered women seeking refuge in shelters (e.g., Rosenbaum & O'Leary, 1981). Complicating data collection, several studies have found great variability in reports of domestic violence among family members, with women partners reporting higher rates of violence and threats of violence than the men themselves report (e.g., Bulcroft & Straus, 1975; Edleson & Brygger, 1986; Jouriles & O'Leary, 1985). Thus, it is only with emergence of treatment programs for battering men that groups of perpetrators have been available for assessment. Although a few studies have attempted to compare battering men with nonbattering men, most have reported only descriptive information. Little observation of spousal

Diane R. Follingstad and **Heather Breiter** • Department of Psychology, University of South Carolina, Columbia, South Carolina 29208.

Handbook of Prescriptive Treatments for Adults, edited by Michel Hersen and Robert T. Ammerman. Plenum Press, New York, 1994.

interaction has been conducted to assess communication, problem-solving, and negotiation skills (Bagarozzi & Giddings, 1983). Thus, information concerning men who are violent in their significant relationships often remains speculative.

Etiology

Unfortunately, most of the studies of violence in male–female relationships have utilized only frequency counts, percentages, and correlations (Bagarozzi & Giddings, 1983). It has yet to be determined whether the observed characteristics of the perpetrator, environment, or relationship play a causal role in the violence or outcomes of the violence (Tolman & Bennett, 1990). When examining the research on characteristics of battering men, one must be judicious in the interpretation of the importance of a causal factor once it is identified (Gelles, 1980) to avoid mistaking "a benign element for a causal one" (Tolman & Bennett, 1990, p. 87).

Although it is difficult to determine which factors are causal in the perpetration of relationship abuse, there exists a body of literature of factors associated with battering in general. Violence by males toward intimates does not appear to be linearly predictable, but seems multifaceted. Most theories that have been proposed have been psychological/psychopathological, interpersonal, or sociological.

Psychological Theories. Psychoanalytic theory provided the earliest explanation for wife assault. Early development of specific traits was postulated to predispose individuals to using violence. Early writers in the field of spouse abuse promoted the idea that batterers possessed particular personality traits, influenced by early development, that caused their use of violence toward their marital partners (e.g., Roy, 1977).

Another psychological theory hypothesizes that psychopathology is at the root of violent behavior toward a spouse. According to this theory, the aberrant traits of wife abusers can be linked to some type of psychological disorder. Some authors have attempted to apply diagnostic criteria to battering men, suggesting presence of antisocial, passive-aggressive, paranoid, borderline, or obsessive-compulsive personality disorders (e.g., Deschner, 1984; Faulk, 1974). Although evidence suggests that abusive males possess traits consistent with diagnoses of borderline and antisocial personality disorders, there have also been other, nonpathological traits consistently associated with battering (Hotaling & Sugarman, 1986). Most researchers assessing battering men have agreed that there is a lack of homogeneity in personality and behavioral factors.

Social learning theories have long viewed violence as a learned behavior rather than a behavior emerging from personality deficits or psychiatric disorders. Specifically, modeling of abusive behavior in the family of origin has been singled out by social learning theorists as an important element of the intergenerational transmission of violence. Operant conditioning comes into play when the aggressor learns that violence is reinforced through the victim's compliance and submission and that no sanctions follow violence.

Interpersonal Theories. Systems theory views marital violence as resulting from circular causality and reciprocal interactions between the couple that maintain the violent system (Bograd, 1984). Specifically, violence is seen as "an aspect of the couple's homeostatic patterns that maintains relationship rules and prevents change" (Weitzman & Dreen, 1982, p. 259). The assumption that the woman shares responsibility for violent incidents in a marriage is considered by some to be present in this theory (Bograd, 1984). Some authors have criticized the systems theory approach because it appears to blame the victim, shifts responsibility from the husband, fails to acknowledge the fact that severe abuse is perpetrated mainly toward women, and fails to address the complexity of the issue (e.g., Bograd, 1984; Libow, Raskin, & Caust, 1982). These same authors have also pointed out that systems theory fails to consider the social, economic, and political climate in which these systems are embedded.

Sociological Theories. The sociological perspective focuses on cultural norms that create the structure for families, which in turn promote and maintain the existence of marital violence (Bagarozzi & Giddings, 1983). These norms may exist throughout a particular culture, or in varying degrees within subcultures. Thus, this perspective views the structure of marriages, the historical isolation of nuclear families, the proliferation of violence in our society, and sex-role socialization as creating a climate for violence within marriages.

Feminist perspectives focus even more specifically on the social structure of American culture as being patriarchal (Bograd, 1984). The feminist conceptualization of wife abuse assumes that men are socialized to be in control and dominant and that battering emerges as a result. According to feminist theorists, when the greater culture functions as a patriarchal society, it is not surprising to see smaller units of that society (i.e., the family unit) mirroring those values (Gondolf, 1985). Gondolf suggested that lack of resources and the historical lack of institutional response on behalf of abused women have also contributed to the problem.

Assessment Strategies

It is unusual to hear of a treatment program for abusive men that conducted assessment measures prior to treatment for the purpose of treatment planning. Rather, data collection has typically been used for research purposes. Additionally, because formats have typically been group oriented, individualized "assessment" of maritally violent men does not have the history and degree of information and measures which are usually found in the assessment of psychopathology.

For research purposes, a measure of violent behavior is typically given to men in treatment programs to ensure that they belong in the program, as well as to assess changes in violent behavior. Men have also been deemed appropriate for treatment as battering spouses when they volunteer for or are court mandated to treatment. Other measures given to the abusing men are then a function of whatever research questions are of interest to the investigator. Saunders (1992) detailed a variety of measures that could be used to assess specific dimensions of the battering men (e.g., anger, depression, jealousy, assertiveness).

The Conflict Tactics Scale (CTS) (Straus, 1979) has most frequently been administered to assess the presence of physical abuse. Criticisms of the CTS have included its inability to distinguish between initiated violence and violence used in self-defense, its inability to determine level of injury, and its inability to measure motives for violence. Hudson and McIntosh (1981) have developed an Index of Spouse Abuse, but only 4 of the 11 items pertain to physical abuse. Similarly, Lewis's (1983) Wife Abuse Inventory contains only 2 of 31 items focused specifically on physical abuse. Because of the shortcomings of other measures, the CTS is most often used and cited in the literature.

Research about battering men yields potentially useful information for treatment planning and purposes. Such information falls under several categories: (a) psychosocial demographics; (b) personality traits and characteristics; (c) attitudes and beliefs; (d) psychopathology; (e) typologies of the abusing men; and (f) relationship characteristics.

Psychosocial Demographics

Roberts (1987) found that wife battering was more prevalent among males under age 40 (when age was investigated as a factor) in a large urban sample. Surprisingly, Roberts identified almost half of the sample as cohabitating, with most of the others married, and only a small portion separated. Researchers have generally found spouse abuse in all socioeconomic levels (SES), although Saunders (1982) and Sugarman and Hotaling (1989) reported wife abuse to be more prevalent in lower SES groups. Potentially affecting SES demographics of batterers is the frequent finding that unemployment is much higher for battering men than nonbattering men (Fitch & Papantonio, 1983; Gaguin, 1978; Roberts, 1987). Fleming (1979) found economic stress to be associated with battering, possibly because many of the battering men were employed as blue-collar workers (Roberts, 1987).

Coexisting problem behaviors in battering men have been cited by a number of researchers. Sonkin, Martin, and Walker (1985) found higher rates of early discharge from the military for violence, alcohol and drug problems, or desertion. Roberts (1987) found that 60% of battering men he sampled had some other criminal history, mostly less serious offenses. Support for this finding comes from Fagan, Stewart, and Hansen (1983), who found that men with the most serious assaults on a partner were more likely to have prior court involvement for stranger assault. Many studies have found high percentages of abusing men in their samples who had witnessed interparental aggression, had been physically abused themselves, or both. However, Browning (1983) did not find any differences in levels of childhood abuse or parental violence in the family of origin when batterers were directly compared to nonbatterers.

Personality Traits and Characteristics

There has been strong research support for the idea that battering men have low self-esteem (e.g., Hale, Zimostrad, Duckworth, & Nicholas, 1988; Maiuro, Cahn, Vitaliano, Wagner, & Zegree, 1988; Sugarman & Hotaling, 1989). Goldstein and Rosenbaum (1985) found that abusive men perceived their wives' behavior and other life situations as more of a threat to their self-concept than did nonabusive men, suggesting that low self-esteem is not just self-condemnation resulting from the men's abusive behavior. Several studies have reported that abusive men feel inadequate as males (e.g., Rosenbaum, 1986; Star, 1983), and Tolman and Bennett's (1990) review reported that the men "view themselves as both low in masculinity and low in positive traits stereotypically associated with either gender" (p. 96).

Researchers hypothesize that this poor self-concept feeds into the strong emotional dependency reported by other researchers (e.g., Elbow, 1977; Faulk, 1974; Ponzetti et al., 1982). Other writers have termed this phenomenon "dependency conflict," reflecting the view that abusive men typically resent and reject their feelings of dependency while also feeling the need to have someone upon whom to be emotionally dependent (e.g., Coleman, 1980; Star, 1983; Weitzman & Dreen, 1982).

The inordinate need of battering men to control and possess their partners may be seen as resulting from dependency and the fear of losing them (Ganley, 1981). Researchers have used different concepts to express this idea. Rouse (1990) reported research findings on the need for dominance. Jealousy and possessiveness have been cited by many authors (e.g., Bernard & Bernard, 1984; Maiuro et al., 1988), and other researchers have more directly discussed the concept of control (e.g., Gondolf, 1985; Weitzman & Dreen, 1982). Battering men's need for control often makes them appear highly rigid (Elbow, 1977) and resistant to change (Waldo, 1987).

Although battering men have a strong need to control others, they also appear to have impulse control problems (Ganley, 1981; Hale et al., 1988) and low frustration tolerance (Star, 1983). In stressful situations, battering men seem less able to use reasoning processes (Dutton & Browning, 1988). Lohr, Hamberger, and Bonge (1988) found abusive men to have higher scale scores on the Problem Avoidance and Helplessness for Change subscales of the Irrational Beliefs Test. Eisikovits, Edleson, Guttman, and Sela-Amit (1991) also found abusing men to possess fewer rational beliefs.

A number of factors add to the difficulty abusing men have in finding suitable alternate methods for handling feelings and conflicts. Gondolf (1985) viewed these men as detached from their feelings and having underdeveloped communication skills. Ponzetti et al. (1982) reported battering men to be inexpressive, suggesting an inability to accurately and richly describe their internal lives; as a result, they resort to violence. Assessment of assertiveness skills has almost always indicated a deficit in this area for battering men (e.g., Maiuro et al., 1988).

On most measures of hostility and anger (with the exception of the Novaco Anger Scale), abusive men receive higher scores (e.g., Maiuro et al., 1988). Dutton and Browning (1988) found higher self-reported anger levels in battering men who viewed videotapes of marital situations, and an observational study indicated that physically abusive men expressed more negative affect and anger (Margolin, John, & Gleberman, 1988).

Once anger has been expressed through physical violence, battering men tend to deny, minimize, or lie about their actions, and they also tend to externalize blame and responsibility for their difficulties (Ganley, 1981; Waldo, 1987). To complicate matters, abusive men are often socially isolated or have only superficial interpersonal contacts (Benjamin & Walz, 1983). This keeps them from receiving corrective feedback or support for expression of feelings that might prevent violent episodes.

Attitudes and Beliefs

Eisikovits et al. (1991) cautioned that there is insufficient evidence to conclude that abusing men possess similar attitudes or that attitudes are in any way predictive of their use of physical force. However, attitudes and beliefs of battering men have been investigated in depth. For example, sex-role attitudes have been investigated frequently, and Hotaling and Sugarman's (1986) review reported inconsistent results in the literature. Some articles indicated that battering men had more traditional sex-role attitudes, whereas other studies found no differences between battering and nonbattering men.

Saunders (1982) specifically assessed battering men's attitudes toward use of violence against women and found them to possess attitudes that justify the use of force. However, Saunders, Lynch, Grayson, and Linz (1987) later found that abusing men were different from male college students on only half of the subscales of their inventory. Eisikovits et al. (1991), in contrast, found battering men to be *less* likely than nonbattering men to believe the use of force in relationships was justified.

Beliefs regarding control were investigated by Eisikovits et al. (1991), who found abusing men to have a somewhat stronger belief in the control of powerful others. This study also found that battering men tended to see themselves as having more control over their own lives than nonabusing men. Hale et al. (1988) found abusing men as a group to have a lack of respect for social standards.

Psychopathology

Several studies specifically focused on clinical psychopathology in male batterers, as defined by psychological testing profiles and DSM-III criteria. Almost all these studies investigated battering men in treatment settings.

Hamberger and Hastings (1988) postulated that psychopathology typically had been minimized in explanations of the etiology of spousal violence, and they believed that failure to consider this aspect could result in artificial limitations on the choice and application of treatment techniques. Using the Millon Clinical Multiaxial Inventory (MCMI), Hamberger and Hastings (1985, 1986) investigated presence of personality disorders in batterers. The original results were replicated one year later using a similar sample of men attending a violence abatement program. Factor analysis of scores on the personality disorder scales of the MCMI resulted in three factors (schizoidal/borderline, narcissistic/antisocial, and passive dependent/compulsive), yielding eight groups when the possible combinations of high and low factor scores were utilized. Only 12 of the 99 men participating in the replication study (Hamberger & Hastings, 1986) showed no evidence of personality disorder. Because battering men in their sample fell into all eight combinations of the three factors, there was support for Hamberger and Hastings's idea that there are a number of types of batterers, rather than just one profile for these men.

When comparing batterers with nonbatterers, Hastings and Hamberger (1988) found that: nonabusers were "less alienated, less in need of approval, less sensitive to rejection, less moody and negativistic, less passive-aggressive and more conforming and conventional. Nonbatterers showed fewer and less intense borderline characteristics than did batterers, as well as less anxiety, depression, somatic complaints and problems with alcohol or other drugs" (p. 768).

In one of the best-controlled studies to date, Hamberger and Hastings (1991) found that batterers who were referred for treatment, whether or not they were alcoholic, and had significantly more borderline characteristics when compared with community-identified batterers and nonviolent men. Alcoholic batterers also had the highest MCMI elevations. Hamberger and Hastings found community-identified batterers to be similar on test data to nonviolent married men.

Three articles measured psychopathology using the Minnesota Multiphasic Personality Inventory (MMPI). Caesar (1986) found that 13 of 20 batterers showed a significant elevation on Scale 4 (psychopathic deviate) of the MMPI. In addition, Scale 4 was most likely elevated in conjunction with Scale 3 (hysteria) and Scale 6 (paranoia). Although batterers' scores were not statistically different from those of nonbatterers, their mean score across all scales was $T = 71$, which suggests the presence of psychopathology. Geffner, Kraeger-Cook, and Sharne (1986) also found significantly elevated Scale 4 scores on the mean profile for 50 abusers, providing additional support for the idea that battering men have personality disorders. Hale et al. (1988) gave the MMPI to 67 men who had voluntarily entered treatment because of abuse. No analysis was performed to control for severity or frequency of abusive events. The highest elevations for these men were on Scale 4 and Scale 2 (depression), with slight elevations on Scale 7 (psychasthenia) and Scale 8 (schizophrenia). The most common 2-point codes were, respectively, 24/42, 48/84, 49/94, and 34/43. In 56% of the profiles, Psychopathic deviate (4) was one of the top two scales. Scores on research scales indicated low ego strength, dependency, and the likelihood of alcohol addiction (68% of scores above the cutoff point).

In a study utilizing interviews with either the batterer or his partner, Stewart and deBlois (1981) found more psychopathology among abusers than nonabusers: spouse abusers were twice as likely to be diagnosed with antisocial personality disorder or alcoholism than nonabusers. Another interview study of abusers who were taken into custody reported that 61% could be diagnosed with a psychological disorder, the most common of which were depression and delusional jealousy, followed by anxiety disorders, personality disorders, dementia, and post-head-injury syndrome (Faulk, 1974).

Typologies

In addition to the typologies of Hamberger and Hastings (1988), several other investigators have attempted to determine whether batterers clustered in recognizable types. In a review of the literature, Tolman and Bennett (1990) echoed the idea that evidence suggests abusers are a heterogeneous mixture. However, they concluded that it is currently unclear whether typologies are relevant for treatment.

Elbow (1977) organized abusers into four groups: the controller, the incorporator, the approval-seeker, and the defender. Each type is hypothesized to have different motivations for engaging in violence. The controller uses violence to reestablish control, the incorporator uses it to prevent the loss of the person without whom he could not feel complete, the approval-seeker uses violence in response to a perception of rejection, and the defender uses it to keep the partner in an inferior role. Faulk (1974) used traits to identify types of batterers most evident to him after clinical interviews: dependent and passive; dependent and suspicious; violent and bullying; successful and domineering; and stable and normally affectionate.

Deschner (1984), borrowing from models of child abusers, suggested eight types of maritally violent abusers: (1) social chaos/deprivation type; (2) child-parent type; (3) obsessive-compulsive type; (4) type which responds abnormally to crying and loud complaining; (5) special scapegoat type; (6) pathologically jealous type; (7) mentally ill type; and (8) mental disturbance type. Gondolf (1988), using reports of battered women in shelters, found that 7% of abusing men were "sociopathic," with histories of being the most severely violent and having prior arrests. He considered 41% "antisocial," also extremely abusive men but less likely as a group to have a prior history of arrest. The remainder (52%) were considered "typical" in that they engaged in less severe violence, were likely to be apologetic after an episode, and were unlikely to have been arrested.

Saunders (1987) based his groupings of battering men on research data. The first group scored high on emotional variables (i.e., anger, depression, jealousy). These men engaged in moderate use of violence and alcohol. A second type was most likely to have been violent only at home, had the greatest degree of marital satisfaction of the three groups, and had the least rigid sex-role stereotyping. The final group was likely to have been violent outside the home, had the worst history of violence and alcohol abuse, and was most likely to have a history of being abused as a child.

Hershorn and Rosenbaum (1991) were specifically interested in applying Megargee, Cook, and Mendlesohn's (1967) concept of over- and undercontrolled hostility to batterers. Men who were abusive and who scored high on overcontrolled hostility had less frequent but highly explosive, severe aggressive episodes. The wives were the sole target of these men's aggression. Battering men who were rated as showing undercontrolled hostility were more generally and frequently aggressive. They were more likely to have seen interparental violence and to have had rejecting mothers.

Three clusters found by Hale et al. (1988) were based on MMPI data. The first cluster of battering men included those who were either exaggerating symptomatology or were seriously disturbed, in that they showed high elevations on almost all clinical scales. The second cluster was very different from the first, showing no elevations on clinical scales. The third group of abusing men showed a typical code type of 24/42, with lesser elevations on Scales 7 and 8, a pattern similar to the mean profile of the entire sample. This third profile indicated psychopathic tendencies with depression, some elevation of trait anxiety, and possibly some thought disturbance or feelings of alienation.

Relationship Characteristics

Edleson, Eisikovits, Guttman, and Sela-Amit (1991) reported that battering men and their wives showed low levels of marital adjustment and high levels of conflict over children. In their analysis of risk markers, Sugarman and Hotaling (1989) found that battering men have a significantly larger number of issues over which they are in conflict with their wives. Two different studies (Hanks & Rosenbaum, 1977; Weitzman & Dreen, 1982) reported that relationship rules are rigid between partners when the man is an abuser.

Two additional studies looked at the abusive husband's communication with and reactions to his wife. Rosenbaum and O'Leary's (1981) observational study resulted in findings that batterers are less assertive with their wives than nonabusive husbands. Waldo (1987) asserted that abusive men have difficulty viewing their wives as separate human beings, with the result that they experience outrage if the women do anything contrary to their desires.

Intervention Strategies

Evidence for Prescriptive Interventions

Three main modalities of intervention have been reported for treatment of battering men: individual therapy, couples' therapy, and men's groups. There are very few articles on results of individual therapy efforts with maritally violent men. In addition, treatment approaches are typically not based on an assessment of the individual man, his needs, or his experiences. A 1989 review of the existing literature on interventions with battering men identified only two efforts to intervene at an individual therapy level, both utilizing cognitive-behavioral or behavioral techniques to address isolated aspects of the men's problems (focusing on obsessive violent thoughts and focusing on generalized violent behavior) (Eisikovits & Edleson, 1989).

One unique program focusing on long-term, insight-oriented individual therapy is offered by the Abused Women's Aid in Crisis (AWAIC) (Garnet & Moss, 1982). Although most of their services are directed toward victims' needs, AWAIC offers individualized treatment to men who volunteer.

Therapy approaches to address battering with couples are often based on family systems theory, social learning theory, or an anger control model (Eisikovits & Edleson, 1989). Couples' therapy has been used with individual couples as well as groups of couples. A pioneering treatment program for batterers included the abused women in the treatment because the directors of the program found that many of the women returned to their partners (Geller & Walsh, 1977–1978). The Victims' Information Bureau of Suffolk County, New York (VIBS), began offering conjoint therapy that focused on acceptance of anger and conflict and taught modes of acceptable expression of those feelings. Geller and associates claimed that more than 250 couples were successfully treated in conjoint therapy over a 4-year period (Geller & Wasserstrom, 1984). Another well-known program for treating couples was begun by Neidig and Friedman (1984), who saw couples in groups. They used a psychoeducational format focusing on anger control, stress reduction, communication, and appropriate expression of conflict. This couples' program also addressed jealousy, sex-role stereotyping, and marital dependency.

Men's groups appear to be the most frequently used form of treatment available to battering men. Reasons for this prevalence include the ability to treat larger numbers of clients at one time, financial expediency, the existence of programs specifically designed to address abuse, and utilization of all group members to address denial and minimization on the part of individual clients. Men's groups have a variety of theoretical underpinnings, including cognitive-behavioral, ecological, gender-role socialization, and anger control models (Eisikovits & Edleson, 1989; Tolman & Bennett, 1990). Profeminist viewpoints, such as explanations of the impact of socialization on gender roles, are occasionally included in the group format as well (Tolman & Bennett, 1990). Techniques used in men's groups vary according to the program's theoretical approach to treatment and may include the following: modeling, communication skills training, anger control training, consciousness raising, stress reduction training, assertiveness training, skills for coping with depression, alcohol and drug abuse education, self-esteem training, sex role education, and cognitive restructuring (Eisikovits & Edleson, 1989).

By far the most common theoretical approach to treatment for battering men is cognitive-behavioral. Most group treatments tend to adopt a preplanned, general format that includes psychoeducational skill-building modules adapted from other fields (Eisikovits & Edleson, 1989). No attempt is made to tailor sessions to individual clients' needs; rather, use of a general package is expected to address all possible etiological aspects. For example, if one man uses violence because he is unaware of his feelings, another uses violence to reduce tension, and another uses violence because he feels the need to control his wife, all of these causal factors are likely to be addressed by the general program.

Several prototypical programs have emerged over the years. One of the most commonly cited programs is EMERGE, which was developed in 1977 as the first program solely for the purpose of treating battering men (Adams & McCormick, 1982). After utilizing several treatment formats, including individual and couples' therapy, EMERGE chose to offer men's groups only (Jennings, 1987). This approach takes a consciousness-raising, self-help orientation that attempts to increase awareness about sex-role attitudes, emotional experiences, and individual responsibility. EMERGE has served as the basis for many group treatment programs for battering men around the country.

Several other approaches developed in the late 1970s that emphasized group formats for consciousness raising and skill building. The Stop Abuse by Males (SAM) program chose the group format as the most appropriate and effective forum (Boyd, 1978). The Abusive Men Exploring New Directions (AMEND) program used the group format to teach abilities such as communication skills and anger management, while also including discussions of sex-role stereotyping and the cycle of violence (Roberts, 1984). The Domestic Violence Program (DVP) used supportive men's groups in combination with skill instruction to increase awareness of the causes of violence and alternatives to it (Roberts, 1984). The Volunteer Counseling Service in New York (Roberts, 1982), the Men and Stress Control Group (Steinfeld, 1980), and the Men's Group for Temper Control (Barnhill, Bloomgarten, Berghorn, Squires, & Siracusa, 1980) all used the group format to address both the educational and support needs of batterers. More recently, a structured, skill-training, cognitive-behavioral approach has been taken in Alternatives to Aggression (ATA) (Saunders, 1984).

Although Eisikovits and Edleson (1989) claim that research on abuse is rarely driven by etiological considerations, approaches to the treatment of battering men are generally based on some theory of battering and the best way to treat it. After reviewing current programs, Jennings (1987) made a case for a more individualized, unstructured approach for interventions. He made the point that an unconditional acceptance of the packaged, cognitive-behavioral approach for treating battering men is unfounded, because it lacks the support of well-controlled studies demonstrating the superiority of the cognitive-behavioral approach as the treatment of choice. However, the state of the art is such that many of the original, pioneering approaches serve as bases for the men's battering treatment programs seen today.

Selecting Optimal Intervention Strategies

Defining the optimal treatment approach is difficult because of methodological problems in research studies. For example, there is little consistency across studies in definitions of successful outcomes (Eisikovits & Edleson, 1989; Russell, 1988). Many of the studies base their evaluations only on clients' self-reports, which is a questionable procedure in this area of study if the men's self-reports are never validated by other sources (Russell, 1988). The length of time between intervention and follow-up varies among studies, making it difficult to determine if lasting changes in behavior were accomplished by many interventions (Eisikovits & Edleson, 1989; Russell, 1988). The paucity of data on treatment dropouts is another flaw, as is the failure to include control groups in many of the studies (Russell, 1988).

Because of the dearth of empirical information on individual therapeutic treatment for battering men, it is difficult to judge the success or potential for success of this type of intervention. In general, individual treatment is not the most commonly used treatment approach for battering men, and there are no recent articles to support its use as the treatment of choice.

More research has been published on interventions with couples including battering men and their partners, but the methodological flaws mentioned above are prevalent here (Eisikovits & Edleson, 1989; Russell, 1988; Tolman & Bennett, 1990). Six studies were conducted on the effectiveness of interventions with couples between 1983 and 1986. All but one of these studies reported successful outcomes, but the quality and clarity of their definitions of success varied. Detailed discussions of the empirical studies on interventions with couples, their results, and their shortcomings can be found in reviews by Eisikovits and Edleson (1989) and Tolman and Bennett (1990). Although case study and anecdotal reports appear to be encouraging, results from these studies must be considered inconclusive.

By far the most extensively researched type of intervention for battering men are groups specifically designed to address the issue of abuse. Approximately 20 outcome evaluation studies were published between 1981 and 1989. Reported success rates of men's groups varied between approximately 55 and 85%, and changes in associated behaviors and attitudes are reported to be extensive (e.g., decreases in depression and negative attitudes toward women, increases in assertiveness). As with the literature on couples' interventions, the empirical literature on battering men's groups suggests efficacy, but conclusions are tentative because of methodological flaws. For a more complete discussion of the effectiveness of men's groups according to empirical studies, refer to reviews by Eisikovits and Edleson (1989) and Tolman and Bennett (1990).

Despite mixed empirical results, men's groups are typically the treatment of choice for battering men. Several reasons for choosing the group format instead of couples' therapy have been cited by experts in the field. Many professionals believe the group format is necessary to address the support and interpersonal needs of the batterer (Ganley, 1981; Saunders, 1980). Others recommend group therapy over couples' treatment in order to convey to the man the importance of individual responsibility and to avoid compromising the woman's safety (Pressman, 1989; Willbach, 1989). Although most experts agree that men's groups are important for accomplishing initial treatment objectives, several have concluded that a more comprehensive, multilevel intervention is required to address the complexity of the issues involved in battering (Eisikovits & Edleson, 1989; Tolman & Bennett, 1990). Such intervention may take the form of conjoint sessions conducted after both parties have participated in same-sex support groups (Pressman, 1989).

Problems in Carrying Out Interventions

Most of the literature addressing problems in carrying out interventions for battering has been focused on group approaches to treating men. Problems in carrying out interventions with men who batter have been identified as predominantly involving the elicitation of initial treatment participation and the control of dropout rates.

Battering men come to groups through individual initiative, referrals from various sources (e.g., military bases, physicians, clergy), or court mandates. Attracting men to programs that address their battering is difficult for many reasons, including denial of the problem, lack of motivation, fear of social stigma, financial considerations, and reluctance to publicly acknowledge their violent behavior.

Once men attend a group for batterers, there are often significant difficulties getting them to stay in the program. Attrition rates have been estimated to be as high as 40% (Pirog-Good & Stets, 1986) in some programs. Attempts have been made to identify programmatic aspects that may reduce dropout rates and to identify characteristics of men who are most likely to complete batterers' group programs. Orientation and preparation sessions conducted prior to groups have been hypothesized to prevent high dropout rates. A recent study conducted by Tolman and Bhosley (1989) looked at the effects of a pregroup preparation workshop designed to reduce dropout from men's groups. The authors concluded that there appeared to be a positive effect in preventing dropout in early sessions associated with an intensive preparation effort, but that the workshop may not serve to prevent dropout over the long term. Pirog-Good and Stets (1986) examined programmatic aspects influencing dropout rates and found that high completion rates were associated with programs adopting a short-term treatment approach, programs that accepted referrals from law enforcement or judicial officials, and programs that did not levy a fee on attendees.

Several researchers have investigated the characteristics of men who complete groups for battering men. One study conducted on both men and women completing a 4-week group (Faulkner, Cogan, Nolder, & Shooter, 1991) found that completers tended to have lower levels of substance abuse (according to the MCMI) and that they were court-referred. Two other studies, however, found no significant differences in completion rates of men who were court-referred and men who were not (Grusznski & Carrillo, 1988; Saunders & Parker, 1989). Other findings indicate that better-educated men (Grusznski & Carrillo, 1988; Saunders & Parker, 1989), older men (DeMaris, 1989; Saunders & Parker, 1989), and men without a prior conviction are more likely to complete treatment (DeMaris, 1989). According to Grusznski and Carrillo (1988), completers tend to be employed, to have children, to make fewer threats before intake in the program, to have witnessed abuse as children, and to have greater expressed control. Minority men and men who were not employed were found by Saunders and Parker (1989) to be less likely to complete batterers' groups.

Relapse Prevention

Rates of recidivism in completers of men's groups have been reported to be as low as 4% after 3 years (Dutton, 1986) and as high as 66 to 75% (Gondolf, 1987) one year after completion of a program. Unfortunately, many of these studies do not report rates of recidivism for dropouts or those in control groups for purposes of comparison. Although rates of violence posttreatment are usually set as a criterion for success of programs, there is little literature actually addressing the prevention of recidivism in such men who batter. What little information does exist on recidivism and the associated characteristics of men has been gathered only from those who participated in groups for battering men.

DeMaris and Jackson (1987) conducted a follow-up investigation of 53 men who completed counseling programs for their battering and found a 35% rate of recidivism. Associated factors included observation of parental violence and presence of an alcohol problem. Men questioned by Demaris and Jackson reported that they successfully avoided using violence after treatment by phoning a counselor, using self-monitoring techniques to control their anger, or leaving their homes when confrontation was imminent. Another study by Hamberger and Hastings (1990) investigated the demographic and personality correlates of recidivism in 106 men who completed a program designed to reduce abuse. They found that men who had higher rates of substance abuse both before and after treatment were more likely to recidivate. Additionally, they found that men who scored higher on the Narcissistic, Gregarious, and Aggressive scales of the MCMI tended to recidivate more. Hamberger and Hastings (1990) did not find that self-referral decreased likelihood of recidivism, and they were unable to distinguish between those who recidivated and those who did not on the basis of past criminal record.

In a discussion of prevention of recidivism, Tolman and Bennett (1990) conclude that multifaceted interventions involving the batterer, associated institutions, and the victim may well be the most effective approach to preventing recidivism. Substance abuse and a history of having witnessed aggression appear to be strongly associated with recidivism. Procedures addressing these issues (e.g., concurrent participation in a substance abuse group) may help reduce recidivism after violent men complete a battering men's group.

Case Illustration

Case Description

William Stone is a 54-year-old, married, African-American man with three grown children. He is an attractive man with a pleasant demeanor whose conversation was punctuated with smiles and some laughter. He talked quite openly about most topics, with the exception of specifics of the physical abuse toward his current wife and past wife.

Mr. Stone was the oldest of nine children in an intact family from New York City, although he reported that his father also had a number of children "in the street." Mr. Stone reported that in his family of origin, physical abuse directed by his father toward his mother was an almost daily occurrence. His first memory of his father's violence was at the age of 7 or 8, when he would hear crying in the night and see injuries on his mother the next morning. Although the children were also physically abused at times, it appears most of the abuse was directed at his mother. Mr. Stone remembers that his own difficulties handling anger began at about 7 or 8 years of age. He began to get into fights in school and around the neighborhood. He remembers thinking that his mother was constantly being taken advantage of and that he was not going to let anybody do the same to him. He would not argue with others but, rather, would "just go and get a stick or brick." He experienced much confusion throughout his life in that he did not want to be like his father, but had a stronger feeling that he did not want anybody to take advantage of him.

At 14 years of age, William left home to live with a friend of his mother's in order to escape the home situation. He quit school at age 16 in order to enter the military because he was "worried he would kill his father" if he did not remove himself from the family. Entering the military was a difficult adjustment for Mr. Stone, and he remembers crying many nights because he wanted to be back home. In the military, he received his GED and took some college courses but frequently got into trouble for physical violence. He was violent toward other servicemen and was considered to be a "troublemaker" by some commanders. His violence frightened him, and he worried frequently that he might kill someone who treated him badly. Mr. Stone retired from the military after 20 years and currently works as a records clerk at a university hospital.

Mr. Stone married for the first time at age 18 and remained married for approximately 7 years to his first wife. William reported that his first wife drank a lot, did not maintain the house, had a reputation for having affairs, and never liked going overseas with him. They were separated for $2\frac{1}{2}$ years during the marriage and were divorced when Mr. Stone realized he might kill her. Physical violence was frequent, and a major episode involved his pushing her down a flight of steps, for which she required hospitalization. William would feel remorse following physically violent episodes and promise never to be violent again, but abuse would always resume after some time.

Several years after his divorce from his first wife, Mr. Stone remarried after a brief courtship and has remained married. Even though he engaged in less physical violence in the second marriage than in his first, he reported that he engaged in verbal abuse, which he felt was also hurtful. He attributed the initial decrease in physical abuse to the sanctions, both personal and financial, that the military placed on him for his violent behavior. In his second marriage, William reported that he had a strong need for control and felt very jealous and possessive of his wife. For example, he would check the mileage on the car to see how far she had driven that day. Looking back, Mr. Stone feels his views toward relationships were "old-fashioned." William reported that alcohol was not a precipitant of violent episodes, but stress in his life was definitely a factor that led to his feeling out of control. In addition, he felt that his anger level was always extremely high. He reported being angry at everybody who "looked at him wrong" and kept a gun in his car. On one occasion, Mr. Stone pointed the gun at a man who was angry because Mr. Stone would not move his car. Looking back, Mr. Stone feels that there was a high likelihood he could have killed somebody along the way.

William reported that his second marriage has been difficult and that he and his wife still disagree a great deal. However, he feels that he has come to a point where he does not feel as much anger, and he uses no physical force. Early on, Mr. Stone was motivated to remain in the marriage primarily because he wanted contact with his children. After 17 years of marriage, he separated from his wife for 11 months, and it was at this time that he entered a treatment program for battering men. A friend had seen a newspaper article about the program and told William that he needed to inquire about it. He decided to participate in treatment because he acknowledged that he was not happy, was taking his anger out on his children, and thought the program might help his marriage.

Assessment

The treatment program that Mr. Stone entered had no formal assessment procedures. Initially, a one-hour interview was conducted by a counselor who was not involved in the treatment. The interview was devoted to collecting information on the client's history of abuse, his current relationship, and his family of origin. Information of this nature is used in an informal way to alert the group leaders to possible issues for the client and is limited in usefulness by the degree of honesty of the client.

Intervention Selection

William Stone entered the only treatment program in the city in which he lived that focused on male violence toward intimates. Because the program was advertised as having this focus, Mr. Stone thought that it was an appropriate one for his problems. He did not consider any other form of treatment.

Intervention Course and Problems in Carrying Out Interventions

Mr. Stone stayed in the treatment program as a client for more than 3 years. He remembers initially not liking the group program because he was asked questions about his background and believed it was "none of their business." William also questioned the genuineness of the group leaders in the beginning, but he remained in the program because he agreed with them that regardless of what happened to his current marriage, he would take his problematic feelings into other relationships. The longer he stayed in the group, the more he felt he was there for his own needs. Because the group had no minimum or maximum length of participation and new group members entered periodically, Mr. Stone continued to participate because he wanted to make sure he "had a handle on his anger and feelings" before terminating. Sometimes, he would be the only African-American man in the group, but he kept telling himself to be concerned only about what he was learning from the group. He participated in the group for longer than the group leaders thought he needed to attend, but Mr. Stone believed it took a very long time to change his thinking processes.

The group itself was run in an unstructured manner, emphasizing the importance of members' talking openly about themselves and their problems. The group leaders had a repertoire of exercises that they tailored to particular men's difficulties. The group was broadly focused in content, covering such topics as anger expression and management, identification and expression of feelings, need for control, insecurity, and sex roles. Group leaders encouraged members to generate alternatives to old behaviors. Confrontation was a tactic used by group leaders when they believed members were minimizing events or engaging in denial. Emphasis was placed on group members' supporting one another, except in the area of violence.

Mr. Stone found that aspects of the group facilitated his trust and personal progress. Group leaders seemed very genuine in their concern and in the faith they placed in him. Confidentiality on the part of the group leaders was crucial to Mr. Stone because of negative experiences he had had in the military with people gossiping about servicemen's difficulties. Repetition of the idea that "nobody can make you mad—they can do things you don't like, but they can't make you angry" was important for implanting that notion firmly in his mind. He also benefitted from emphasis on the idea that a person had to take responsibility for his or her own actions.

Outcome and Termination

Mr. Stone remained in the treatment group longer than the leaders felt was necessary. At the end of 3 years, he felt that the treatment program's ideas were firmly implanted in his mind and that he would not be violent again. At that time Mr. Stone decided to stop attending group sessions. He was interested in conjoint sessions with his wife when he felt he had reached the point of taking responsibility for his own actions. However, his wife was not interested, maintaining that violence was his problem. Thus, there was no conjoint treatment.

Follow-Up and Maintenance

Shortly after Mr. Stone left the treatment group, one of the leaders asked him to consider a trial period of being a group leader. The group leader perceived William as having a way of talking to people that was effective in getting them to understand. Mr. Stone initially had no interest in this idea but was convinced to try it for 30 days to see if he could help just one person. Four years later, he is still a group leader once a week for the battering men's treatment program. In reality, his commitment to the program and the clients extends beyond the once-a-week session—he may receive up to 20 calls from group members in a week, because the men seem drawn to him for support. William encourages group members to call him if they feel the need to talk and extends that courtesy to families of the group members as well. When queried, Mr. Stone noted that he does not feel that his role as group leader is necessary to maintain his nonviolent status. Indeed, William maintains that he will never again be violent, feeling that he has replaced the expression of anger with positive assertion and that he has the coping skills to mitigate the anger and rage he once felt. To date, he has never again used physical force in his marital relationship, nor has he been violent outside the marriage.

Summary

Only in the last decade have those studying battering men been able to use information collected directly from the men themselves. Typically, battering men in research studies are either self-referred or court mandated to treatment programs where assessment has been conducted, and there is almost no knowledge of whether such men who have been in treatment are similar to or different from the greater population of battering men. Theories from the fields of psychology, sociology, and psychopathology have been advanced to explain marital violence.

Individual therapy, couples' therapy, and men's group have been the modalities of intervention reported in treatment literature. However, very little anecdotal or research information is available as to individual assessment of and therapy with battering men. Couples' therapy is more common than individual treatment, and several prototypical programs have begun. A number of studies involving couples in therapy in which abuse was the major issue have reported successful outcomes, but methodological flaws do not allow for solid conclusions at this time. The most popular format for treatment of battering men is men's groups designed to address abuse. Although groups for battering men have the usual benefits of such treatment, many experts believe that focusing on the men without their partners present also addresses denial, minimization, and externalization of blame by the men about the abuse. Treatment groups focus on the men, their attitudes, and their skills to work toward violence-free outcomes. Most groups tend to adopt a preplanned general format that includes psychoeducational modules adapted from other fields. Success rates have been reported to range from 55 to 85%, although the data are typically given for completers of the programs. Some experts have recommended later conjoint sessions as a way to use a comprehensive, multilevel approach to address a complex issue.

Major problems in carrying out interventions center around difficulty in initially attracting battering men to treatment and keeping them in treatment after they begin. Recidivism rates have varied across studies, but several demographic and personality correlates associated with recidivism have been identified. Multifaceted interventions have been recommended for prevention of recidivism.

References

Adams, D., & McCormick, A. (1982). Men unlearning violence: A group approach based on the collective model. In M. Roy (Ed.), *The abusive partner*. New York: Van Nostrand Reinhold.

Bagarozzi, D. A., & Giddings, C. W. (1983). Conjugal violence: A critical review of current research and clinical practices. *American Journal of Family Therapy, 11*, 3–15.

Barnhill, L., Bloomgarten, R., Berghorn, G., Squires, M., & Siracusa, A. (1980). Clinical and community interventions in violence in families. In L. Wolberg & M. Aronson (Eds.), *Group and family therapy— 1980*. New York: Stratton Medical Book.

Benjamin, L., & Walz, E. (1983). *Violence in the family: Child and spouse abuse*. Ann Arbor, MI: ERIC/CAPS.

Bernard, J. L., & Bernard, M. L. (1984). The abusive man seeking treatment: Jekyll and Hyde. *Family Relations, 33*, 543–547.

Bograd, M. (1984). Family systems approaches to wife battering: A feminist critique. *American Journal of Orthopsychiatry, 54*, 558–568.

Boyd, V. (1978, August). *Domestic violence: Treatment alternatives for the male batterer*. Paper presented at the meeting of the American Psychological Association, Toronto.

Browning, J. J. (1983). *Violence against intimates: Toward a profile of wife assaulters*. Unpublished doctoral dissertation, University of British Columbia, Vancouver.

Bulcroft, R. A., & Straus, M. A. (1975). *Validity of husband, wife and child reports of intrafamily violence and power*. Unpublished manuscript, University of New Hampshire.

Caesar, P. L. (1986, August). *Men who batter: A heterogeneous group*. Paper presented at the Meeting of the American Psychological Association, Washington, DC.

Coleman, K. H. (1980). Conjugal violence: What 33 men report. *Journal of Marriage and Family Therapy, 6*, 207–213.

DeMaris, A. (1989). Attrition in batterers' counseling: The role of social and demographic factors. *Social Service Review, 63*, 142–154.

DeMaris, A., & Jackson, J. K. (1987). Batterers' reports of recidivism after counseling. *Social Casework, 68*, 458–465.

Deschner, J. P. (1984). *The hitting habit: Anger control for battering couples*. New York: Free Press.

Dutton, D. G. (1986). The outcome of court-mandated treatment for wife assault: A quasi-experimental evaluation. *Violence and Victims, 1*, 163–175.

Dutton, D. G., & Browning, J. J. (1988). Concern for power, fear of intimacy and aversive stimuli for wife assault. In G. T. Hotaling, D. Finkelhor, J. T. Kirkpatrick, & M. A. Straus (Eds.), *Family abuse and its consequences* (pp. 163–175). Newbury Park, CA: Sage.

Edleson, J. L., & Brygger, M. P. (1986). Gender differences in reporting of battering incidents. *Family Relations, 35*, 377–382.

Edleson, J. L., Eisikovits, Z. C., Guttman, E., & Sela-Amit, M. (1991). Cognitive and interpersonal factors in woman abuse. *Journal of Family Violence, 6*, 167–182.

Eisikovits, Z. C., & Edleson, J. L. (1989, September). Intervening with men who batter: A critical review of the literature. *Social Service Review, 63*, 384–414.

Eisikovits, Z. C., Edleson, J. L., Guttman, E., & Sela-Amit, M. (1991). Cognitive styles and socialized attitudes of men who batter: Where should we intervene? *Family Relations, 40*, 72–77.

Elbow, M. (1977). Theoretical considerations of violent marriages. *Social Casework, 58*, 515–526.

Fagan, J., Stewart, D. K., & Hansen, H. (1983). Violent men or violent husbands? Background factors and situational correlates. In D. Finkelhor (Ed.), *The dark side of families* (pp. 49–68). Beverly Hills, CA: Sage.

Faulk, M. (1974). Men who assault their wives. *Medicine, Science and the Law, 14*, 180–183.

Faulkner, K. K., Cogan, R., Nolder, M., & Shooter, G. (1991). Characteristics of men and women completing cognitive/behavioral spouse abuse treatment. *Journal of Family Violence, 6*, 243–254.

Fitch, F. J., & Papantonio, A. (1983). Men who batter: Some pertinent characteristics. *Journal of Nervous and Mental Disorders, 171*, 190–192.

Fleming, J. B. (1979). *Stopping wife abuse*. New York: Anchor.

Gaguin, D. (1978). Spouse abuse: Data from the national crime survey. *Victimology: An International Journal, 2*, 635.

Ganley, A. L. (1981). *Court mandated counseling for men who batter: A three-day workshop for mental health professionals: Participant's manual*. Washington, DC: Center for Men's Policy Studies.

Garnet, S., & Moss, D. (1982). How to set up a counseling program for self-referred batterers: The AWAIC model. In M. Roy (Ed.), *The abusive partner*. New York: Van Nostrand Reinhold.

Geffner, R., Kraeger-Cook, S., & Sharne, K. (1986, October—November). *Batterer and victim characteristics: Implications for treatment*. Paper presented at the Meeting of the American Society of Criminology, Atlanta.

Geller, J., & Walsh, J. (1977–1978). A treatment model for the abused spouse. *Victimology: An International Journal, 1*, 627–632.

Geller, J. A., & Wasserstrom, J. (1984). Conjoint therapy for the treatment of domestic violence. In A. R. Roberts (Ed.), *Battered women and their families: Intervention strategies and treatment programs*. New York: Springer.

Gelles, R. J. (1980). Violence in the family: A review of research in the 70s. *Journal of Marriage and the Family, 42*, 873–885.

Goldstein, D., & Rosenbaum, A. (1985). An evaluation of the self-esteem of maritally violent men. *Family Relations, 34*, 425–428.

Gondolf, E. W. (1985). Fighting for control: A clinical assessment of men who batter. *Social Casework: The Journal of Contemporary Social Work, 66*, 48–54.

Gondolf, E. W. (1987). Evaluating programs for men who batter: Problems and prospects. *Journal of Family Violence, 2*, 95–108.

Gondolf, E. W. (1988). Who are those guys? Toward a behavioral typology of batterers. *Violence and Victims, 3*, 187–203.

Grusznski, R. J., & Carrillo, T. P. (1988). Who completes batterers' treatment groups? An empirical investigation. *Journal of Family Violence, 3*, 141–150.

Hale, G., Zimostrad, S., Duckworth, J., & Nicholas, D. (1988). Abusive partners: MMPI profiles of male batterers. *Journal of Mental Health Counseling, 10*, 214–224.

Hamberger, L. K., & Hastings, J. E. (1985, March). *Personality correlations of men who abuse their partners: Some preliminary data*. Paper presented at the meeting of the Society of Personality Assessment, Berkeley, CA.

Hamberger, L. K., & Hastings, J. E. (1986). Personality correlates of men who abuse their partners: A cross-validation study. *Journal of Family Violence, 1*, 323–341.

Hamberger, L. K., & Hastings, J. E. (1988). Characteristics of male spouse abusers consistent with personality disorders. *Hospital and Community Psychiatry, 39*, 763–770.

Hamberger, L. K., & Hastings, J. E. (1990). Recidivism following spouse abuse abatement counseling: Treatment program implications. *Violence and Victims, 5*, 157–170.

Hamberger, L. K., & Hastings, J. E. (1991). Personality correlates of men who batter and nonviolent men: Some continuities and discontinuities. *Journal of Family Violence, 6*, 131–147.

Hanks, S. E., & Rosenbaum, C. P. (1977). Battered women: A study of women who live with violent alcohol abusing men. *American Journal of Orthopsychiatry, 47*, 291–306.

Hastings, J. E., & Hamberger, L. K. (1988). Personality characteristics of spouse abusers: A controlled comparison. *Violence and Victims, 3*, 31–48.

Hershorn, M., & Rosenbaum, A. (1991). Over- versus undercontrolled hostility: Application of the construct to the classification of maritally violent men. *Violence and Victims, 6*, 151–158.

Hotaling, G. T., & Sugarman, D. B. (1986). An analysis of risk markers in husband to wife violence: The current state of knowledge. *Violence and Victims, 1*, 101–124.

Hudson, W. W., & McIntosh, S. R. (1981). The assessment of spouse abuse: Two quantifiable dimensions. *Journal of Marriage and the Family, 11*, 873–888.

Jennings, J. L. (1987). History and issues in the treatment of battering men: A case for unstructured group therapy. *Journal of Family Violence, 2*, 193–213.

Jouriles, E. N., & O'Leary, K. D. (1985). Interspousal reliability of reports of marital violence. *Journal of Consulting and Counseling Psychology, 53*, 419–421.

Lewis, B. Y. (1983). The Wife Abuse Inventory: A screening device for the identification of abused women. *Social Casework, 30*, 32–36.

Libow, J. A., Raskin, P. A., & Caust, B. L. (1982). Feminist and family systems therapy: Are they irreconcilable? *American Journal of Family Therapy, 10*, 3–12.

Lohr, J. M., Hamberger, L. K., & Bonge, D. (1988). The nature of irrational beliefs in different personality clusters of spouse abusers. *Journal of Rational Emotive and Cognitive Behavior Therapy, 6*, 273–285.

Maiuro, R. D., Cahn, T. S., Vitaliano, P. P., Wagner, B. C., & Zegree, J. B. (1988). Anger, hostility and depression in domestically violent versus generally assaultive men and nonviolent control subjects. *Journal of Consulting and Clinical Psychology, 56*, 17–23.

Margolin, G., John, R., & Gleberman, L. (1988). Affective responses to conflictual discussions in violent and nonviolent couples. *Journal of Consulting and Clinical Psychology, 56*, 24–33.

Megargee, E. J., Cook, P. E., & Mendelsohn, G. A. (1967). Development and validation of an MMPI scale of assaultiveness in overcontrolled individuals. *Journal of Abnormal Psychology, 72*, 519–528.

Neidig, P. H., & Friedman, D. H. (1984). *Spouse abuse: A treatment program for couples*. Champaign, IL: Research Press.

Pirog-Good, M. A., & Stets, J. (1986). Programs for abusers: Who drops out and what can be done. *Response to the Victimization of Women and Children, 9*, 17–19.

Ponzetti, J. J., Cate, R. M., & Koval, J. E. (1982). Violence between couples: Profiles of the male abuser. *Personnel and Guidance Journal, 61*, 222–224.

Pressman, B. (1989). Wife-abused couples: The need for comprehensive theoretical perspectives and integrated treatment models. *Journal of Feminist Family Therapy, 1*, 23–43.

Roberts, A. R. (1982). A national service for batterers. In M. Roy (Ed.), *The abusive partner*. New York: Van Nostrand Reinhold.

Roberts, A. R. (1984). Intervention with the abusive partner. In A. Roberts (Ed.), *Battered women and their families*. New York: Springer.

Roberts, A. R. (1987). Psychosocial characteristics of batterers: A study of 234 men charged with domestic violence offenses. *Journal of Family Violence, 2*, 81–93.

Rosenbaum, A. (1986). Of men, macho and marital violence. *Journal of Family Violence, 1*, 121–129.

Rosenbaum, A., & O'Leary, K. D. (1981). Marital violence: Characteristics of abusive couples. *Journal of Consulting and Clinical Psychology, 49*, 63–71.

Rouse, L. (1990). The dominance motive in abusive partners: Identifying couples at risk. *Journal of College Student Development, 31*, 330–335.

Roy, M. (1977). A current survey of 150 cases. In M. Roy (Ed.), *Battered women*. New York: Van Nostrand Reinhold.

Russell, M. (1988). Wife assault theory, research, and treatment: A literature review. *Journal of Family Violence, 3*, 193–208.

Saunders, D. G. (1980). A model for the structured group treatment of male-to-female violence. *Behavioral Group Therapy, 2*, 2–9.

Saunders, D. G. (1982). Counseling the violent husband. In P. A. Keller & L. G. Ritt (Eds.), *Innovations in clinical practice*. Sarasota, FL: Professional Resource Exchange.

Saunders, D. G. (1984). Helping husbands who batter. *Social Casework, 65*, 347–353.

Saunders, D. G. (1987, July), *Are there different types of men who batter? An empirical study with possible implications for treatment*. Paper presented at the Third National Conference for Family Violence Researchers, University of New Hampshire, Durham, NH.

Saunders, D. G. (1989, October). *Who hits first and who hurts most? Evidence for the greater victimization of women*. Paper presented at the annual meeting of the American Society of Criminology, Reno, NV.

Saunders, D. G. (1992). Woman battering. In R. T. Ammerman & M. Hersen (Eds.), *Assessment of family violence*. New York: Wiley.

Saunders, D. G., Lynch, A. B., Grayson, M., & Linz, D. (1987). The Inventory of Beliefs about Wife Beating: The construction and initial validation of a measure of beliefs and attitudes. *Violence and Victims, 2*, 39–57.

Saunders, D. G., & Parker, J. C. (1989). Legal sanctions and treatment follow-through among men who batter: A multi-variate analysis. *Social Work Research's Abstracts, 25*, 21–29.

Sonkin, D. J., Martin, D., & Walker, L. E. (1985). *The male batterer: A treatment approach*. New York: Springer.

Star, B. (1983). *Helping the abuser*. New York: Family Services Association of America.

Steinfeld, G. (1980). *Progress report: Men and stress control*. Unpublished manuscript. Bridgeport, CT: Bridgeport Division of the YMCA.

Stewart, M. A., & deBlois, C. S. (1981). Wife abuse among families attending a child psychiatry clinic. *Journal of the American Academy of Child Psychiatry, 20*, 845–862.

Straus, M. A. (1977). Wife beating: How common and why? *Victimology, 2*, 443–458.

Straus, M. A. (1979). Measuring intrafamily conflict and violence: The Conflict Tactics Scale. *Journal of Marriage and the Family, 41*, 75–88.

Straus, M. A. (1980). Wife beating: How common and why? In M. A. Straus & G. T. Hotaling (Eds.), *The social causes of husband–wife violence*. Minneapolis: University of Minnesota Press.

Sugarman, D. B., & Hotaling, G. T. (1989). Violent males in intimate relationships: An analysis of risk markers. *Journal of Applied Social Psychology, 19*, 1034–1048.

Tolman, R. M., & Bennett, L. W. (1990). A review of quantitative research on men who batter. *Journal of Interpersonal Violence, 5*, 87–118.

Tolman, R. M., & Bhosley, G. (1989). A comparison of two types of pregroup preparation for men who batter. *Journal of Social Service Research, 13*, 33–43.

Waldo, M. (1987). Also victims: Understanding and treating men arrested for spouse abuse. *Journal of Counseling and Development, 65*, 385–388.

Weitzman, J., & Dreen, K. (1982). Wife beating: A view of the marital dyad. *Social Casework, 63*, 259–265.

Willbach, D. (1989). Ethics and family therapy: The case management of family violence. *Journal of Marital and Family Therapy, 15*, 43–52.

Index